SCHEUER'S
Liver Biopsy Interpretation

Content Strategist: *Michael Houston*
Content Development Specialist: *Joanne Scott*
Project Manager: *Andre Riley*
Design: *Miles Hitchen*
Illustration Manager: *Lesley Frazier*
Illustrator: *Deborah Maizels*
Marketing Manager(s) (UK/USA): *Veronica Short*

SCHEUER'S
Liver Biopsy Interpretation

NINTH EDITION

Jay H. Lefkowitch

Professor of Clinical Pathology and Cell Biology
College of Physicians and Surgeons of Columbia University
New York

ELSEVIER Edinburgh London New York Oxford Philadelphia St Louis Sydney Toronto 2016

ELSEVIER

First edition 1968
Second edition 1973
Third edition 1980
Fourth edition 1988
Fifth edition 1994
Sixth edition 2000
Seventh edition 2005
Eighth edition 2010

Notices

Knowledge and best practice in this field are constantly changing. As new research and experience broaden our understanding, changes in research methods, professional practices, or medical treatment may become necessary. Practitioners and researchers must always rely on their own experience and knowledge in evaluating and using any information, methods, compounds, or experiments described herein. In using such information or methods they should be mindful of their own safety and the safety of others, including parties for whom they have a professional responsibility.

With respect to any drug or pharmaceutical products identified, readers are advised to check the most current information provided (i) on procedures featured or (ii) by the manufacturer of each product to be administered, to verify the recommended dose or formula, the method and duration of administration, and contraindications. It is the responsibility of practitioners, relying on their own experience and knowledge of their patients, to make diagnoses, to determine dosages and the best treatment for each individual patient, and to take all appropriate safety precautions.

To the fullest extent of the law, neither the Publisher nor the authors, contributors, or editors, assume any liability for any injury and/or damage to persons or property as a matter of products liability, negligence or otherwise, or from any use or operation of any methods, products, instructions, or ideas contained in the material herein.

ISBN: 978-0-7020-5548-5
E-ISBN: 978-0-7020-6655-9
Inkling ISBN: 978-0-7020-6654-2

 your source for books, journals and multimedia in the health sciences
www.elsevierhealth.com

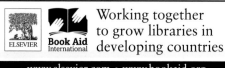

Printed in China

Last digit is the print number: 9 8 7 6 5 4 3 2 1

The publisher's policy is to use **paper manufactured from sustainable forests**

Contents

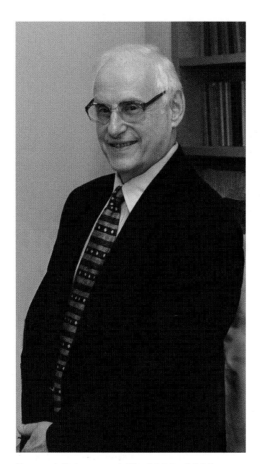

In memory of Peter J. Scheuer, M.D.

'a man of an angel's wit and singular learning. I know not his fellow. For where is the man of that gentleness, lowliness and affability? And, as time requireth, a man of marvellous mirth and pastimes, and sometime of as sad gravity. A man for all seasons'.

Robert Whittington (1520)

Peter J Scheuer, MD, 1928–2006.
(Photograph by Charles Manley, Columbia University.)

Peter J Scheuer attended the Royal Free Hospital School of Medicine in London, UK, where he later became Professor of Pathology and Chairman of the Department of Histopathology. The first edition of Professor Scheuer's *Liver Biopsy Interpretation* was published in 1968, only a decade after Menghini first introduced the technique of needle liver biopsy. Professor Scheuer's many publications on hepatobiliary disease included seminal papers on primary biliary cirrhosis, histological grading of hepatic iron and the classification of chronic hepatitis. He collaborated extensively with his esteemed colleague Professor Dame Sheila Sherlock and the clinical Liver Unit, further establishing the Royal Free Hospital as a major international destination for patients with liver disease and for trainees in clinical hepatology and liver pathology.

Preface

This edition of *Scheuer's Liver Biopsy Interpretation* marks the passage of 47 years since the first edition appeared in 1968. At nearly half a century, there have been landmark changes in the field of hepatology, from an expanded lexicon of hepatitis viruses (A–E) to worldwide life-saving successes in liver transplantation to the current pervasiveness of obesity and diabetes and their manifestations in the form of non-alcoholic fatty liver disease. In the interval since the eighth edition, numerous studies have emerged which have an impact on what the pathologist sees down the microscope when examining a specimen of liver tissue. This ninth edition, accordingly, has many new images, descriptions, references and perspectives which have specifically been assembled so as to provide the reader with the breadth (and nuance) for contemporary interpretation of liver biopsy material. Pathologists whose practices routinely include liver biopsies will almost certainly encounter macrovesicular steatosis and they should therefore be prepared to recognise when steatohepatitis is present, in both its early and progressive forms, and to know the value of connective tissue, iron and several possible immunohistochemical stains in this setting. This is one of many topics which have been substantially updated in this edition. Immunohistochemistry continues to figure prominently in the evaluation of primary and secondary liver tumours and has received expanded coverage. The genomic work-up of neoplasms through genome-wide studies, *in situ* hybridisation, sequencing and other molecular diagnostic techniques has become more readily available and technically feasible. The methodology for these studies is applicable to a variety of liver specimens, even including archived formalin-fixed, paraffin-embedded liver biopsy samples. As a result, the pathologist's role in diagnosing hepatic neoplasms has been greatly augmented beyond strict morphology to also involve determination of the mutational status of certain oncogenes, numbers of gene copies, deletions and translocations and establishing their significance in targeted therapy. This important area clearly benefits from collaborative efforts within departmental subdivisions as well as between departments and institutions. It is an exciting field which is likely only to increase in importance in coming years.

The major goal of the ninth edition (the advances cited above notwithstanding) remains identical to that of previous editions: a practical and concise 'bench book' for use by the microscope. I am hopeful that Professor Scheuer would have looked favourably on and encouraged the inclusion of new material in this edition, while keeping to the fore a focus on the basic organising principles by which we evaluate liver biopsies.

Jay H. Lefkowitch

Acknowledgements

This edition has benefited greatly from the difficult and challenging questions about liver biopsies posed by my colleagues in pathology and in clinical hepatology at Columbia University Medical Center and by many referring pathologists and clinicians at other institutions. Thanks are due to them, particularly to those individuals who have generously contributed illustrative material for the ninth edition. Our pathology residents, fellows and younger faculty have been an additional helpful resource in guiding the writing and selection of images for this edition. Special mention in this regard is owed to my junior departmental colleagues Dr Marcela Salomao and Dr Stephen Lagana. Ms Casey Schadie has provided invaluable and expert administrative assistance with unfailing good humour. Welcome and much-appreciated assistance in patient-related matters was given by Griselle Vicioso and Janelle Dryer in our Center for Liver Disease and Transplantation. The exceptionally fine histopathology laboratory in our department continues to thrive under the outstanding supervision of Sunilda Valladares-Silva. Thanks also go to Doreen Hebert for database searches and multitasking beyond the call of duty. Jackie Lewin of the Electron Microscopy Unit of the Royal Free Hospital, University College London, is now retired but happily still serves as an expert sounding board for my questions about liver ultrastructure.

The prospect of a new edition of *Scheuer's Liver Biopsy Interpretation* was greatly enhanced by the opportunity of working again with Michael Houston at Elsevier, who has provided his encouragement and long-time publishing expertise to the process. I am also fortunate in again having on board Joanne Scott, Deputy Content Development Manager, whose personal style and acumen in medical textbook preparation have made my work all the more pleasurable. Andrew Riley, as Project Manager based in Oxford, has been enormously helpful throughout the final production stage of this edition. Louise Scheuer's academic and personal advice and support have been and continue to be enormously appreciated. Although it is astonishing to contemplate that nearly half a century has passed since Peter Scheuer wrote the first edition of this textbook, his ethos was very much at hand during the preparation of the ninth edition, along with fond memories of other esteemed teachers and mentors, including Hans Popper, Kamal Ishak and Dame Sheila Sherlock.

General Principles of Biopsy Assessment

Introduction

Liver biopsy is one of many diagnostic tools used in the evaluation and management of patients with liver disease. It continues to play an important role because the concepts and classifications of liver disease are rooted in morphology. Moreover, looking at a liver biopsy specimen through the microscope is a very direct way of visualising the morphological changes that affect the liver in disease. The pathologist's interpretation (rather than mere enumeration) of these changes is used to answer important clinical questions such as disease causation and activity, and is important in therapeutic decision making.[1] A thorough and informed interpretation of liver biopsy findings therefore stands to have substantial impact on patient care. It bears emphasising that the evidence base[2] for much of liver biopsy interpretation rests on the large body of important observations reported in the pathology literature during the past 60 years, since Menghini in 1958 first introduced the technique of percutaneous needle biopsy.[3] Questions of a more basic pathobiological nature can also be addressed by applying contemporary techniques of molecular and genomic medicine to liver biopsy material.

There are many reasons for liver biopsy (**Box 1.1**), as will be apparent from the contents of this book. Establishing a tissue diagnosis of neoplastic disease, evaluation of jaundice of uncertain cause and assessment of pyrexia of unknown aetiology continue to be common diagnostic problems. In the present era of emerging personalized and precision medicine, liver biopsy for tumour diagnosis (especially for hepatocellular carcinoma) optimizes the possibility of genetic and molecular analysis for targeting therapy.[3a,3b] Pathologists are well familiar with the need for formal grading and staging of chronic hepatitis (covered in **Ch. 9**). The ubiquitous 'elevated liver function tests' inscribed on biopsy requisitions are now very often explained by steatosis, steatohepatitis or related conditions (**Ch. 7**) stemming from the wide prevalence of obesity, diabetes, hyperlipidaemia and metabolic syndrome. Indeed, in evaluating abnormal liver function tests in patients with negative serological studies,

Box 1.1 Reasons for liver biopsy
Evaluation of abnormal liver function tests
Investigation of pyrexia of unknown aetiology
Diagnosis of neoplasms
Evaluation of ascites and portal hypertension
Grading and staging of chronic hepatitis
Documentation of steatosis and its possible complications
Evaluation of liver dysfunction after liver, kidney and bone marrow transplantation
Investigation of jaundice of unclear aetiology
Determination of the effects of therapy

liver biopsy is rarely normal.[4] The work-up of liver dysfunction following liver, kidney or haematopoietic cell transplantation is also reliant on information from liver biopsies, which must be reported promptly and with due consideration that the pathological changes in these patients may reflect more than one aetiological factor.

Box 1.2 Liver biopsy techniques and routes

Percutaneous
    Suction (e.g. Menghini, Klatskin, Jamshidi needles)
    Cutting (e.g. Vim–Silverman, TruCut needles)
    Spring-loaded

Transjugular
Thin-needle with ultrasound/computed tomography guidance
Laparoscopic
Operative wedge
Fine-needle aspiration

Type and adequacy of liver biopsy specimen

Several liver biopsy techniques and routes are now available for use (**Box 1.2**), each with inherent diagnostic advantages and disadvantages.[1] Liver biopsy is an invasive technique which requires a skilled operator and all possible safeguards to minimise the risk of complications. Precise guidelines vary from one centre to another.[5] Following the biopsy procedure the needle track may be plugged with gelatin sponge (**Fig. 1.1**) or other materials[6] (**Fig. 1.2**) to prevent bleeding.[7] The standard percutaneous suction needle biopsy popularised by Menghini[3] continues to be in active use, while biopsy samples obtained with thin needles under computed tomography guidance and by the transjugular route are now seen more often. Whatever method is chosen, the operator should carefully consider whether the specimen obtained is likely to be adequate for the intended purpose. For example, a small needle specimen obtained with a small-bore needle guided by ultrasound imaging may be adequate for the diagnosis of hepatocellular carcinoma, but not necessarily suitable for the diagnosis and histological evaluation of chronic hepatitis.[8] With needles of the Menghini type the biopsy core is aspirated and may fragment if the liver is cirrhotic. This is discussed further in **Chapter 10**. Cutting needles have been reported to produce better specimens,[9] but in patients with

Figure 1.1
Foreign material. This is absorbable gelatin which was used to plug a needle track. A small amount of liver tissue is seen at the point of the arrow. (Needle biopsy, H&E.)

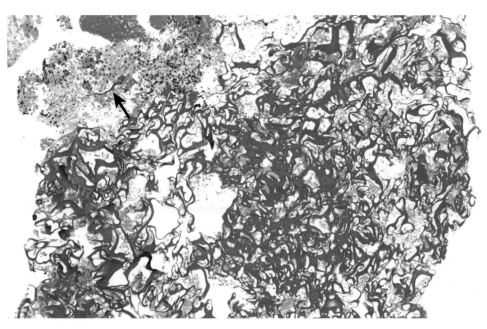

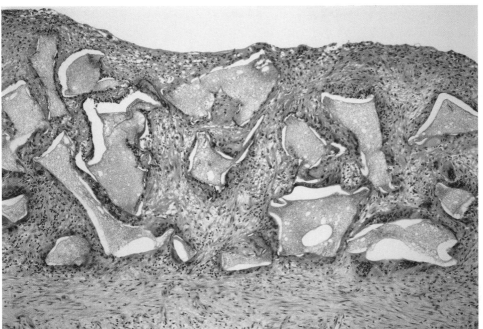

Figure 1.2
Foreign material.
Material used to plug a needle track has here escaped and produced a peritoneal foreign-body giant-cell reaction.[6] (H&E.)

focal lesions aspiration needles often sample both the lesion itself and the adjacent liver; this is helpful in planning treatment.

Biopsy pathology differs from autopsy pathology in that there are pitfalls peculiar to small samples. A needle biopsy specimen of liver represents perhaps one fifty-thousandth of the whole organ and there is thus an obvious possibility of sampling error. Some diseases of the liver are diffuse and involve every acinus, so that sampling error is unlikely; these can be diagnosed with confidence even in small specimens. A diagnosis of acute viral hepatitis can be established in a needle specimen only a few millimetres long, whereas a specimen of similar size may not be adequate for the accurate diagnosis and evaluation of chronic liver disease, for assessment of bile duct numbers, for assessing the full extent of steatosis[10] or for the detection of focal lesions such as tumour deposits or granulomas. Focal or unevenly distributed lesions cannot be entirely excluded on the basis of their absence from an unguided needle biopsy specimen. When focal lesions are suspected, multiple biopsies may help to reduce sampling error.

Chronic hepatitis and cirrhosis present particular sampling problems. In some patients with hepatitis there is a zone of extensive necrosis immediately adjacent to the capsule, whereas the deeper parenchyma is less severely affected. A small specimen consisting of tissue from the subcapsular zone of the liver would then give a misleadingly pessimistic impression (**Fig. 1.3**). In cirrhosis the structure of a nodule is sometimes very similar to that of normal liver, so that a sample consisting almost entirely of the parenchyma from within a nodule may present serious diagnostic difficulties (**Fig. 1.4**). These are accentuated by the resistance of dense fibrous tissue; in a patient with cirrhosis an aspiration biopsy needle may glance off fibrous septa and selectively sample the softer nodular parenchyma. For this reason, some clinicians prefer to use cutting needles in patients with suspected cirrhosis.[11]

Abnormalities in a liver biopsy may represent changes remote from a pathological lesion rather than the lesion itself. In large bile-duct obstruction, for example, the results of the obstruction are clearly seen in the biopsy sample, whereas the cause of the obstruction is usually not visible. The biopsy may be taken from the vicinity of a focal liver lesion such as metastatic carcinoma, and present one or more of a range of pathological features,

3

**Figure 1.3
Subcapsular
necrosis.**
There is a zone of
multiacinar necrosis
immediately deep to
the liver capsule
(right) in this patient
with chronic
hepatitis. The
changes are less
severe in the deeper
tissue to the left. A
small superficial
sample would have
presented problems
of interpretation.
(Needle biopsy, H&E.)

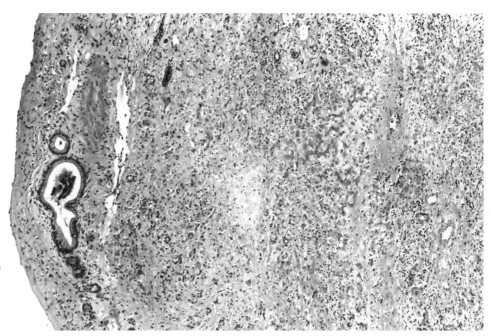

**Figure 1.4
Cirrhosis.**
Appearances are
nearly normal
because the sample
is from the centre of
a nodule and does
not include septa. A
portal tract (at right,
below centre) is
small and poorly
formed. (Needle
biopsy, H&E.)

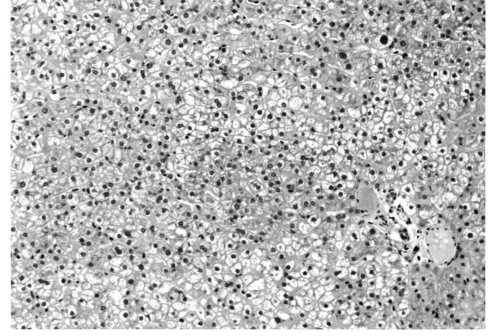

often puzzling to the interpreter (**Fig. 1.5**). Similarly, disease elsewhere in the body may give rise to reactive changes in the liver; biopsy appearances are not normal, but at the same time do not indicate primary liver disease.

Biopsies reveal lesions or diseases rarely seen at autopsy because of their relatively benign course, such as sarcoidosis. In other conditions the evolution of a disease to an end stage means that the earlier and more characteristic pathological features are rarely

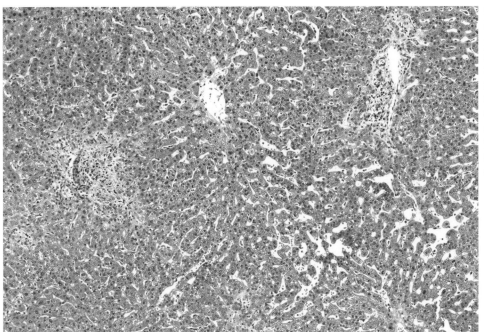

Figure 1.5
Changes near metastatic tumour.
Portal changes like those of biliary obstruction are seen (left, and top right), and there is sinusoidal dilatation in the perivenular area (bottom right). (Needle biopsy, H&E.)

seen at autopsy or even at liver transplantation. In such cases liver biopsies provide valuable insights into the pathology of the disease.

Liver biopsy does not always provide a final or complete diagnosis. Sometimes it even fails to give helpful information. In most cases, however, an adequate and properly processed biopsy is an important item among the diagnostic tests to which the patient is subjected. The relatively limited range of morphological reactions of the liver to injury determines a need for full clinical, biochemical, immunological and imaging data to complement the biopsy findings. Pathologists need this information in order to avoid writing clinically unhelpful, or even misleading, reports, though they may prefer to read the slides before the clinical data to avoid bias.[12] Conversely, it is important that pathologists should produce clear and full reports on the biopsy findings for their clinical colleagues. Every report should attempt to answer one or more clinical questions, whether or not these are explicitly stated on the request form. The use of a standardised checklist has been advocated as a means of ensuring that no potentially useful information is omitted.[13] However, most pathologists currently write unstructured reports. These can be supplemented by a summary giving the essential message which the pathologist wants to convey.

The specimen at the bedside and in the laboratory

Before a liver biopsy is undertaken, the clinician may wish to discuss with the pathologist the need for any special treatment of the specimen, such as freezing part of the specimen or taking tissue for electron microscopy.[12] Accurate assessment of the often subtle changes in a liver biopsy requires sections of high quality. The pathologist is usually aware of possible artefacts in liver biopsy material, as in any histological specimen. Artefacts should obviously be avoided whenever possible, and recognised as such when they do occur. A biopsy of adequate size may be made undiagnosable by rough handling (**Fig. 1.6**), poor fixation, overheating, poor microtome technique and bad staining, all of which can

**Figure 1.6
Traumatic artefact.**
The triangular spaces, which slightly resemble blood vessels, are artefacts caused by rough packing of the specimen between pieces of foam sponge. (H&E.)

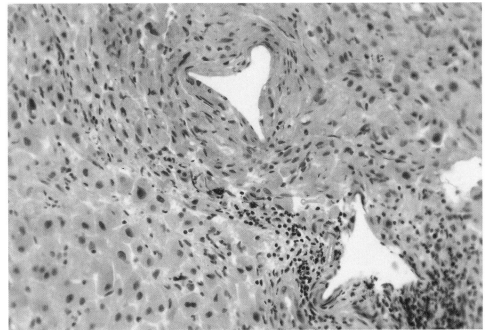

**Figure 1.7
Fixation artefact.**
Hepatocytes in the central part of the specimen are swollen and pale-staining because of poor fixation. Prolonged saline immersion has separated and created widened spaces between hepatocytes. (Needle biopsy, H&E.)

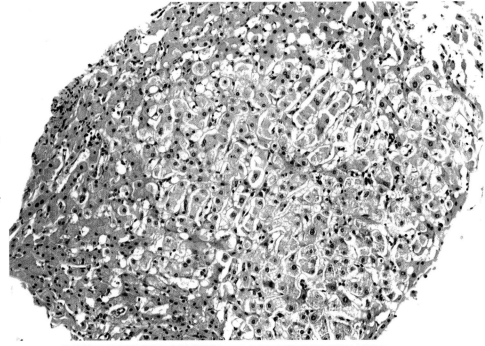

obscure the criteria on which histological diagnoses are based. Poor fixation coupled with prolonged saline immersion sometimes leads to potentially confusing liver-cell swelling and widespread separation of hepatocytes and distortion of the liver-cell plate structure (**Fig. 1.7**). False-positive staining for iron is unrelated to particular cells or structures, or is in a different focal plane from the tissue. Foreign materials injected radiologically may

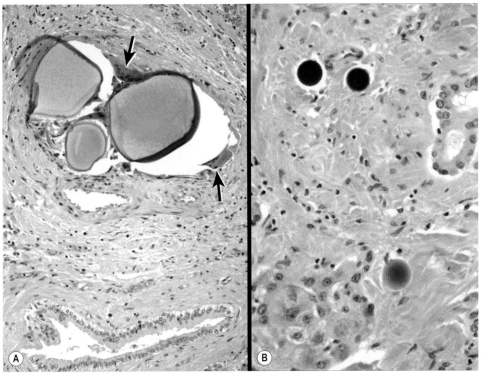

Figure 1.8
Chemoembolic gels and Yttrium 90 microspheres.
A: Chemoembolic gels are present within a medium-size hepatic artery branch. Foreign-body giant cells have gathered around the gels (arrows). **B:** Yttrium 90 microspheres are present within microvessels in and adjacent to the portal tract. (Explant livers, H&E.)

appear puzzling to the pathologist due to unfamiliarity or because of localisation in unexpected organs which have been unintentionally embolised. Primary and metastatic tumours of the liver are often treated with drug-eluting chemoembolic gels via transarterial chemoembolism (TACE) or by Yttrium 90 microspheres in selective internal radiation therapy (SIRT). TACE gels are large (300 μm) and typically lodge within medium-size hepatic artery branches within portal tracts,[14] while Yttrium 90 microspheres, due to their considerably smaller size (30–40 μm), may migrate from portal tract arteries to small portal microvessels, periportal inlet vessels and sinusoids[15] (**Fig. 1.8**).

This book is mainly about changes seen in conventionally stained paraffin sections and cytological preparations. There are many other ways of looking at or investigating a tissue sample, some of them helpful in routine diagnosis. Immunohistochemistry is frequently an essential aspect of liver biopsy evaluation. Its value in individual diseases is covered in the subsequent chapters. One example is use of immunostains to address the functional heterogeneity and 'zonation' of the normal liver lobule or acinus (which is based upon oxygenation[16] and Wnt/β-catenin signalling[17,17a]). The liver's zonation can be demonstrated using immunohistochemical stains for enzymes localised to particular acinar zones. A striking example is glutamine synthetase, which is involved in ammonia metabolism and is only present in the several layers of hepatocytes surrounding efferent venules (**Fig. 1.9**). Demonstration of the ductular reaction using antibody to cytokeratin 7 (or 19) (**Fig. 1.10**) is important in several chronic biliary tract diseases, in fibrosing cholestatic hepatitis after liver transplantation, and in the progression of fibrosis in steatohepatitis and other conditions.[18] Immunostains are useful in demonstrating viral hepatitis antigens (**Ch. 9**) and are the most accurate way of diagnosing α_1-antitrypsin deficiency morphologically. Immunohistochemistry is used extensively in the evaluation of primary and secondary tumours of the liver (**Ch. 11**). Electron microscopy has a well-defined place in liver pathology and is dealt with in the final chapter.

Figure 1.9
Immunohisto-
chemistry and the
functional
heterogeneity of
the liver lobule.
Glutamine
synthetase
immunostain shows
positivity for this
urea cycle enzyme
localised to a rim
of perivenular
hepatocytes, while
the mid-zone and
periportal regions
are negative. P,
portal tract.

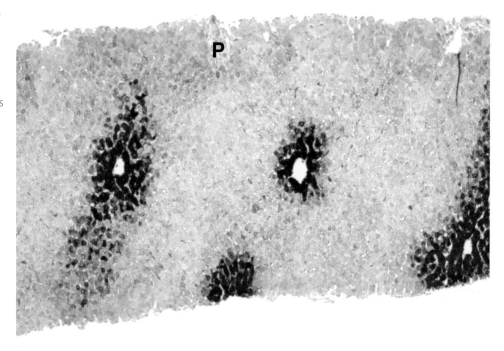

Figure 1.10
Cytokeratin 7
immunostain in
biliary tract
disease.
A vigorous ductular
reaction has
developed in this
case of primary
sclerosing
cholangitis, as
demonstrated with
cytokeratin 7
immunostain. The
native bile duct (bd)
is also identified with
this method.

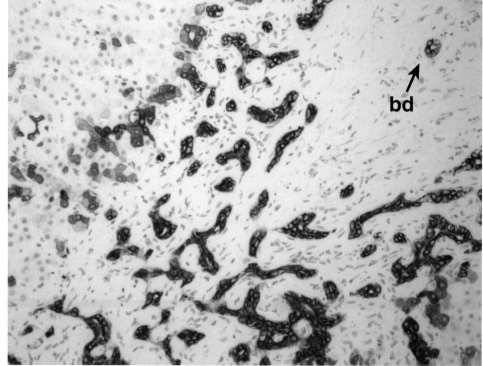

In situ hybridisation has been applied to liver tissue for the identification or assessment of replication of hepatitis viruses and cytomegalovirus. The polymerase chain reaction (PCR) can be applied to liver tissue, and provides more direct evidence of virus infection in the liver than serum PCR. DNA extracted from biopsy tissue can be used in analysis of viral infections and several inherited metabolic diseases.

Part of the biopsy specimen can be analysed for copper, iron or abnormally stored substances, and enzyme activities can be assayed by micromethods. In the case of copper and iron, these measurements can if necessary be made after paraffin embedding, as discussed in **Chapter 14**. Elution of Sirius red from sections provides an accurate method for the measurement of tissue collagen,[19] and this stain is also used for image analysis of collagen.[20,21] *In situ* demonstration of enzymes can be achieved by immunocytochemical methods or by means of enzyme histochemistry, as has been described in the functional zonation of human liver.[22,23]

Well-established techniques of morphometry and image analysis have been applied to tissue sections to obtain data on relative volumes of tissue components in normal human liver[24,25] and in disease. Three-dimensional reconstruction using a computer has helped in the understanding of disease processes and of the relationship between anatomical structures.[26–28]

References

1. Rockey DC, Caldwell SH, Goodman ZD, et al. Liver biopsy. Hepatology 2009;49:1017–44.
2. Crawford JM. Evidence-based interpretation of liver biopsies. Lab Invest 2006;86:326–34.
3. Menghini G. One-second needle biopsy of the liver. Gastroenterology 1958;35:190–9.
3a. Torbenson M, Schirmacher P. Liver cancer biopsy–back to the future?! Hepatology 2015;61:431–3.
3b. Sherman M, Bruix J. Biopsy for liver cancer: how to balance research needs with evidence-based clinical practice. Hepatology 2015;61:433–7.
4. Skelly MM, James PD, Ryder SD. Findings on liver biopsy to investigate abnormal liver function tests in the absence of diagnostic serology. J Hepatol 2001;35:195–9.
5. Sue M, Caldwell SH, Dickson RC, et al. Variation between centers in technique and guidelines for liver biopsy. Liver 1996;16:267–70.
6. Thompson NP, Scheuer PJ, Dick R, et al. Intraperitoneal Ivalon mimicking peritoneal malignancy after plugged percutaneous liver biopsy. Gut 1993;34:16–35.
7. Sawyer AM, McCormick PA, Tennyson GS, et al. A comparison of transjugular and plugged-percutaneous liver biopsy in patients with impaired coagulation. J Hepatol 1993;17:81–5.
8. Petz D, Klauck S, Röhl FW, et al. Feasibility of histological grading and staging of chronic viral hepatitis using specimens obtained by thin-needle biopsy. Virchows Arch 2003;442:238–44.
9. Sada PN, Ramakrishna B, Thomas CP, et al. Transjugular liver biopsy: a comparison of aspiration and Trucut techniques. Liver 1997;17:257–9.
10. Ratziu V, Charlotte F, Heurtier A, et al. Sampling variability of liver biopsy in nonalcoholic fatty liver disease. Gastroenterology 2005;128:1898–906.
11. Gerber MA, Thung SN, Bodenheimer HC Jr, et al. Characteristic histologic triad in liver adjacent to metastatic neoplasm. Liver 1986;6:85–8.
12. Desmet VJ. What more can we ask from the pathologist? J Hepatol 1996;25(Suppl. 1):25–9.
13. Foschini M, Sarti F, Dina RE, et al. Standardized reporting of histological diagnoses for non-neoplastic liver conditions in needle biopsies. Virchows Arch 1995;426:593–6.
14. Panaro F, Ramos J, Gallix B, et al. Hepatic artery complications following liver transplantation. Does preoperative chemoembolization impact the postoperative course? Clin Transplant 2014;28:598–605.
15. Luo D-L, Chan JKC. Basophilic round bodies in gastric biopsies little known by pathologists: iatrogenic Yttrium 90 microspheres deriving from selective internal radiation therapy. Int J Surg Pathol 2013;21:535–7.
16. Jungermann K, Kietzmann T. Oxygen: modulator of metabolic zonation and disease of the liver. Hepatology 2000;31:255–60.
17. Burke ZD, Reed KR, Phesse TJ, et al. Liver zonation occurs through a β-catenin-dependent, c-Myc-independent mechanism. Gastroenterology 2009;136:2316–24.
17a. Yang J, Mowry LE, Nejak-Bowen KN, et al. Beta-catenin signaling in murine liver zonation and regeneration: a Wnt-Wnt situation! Hepatology 2014;60:964–76.
18. Williams MJ, Clouston AD, Forbes SJ. Links between hepatic fibrosis, ductular reaction, and progenitor cell expansion. Gastroenterology 2014;146:349–56.
19. Jimenez W, Pares A, Caballeria J, et al. Measurement of fibrosis in needle liver biopsies: evaluation of a colorimetric method. Hepatology 1985;5:815–18.
20. Pape L, Olsson K, Petersen C, et al. Prognostic value of computerized quantification of liver fibrosis in children with biliary atresia. Liver Transplant 2009;15:876–82.
21. Sandrini J, Boursier J, Chaigneau J, et al. Quantification of portal-bridging fibrosis area more accurately reflects fibrosis stage and liver stiffness than whole fibrosis or perisinusoidal fibrosis areas in chronic hepatitis C. Mod Pathol 2014;27:1035–45.

22 Lamers WH, Hilberts A, Furt E, et al. Hepatic enzymic zonation: a reevaluation of the concept of the liver acinus. Hepatology 1989;10:72–6.

23 Sokal EM, Trivedi P, Cheeseman P, et al. The application of quantitative cytochemistry to study the acinar distribution of enzymatic activities in human liver biopsy sections. J Hepatol 1989;9:42–8.

24 Ranek L, Keiding N, Jensen ST. A morphometric study of normal human liver cell nuclei. Acta Pathol Microbiol Scand [A] 1978;83:467–76.

25 Rohr HP, Luthy J, Gudat F, et al. Stereology: a new supplement to the study of human liver biopsy specimens. In: Popper H, Schaffner F, editors. Progress in Liver Diseases, vol. V, 1st ed. New York, NY: Grune & Stratton; 1976. p. 24.

26 Yamada S, Howe S, Scheuer PJ. Three-dimensional reconstruction of biliary pathways in primary biliary cirrhosis: a computer-assisted study. J Pathol 1987;152:317–23.

27 Nagore N, Howe S, Boxer L, et al. Liver cell rosettes: structural differences in cholestasis and hepatitis. Liver 1989;9:43–51.

28 Ludwig J, Ritman EL, LaRusso NF, et al. Anatomy of the human biliary system studied by quantitative computer-aided three-dimensional imaging techniques. Hepatology 1998;27:893–9.

Laboratory Techniques

Processing of the specimen

As soon as a needle biopsy specimen is obtained from the patient it should be expelled gently into fixative or on to a piece of glass, card or wood. Filter paper is less suitable because fibres tend to adhere to the tissue and may interfere with sectioning. The specimen must be treated with great care and excessive manipulation should be rigorously avoided; distortion of the specimen by rough handling at this stage may seriously interfere with accurate diagnosis, because diagnosis often depends on subtle criteria. At this stage, minute pieces can be put into an appropriate fixative for electron microscopy (**Ch. 17**), preferably by an operator experienced in this technique, and samples taken for chemical analysis or freezing. Frozen sections may be needed for demonstration of lipids. If porphyria is suspected, a very small amount of the unfixed tissue can be examined under ultraviolet light or with a suitable quartz halogen source, either whole or smeared on to a glass slide.

Tissue for paraffin embedding should be transferred to a fixative as soon as possible. When transit to the laboratory is likely to involve much movement, it is helpful to fill the container to the brim with fixative. Buffered formalin and formol saline are both suitable for routine fixation, which is accomplished after 3 h at room temperature or less at higher temperatures (**Table 2.1**). Operative wedge biopsies and larger specimens need longer fixation. Fixatives other than formalin are successfully used in some centres; handbooks of laboratory techniques should be consulted for optimum times and conditions for each fixative.

Minute fragments can be hand-processed more quickly than larger pieces and this also avoids undue shrinkage and hardening. Automated vacuum embedding allows the time of processing of needle specimens to be drastically reduced, as shown in **Table 2.1**; the ultrarapid method by which a good section can be produced in about 2 h has become important because of the need for rapid decisions on treatment in patients who have undergone liver transplantation. Frozen sections, occasionally needed for a decision at surgery, can be cut by a standard method using a cryostat. They are sometimes adequate for diagnosis of obvious lesions such as neoplasms, but are unsuitable for recognition of subtle changes, and can even be dangerously misleading.

The exact number of sections routinely cut from a block varies widely from one laboratory to another. In Scheuer's former laboratory at the Royal Free Hospital in London, 10 or more consecutive sections 3–5 μm thick are cut from each block and alternate sections used for the staining procedures outlined in the next paragraphs. The remaining sections are stored. Step sections are used when discrete lesions such as granulomas or tumour deposits are suspected or for identification of bile ducts when duct paucity is suspected.

Table 2.1 Sample tissue schedules for liver biopsies

Agent	Manual overnight automatic (vacuum)*	Routine overnight automatic	Routine automatic (vacuum)*	Ultrarapid
Buffered formalin	3 h	3 h	2 h	30 min
Formalin–ethanol–water (1:8:1)	Overnight	–	–	–
70% ethanol	–	3 h	1 h	3 min
90% ethanol	–	3 h	1 h	2 min
100% ethanol	2 × 1 h	2 × 2 h	3 × 1 h	3 × 2 min
Xylene	3 × 1 h	3 × 1 h	4 × 1 h	4 × 5 min
Wax (60°C)	2 × 1 h	2 × 1 h	3 × 1 h	3 × 5 min
Total time	24 h	18 h	14 h	1 h 16 min

*All at 50°C except for wax step.

Serial or near-serial sections are helpful when utilising multiple immunohistochemical stains.

Choice of stains

The stains routinely applied to liver biopsies vary according to local custom. The minimum advised is haematoxylin and eosin (H&E) and a reliable method for connective tissue. The author prefers a silver preparation for reticulin as the principal method for showing connective tissue, for reasons discussed below, but trichrome stains also have important applications and can reveal changes not easily seen in a reticulin, such as the pericellular fibrosis of steatohepatitis. Routine staining for iron enables the biopsy to be used to screen for iron storage disease and the periodic acid–Schiff (PAS) stain after diastase digestion (DPAS or PASD) provides a relatively crude, but practicable screening procedure for α_1-antitrypsin deficiency as well as showing activated macrophages and bile-duct basement membranes. Stains for copper-associated protein, elastic fibres and hepatitis B surface antigen are useful and arguably essential additions to the routine list. Some pathologists like to see two H&E-stained sections, one from the beginning and the other from the end of a series of consecutive sections. Other methods are used as required for particular purposes. The extent to which 'special' stains form part of the routine set must be decided by each pathologist.

A **reticulin** preparation is important for accurate assessment of structural changes. Without it, thin layers of connective tissue and hence cirrhosis may be missed, as may foci of well-differentiated hepatocellular carcinoma in which the reticulin structure is often highly abnormal (**see Fig. 11.13**). Counterstaining is sometimes used, but is apt to distract rather than help, bearing in mind that the chief function of the reticulin preparation is to provide a sensitive low-power indicator of structural changes.

Stains for **collagen** such as chromotrope–aniline blue (CAB) are important for the detection of new collagen formation, especially in alcoholic steatohepatitis and its imitators (**Ch. 7**). Collagen staining is therefore advised for any biopsy showing substantial steatosis. It also helps to show blocked veins within scars; these are easily missed on H&E staining. It is therefore wise to use a trichrome stain when vascular disease is suspected.

A stain for **elastic fibres** such as the orcein stain, Victoria blue or elastic–Van Gieson is also useful to identify blocked vessels. The stains often enable the pathologist to distinguish between recent collapse and old fibrosis, since only the latter is positive (**Ch. 6**). Again, this distinction may be very difficult to make on H&E and even with the help of stains for collagen and reticulin. The orcein and Victoria blue also show copper-associated protein and hepatitis B surface material.

Staining for **iron** by Perls' or another similar method enables not only iron but also bile, lipofuscin and other pigments to be evaluated, as discussed in **Chapter 3**. Counterstaining should be light to avoid obscuring small amounts of pigment.

Staining of **glycogen** by means of the PAS method or Best's carmine demonstrates the extent of any liver cell loss, and shows focal areas devoid of hepatocytes such as granulomas. **Glycoproteins** may be demonstrated by the PAS method after digestion with diastase to remove glycogen. This stain serves to accentuate hypertrophied macrophages, such as Kupffer cells filled with ceroid pigment after an acute hepatitis or episode of cholestasis. Alpha$_1$-antitrypsin bodies stain strongly, but the stain is not sufficiently sensitive to enable all examples of α_1-antitrypsin deficiency to be detected.

Staining for **copper** is mainly used in suspected Wilson's disease, although, as explained in **Chapter 14**, it is not always helpful and may even be negative. The rhodanine method is preferred because it is easy to distinguish the orange-red colour of copper from bile, a distinction which is occasionally difficult with rubeanic acid. In Wilson's disease, there is variable correlation between the presence of stainable copper and staining for **copper-associated protein**. In chronic cholestasis, however, the two usually correspond.

Other non-immunological methods useful on occasion include the Ziehl–Neelsen stain for mycobacteria and for the ova of *Schistosoma mansoni*. Specific staining for bilirubin is rarely necessary, but conjugated bilirubin stains a bright green colour by the Van Gieson method. (**see Fig. 4.10**). **Amyloid** is stained by the usual techniques.

For **immunohistochemical staining**, standard techniques are applied. Among antibodies that are helpful in everyday practice are those against components of the hepatitis B virus, the delta agent, cytomegalovirus and α_1-antitrypsin. Neoplasms of doubtful histogenesis or differentiation are investigated by appropriate panels of antibodies, as in any other organ. In hepatocellular carcinoma, bile canaliculi between tumour cells may stain with a polyclonal anti-CEA (carcinoembryonic antigen) antibody, cross-reacting with a canalicular antigen. Assessment of bile-duct loss may require staining of cytokeratins 7 and 19, characteristic of bile-duct rather than liver-cell cytoplasm and of the ductular reaction (**Ch. 4**). The application of immunohistochemistry as well as of other modern techniques is discussed in more detail in **Chapter 17**.

Most of the staining methods mentioned above are used routinely in many laboratories, and can be found in the books listed under General reading at the end of this chapter. A selection of methods is given below (**Box 2.1**).

Box 2.1 Staining methods

Silver impregnation for reticulin fibres (Gordon & Sweets)

1. Bring section to distilled water.
2. Treat with acidified potassium permanganate for 10 min; wash in distilled water.
3. Leave section in 1% oxalic acid until pale (about 1 min). Wash well in several changes of distilled water.
4. Mordant in 2.5% iron alum for 10 min. Wash in several changes of distilled water.

Box 2.1 Continued

5. Treat with silver solution until section is transparent (about 10–15 s). Wash in several changes of distilled water.
6. Reduce in 10% formalin (4% aqueous solution of formaldehyde) for 30 s. Wash in tap water followed by distilled water.
7. Tone if desired in 0.2% gold chloride for 1 min. Rinse in distilled water.
8. Fix in 2.5% sodium thiosulphate for 5 min. Wash several times in tap water.
9. Transfer section to ethanol, clear and mount.

Reticulin appears black. The colour of the collagen varies according to whether step 7 is used; in untoned preparations it is yellow-brown.

Silver solution

To 5 ml of 10% aqueous silver nitrate, add strong ammonia (sp. gr. 0.88) drop by drop until the precipitate which forms is just dissolved. Add 5 ml of 3% sodium hydroxide. Add strong ammonia drop by drop until the resulting precipitate dissolves. The solution does not clear completely. Make up to 50 ml with distilled water. Scrupulously clean glassware should be used throughout.

Acidified potassium permanganate

To 95 ml of 0.5% potassium permanganate, add 5 ml of 3% sulphuric acid.

Chromotrope–aniline blue (CAB) method for collagen and Mallory bodies

(As used at Mount Sinai Hospital, New York; modified from Roque[1] and Churg & Prado[2])
1. Bring section to water.
2. Stain nuclei by the celestine blue–Lillie Mayer sequence or other method. Rinse in distilled water.
3. Immerse in 1% phosphomolybdic acid for 1–3 min. Rinse well in distilled water.
4. Stain with CAB solution for 8 min. Rinse well in distilled water. Blot.
5. Dehydrate quickly, clear and mount.

Collagen is stained blue. Mallory bodies stain blue or sometimes red. Giant mitochondria stain red.

CAB solution

Aniline blue (1.5 g) is dissolved in 2.5 ml HCl and 200 ml distilled water with gentle heat; 6 g chromotrope 2R is added. The pH should be 1.0.

Orcein stain for copper-associated protein, elastic fibres and hepatitis B surface material[3]

1. Bring section to water.
2. Treat with acidified potassium permanganate for 15 min.
3. Rinse in water and decolorise in 2% oxalic acid.
4. Rinse in distilled water, then wash in tap water for 3 min.
5. Stain in commercial orcein solution for 30–60 min, at room temperature.
6. Rinse in water, then differentiate if necessary in 1% HCl in 70% ethanol.
7. Dehydrate, clear and mount.

Elastic fibres, copper-associated protein and hepatitis B surface material (HBsAg) stain brown. The method is less sensitive for HBsAg than immunohistochemical techniques. However, of the components listed, copper-associated protein is often the most difficult to stain reliably. Natural orceins seem to be more satisfactory than synthetic ones, but are difficult or impossible to obtain. In case of difficulty, doubling the concentration of orcein and the amount of HCl may help (Hans Popper, personal communication).

Box 2.1 Continued

Acidified potassium permanganate

To 95 ml of 0.5% potassium permanganate, add 5 ml of 3% sulphuric acid.

Rhodanine stain for copper[4]

1. Bring section to distilled water.
2. Incubate in rhodanine working solution for 18 h at 37°C or 3 h at 56°C.
3. Rinse in several changes of distilled water and stain with Carazzi's haematoxylin for 1 min.
4. Rinse with distilled water and then quickly in borax solution. Rinse well in distilled water.
5. Dehydrate, clear and mount.

Copper deposits stain bright red. Bile stains green. Weakly positive stains tend to fade, but fading can be reduced by staining at the higher temperature and by using certain mounting media (e.g. Ralmount (Raymond A. Lamb), DPX or Diatex). Note the two alternative times and temperatures for the rhodanine working solutions. The staining time can be shortened further.[5]

Rhodanine stock solution

p-Dimethylaminobenzylidene rhodanine	0.2 g
Ethanol	100 ml

The working solution is prepared by diluting 3 ml of the well-shaken stock solution with 47 ml distilled water.

Borax solution

Disodium tetraborate	0.5 g
Distilled water	100 ml

Victoria blue method for copper-associated protein, elastic fibres and hepatitis B surface material[6]

1. Bring section to distilled water.
2. Treat with acidified potassium permanganate (see Gordon & Sweets' reticulin, above) for 5 min.
3. Treat with 4% aqueous sodium metabisulphite for 1 min.
4. Wash in running tap water.
5. Wash well with 70% ethanol.
6. Stain in Victoria blue solution in a Coplin jar for a minimum of 4 h, and preferably overnight.
7. Wash well with 70% ethanol. This is the differentiation step; ensure that the background of the section is clear.
8. Wash in running tap water for 1 min.
9. Stain with nuclear fast red solution for 5 min.
10. Wash in running water for 2 min.
11. Dehydrate, clear and mount.

Copper-associated protein, elastic fibres and HBsAg are stained blue on a pink background.

Victoria blue solution

Distilled water	200 ml
Dextrine	0.5 g
Victoria blue	2 g
Resorcinol	4 g

Box 2.1 Continued

Slowly warm the mixture of the above until it boils. Gradually add 25 ml of boiling 29% ferric chloride solution and boil for a further 3 min. Cool and filter through fine paper. Dry the filtrate on the filter paper to complete dryness in a 56°C oven. Dissolve the filtrate in 400 ml 70% ethanol. Finally add 4 ml concentrated HCl and 6 g phenol. The solution is best left for 2 weeks before use.

Nuclear fast red

Dissolve 0.1 g nuclear fast red in 100 ml warmed 5% aluminium sulphate. Filter when cool.

References

1 Roque AL. Chromotrope aniline blue method of staining Mallory bodies of Laennec's cirrhosis. Lab Invest 1953;2:15–21.
2 Churg J, Prado A. A rapid Mallory trichrome stain (Chromotrope–aniline blue). Arch Pathol 1956;62:505–6.
3 Shikata T, Uzawa T, Yoshiwara N, et al. Staining methods of Australia antigen in paraffin section – detection of cytoplasmic inclusion bodies. Jpn J Exp Med 1974;44:25–36.
4 Lindquist RR. Studies on the pathogenesis of hepatolenticular degeneration. II. Cytochemical methods for the localization of copper. Arch Pathol 1969;87:370–9.
5 Emanuele P, Goodman ZD. A simple and rapid stain for copper in liver tissue. Ann Diagn Pathol 1998;2:125–6.
6 Tanaka K, Mori W, Suwa K. Victoria blue-nuclear fast red stain for HBs antigen detection in paraffin section. Acta Pathol Jpn 1981;31:93–8.

General reading

Bancroft JD, Gamble M, editors. Theory and Practice of Histological Techniques. 5th ed. London: Churchill Livingstone; 2002.
Kiernan JA. Histological and Histochemical Methods: Theory and Practice. 3rd ed. Oxford: Butterworth-Heinemann; 1999.
Lefkowitch JH. Special stains in diagnostic liver pathology. Semin Diagn Pathol 2006;23:190–8.
Polak JM, van Noorden S. Introduction to Immunocytochemistry. 2nd ed. Microscopy Handbooks 37. Oxford: Bios Scientific Publishers; 1997.
Prophet EB, Mills B, Arrington JB, et al., editors. Laboratory Methods in Histotechnology. Washington, DC: American Registry of Pathology; 1992.

The Normal Liver

Structures and components

Functional units and nomenclature

Under the low power of the light microscope, normal liver is seen to have a regular structure based on portal tracts and efferent veins. The smallest portal tracts contain portal venules, hepatic arterioles and small interlobular bile ducts. Blood from both venules and arterioles passes through the sinusoidal system to reach efferent hepatic venules. From these, the blood drains into successively larger veins to reach the inferior vena cava. Bile flows from the smallest ducts into larger ducts, to reach the small intestine by way of the common bile duct.

The functional relationship between these various structures has been the subject of much debate. The most widely used models are the classic lobule and Rappaport's acinus.[1] The lobule has an efferent venule at its centre and portal tracts at its periphery (**Fig. 3.1**). The acinus is based on a terminal portal tract, with blood passing from this, through successively less well-oxygenated parenchymal zones 1, 2 and 3, to efferent venules. It is worth emphasising that both lobules and acini are concepts rather than fixed anatomical structures. Several other models have been proposed, as well as modifications to the original lobular model.[2-4] From a pathologist's point of view, both lobular and acinar concepts have their merits in different situations. To give examples, the sinusoidal congestion of venous outflow obstruction is often more easily understood on the basis of the lobule, with maximum intensity at its centre. Bridging hepatic necrosis, however, is difficult to understand in terms of the lobule and has been explained as death of hepatocytes in acinar zones 3, the zones in which oxygen saturation is relatively low. In everyday practice it seems best to use words compatible with either model as far as possible. In this book we have therefore used the term 'periportal' to describe the part of the parenchyma lying nearest to a small portal tract, and 'perivenular' for the parenchyma near an efferent venule.

Portal tracts

Portal tracts of different size may be seen in biopsies (**see Fig. 4.1**). The smallest represent terminal tracts from which blood enters the parenchyma. Larger portal tracts contain vessels and ducts which convey blood and bile to and from the smaller tracts. Pathological processes do not necessarily affect large and small tracts to the same extent.

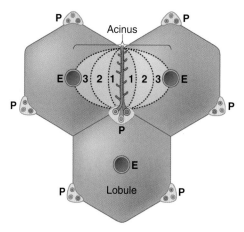

Figure 3.1 Diagrammatic representation of a simple acinus.
It is divided into zones 1, 2 and 3, with three adjacent lobules for comparison. Portal tracts (P) contain
bile ducts, arterioles and venules. E, efferent vein (central vein or terminal hepatic venule).

**Figure 3.2
Normal adult liver.**
A small portal tract
contains a portal
venule (V), arteriole
(A) and interlobular
bile duct (B). (Needle
biopsy, H&E.)

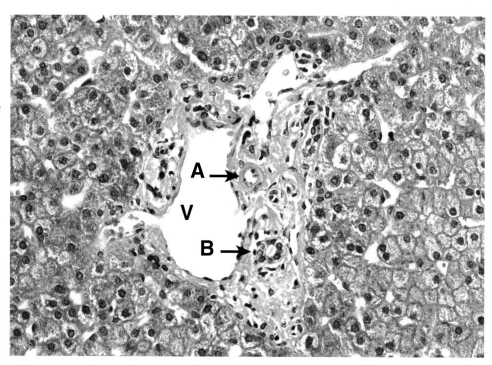

A typical small portal tract contains a bile duct, portal venule, hepatic arteriole and lymphatics, all embedded in connective tissue (**Fig. 3.2**). A few lymphocytes and mast cells may be seen even in normal subjects and nerve fibres can be demonstrated by appropriate staining. The exact contents are variable, however, depending in part on the angle of sectioning. In a study of 16 needle biopsies from normal subjects,[5] 38%, 9% and 7% of tracts did not contain a portal-vein branch, hepatic arteriole or bile duct, respectively. Most, but by no means all, hepatic artery branches are accompanied by bile ducts. These observations have obvious implications for the histological diagnosis of bile duct or blood vessel loss. A confident diagnosis requires examination of several portal tracts.

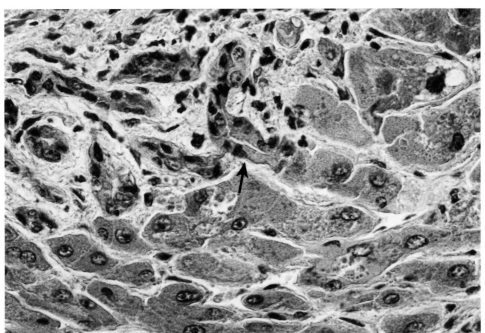

Figure 3.3
Bile ductules and canals of Hering.
These are unusually prominent in this cirrhotic liver. A liver cell plate is seen in continuity with a ductular structure (arrow). (Needle biopsy, H&E.)

Bile ducts

Near or at the margins of the small portal tracts, the bile canaliculi, formed as spaces between adjacent hepatocytes, communicate with the canals of Hering.[6-8] These are lined partly by hepatocytes and partly by biliary epithelial cells. From the canals of Hering, bile drains into bile ductules lined entirely by biliary epithelium (**see Fig. 5.1**). Neither canals of Hering nor ductules are easily seen in normal liver, but they may become apparent in disease (**Fig. 3.3**). The exact location of the junction between the canals of Hering and bile ductules varies, the ductules sometimes having an intraparenchymal portion, seen in two-dimensional sections as apparently isolated ductules among hepatocytes. The canals of Hering and bile ductules have received much attention in recent years, because they appear to be the site of a progenitor-cell compartment which becomes activated when a need for new hepatocytes and bile ducts cannot be adequately met otherwise.[8-10] Progenitor cells can be immunostained for cytokeratins CK7 and CK19, EpCAM (epithelial cell adhesion molecule) and NCAM (neural cell adhesion molecule)[11] and also stain with OV-6, an antibody used on frozen tissue to mark similar cells ('oval cells') in rodents.[11,12] The response to various types of liver injury may also involve participation of hepatoblasts derived from progenitor cells.[12]

The interlobular ducts into which the ductules drain have an internal diameter of less than 100 µm and are more or less centrally located in the small portal tracts. They are lined by cuboidal or low columnar epithelium and have a basement membrane associated with diastase periodic acid–Schiff (DPAS)-positive material. Portal venules and hepatic arterioles usually lie close to these ducts but, as already noted, not all three structures are necessarily seen in a single plane of section. Positive identification of bile ducts in pathological states can be difficult, but is made easier by cytokeratin staining; ducts contain CK7 and CK19 in addition to CK8 and CK18; the latter two are also found in hepatocytes.[13]

Bile drains from the interlobular ducts into septal bile ducts having an internal diameter of more than 100 µm. Septal ducts are lined by tall columnar epithelium, with basally located nuclei. These and larger ducts towards the hepatic hilum are sometimes associated with heterotopic exocrine pancreatic tissue.[14] Around the largest intrahepatic ducts there are peribiliary glands.[14]

Hepatic sinusoids, space of Disse and extracellular matrix

Hepatic sinusoids

The hepatic sinusoids are lined by specialised endothelial cells, which form an incomplete, porous barrier allowing easy exchange of materials between blood and hepatocytes. The endothelial cells are positive for cluster differentiation markers CD4, CD13, CD14, CD16, CDw32, CD36 and CD54 and thus have a different phenotype from capillary endothelium, portal venules and terminal hepatic venules; these stain for CD31 and CD34 and bind *Ulex europaeus* lectin.

Within the sinusoidal lumen lie the Kupffer cells, specialised hepatic macrophages which are demonstrable with immunostain for CD68. These have irregular processes, which may straddle the sinusoidal lumen. They are more numerous near portal tracts. Activated Kupffer cells, unlike endothelial cells, are DPAS- and muramidase-positive. Phenotypically distinct lymphocytes are found both within the sinusoidal lumens and in the portal tracts.[15] Lymphocytes in the lumens include pit cells having natural killer (NK) activity.[16]

Space of Disse

The space of Disse, lying between the sinusoidal endothelium and the hepatocytes, is not conspicuous in paraffin-embedded biopsies, but may be artefactually prominent in autopsy material. It contains components of the extracellular matrix, nerves[17,18] and hepatic stellate cells.

Hepatic stellate cells are members of the myofibroblast family. There is international agreement that the term 'stellate cell' should be used rather than one of many synonyms in the literature[19] (see Glossary). Stellate cells are involved in fibrogenesis and in the control of sinusoidal blood flow.[20,21] They may also act as antigen-presenting cells. In childhood and adolescence, stellate cells are positive for alpha smooth-muscle actin, but thereafter become negative until activated under pathological conditions.[22] Both resting and activated stellate cells are positive for synaptophysin,[23] for vinculin after microwave pretreatment of paraffin sections[24] and for cellular retinol-binding protein-1 (CRBP-1).[25] Difficult to identify in normal liver in routine sections, stellate cells can be recognised in pathological conditions by their vacuolated cytoplasm and consequently scalloped nucleus (**see Fig. 7.6**). It is likely that the hepatic stellate cell is not the only cell type in the liver concerned with collagen synthesis.[26,27]

The extracellular matrix comprises many different components. Collagen types I and III predominate. Types IV, V, VI, VIII, XIV, XVIII and XIX are also present, together with proteoglycans and glycoproteins such as fibronectin and laminin.[28] Type III collagen is the main component of reticulin fibres in the space of Disse (**Fig. 3.4**), while type I is abundant in portal tracts and in the walls of efferent veins. Elastic fibres, abundant in portal tracts, are not demonstrable in sinusoidal walls in normal liver.[29]

Hepatocytes

The hepatocytes are arranged in plates separated by the sinusoidal labyrinth (**Fig. 3.5**). The layer of hepatocytes next to a small portal tract is known as the limiting plate. In adults the hepatocyte plates are one cell thick, but in any one section a few plates will appear thicker because of tangential cutting. Widespread formation of twin-cell plates indicates hyperplasia, recent or current.

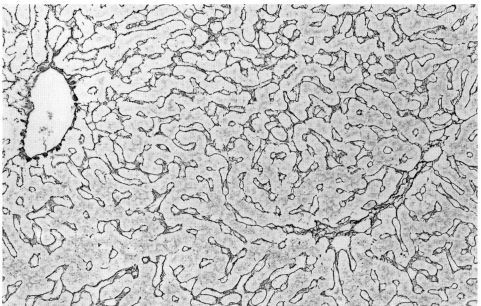

Figure 3.4
Normal adult liver.
There is a regular reticulin network between the portal tract (below right) and the efferent hepatic venule to the left. (Needle biopsy, reticulin.)

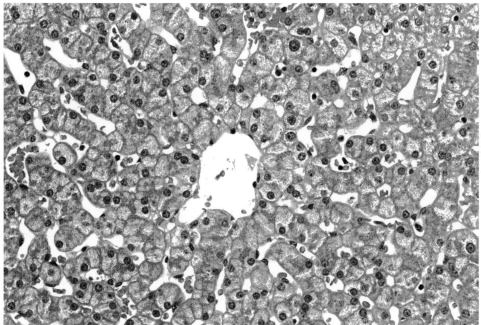

Figure 3.5
Normal adult liver.
Hepatocyte plates, for the most part one cell thick, radiate out from the terminal venule in the centre. (Wedge biopsy, H&E.)

Hepatocytes are polygonal cells with well-defined cell borders. Each cell contains one or more nuclei. Most cells contain one nucleus; a few contain two in normal subjects. Nucleoli are often visible, mitotic figures rare. Most of the nuclei are diploid,[30] but smaller numbers of tetraploid and even larger nuclei are found, especially in older subjects.[31] Polyploidy and variation in nuclear size are therefore normal characteristics of adult human liver. A few periportal nuclei may appear vacuolated because of glycogen accumulation, especially in children and adolescents.

Hepatocyte cytoplasm is normally rich in glycogen. In sections stained with haematoxylin and eosin (H&E) the cytoplasm appears granular and often pale-staining centrally, where glycogen and endoplasmic reticulum predominate. A few fat vacuoles and occasional apoptosis may be seen in the absence of obvious disease. Many different proteins can be demonstrated in or on the hepatocytes, in keeping with the liver's many metabolic functions. These include secreted proteins such as albumin and cell-surface proteins such as adhesion molecules.[32] Structural proteins include cytokeratins 8 and 18. Staining with the antibody Hep Par 1 is positive,[33] but this is not exclusive to hepatocytes.

Between the hepatocytes, their walls formed by two or three cells, are the bile canaliculi, already mentioned. They are usually too small to be readily seen by light microscopy in routine paraffin sections, but are occasionally visible as minute spaces at the biliary poles of the hepatocytes. Bile is rarely seen in normal subjects. The canalicular network can be demonstrated using a polyclonal antibody to carcinoembryonic antigen (CEA), which reacts with the canalicular antigen biliary glycoprotein (**see Fig. 11.15**). Another option is antibody to CD10 (neutral endopeptidase), which is expressed on the surface microvilli of bile canaliculi (**see Fig. 1.8**) and on the apices of cholangiocytes.[34] It should be noted that physiological expression of CD10 on canaliculi develops only after 24 months of age[34] and, consequently, immunostain results will be negative in younger children and neonates.

Hepatocellular pigments (Table 3.1)

Within the hepatocytes, aggregated near the bile canaliculi and most abundant in perivenular areas, there are fine yellow-brown granules of lipofuscin pigment (**Fig. 3.6**).

Table 3.1 Identification of hepatocellular pigments

	Haemosiderin	Lipofuscin	Dubin–Johnson pigment	Bile	Copper-associated protein
Distribution	Periportal	Perivenular	Perivenular, often also in Kupffer cells	Often perivenular; also in canaliculi and Kupffer cells	Periportal in chronic cholestasis
Intracellular site	Pericanalicular	Pericanalicular	Pericanalicular	Pericanalicular or diffuse	Variable
Granule size (approximate)	1 μm	1 μm often	>1 μm	Variable	≤1 μm
Colour	Golden brown, refractile	Yellow brown	Dark brown	Yellow, brown or green	Grey
Perls' stain for iron	+	–	–	–	–
Diastase–PAS stain	–	Variable	Variable	Variable	Often +
Long Ziehl–Neelsen stain	–	+	Often +	–	–
Orcein, Victoria blue stain	–	–	–	–	+

PAS, periodic acid–Schiff.

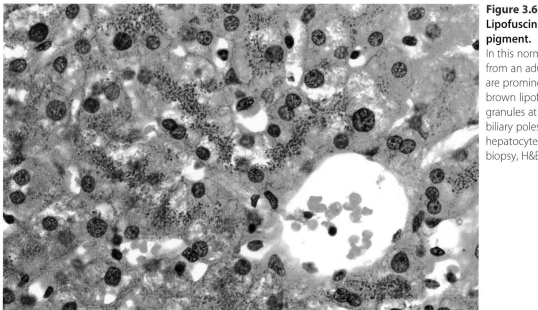

Figure 3.6 Lipofuscin pigment. In this normal liver from an adult there are prominent brown lipofuscin granules at the biliary poles of the hepatocytes. (Wedge biopsy, H&E.)

Lipofuscin is a normal constituent of adult liver, increasing in amount with age but also sometimes found in children. The granules represent lysosomes containing materials which cannot be further degraded. The amount of the pigment varies greatly in normal liver, making assessment of an increase or decrease in disease subject to error in the absence of well-controlled morphometric data. Lipofuscin also varies in its staining properties according to its constituents and age. It is acid-fast, has reducing properties and stains variably with DPAS. Perls' stain for iron is negative.

Large amounts of lipofuscin are difficult to distinguish from Dubin–Johnson pigment by light microscopy alone, but the latter is usually coarser and darker (**see Fig. 13.19**). Intracellular bile can be distinguished from lipofuscin by its bright green staining with Van Gieson's method (**see Fig. 4.10**) and by the almost invariable presence of bile thrombi in canaliculi. An exception to this is liver following transplantation, in which diffuse intracellular bile is common in the absence of bile thrombi.

Normal liver is negative for stainable iron. All but very small amounts should be further investigated by appropriate biochemical and genetic methods. This is because it is important to identify patients with the common and treatable condition of hereditary haemochromatosis (**Ch. 14**).

Copper-associated protein is seen in high copper states as grey-brown or red intracytoplasmic granules, usually in a periportal location. It can be stained with orcein, Victoria blue and DPAS.

Normal appearances in childhood

Haematopoiesis is active during the fetal period (**Fig. 3.7**) and continues until a few weeks after birth. Haemopoietic cells are present in portal tracts and sinusoids (**Fig. 3.8**). Hepatocyte plates are mainly two cells thick until the age of 5 or 6 years, when the adult pattern of single-cell plates is established. Hepatocytes and their nuclei vary little in size. Glycogen vacuolation of nuclei is common until adolescence. Lipofuscin pigment is absent or scanty in the first two decades of life.

Figure 3.7
Liver of fetus at 19 weeks' gestation.
Many haemopoietic cells are seen in sinusoids and in the immature portal tract. A ductal plate at the margin of the tract (arrows) indicates bile-duct formation. (Postmortem liver, H&E.)

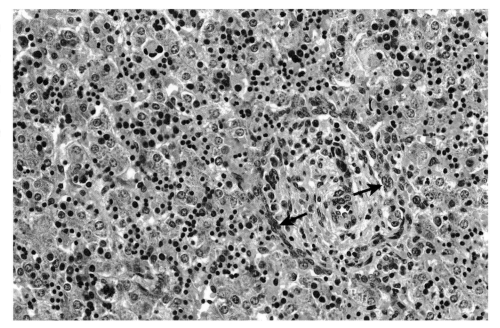

Figure 3.8
Normal liver in a neonate.
Abundant haemopoietic cells are seen in the portal tract and in the sinusoids. (Postmortem liver, H&E.)

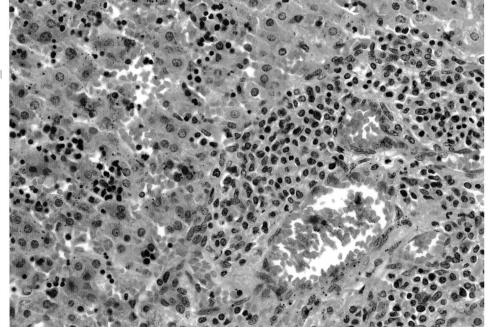

Ageing

The size of hepatocytes and their nuclei becomes more variable with increasing age, most notable in perivenular regions (**Fig. 3.9**). This variation is due to greater numbers of polyploid cells,[31] with large nuclear and cell volumes. Lipofuscin pigment in hepatocytes is often abundant, especially around terminal hepatic venules (**Fig. 3.6**). Portal connective

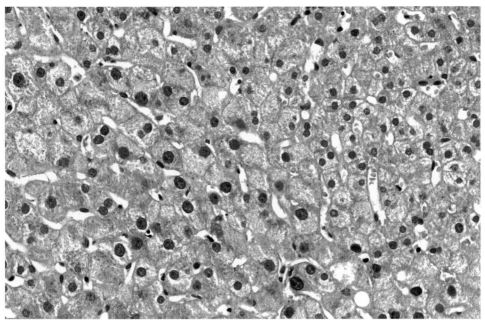

Figure 3.9
Liver in an elderly person.
Hepatocyte nuclei vary considerably in size. (Needle biopsy, H&E.)

tissue becomes denser, and arteries may be thick-walled, even in normotensive subjects.[35] Pseudocapillarisation of the sinusoidal lining with loss of permeability may have important consequences for lipid metabolism and vascular disease.[36]

Biopsy of the normal liver

Percutaneous liver biopsies are necessarily taken though the liver capsule, which may be seen at one end of the core or as a separate piece. It sometimes contains vessels and bile ducts, but can be distinguished from a pathological septum by the density and maturity of the connective tissue. Deeper in the core, pathological septa must also be distinguished from longitudinally cut portal tracts (**Fig. 3.10**). The length and width of the liver core are often critical for diagnosis, as discussed under the heading of grading and staging in **Chapter 9**. Short pieces or slender cores taken with narrow needles may be inadequate for the diagnosis of unevenly distributed, non-neoplastic lesions.

Other organs and tissues, especially skin, pleura and intercostal muscle, are sometimes included in the specimen. Close apposition to the liver core of fibrous tissue or of tumour does not necessarily reflect hepatic fibrosis or tumour within the liver.

Transjugular biopsy is now often used and usually provides ample-sized specimens, sometimes including longitudinally cut portions of efferent vein walls.

Surgical biopsies taken from the inferior margin of the liver are in the form of wedges covered on two aspects by capsule. The structure of the immediately subcapsular zone differs somewhat from the deeper tissue (**Fig. 3.11**), but there is good correlation between the volume fraction of non-parenchymal components in subcapsular and deeper zones.[37] Appearances mimicking cirrhosis do not usually extend for more than 2 mm into the liver, and confusion is unlikely except with very small superficial samples.

In surgical biopsies taken some time after the beginning of an operation, neutrophil leukocytes accumulate under the capsule and in portal tracts, around terminal venules and focally within the parenchyma (**Fig. 3.12**). Here, there is focal loss of hepatocytes. Similar parenchymal changes have been reported after heavy sedation without full anaesthesia.[38] They are also found in patients infected with cytomegalovirus (**Ch. 15**).

**Figure 3.10
Normal adult liver.**
Two normal portal tracts (P), cut longitudinally, mimic septa. Between them is an efferent hepatic venule (V). (Needle biopsy, reticulin.)

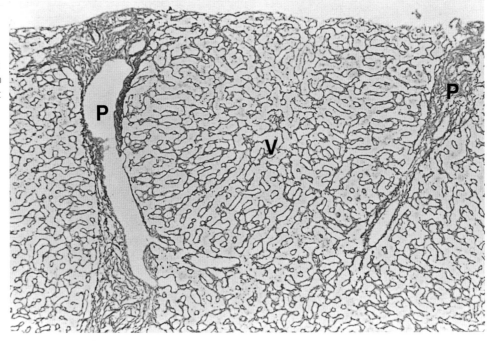

**Figure 3.11
Normal adult liver.**
The capsule is thick and portal tracts are prominent. (Postmortem liver, trichrome.)

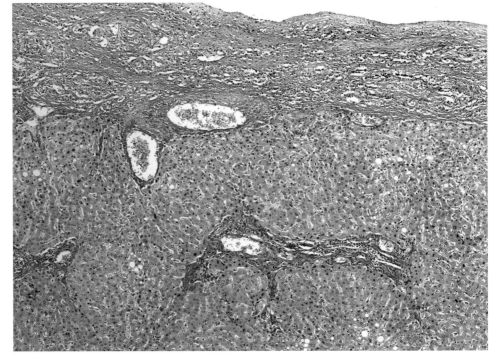

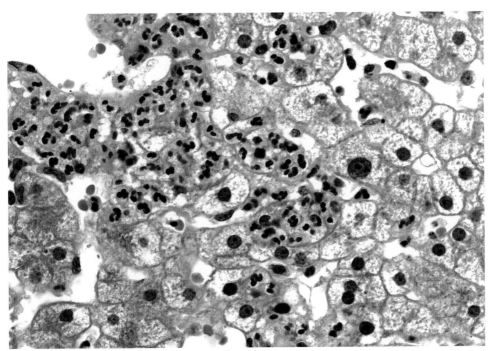

**Figure 3.12
Operative wedge biopsy.**
Clumps of neutrophils mark sites of hepatocellular necrosis, resulting from the procedure. Part of an efferent venule is seen (top left). (Wedge biopsy, H&E.)

References

1   Rappaport AM. The microcirculatory acinar concept of normal and pathological hepatic structure. Beitr Pathol 1976;157:215–43.

2   Saxena R, Theise ND, Crawford JM, et al. Microanatomy of the human liver – exploring the hidden interfaces. Derivation of hepatocytes from bone marrow cells in mice after radiation-induced myeloablation. Hepatology 1999;30:1339–46.

3   Roskams T, Desmet VJ, Verslype C. Development, structure and function of the liver. In: Burt AD, Portmann BC, Ferrell LD, editors. MacSween's Pathology of the Liver. 5th ed. Edinburgh: Churchill Livingstone/Elsevier; 2007. p. 1–74.

4   Reuben A. Now you see it, now you don't. Hepatology 2003;38:781–4.

5   Crawford AR, Lin X-Z, Crawford JM. The normal adult human liver biopsy: a quantitative reference standard. Hepatology 1998;28:323–31.

6   Theise ND, Saxena R, Portmann BC, et al. The canals of Hering and hepatic stem cells in humans. Hepatology 1999;30:1425–33.

7   Saxena R, Theise N. Canals of Hering: recent insights and current knowledge. Semin Liver Dis 2004;24:43–8.

8   Roskams TA, Theise ND, Balabaud C, et al. Nomenclature of the finer branches of the biliary tree: canals, ductules, and ductular reactions in human livers. Hepatology 2004;39:1739–45.

9   Roskams TA, Libbrecht L, Desmet VJ. Progenitor cells in diseased human liver. Semin Liver Dis 2003;23: 385–96.

10 Kuwahara R, Kofman AV, Landis CS, et al. The hepatic stem cell niche: identification by label-retaining cell assay. Hepatology 2008;47:1994–2002.

11 Roskams T, De Vos R, van Eyken P, et al. Hepatic OV-6 expression in human liver disease and rat experiments: evidence for hepatic progenitor cells in man. J Hepatol 1998;29:455–63.

12 Zhang L, Theise N, Chua M, et al. The stem cell niche of human livers: symmetry between development and regeneration. Hepatology 2008;48:1598–607.

13 van Eyken P, Desmet VJ. Cytokeratins and the liver. Liver 1993;13:113–22.

14 Terada T, Nakanuma Y, Kakita A. Pathologic observations of intrahepatic peribiliary glands in 1000 consecutive autopsy livers. Heterotopic pancreas in the liver. Gastroenterology 1990;98:1333–7.

15 Norris S, Collins C, Doherty DG, et al. Resident human hepatic lymphocytes are phenotypically different from circulating lymphocytes. J Hepatol 1998;28:84–90.

16 Nakatani K, Kaneda K, Seki S, et al. Pit cells as liver-associated natural killer cells: morphology and function. Med Electron Microsc 2004;37:29–36.

17 Tiniakos DG, Lee JA, Burt AD. Innervation of the liver: morphology and function. Liver 1996;16:151–60.

18 Akiyoshi H, Gonda T, Terada T. A comparative histochemical and immunohistochemical study of aminergic, cholinergic and peptidergic innervation in rat, hamster, guineapig, dog and human livers. Liver 1998;18:352–9.

19 International Consensus Group. Hepatic stellate cell nomenclature. Hepatology 1996;23:193.

20 Pinzani M. Hepatic stellate (Ito) cells: expanding roles for a liver-specific pericyte. J Hepatol 1995;22:700–6.

21 Rockey DC. Hepatic blood flow regulation by stellate cells in normal and injured liver. Semin Liver Dis 2001;21:337–49.

22 Schmitt-Graff A, Kruger S, Bochard F, et al. Modulation of alpha smooth muscle actin and desmin expression in perisinusoidal cells of normal and diseased human livers. Am J Pathol 1991;138:1233–42.

23 Cassiman D, van Pelt J, De Vos R, et al. Synaptophysin: a novel marker for human and rat hepatic stellate cells. Am J Pathol 1999;155:1831–9.

24 Kawai S, Enzan H, Hayashi Y, et al. Vinculin: a novel marker for quiescent and activated hepatic stellate cells in human and rat livers. Virchows Arch 2003;443:78–86.

25 Lepreux S, Bioulac-Sage P, Gabbiani G, et al. Cellular retinol-binding protein-1 expression in normal and fibrotic/cirrhotic human liver: different patterns of expression in hepatic stellate cells and (myo)fibroblast subpopulations. J Hepatol 2004;40:774–80.

26 Cassiman D, Roskams T. Beauty is in the eye of the beholder: emerging concepts and pitfalls in hepatic stellate cell research. J Hepatol 2002;37:527–35.

27 Ramadori G, Saile B. Mesenchymal cells in the liver: one cell type or two? Liver 2002;22:283–94.

28 Schuppan D, Ruehl M, Somasundaram R, et al. Matrix as a modulator of hepatic fibrogenesis. Semin Liver Dis 2001;21:351–72.

29 Porto LC, Chevallier M, Peyrol S, et al. Elastin in human, baboon, and mouse liver: an immunohistochemical and immunoelectron microscopic study. Anat Rec 1990;228:392–404.

30 Deprez C, Vangansbeke D, Fastrez R, et al. Nuclear DNA content, proliferation index, and nuclear size determination in normal and cirrhotic liver, and in benign and malignant primary and metastatic hepatic tumors. Am J Clin Pathol 1993;99:558–65.

31 Kudryatsev BN, Kudryatseva MV, Sakuta GA, et al. Human hepatocyte polyploidization kinetics in the course of life cycle. Virchows Arch B Cell Pathol 1993;64:387–93.

32 Hinchliffe SA, Woods S, Gray S, et al. Cellular distribution of androgen receptors in the liver. J Clin Pathol 1996;49:418–20.

33 Wennerberg AE, Nalesnik MA, Coleman WB. Hepatocyte paraffin 1: a monoclonal antibody that reacts with hepatocytes and can be used for differential diagnosis of hepatic tumors. Am J Pathol 1993;143:1050–4.

34 Byrne JA, Meara NJ, Rayner AC, et al. Lack of hepatocellular CD10 along bile canaliculi is physiologic in early childhood and persistent in Alagille syndrome. Lab Invest 2007;87:1138–48.

35 Fiel MI, Deniz K, Elmali F, et al. Increasing hepatic arteriole wall thickness and decreased luminal diameter occur with increasing age in normal livers. J Hepatol 2011;55:582–6.

36 Le Couteur DG, Fraser R, Cogger VC, et al. Hepatic pseudocapillarisation and atherosclerosis in ageing. Lancet 2002;359:1612–15.

37 Ryoo JW, Buschmann RJ. Comparison of intralobular non-parenchyma, subcapsular non-parenchyma, and liver capsule thickness. J Clin Pathol 1989;42:740–4.

38 McDonald GS, Courtney MG. Operation-associated neutrophils in a percutaneous liver biopsy: effect of prior transjugular procedure. Histopathology 1986;10:217–22.

General reading

Crawford AR, Lin X-Z, Crawford JM. The normal adult human liver biopsy: a quantitative reference standard. Hepatology 1998;28:323–31.

Crawford JM, Burt AD. Anatomy, pathophysiology and basic mechanisms of disease. In: Burt AD, Portmann BC, Ferrell LD, editors. MacSween's Pathology of the Liver. 6th ed. Edinburgh: Churchill Livingstone/Elsevier; 2012. p. 1–78.

Dollé L, Best J, Mei J, et al. The quest for liver progenitor cells: a practical point of view. J Hepatol 2010;52:117–29.

Friedman SL. Mechanisms of hepatic fibrogenesis. Gastroenterology 2008;134:1655–69.

Geerts A. History, heterogeneity, developmental biology, and functions of quiescent hepatic stellate cells. Semin Liver Dis 2001;21:311–35.

Lemaigre FP. Mechanisms of liver development: concepts for understanding liver disorders and design of novel therapies. Gastroenterology 2009;137:62–79.

Reuben A. Now you see it, now you don't. Hepatology 2003;38:781–4.

Roskams TA, Libbrecht L, Desmet VJ. Progenitor cells in diseased human liver. Semin Liver Dis 2003;23:385–96.

Roskams TA, Theise ND, Balabaud C, et al. Nomenclature of the finer branches of the biliary tree: canals, ductules, and ductular reactions in human livers. Hepatology 2004;39:1739–45.

Si-Tayeb K, Lemaigre FP, Duncan SA. Organogenesis and development of the liver. Dev Cell 2010;18:175–89.

Zhang L, Theise N, Chua M, et al. The stem cell niche of human livers: symmetry between development and regeneration. Hepatology 2008;48:1598–607.

Assessment and Differential Diagnosis of Pathological Features

Initial examination and reporting

Naked-eye examination and description of biopsy specimens

Although naked-eye examination and description are of limited diagnostic value, they reduce the possibility of specimen identification error. The pathologist should make sure that the whole specimen has been adequately sectioned by comparing the size of the sectioned and stained tissue with the measurement recorded on macroscopic examination. Naked-eye examination also helps in the selection of suitable areas for electron microscopy. The contour and colour of needle biopsy specimens in the fixative container, in the paraffin block or on the glass slide itself may provide some preliminary diagnostic impressions, barring any technical artefacts imposed by unusual specimen handling or staining. Normal liver gives rise to cylinders of even colour and thickness, which do not fragment easily. By this standard, needle biopsies can usually be categorised as one of the following three types, based on their contours (**Fig. 4.1**): (1) *normal contour* (suggesting relatively intact architecture without advanced fibrosis, although significant pathology such as hepatitis, cholestasis or other findings may nonetheless be present); (2) *irregular contour* (suggesting the presence of chronic disease, with focal regions of narrowing due to substantial fibrosis or cirrhosis); and (3) *fragmented biopsy* (consistent with cirrhosis, primary hepatocellular carcinoma or metastatic tumour). Such impressions obviously require further confirmation on microscopy. Cholestasis imparts a green colour, whereas fatty liver is pale brown or yellow and may float in the fixative. In cholesterol ester storage disease and Wolman's disease the specimen is bright orange; this should warn the pathologist of the need to keep some tissue for frozen sectioning and electron microscopy. A black or very dark brown colour is characteristic of the Dubin–Johnson syndrome. Metastatic tumour, like fibrous tissue, is often white. Congested liver is deep red in colour.

Routine microscopy

Routine microscopy of liver biopsies should include systematic assessment of overall structure, portal tracts and their contents, terminal hepatic venules, hepatocytes and sinusoidal cells. Some pathologists use a pro forma or checklist in order to avoid omitting relevant data.[1]

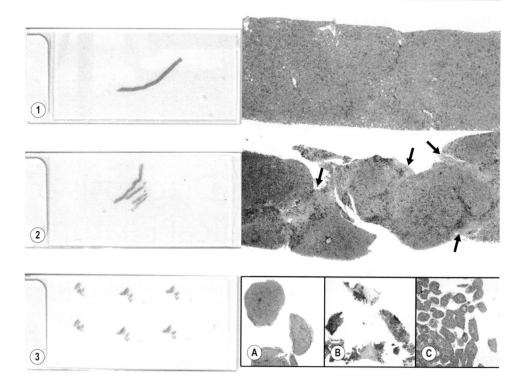

Figure 4.1 Variations in needle liver biopsy specimens.
The contours of the needle biopsy cores on the glass slide may offer some preliminary diagnostic impressions, usually falling into one of the following three categories: (1): normal contour (suggesting relatively preserved architecture without extensive fibrosis, although chronic hepatitis, steatosis or other disease may be present); (2) irregular contour, where fibrosis or cirrhosis has resulted in focal narrowing (fibrotic portal tracts shown at arrows); and (3) fragmentation, usually due to one of three conditions: cirrhosis (**A**), metastatic tumour (**B**) or primary hepatocellular carcinoma (**C**). (Needle biopsies, H&E).

The following sections are intended to help in the evaluation of pathological changes. Most of the information is also found in other parts of the book, under individual diseases. There is inevitably some repetition, because many of the listed features are found in combination. The final part of the chapter contains guidance on the differential diagnosis of a number of specific pathological findings.

Basic patterns of injury

Structural changes, collapse and fibrosis

Minor structural changes are difficult to assess in sections stained with haematoxylin and eosin (H&E), and may indeed be missed altogether. Examination of a connective tissue preparation is therefore often important. Normal liver tissue shows a hierarchy of ramifying portal tracts of varied sizes which are present in needle and wedge biopsy samples (**Fig. 4.2**). The subdivisions of these portal tracts parallel the hierarchy of hepatic artery and portal vein branches and bile ducts as they distribute throughout the liver and can thereby be roughly subdivided into segmental, area, conducting (septal) and terminal

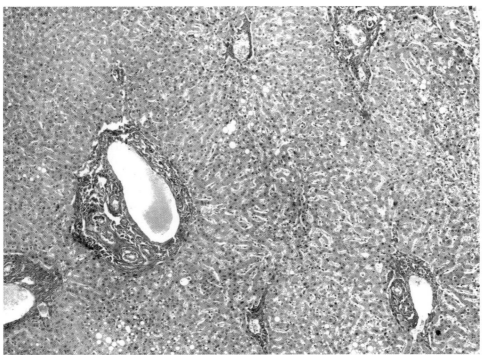

Figure 4.2
Portal tract size variations.
Biopsies contain portal tracts ranging in size from larger conducting tracts (at left) to the small terminal tracts (right top and bottom) from which blood enters the parenchyma. (Wedge biopsy, chromotrope–aniline blue.)

portal tract units (**see Fig. 5.1**). For detection of the most minor abnormalities an uncounterstained silver impregnation for reticulin is generally best, although pericellular fibrosis is most easily detected in sections stained for collagen.

Using these methods, an impression may be gained that, although portal tracts and terminal venules are normally related to each other, the portal tracts are enlarged and perhaps even linked by fibrous septa. This is consistent with mild chronic viral hepatitis or with one of the conditions in which portal changes typically predominate; these include biliary tract disease, haemochromatosis, congenital hepatic fibrosis and schistosomiasis. If on the other hand the reticulin framework of the parenchyma is distorted, lesions characterised by lobular damage should be considered. These include acute and chronic hepatitis as well as forms of biliary disease in which there is also hepatocellular damage, notably primary biliary cirrhosis. Venous congestion leads to regular condensation of perivenular reticulin.

Recent collapse and fibrosis are sometimes difficult to distinguish, even with the help of good collagen stains. A stain for elastic tissue can help to resolve this problem because the presence of elastic fibres outside the portal tracts is an indication of long-standing disease. Collagen stains are helpful for the recognition of blocked veins, for example in necrotic areas, alcoholic liver disease, venous outflow obstruction and epithelioid haemangioendothelioma. Collagen staining is important for the detection of pericellular fibrosis, as already indicated, and should therefore be used whenever there is substantial steatosis or a suspicion of steatohepatitis.

The histological diagnosis of cirrhosis is fully discussed in **Chapter 10**. Once cirrhosis has developed, the pattern of fibrosis is one of the features that may help to determine its cause. In primary or secondary biliary cirrhosis, for example, fibrosis expanding and linking the portal tracts is a more important early factor in pathogenesis than hepatocellular regeneration; this is reflected in the morphological picture of broad perilobular septa surrounding irregularly shaped islands of parenchyma (**see Fig. 5.11**). In hereditary haemochromatosis and chronic venous outflow obstruction the impression is also of fibrosis rather than regeneration as the principal pathogenetic factor. In these diseases with a long precirrhotic phase of fibrosis, transected parenchymal peninsulas may be mistaken for true regenerative nodules. This is particularly common just deep to the liver capsule. Isolated subcapsular nodules in an otherwise not nodular biopsy should therefore be interpreted with caution.

Hepatocellular damage

There is a broad histological spectrum of possible hepatocellular damage, ranging from subtle changes affecting the appearance of the cytoplasm or specific organelles to obvious hepatocyte ballooning, apoptosis or necrosis. Normal hepatocytes are polygonal in shape, with abundant pale-staining granular cytoplasm rich in glycogen. An occasional **apoptotic body** (acidophil body) may be seen in normal liver. When present, apoptotic bodies are typically seen within sinusoidal spaces following extrusion from liver-cell plates (**Fig. 4.3**). These ovoid bodies are highly eosinophilic and sometimes require through-focusing on microscopic examination because their thickness is not confocal with the surrounding tissue. In cholestasis from any cause, and in donor livers shortly after transplantation, there is often an increase in the number of apoptotic bodies as well as in mitotic figures in

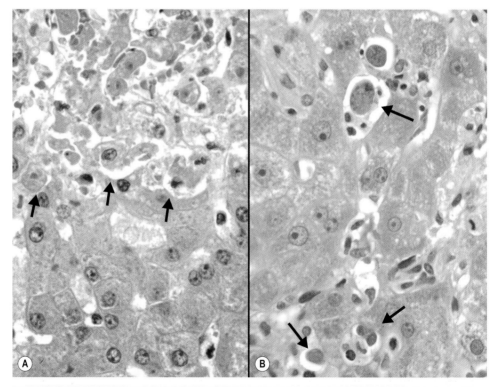

Figure 4.3 Coagulative necrosis vs apoptosis.
A: The hepatocytes above the arrows have undergone coagulative necrosis and are sharply delimited from the viable hepatocytes below. Necrosis was initiated by ischaemia due to hepatic artery thrombosis after liver transplantation. The necrotic hepatocytes show hypereosinophilia, nuclear pyknosis and discohesion. (Explant liver, H&E.) **B:** Multiple apoptotic bodies of different sizes are seen within sinusoids (arrows). The accentuated hepatocellular apoptosis was due to early recurrence of hepatitis C virus infection 2 months after transplantation. (Allograft needle biopsy, H&E.)

hepatocytes. Abundant apoptotic bodies are found in acute hepatitis from any cause.[2] They were first described by Councilman in yellow fever, so that the term 'Councilman body' should strictly speaking be confined to that disease (**see Ch. 6**).

Hepatocytes may demonstrate cytoplasmic '**ground-glass' change** in a variety of conditions[3] (**Table 4.1**). The affected liver cells have a pale pink homogeneous appearance resembling frosted glass (**Fig. 4.4**). The change may involve all or a portion of the hepatocyte cytoplasm or may be in the form of a rounded or crescentic inclusion, sometimes with a surrounding artefactual empty white space. A common example is the hepatitis B surface antigen-containing ground-glass inclusion seen in individuals with chronic hepatitis B (**Fig. 4.4A, and see Fig. 9.13**). Such inclusions are scattered randomly through the lobular parenchyma but sometimes are numerous. Use of certain medications (e.g. barbiturates) and occasionally hepatocellular cholestasis[4] can result in similar appearances, but confined to perivenular hepatocytes (**Figs 4.4B, 4.4D**) (**see Fig. 8.1**), where it is referred to as 'pseudo-ground-glass' change. Recipients of transplants (liver, cardiac, bone marrow) may also show ground-glass-like inclusions containing an abnormal type of glycogen[5–7] (**Fig. 4.4C**). These have a predilection for periportal hepatocytes, as do the ground-glass inclusions of Lafora's disease (myoclonus epilepsy. Assessment of the clinical setting together with the staining methods shown in **Table 4.1** usually clarifies the cause of the ground-glass change.

Table 4.1 Differential diagnosis of ground-glass hepatocytes

Condition	Staining method(s)
Chronic hepatitis B	Orcein, Victoria blue Immunostain for HBsAg
Medication (e.g. barbiturate)	–
Cyanamide alcohol aversion therapy	Diastase–PAS
Lafora's disease (myoclonus epilepsy)	PAS, colloidal iron
Type IV glycogenosis	PAS
Transplant recipients	PAS

HBsAg, Hepatitis B surface antigen; PAS, periodic acid–Schiff.

Moderate **hepatocyte swelling** is sometimes due to adaptive hyperplasia of smooth endoplasmic reticulum in response to drugs or, occasionally, is due to cholestasis. Perivenular hepatocyte swelling may be seen in allograft biopsies soon after liver transplantation due to preservation injury of the donor liver (**see Fig. 16.2**). More severe swelling with rounding of the cell outlines is a feature of cell damage (**Fig. 4.5A**). It may accompany canalicular cholestasis (**see Fig. 5.2 and Fig. 16.9**), but is most characteristically found in various forms of hepatitis (**Fig. 4.5A and see Fig. 6.2**) where it is recognized by disruption of the liver-cell plates and by accompanying inflammatory cell infiltration. The liver-cell swelling seen in viral, drug and autoimmune hepatitis differs from that seen in **hepatocellular ballooning** of steatohepatitis where the liver cells have a clarified appearance and wisp-like strands of rarefied cytoplasm, sometimes with Mallory–Denk bodies (**Fig. 4.5B and see Fig. 7.8**). The term *hepatocyte ballooning* therefore has taken on a special significance when examining liver biopsies for evidence of steatohepatitis, as is further discussed in **Chapter 7**. In microvesicular steatosis, the cytoplasm of hepatocytes is expanded by minute fat droplets which are sometimes too small to resolve by routine microscopy. The frequent presence of larger fat vacuoles and the clinical context should help to make the diagnosis. Another type of hepatocyte swelling is seen in **feathery degeneration** (**Fig. 4.5C**), where intracellular cholestasis with retention of bile and bile salts results in mild hepatocyte enlargement and pale, rarefied and reticular, often vacuolated cytoplasm. Feathery degeneration is most often seen in association with large bile-duct obstruction.

Death of individual hepatocytes or small groups of these cells is loosely called **focal necrosis** (**Fig. 4.6**), although the mechanism may in fact be apoptosis, or even a combination of both (*necroapoptosis*[8]). The distinction cannot always be made easily by routine microscopy unless apoptotic bodies are seen. Focal necrosis is associated with accumulation of inflammatory cells of various types, including macrophages. **Spotty necrosis** (**Fig. 4.6**) is a term used for the same lesion in the context of acute hepatitis. Focal necrosis is a common finding which does not in itself indicate primary disease of the liver, because

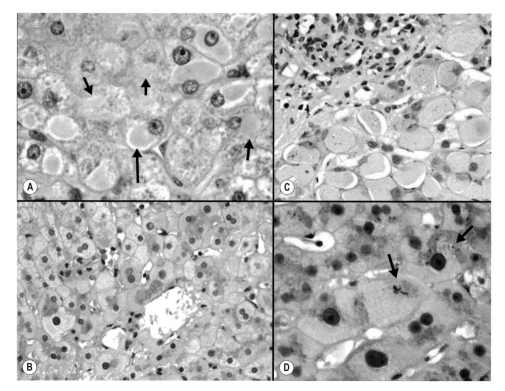

Figure 4.4 Ground-glass and ground-glass-like hepatocytes.
A: Numerous ground-glass cytoplasmic inclusions are seen within hepatocytes (large arrows) in this case of chronic hepatitis B. The inclusions represent hepatitis B virus surface antigen. Some inclusions are separated from the hepatocyte cell membrane by an artefactual empty or white halo. Even small inclusions show distinctive pale pink homogeneity (arrows). **B:** Hepatocytes around the terminal venule show pseudo-ground-glass change (induction of smooth endoplasmic reticulum) due to medication. Compare with the normal granular-appearing hepatocytes in the upper left-hand field. **C:** Liver biopsy from a bone marrow transplant recipient. There are also numerous periportal ground-glass-like inclusions. The inclusions resemble glycogen, and are thought to be a result of the many medications used in the posttransplantation clinical setting. **D:** Portions of the cytoplasm of the several hepatocytes at centre show pseudo-ground-glass change due to intracellular cholestasis (arrows). (Needle biopsies, H&E.)

it is often part of a non-specific reaction to disease elsewhere in the body. While degenerating hepatocytes or cell fragments are sometimes seen within the focal inflammatory infiltrate, the inflammatory reaction is usually more obvious than the necrosis, and the latter is assumed to have taken place because of a gap in a liver-cell plate (liver-cell 'dropout').

Hepatocyte death by **coagulative necrosis** (**Fig. 4.3**) is usually clear from its perivenular location and involvement of a contiguous group of hepatocytes in the zone of diminished perfusion. Necrotic hepatocytes show distinctive cytoplasmic eosinophilia, abnormal sizes and contours and nuclear pyknosis and karyorrhexis. Perivenular (centrilobular, acinar zones 3) coagulative necrosis is usually seen following hypotensive or septic shock, or after hypoperfusion due to left ventricular failure or hepatic artery thrombosis. If several days have elapsed since the episode(s) of liver hypoperfusion, there sometimes is a reactive sinusoidal neutrophil infiltrate adjacent to the necrotic hepatocytes, particularly if the patient has been maintained on pressor agents.[9]

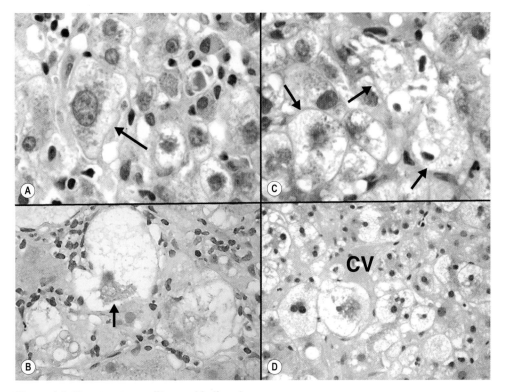

Figure 4.5 Hepatocyte swelling and ballooning.
A: A swollen and enlarged hepatocyte (arrow) is seen near lymphocytes and ceroid-laden Kupffer cells in this case of acute hepatitis. Compare the swollen liver cell to the more normal glycogenated hepatocytes at lower right. **B:** Hepatocyte ballooning in this case of non-alcoholic steatohepatitis (NASH) shows distinctive cytoplasmic rarefaction and wisp-like strands of cytoplasm. One affected hepatocyte also contains clumped eosinophilic Mallory–Denk body material (arrow). **C:** Feathery degeneration with retention of bile salts and visible bile is seen in these ballooned hepatocytes (arrows). **D:** Liver allograft biopsy obtained 1 week after transplantation because of abnormal serum liver tests. Hepatocytes around the central vein (CV) are swollen because of preservation injury. (Needle biopsies, H&E.)

Confluent necrosis

Confluent necrosis (**see Fig. 8.4**) refers to substantial areas of liver-cell death. The most common cause of this type of necrosis in biopsy material is hepatitis, whether viral, drug-related or autoimmune, in which case the necrosis is accompanied by an inflammatory reaction. Confluent necrosis with little or no inflammation is seen in hypoperfusion of the hepatic parenchyma (**Fig. 4.6**), as in shock or left ventricular failure, and in heatstroke (**see Fig. 12.2**). Paracetamol (acetaminophen) poisoning produces a similar lesion (**see Fig. 8.4**). In all the above examples the necrosis is typically perivenular. A predilection for mid-zonal (acinar zones 2) necrosis is seen with yellow fever (**see Fig. 6.3**) and dengue virus infections. Some poisons, including ferrous sulphate and phosphorus,[10] typically cause periportal (zone 1) necrosis. Haphazardly distributed areas of necrosis are found in disseminated herpesvirus infections (e.g. herpes simplex, varicella) (**see Fig. 15.4**) and in mycobacterial diseases. Tumour necrosis may be so extensive that no recognisable tumour tissue is present in the section; in such cases the reticulin pattern may help to establish a diagnosis.

Figure 4.6
Focal necrosis vs. spotty necrosis.
A: Focal necrosis (at arrow) is seen in this otherwise quiescent lobular parenchyma. The liver-cell plates are interrupted by a collection of lymphocytes and Kupffer cells where there appears to be 'liver-cell dropout'.
B: This case of acute viral hepatitis shows 'spotty necrosis' with numerous necroinflammatory foci throughout the lobule. (Needle biopsies, H&E.)

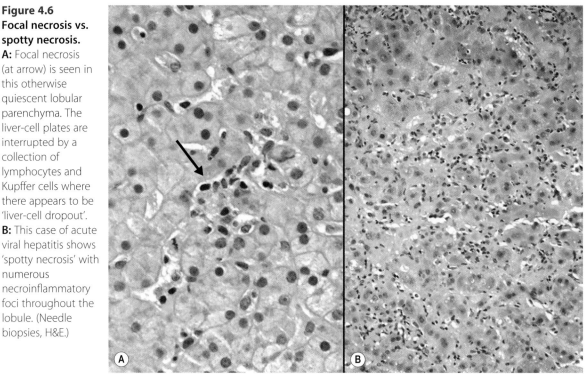

If severe and extensive, confluent necrosis may form bridges linking vascular structures and is referred to as **bridging necrosis**. Linking of portal tracts to each other is common in conditions in which portal tracts are widened, for example by chronic hepatitis or biliary tract disease. Linking of perivenular areas to each other is found in some examples of parenchymal hypoperfusion and venous outflow obstruction (**Fig. 4.6**).

Bridging hepatic necrosis linking terminal hepatic venules (centrilobular veins) to portal tracts (**Figs 4.7 and 4.8**) deserves specific notation by the pathologist because of its potential association with more severe disease.[11] Central-to-portal bridging necrosis is a fairly common feature of acute hepatitis of viral type; in such cases the bridges show inflammation, loss of hepatocytes and reticulin condensation, without significant fibrosis or elastic fibres. It is also seen in exacerbations of chronic hepatitis. Old bridges contain elastic fibres as well as collagen fibres. Such bridging fibrosis is an important component of the more severe examples of both chronic viral and autoimmune hepatitis. Contraction of collagen-rich bridges may produce rapid and severe distortion of the normal hepatic microstructure, with correspondingly rapid progression to cirrhosis.

Panlobular (panacinar) and multilobular (multiacinar) necrosis (see Fig. 6.11) are terms used to describe confluent necrosis involving entire single lobules or several adjacent lobules respectively. They are further discussed in **Chapter 6**. **Massive hepatic necrosis** describes loss of virtually all hepatic parenchyma and is characteristically seen in *acute liver failure* of viral, drug, autoimmune or unknown causation. Histologically there is widespread hepatocyte loss with collapse of reticulin accompanied by outgrowth of periportal bile ductular structures ('neocholangioles') derived from activated hepatic progenitor cells. Such livers grossly are reduced in size and show capsular wrinkling due to loss of subcapsular parenchyma. The term **submassive necrosis** is used in certain cases which present clinically as acute liver failure to describe severe loss of liver parenchyma (as in massive hepatic necrosis), but accompanied by foci of regenerative hyperplasia and nodules that are visible on both gross and histological examination (**Fig. 4.9**). The presence of

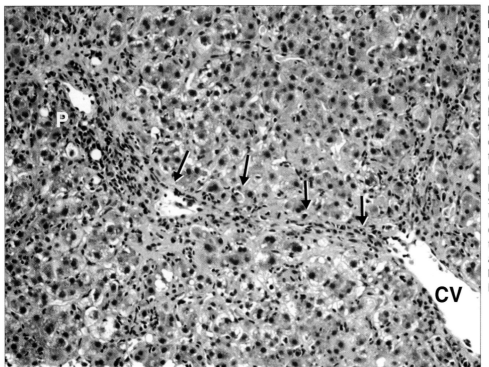

**Figure 4.7
Bridging hepatic
necrosis.**
A narrow bridge of
hepatocyte loss and
inflammation
(arrows) extends
between the portal
tract (P) and the
central vein (CV) in
this case of acute
hepatitis. The liver
parenchyma nearby
shows extensive
unrest and lobular
disarray. Compare to
the reticulin stain of
a similar example in
Figure 4.8. (Needle
biopsy, H&E.)

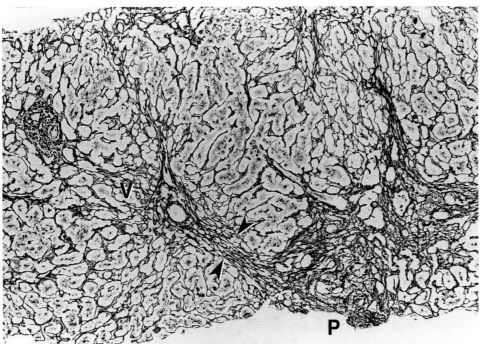

**Figure 4.8
Acute hepatitis
with bridging
necrosis.**
Collapsed reticulin
here gives a false
impression of
chronic liver disease.
A bridge or passive
septum (arrowheads)
links an expanded
portal tract (P) with a
terminal hepatic
venule (V). (Needle
biopsy, reticulin.)

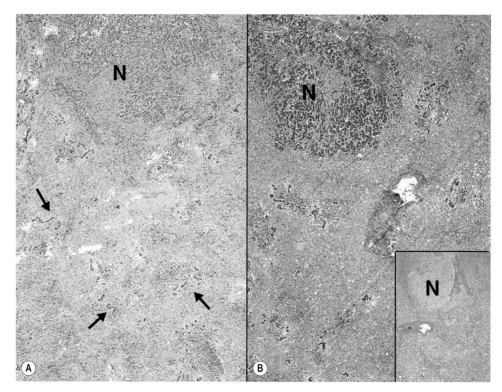

Figure 4.9 Submassive necrosis.
A: In this case of fulminant hepatitis, nearly all the liver parenchyma has disappeared due to massive necrosis. A ductular reaction is prominent (arrows). A few regenerative nodules were evident on gross examination of the explant liver and are also evident microscopically (N). **B:** Trichrome connective tissue stain highlights the extent of parenchymal necrosis, the ductular reaction, native portal tracts (bright blue) and very early fibrosis (light grey-blue) in the regions of collapse. An emerging regenerative nodule is present at top (N). Inset: Reticulin stain of the same field shown in **A** and **B** contrasts the reticulin collapse and condensation below and the regenerative nodule (N) at top. (Explant liver; **A**: H&E; **B**: trichrome stain; inset: reticulin stain.)

regenerative nodules and, depending on the individual case, evidence of early fibrosis are consistent with a more protracted time course, possibly of several months, during which the hepatitis may have been subclinical.

Interface hepatitis (piecemeal necrosis)

Interface hepatitis (piecemeal necrosis) (**see Figs 9.3 and 9.4**) is a process of inflammation and erosion of the hepatic parenchyma at its junction with portal tracts or fibrous septa. The term 'interface hepatitis' was introduced because the death of hepatocytes probably involves apoptosis rather than, or as well as, necrosis,[12–14] and because it takes place at the parenchymal–connective tissue interface. It is common in chronic viral hepatitis but is also found in other conditions (**see Box 9.2**). The inflammatory infiltrate is composed mainly of lymphocytes, with or without recognisable plasma cells, and is accompanied by fibrosis of the affected areas with new formation of collagens and other extracellular matrix components.[15] The process is sometimes referred to as classical or lymphocytic piecemeal necrosis in order to distinguish it from biliary, ductular and fibrotic piecemeal necrosis, processes found in chronic biliary tract disease and described in the section on primary biliary cirrhosis in **Chapter 5**.

Cholestasis

In morphological terms, cholestasis is the presence of visible bile in tissue sections. It is also known as bilirubinostasis because the main component seen by light microscopy is bilirubin. Bile is rarely seen in normal liver, and then only in minute amounts; cholestasis should therefore be regarded as pathological. The location of the bile varies. The most common is in dilated bile canaliculi between hepatocytes. This canalicular form of cholestasis, sometimes called **acute cholestasis,** may be accompanied by bile accumulation in the cytoplasm of hepatocytes and Kupffer cells. Canalicular cholestasis is typically perivenular. In contrast, in patients with chronic biliary tract disease, bile may accumulate in periportal hepatocytes. This is also known as cholate stasis because abnormal bile salts are thought to contribute to its pathogenesis.

In large bile-duct obstruction in adults, bile is not usually visible under the microscope within canals of Hering, bile ductular structures or bile ducts, even though the biliary tree may be dilated. The most common cause of ductular cholestasis is sepsis. Dense bile is also visible in ductules and ducts in different forms of ductal plate malformation and in extrahepatic biliary atresia.

Canalicular cholestasis takes the form of bile plugs (bile thrombi) in dilated canaliculi (**see Fig. 5.2**). There is often brown or yellow pigment in nearby hepatocytes and Kupffer cells, but the distinction of this pigment from others such as lipofuscin and ceroid is not a serious practical problem; this is because the presence of bile in the canaliculi makes the diagnosis of cholestasis obvious. In general, cholestasis should only be diagnosed with great caution in the absence of bile plugs in canaliculi, although cytoplasmic liver-cell bilirubinostasis without canalicular bile is quite common after liver transplantation. The perivenular location of canalicular cholestasis is partly an artefact of paraffin embedding, but also reflects real functional differences between the various parts of the acinus.

The colour of bile under the microscope varies according to pigment concentration and the degree of oxidation. It may be dark brown, green or yellow, and is occasionally so pale as to make detection difficult at first glance. The van Gieson stain, which stains bilirubin green, may then be helpful (**Fig. 4.10**). Pale counterstaining, as commonly used in Perls' and Prussian blue methods for iron, also makes bile easier to see. Specific histochemical methods for bilirubin are rarely necessary in ordinary diagnostic work.

When acute cholestasis is prolonged, the relationship of hepatocytes to each other may undergo focal change. Instead of the normal arrangement of two or three hepatocytes around a small bile canaliculus, the number of cells is increased and the lumen of the canaliculus considerably enlarged. The new structures are called cholestatic rosettes (**Fig. 4.11**). The lumens of the rosettes are part of the biliary tree, but the bile may be lost during processing. Even apparently empty rosettes should therefore be regarded as an indication of cholestasis. Other hepatocellular changes in cholestasis are described in **Chapter 5**, in the section on large bile-duct obstruction. Very occasionally prolonged canalicular cholestasis is associated with the accumulation of copper and copper-associated protein, but this is much more characteristic of the chronic periportal form of cholestasis, discussed below. Canalicular cholestasis in perivenular areas is mainly seen in the conditions listed in **Boxes 4.1 and 4.2**. Cholestasis of less regular distribution is common in chronic liver diseases with severe hepatocellular dysfunction or with associated sepsis.

Box 4.1 Common causes of canalicular cholestasis
Obstruction to major bile ducts
Acute hepatitis
Cholestatic drug jaundice
Sepsis
Cholestatic syndromes

Box 4.2 Main causes of bland intrahepatic cholestasis
Drugs (e.g. contraceptive steroids)
Sepsis
Benign recurrent intrahepatic cholestasis
Cholestasis of pregnancy
Posttransplant bile flow impairment or rejection
Lymphomas

**Figure 4.10
Cholestasis.**
Bile thrombi in
dilated canaliculi are
stained bright green.
The red material is
collagen. (Needle
biopsy, haematoxylin
& van Gieson.)

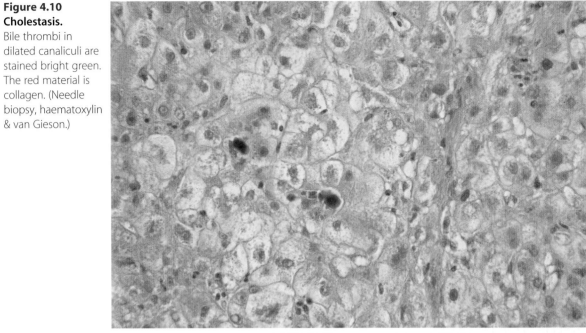

**Figure 4.11
Cholestasis.**
Several liver-cell
rosettes, glandular
formations around
prominent lumens,
are marked by
arrowheads. (Wedge
biopsy, H&E.)

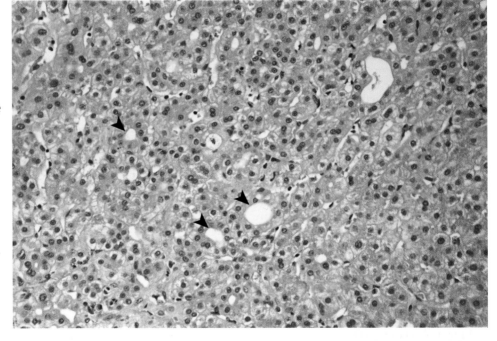

Once cholestasis is identified, the pathologist's main concern should be determining its likely cause. Pertinent questions for consideration are listed in **Box 4.3**. The aetiology usually rests among four diagnostic categories: (1) large bile-duct obstruction; (2) disorders which affect the small, intrahepatic bile ducts; (3) hepatitis; and (4) conditions associated with bland cholestasis (e.g. sepsis, bile-salt transporter mutations). These can usually be distinguished by careful and methodical examination of abnormalities in the lobules and in the portal tracts (**Fig. 4.12**). Accurate histological diagnosis is important because correct treatment may depend upon it, and a wrong answer can lead to dangerous mismanagement. It has to be admitted, however, that the pathologist cannot always give a clear answer to the questions put by the clinician.

> **Box 4.3** Decisions in the acutely jaundiced patient
>
> - Are the patient's major bile ducts obstructed?
> - Does the patient have an acute viral or drug-related hepatitis?
> - Is there evidence for a diagnosis of sepsis?
> - Does the patient have one of the intrahepatic conditions listed in **Box 4.2**?
> - Does the patient have steatohepatitis?
> - Does the patient have chronic liver disease with an acute exacerbation rather than acute liver disease?

Ductular reaction

Since large bile-duct obstruction may require a surgical or endoscopic intervention, biopsies with cholestasis require careful inspection of the portal tracts for the triad of changes[16] that typically develops within several days of obstruction, collectively referred to as the **ductular reaction**: oedema of the portal tract connective tissue; proliferation of bile ductular structures at the edges of the oedematous portal tract stroma; and scattered neutrophil infiltrates. The ductular structures which develop as a prominent feature in a variety of biliary and other conditions are believed to arise from periportal progenitor cells located in the canals of Hering[16a,16b] or possibly from bile duct cells or transdifferentiated hepatocytes (**see Ch. 5**).[16c] The ductular reaction can be viewed as a stereotypical periportal response to injury[17-19] which is exemplified by acute biliary obstruction, but which also occurs in several other pathological settings.

Certain features help in interpreting the diagnostic significance of the ductular reaction. In acute biliary obstruction, the ductular structures are arranged in parallel to the portal–parenchymal interface, associated with the portal oedema and scattered neutrophils previously mentioned (**Fig. 4.13A**). In chronic biliary tract diseases such as primary biliary cirrhosis, the ductular profiles may lie at an angle to the interface or form convoluted tangles (**Fig. 4.13B**). Hepatocellular diseases may also act as a stimulus for the ductular reaction. In a minority of patients with acute hepatitis with much cholestasis, as seen for example in hepatitis A, a ductular reaction may accompany portal infiltrates of lymphocytes and plasma cells.[20] The picture can mimic that of biliary obstruction, and the distinction requires careful consideration of the lobular changes. Ductular reaction is virtually always associated with neutrophils, so that the presence of these cells is not in itself evidence of bile-duct obstruction. Ductular reaction also is seen in some examples of non-biliary cirrhosis in which the ductular structures are not necessarily limited to the margins of portal tracts or the septal–parenchymal interface, but extend to greater distances into the fibrous tissue (**Fig. 4.13C**). However, extensive ductular reaction accompanied by other features of chronic cholestasis suggests cirrhosis of biliary origin.

In panlobular necrosis (seen, for example, in patients with fulminant or subacute viral hepatitis, in severe drug hepatotoxicity or in autoimmune hepatitis), extensive loss of hepatocytes is often associated with an exuberant ductular reaction extending from periportal regions further inward and toward the centres of lobules (**Fig. 4.13D**). The ductular reaction is now considered a major participant in the process of bridging and more progressive fibrosis in chronic liver diseases, including chronic hepatitis B and C,[21-23] steatohepatitis[24] and haemochromatosis[25] (**see Fig. 9.7**). The ductular reaction may be unusually prominent in fibrosing cholestatic hepatitis, which develops in a minority of patients with

Figure 4.12 Algorithmic approach to cholestasis.
Once the site of cholestasis is identified pathologically, careful assessment of portal tracts and acinar changes allows the major differential diagnosis to be established. *In primary biliary cirrhosis (PBC), morphological cholestasis is usually only apparent in later, advanced disease. PSC, primary sclerosing cholangitis.

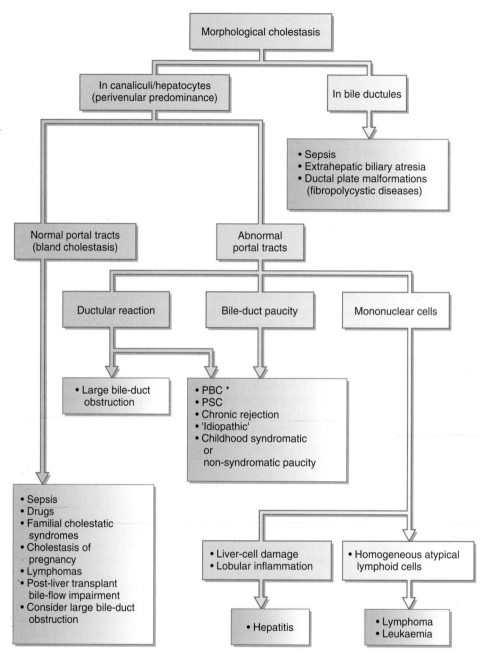

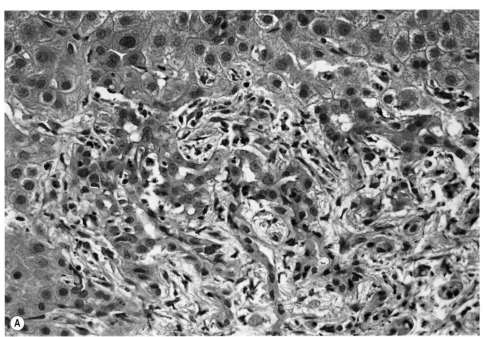

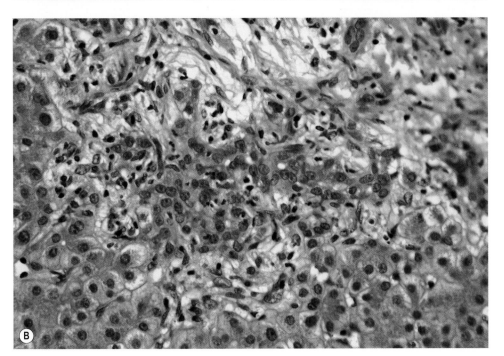

Figure 4.13 The ductular reaction in different diseases.
A: Ductular structures at the edge of the portal tract in bile-duct obstruction.
B: Tangle of ductules in primary biliary cirrhosis.

Figure 4.13, cont'd
C: Non-biliary cirrhosis: ductular structures near the edge of the nodule and within the fibrotic portal tract.
D: Multilobular necrosis: the duct-like structures probably reflect progenitor-cell activity in the absence of adequate hepatocellular regeneration. (H&E.)

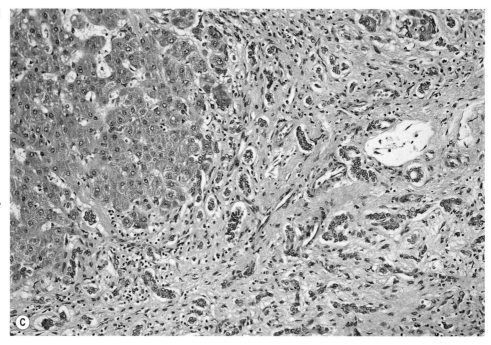

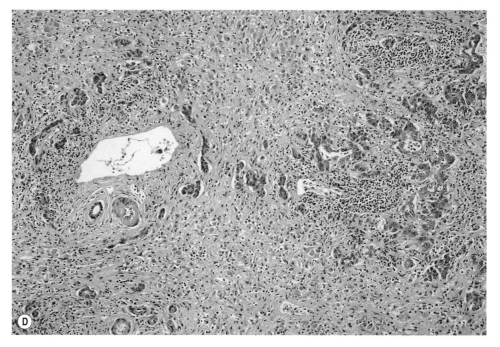

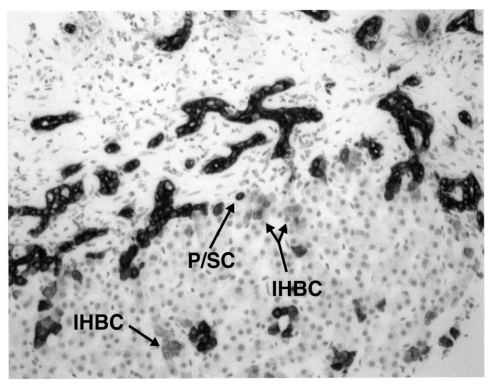

Figure 4.14 The ductular reaction with cytokeratin 7 immunohistochemistry.
In this case of primary sclerosing cholangitis (P/SC) numerous bile ductular structures have developed and are more or less parallel to the portal–parenchymal interface. A few periportal cells with less intense staining more closely resemble hepatocytes and represent intermediate hepatobiliary cells (IHBC), also termed 'biliary hepatocytes'. Small, round and darkly stained periportal cells are likely hepatic progenitor cells. (Needle biopsy, specific immunoperoxidase.)

recurrence of hepatitis B or C after liver transplantation (**see Figs 16.14 and 16.15**). In any situation in which the relative diagnostic importance of the ductular reaction must be established, immunostains for cytokeratin 7 or 19 are useful for highlighting the ductular structures (**Fig. 4.14 and see Figs 5.24 and 5.25**).

Chronic cholestasis (cholate stasis, pseudoxanthomatous change, precholestasis; **see Fig. 5.10**) is seen in chronic liver diseases, especially those involving the biliary tree, and is the result of interference with bile flow at the level of the portal tracts. Bile (i.e. bilirubinostasis) may or may not be obvious, and the lesion is more easily recognised by periportal hepatocellular swelling and pallor, and by the accumulation of copper and copper-associated protein in the affected cells. Mallory–Denk bodies may also be present. In some instances these are associated with an infiltrate of neutrophils, in which case the distinction from steatohepatitis must be made on the overall appearances, the periportal location and clinical context. The connective tissue adjacent to an area of chronic cholestasis is often oedematous. It may show a ductular reaction with mixed acute and chronic inflammatory cells which sometimes disrupts the limiting plates of hepatocytes around the portal tracts. The blurring of this margin has been likened to the features seen in classical interface hepatitis of chronic hepatitis (where a lymphoplasmacytic infiltrate blurs the portal tract-limiting plate margin), and has been referred to with terms such as 'biliary interface hepatitis' (formerly 'ductular piecemeal necrosis'). In chronic biliary tract disease, the ductular structures and associated neutrophils are helpful for recognising the presence and role of the ductular reaction. Chronic cholestasis, unlike acute canalicular cholestasis, is not necessarily associated with clinical jaundice or a high level of serum bilirubin, but the serum alkaline phosphatase level is characteristically raised.

Loss of interlobular bile ducts is a key feature of several diseases in childhood and adult life. These are sometimes referred to as *vanishing bile-duct syndromes.* The principal causes in children are syndromatic and non-syndromatic paucity of intrahepatic bile ducts, α_1-antitrypsin deficiency and early-onset sclerosing cholangitis. Some uncommon familial cholestatic syndromes and Langerhans-cell histiocytosis should also be considered. In adults (**see Table 5.1**) the most common causes are primary biliary cirrhosis, primary sclerosing cholangitis, graft-versus-host disease and chronic liver graft rejection.

In assessing duct loss it is important to bear in mind that not every small portal tract is seen to contain a bile duct in the plane of section. In a study of normal human liver biopsies,[26] 7% of sectioned portal tracts did not contain a bile duct. For confident assessment of duct numbers a biopsy must therefore contain several portal tracts. Loss of ducts is accompanied in many, but not all, cases by the features of chronic cholestasis outlined above. This depends on the extent of duct loss, the underlying aetiology and the degree of fibrosis. A significant ductular reaction develops in some conditions of bile-duct loss (primary biliary cirrhosis, primary sclerosing cholangitis) but not others (Alagille's syndrome in children,[27] chronic liver graft rejection[28]).

Granules of the **copper-associated protein** metallothionein can be stained by several methods, including orcein and Victoria blue. They are usually positive with periodic acid–Schiff (PAS) staining after diastase digestion. Their most common location is in periportal hepatocytes or, in cirrhotic livers, in hepatocytes at the periphery of nodules. This reflects the inability of the hepatocytes to excrete copper efficiently. Some granules can be seen in cirrhosis of any cause, but large amounts should lead to a suspicion of chronic biliary tract disease or intrahepatic cholestasis.[29] Copper itself is usually demonstrable in the same location, and there may be other features of chronic cholestasis, such as ductular proliferation, neutrophils, intercellular fibrosis and oedema. A few granules of copper-associated protein are sometimes seen deeper within the acini in prolonged acute cholestasis.

Copper-associated protein also accumulates in Wilson's disease, as discussed in **Chapter 14**. As a rule neither the protein nor copper itself is demonstrable by staining in the early stages of the disease. When cirrhosis develops in Wilson's disease some nodules may be rich in copper-associated protein and copper (although one may be demonstrable without the other), while others are negative. The copper and the protein are usually diffusely distributed throughout a nodule, in contrast to their location in chronic cholestasis.

Differential diagnosis of individual findings

The selected features illustrated and described below are discussed in other chapters of this book but occur with sufficient frequency or in distinctive contexts as to merit highlighting here.

Bile-duct damage

The presence of damage to intrahepatic bile ducts is usually signalled by the presence of duct epithelial changes accompanied by adjacent portal tract inflammatory cell infiltrates. Damage to intrahepatic bile ducts has many

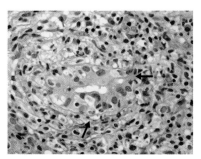

possible causes; prominent examples include primary biliary cirrhosis, idiosyncratic drug toxicity and acute cellular rejection following liver transplantation. Injured bile ducts demonstrate a variety of epithelial abnormalities, including intraepithelial inflammatory cells, epithelial stratification, vacuolisation, necrosis and attenuation, and altered nuclear polarity (**Fig. 4.15**). The inflammation is chiefly lymphocytic, with variable numbers of plasma cells and occasional neutrophils. Eosinophils may be prominent, particularly in primary biliary cirrhosis and with certain hepatotoxic drugs. The most extreme damage may result in complete destruction of the duct epithelium resulting in widespread bile duct loss (*ductopenia*).

Figure 4.15 Bile-duct damage.
The epithelium of the bile duct at centre is infiltrated by lymphocytes and shows altered nuclear polarity, focal vacuolisation and nuclear stratification. The affected bile duct is an example of a 'florid bile duct lesion' seen in primary biliary cirrhosis. The pink basement membrane surrounding the duct has ruptured (arrow below) and has been breached by lymphocytes (arrow at 3 o'clock). (Needle biopsy, H&E.)

Bile-duct plate

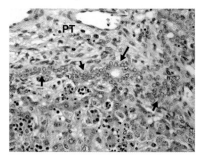

The bile-duct plate is a normal feature of intrahepatic bile-duct tubulogenesis in the growing fetal liver.[30] It may take the form of a single- or double-layered flattened cuboidal epithelial layer surrounding all or part of the loosely organised stroma of the developing portal tracts (**Fig. 4.16**). Its significance lies in its recognition in fetal liver specimens and in understanding its relationship to liver diseases characterised by ductal plate malformations such as congenital hepatic fibrosis (**see Ch. 13**) which represent abnormalities of bile-duct plate remodelling.

Figure 4.16 The bile-duct plate.
In this 19-week fetus the flattened cuboidal epithelium of the bile-duct plate (small arrows) surrounds the circumference of the portal tract (PT) seen at top. Early bile-duct tubulogenesis has been initiated (large arrow). (Postmortem liver, H&E.)

Bile ductular cholestasis

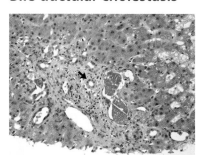

In adults, inspissated concretions of bile localised within periportal bile ductular structures is chiefly seen in sepsis (**Fig. 4.17**). Many, if not most, portal tracts are affected but the native bile ducts usually do not contain bile. In the neonatal liver biopsy this lesion may be seen in extrahepatic biliary atresia and in α_1-antitrypsin deficiency (although in these disorders the ductular bile may be very focal and is usually in smaller bile plugs or inspissates).

Figure 4.17 Bile ductular cholestasis.
Pools of inspissated bile are present in dilated periportal bile ductular structures. This distribution of cholestasis is characteristically seen in sepsis. Note that the native bile duct (arrow) does not contain bile. (Needle biopsy, H&E.)

Ceroid-laden Kupffer cells

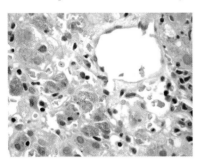

Recent hepatic necroinflammatory activity (e.g. acute or chronic hepatitis or ischaemic injury) is often associated with intrasinusoidal collections of tan-brown-staining, ceroid-laden Kupffer cells (**Fig. 4.18**). The pigment is rich in oxidised lipids, is found within Kupffer cell lysosomes and represents phagocytic debris derived from the cell membranes and other organelles of necrotic hepatocytes. Ceroid-laden Kupffer cells are typically more prominent in centrilobular regions (acinar zones 3), stain positively with diastase-PAS and retain their tan-brown colour on iron stain. The pigment should not be misconstrued as haemosiderin (which on H&E stain appears more glassy and refractile), although small amounts of haemosiderin are sometimes present in acute hepatitis. Recent episodes of obstructive jaundice with cholestasis occasionally lead to similar-appearing pigment in Kupffer cells.

Figure 4.18 Ceroid-laden Kupffer cells.
Recent necroinflammatory activity near the efferent vein at top has resulted in liver-cell dropout and intrasinusoidal collections of enlarged Kupffer cells with tan, granular pigment (phagocytic debris in lysosomes). (Needle biopsy, H&E.)

Sinusoidal congestion

Sinusoidal congestion is often centrilobular (acinar zone 3) due to obstruction of efferent venous outflow returning to the heart in patients with heart failure (**Fig. 4.19**) (the so-called 'nutmeg' liver on gross examina-

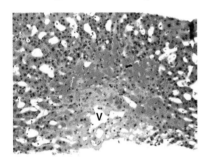

tion), or other causes of *hepatic venous outflow obstruction* (**see Ch. 12**). Sinusoidal dilatation with liver-cell plate atrophy may accompany the congestion, and if obstruction is chronic, there may also be perivenular and perisinusoidal fibrosis ('*cardiac sclerosis*'). In the liver allograft biopsy following liver transplantation, centrilobular congestion with associated lymphocytic central vein and sinusoidal endotheliitis, hepatocyte dropout and variable mild sinusoidal dilatation is diagnostic of *central perivenulitis* as a manifestation of acute cellular rejection. Diffuse sinusoidal congestion is seen in the '*congestive hepatopathy*' of sickle-cell disease, while periportal congestion, haemorrhage, fibrin thrombi and hepatocyte necrosis are features seen in eclampsia (**see Ch. 15**).

Figure 4.19 Sinusoidal congestion.
Sinusoids near the efferent vein (V) are congested and dilated in this biopsy from a patient with long-standing history of heart failure. Mild fibrosis is seen above the vein lumen, consistent with chronic venous outflow obstruction. (Needle biopsy, H&E.)

Erythrophagocytosis

Kupffer cell erythrophagocytosis (**Fig. 4.20**) is an unusual histological finding seen most often in systemic viral

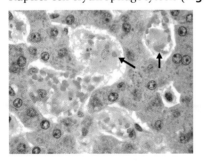

infections and in association with haemophagocytic lymphohistiocytosis[31] (HLH) and its variant form macrophage activation syndrome (MAS). HLH and MAS usually develop in the setting of an underlying acquired condition such as rheumatic disease, systemic viral infection (herpes simplex and Epstein–Barr virus commonly) or malignant lymphoma, or there may be a known genetic cause,[32] with defective inflammatory cell granule function and/or release. Activated lymphocytes in HLH and MAS may infiltrate the portal tracts and sinusoids, sometimes causing bile-duct damage or histological changes resembling chronic hepatitis, including formation of apoptotic bodies (**see Ch. 15**).

Figure 4.20 Erythrophagocytosis.
Erythrocytes are readily seen within sinusoidal Kupffer cells (arrows) in this case of suspected haemophagocytic lymphohistiocytosis. (Needle biopsy, H&E.)

Extramedullary haemopoiesis (EMH)

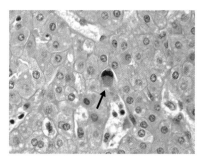

EMH is often present in neonatal liver biopsies and may be seen in adults when bone marrow is replaced by neoplasm or in myelofibrosis. Certain primary liver tumours also feature EMH, particularly hepatoblastoma and hepatocellular adenoma. Congested liver and allograft liver biopsies following liver transplantation are other settings for EMH. **Isolated megakaryocytes** may be seen in any of the preceding conditions (**Fig. 4.21**). They are also occasionally identified in cirrhosis or nodular regenerative hyperplasia. Dysmature sinusoidal megakaryocytes are seen in transient abnormal myelopoiesis associated with Down syndrome.[33]

Figure 4.21 Isolated sinusoidal megakaryocyte.
A solitary megakaryocyte (arrow) is present in a sinusoidal space in this biopsy specimen of hepatocellular adenoma. The constituent hepatocytes of the tumour appear benign and grow in thickened plates. (Needle biopsy, H&E.)

Perisinusoidal fibrosis

Fibrosis within the space of Disse (perisinusoidal fibrosis) in centrilobular regions (acinar zones 3) may be seen in steatohepatitis (**see Ch. 7**) or, in the absence of steatosis, hepatocyte ballooning or evidence of steatohepatitis, as late residua following prior episodes of steatohepatitis. The histological differential diagnosis

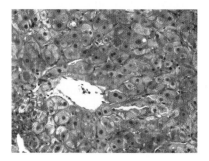

includes long-standing cardiac failure (*'cardiac sclerosis'*) and other conditions associated with chronic hepatic venous outflow obstruction (**Fig. 4.22**); previous episodes of centrilobular necroinflammation in the variant histological form of autoimmune hepatitis (**see Fig. 9.20**); and in liver allografts after liver transplantation, as sequelae of previous episodes of rejection central perivenulitis (**see Ch. 16**). Non-zonal perisinusoidal fibrosis may be seen in certain diabetics with *diabetic* hepatosclerosis (**see Ch. 7**). In liver transplant recipients with recurrent hepatitis C virus infection, perisinusoidal fibrosis in periportal[34] and lobular[35] regions may be associated with more severe disease, including fibrosing cholestatic hepatitis[35] (**see Ch. 16**).

Figure 4.22 Perisinusoidal fibrosis.
The central vein shows a surrounding network of perisinusoidal and pericellular fibrosis typical of the 'chicken-wire' fibrosis associated with alcoholic and non-alcoholic steatohepatitis. Residual fibrosis of this type may be present after resolution of steatosis and steatohepatitis. (Needle biopsy, H&E.)

Inflammatory cell infiltration
Neutrophils

Neutrophils are most numerous in portal tracts in large bile-duct obstruction, and in any condition in which there is an extensive ductular reaction (see above). In ascending cholangitis they are found in the lumens and walls of bile ducts. In intrahepatic or extrahepatic sepsis there may be neutrophils around ducts and bile within their lumens. Neutrophils are also seen in the sinusoids. A few neutrophils in a predominantly lymphocytic–plasmacytic portal infiltrate are common in acute hepatitis from any cause, but predominance of neutrophils suggests possible drug-related liver injury.

Diffuse infiltration of the parenchyma by neutrophils is unusual. It may represent a classical acute inflammatory response to extensive tissue destruction from any cause. Localised infiltrates are found in steatohepatitis, especially when alcohol-related. However, a mainly lymphocytic infiltrate does not exclude the diagnosis if other features are present (**see Ch. 7**). Focal accumulations of neutrophils (microabscesses) are a feature of cytomegalovirus infection (**see Fig. 16.13**) and of perfusion injury in liver grafts. They are also seen in many other complications of liver transplantation, though usually in smaller numbers than in cytomegalovirus infection.[36] Clusters of neutrophils may be found within sinusoids in any wedge biopsies taken in the course of surgery (**see Fig. 3.12**), and should not then be taken as indicating specific hepatic pathology.

Eosinophils

Portal infiltrates in many different liver diseases include occasional eosinophils, and their presence does not necessarily imply drug hypersensitivity or toxicity. Portal tracts often show a few eosinophils accompanying lymphocytes and plasma cells in chronic viral and autoimmune hepatitis. They are common in primary biliary cirrhosis and are occasionally abundant.[37] After liver transplantation they are one of the manifestations of cellular rejection.[38] An infiltrate with very prominent eosinophils suggests drug toxicity, systemic conditions with eosinophilia, parasitic disease or eosinophilic gastroenteritis.[39] Focal accumulations of eosinophils are seen in the parenchyma within some granulomas, notably those due to parasites. Neonatal liver biopsies may show abundant eosinophils within portal tracts and periportal sinusoids as constituents of normal EMH.

Plasma cells

Portal and acinar plasma cell infiltrates are often striking in autoimmune hepatitis, but they may also be seen in acute or chronic viral hepatitis. They are sometimes abundant in hepatitis A. Plasma cells form an important component of the portal infiltrates of primary biliary cirrhosis. Numerous plasma cells in portal tracts with features of biliary tract obstruction, including periductal 'onion-skin' fibrosis, should raise the possibility of IgG4-related sclerosing cholangitis (**see Ch. 5**). Large numbers of plasma cells in liver allograft biopsies may be seen in recurrent autoimmune hepatitis, de novo autoimmune hepatitis and in severe 'alloimmune' rejection lesions in certain transplant recipients with recurrent hepatitis C (**see Ch. 16**).

Lymphoid aggregates and follicles

Lymphoid structures (aggregates and follicles) may develop within portal tracts in several chronic liver diseases; the chief differential diagnosis includes chronic hepatitis, primary biliary cirrhosis and primary sclerosing cholangitis. Lymphoid aggregates are found considerably more often than follicles with germinal centres. Lymphoid aggregates are usually evident on low power as discrete, dense collections of lymphocytes that are

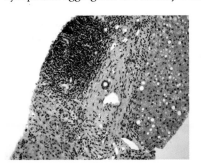

distinct from the more dispersed inflammation in the remainder of the portal tract (**Fig. 4.23**). In chronic hepatitis, aggregates are most often located adjacent to interlobular bile ducts, or they may surround ducts, occasionally with resultant duct injury, but without bile duct loss. They are very common in chronic hepatitis C,[40] but less often present in chronic hepatitis B and autoimmune hepatitis. In primary biliary cirrhosis they represent the 'tombstones' at sites of prior bile duct destruction. In primary sclerosing cholangitis they are a component of the ongoing acute and chronic periductal inflammation involving the large and small bile ducts. Diffuse, multifocal portal tract lymphoid structures may require further investigations to exclude lymphoma.

Figure 4.23 Portal lymphoid aggregate.
This case of chronic hepatitis C shows a dense lymphoid aggregate in the portal tract, to the left of the interlobular bile duct. A much milder and dispersed lymphocytic infiltrate is present in the remainder of the portal connective tissue. (Needle biopsy, H&E.)

Abnormal macrophage pigment

Tan Kupffer cell pigment within sinusoidal Kupffer cells may represent phagocytic debris following recent necroinflammatory activity, as discussed earlier, or may represent biliary material after an episode of cholestasis, or haemosiderin derived from erythrocyte breakdown. The latter pigment is positive on iron stain, while the former pigments usually are diastase PAS-positive. Granular black haemozoin pigment (derived from haemoglobin breakdown) within sinusoidal Kupffer cells and/or portal macrophages is seen in malaria and in schistosomiasis (**see Ch. 15**). A similar black pigment occasionally is seen in individuals who have received gold salts or total knee or hip titanium–aluminium prosthetic replacements.[41]

References

1 Foschini M, Sarti F, Dina RE, et al. Standardized reporting of histological diagnoses for non-neoplastic liver conditions in needle biopsies. Virchows Arch 1995;426:593–6.

2 Yoon J-H, Gores GJ. Death receptor-mediated apoptosis and the liver. J Hepatol 2002;37:400–10.

3 Vázquez JJ. Ground glass hepatocytes: light and electron microscopy. Characterization of the different types. Histol Histopathol 1990;5:379–86.

4 Popper H, Schaffner F. Pathophysiology of cholestasis. Hum Pathol 1970;1:1–24.

5 Lefkowitch JH, Lobritto SJ, Brown RS Jr, et al. Ground-glass, polyglucosan-like hepatocellular inclusions: a 'new' diagnostic entity. Gastroenterology 2006;131:713–18.

6 Wisell J, Boitnott J, Haas M, et al. Glycogen pseudoground glass change in hepatocytes. Am J Surg Pathol 2006;30:1085–90.

7 Bejarano PA, Garcia MT, Rodriguez MM, et al. Liver glycogen bodies: ground-glass hepatocytes in transplanted patients. Virchows Arch 2006;449:539–45.

8 Lemasters JJ. Dying a thousand deaths: redundant pathways from different organelles to apoptosis and necrosis. Gastroenterology 2005;129:351–60.

9 Lefkowitch JH, Mendez L. Morphologic features of hepatic injury in cardiac disease and shock. J Hepatol 1986;2:313–27.

10 Salfelder K, Doehnert HR, Doehnert G, et al. Fatal phosphorous poisoning: a study of forty-five autopsy cases. Beitr Pathol 1972;147:321–40.

11 Boyer JL, Klatskin G. Pattern of necrosis in acute viral hepatitis. Prognostic value of bridging (subacute hepatic necrosis). N Engl J Med 1970;283:1063–71.

12 Kerr JFR, Searle J, Halliday WJ, et al. The nature of piecemeal necrosis in chronic active hepatitis. Lancet 1979;ii:827–8.

13 Hiramatsu N, Hayashi N, Katayama K, et al. Immunohistochemical detection of Fas antigen in liver tissue of patients with chronic hepatitis C. Hepatology 1994;19:1354–9.

14 Takahara T, Nakayama Y, Itoh H, et al. Extracellular matrix formation in piecemeal necrosis: immuno-electron microscopic study. Liver 1992;12:368–80.

15 Portmann B, Popper H, Neuberger J, et al. Sequential and diagnostic features in primary biliary cirrhosis based on serial histologic study in 209 patients. Gastroenterology 1985;88:1777–90.

16 Christoffersen P, Poulsen H. Histological changes in human liver biopsies following extrahepatic biliary obstruction. Acta Pathol Microbiol Scand 1970; 212:150–7.

16a Tsuchiya A, Lu WY, Weinhold B, et al. Polysialic acikd/neural cell adhesion molecule modulates the formation of ductular reactions in liver injury. Hepatology 2014;60:1727–40.

16b Strazzabosco M, Fabris L. Neural cell adhesion molecule and polysialic acid in ductular reaction: the puzzle is far from completed, but the picture is becoming more clear. Hepatology 2014;60:1469–72.

16c Nagahamna Y, Sone M, Chen X, et al. Contributions of hepatocytes and bile ductular cells in ductular reactions and remoderling of the biliary system after chronic liver injury. Am J Pathol 2014;184:3001–12.

17 Roskams T, Desmet V. Ductular reaction and its diagnostic significance. Semin Diagn Pathol 1998;15:259–69.

18 Roskams T. Progenitor cell involvement in cirrhotic human liver diseases: from controversy to consensus. J Hepatol 2003;39:431–4.

19 Gouw ASH, Clouston AD, Theise ND. Ductular reactions in human liver: diversity at the interface. Hepatology 2011;54:1853–63.

20 Teixeira MR Jr, Weller IVD, Murray AM, et al. The pathology of hepatitis A in man. Liver 1982;2: 53–60.

21 Fotiadu A, Tzioufa V, Vrettou E, et al. Progenitor cell activation in chronic viral hepatitis. Liver Int 2004;24:268–74.

22 Eleazar JA, Memeo L, Jhang JS, et al. Progenitor cell expansion: an important source of hepatocyte regeneration in chronic hepatitis. J Hepatol 2004;41:983–91.

23 Gadd VL, Melino M, Roy S, et al. Portal, but not lobular, macrophages express matrix metalloproteinase-9: association with the ductular reaction and fibrosis in chronic hepatitis C. Liver Int 2013;33:569–79.

24 Gadd VL, Skoien R, Powell EE, et al. The portal inflammatory infiltrate and ductular reaction in human non-alcoholic fatty liver disease. Hepatology 2014;59:1393–405.

25 Wood MJ, Gadd VL, Powell LW, et al. Ductular reaction in hereditary hemochromatosis: the link between hepatocyte senescence and fibrosis progression. Hepatology 2014;59:848–57.

26 Crawford AR, Lin X-Z, Crawford JM. The normal adult human liver biopsy: a quantitative reference standard. Hepatology 1998;28:323–31.

27 Fabris L, Cadamuro M, Guido M, et al. Analysis of liver repair mechanisms in Alagille syndrome and biliary atresia reveals a role for Notch signaling. Am J Pathol 2007;171:641–53.

28 International Panel. Update of the international Banff schema for liver allograft rejection: working recommendations for the histopathologic staging and reporting of chronic rejection. Hepatology 2000;31:792–9.

29 Guarascio P, Yentis F, Cevikbas U, et al. Value of copper-associated protein in diagnostic assessment of liver biopsy. J Clin Pathol 1983;36:18–23.

30 Strazzabosco M, Fabris L. Development of the bile ducts: essentials for the clinical hepatologist. J Hepatol 2012;56:1159–70.

31 Janka GE, Lehmberg K. Hemophagocytic lymphocytic lymphohistiocytosis: pathogenesis and treatment. Hematology Am Soc Hematol Educ Program 2013;2013:605–11.

32 Zhang M, Behrens EM, Atkinson TP, et al. Genetic defects in cytolysis in macrophage activation syndrome. Curr Rheumatol Rep 2014;16:439–46.

33 Ishigaki H, Miyauchi J, Yokoe A, et al. Expression of megakaryocytic and myeloid markers in blasts of transient abnormal myelopoiesis in a stillbirth with Down syndrome: report of histopathological findings of an autopsy case. Hum Pathol 2011;42:141–5.

34 Mariňo Z, Mensa L, Crespo G, et al. Early periportal sinusoidal fibrosis is an accurate marker of accelerated HCV recurrence after liver transplantation. J Hepatol 2014;61:270–7.

35 Dixon LR, Crawford JM. Early histologic changes in fibrosing cholestatic hepatitis C. Liver Transplant 2007;13:219–26.

36 MacDonald GA, Greenson JK, DelBuono EA, et al. Mini-microabscess syndrome in liver transplant patients. Hepatology 1997;26:192–7.

37 Terasaki S, Nakanuma Y, Yamazaki M, et al. Eosinophilic infiltration of the liver in primary biliary cirrhosis: a morphological study. Hepatology 1993;17:206–12.

38 Datta Gupta S, Hudson M, Burroughs AK, et al. Grading of cellular rejection after orthotopic liver transplantation. Hepatology 1995;21:46–57.

39 Schoonbroodt D, Horsmans Y, Laka A, et al. Eosinophilic gastroenteritis presenting with colitis and cholangitis. Dig Dis Sci 1995;40:308–14.

40 Scheuer PJ, Ashrafzadeh P, Sherlock S, et al. The pathology of hepatitis C. Hepatology 1992;15:567–71.

41 Brenard R, Dumortier P, Del Natale M, et al. Black pigments in the liver related to gold and titanium deposits. A report of four cases. Liver Int 2007;27:408–13.

General reading

Ludwig J, Batts K. Practical Liver Biopsy Interpretation: Diagnostic Algorithms. 2nd ed. Chicago, IL: ASCP Press; 1998.

Odze RD, Goldblum JR, editors. Surgical Pathology of the GI Tract, Liver, Biliary Tract and Pancreas. 2nd ed. Philadelphia: Saunders Elsevier; 2009.

Roskams T, Desmet VJ. Ductular reaction and its diagnostic significance. Semin Diagn Pathol 1998;15:259–69.

Biliary Disease

Introduction

There are many sites along the biliary tree where bile flow may be interrupted, from the bile canaliculi and smallest intrahepatic ducts to the large bile ducts and duodenum (**Fig. 5.1**). Damage or obstruction at these various sites may result in visible bile in histological sections (cholestasis), altered bile-duct morphology, changes within the portal tracts and periportal parenchyma, or combinations of these. Diseases of the larger ducts must be distinguished from diffuse intrahepatic diseases because of different clinical management, and liver biopsy is often helpful in this respect. However, diseases of large bile ducts, outside and within the liver, share pathological features and may be amenable to similar forms of treatment; for this reason the term 'extrahepatic biliary obstruction' is not used in this chapter. Carcinoma of the main hepatic ducts, for example, may be situated wholly within the liver, yet lead to the changes of large-duct obstruction. This chapter discusses these changes as well as the pathology of primary biliary cirrhosis (PBC) and primary sclerosing cholangitis (PSC), the diagnostic problem of overlap with autoimmune hepatitis (AIH) and several bile-duct paucity disorders.

Cholestasis

The term *cholestasis* in clinical and pathological usage refers to impairment of bile flow. Under the light microscope, cholestasis (sometimes called *bilirubinostasis*) is defined as the presence of bile pigment within bile canaliculi, hepatocytes and other sites. It is the morphological correlate of clinical jaundice. Cholestasis is an important finding in large bile-duct obstruction or in extensive intrahepatic bile-duct disease, but may also accompany the parenchymal damage in certain types of hepatitis. Pure (bland) cholestasis as an isolated lesion requires consideration of several possible aetiologies (**Box 5.1**), which may not be distinguishable by light microscopy alone. For example, in neonatal and childhood jaundice, cholestasis may result from mutations in bile-salt transport proteins on the canalicular membrane[1] or from mitochondriopathies,[2] problems discussed further in **Chapter 13**. In adults, drug hepatotoxicity, circulating endotoxin in

Box 5.1 Causes of intrahepatic cholestasis
Septicaemia
Drug hepatotoxicity
Bile-salt transporter mutations (e.g. Byler disease)
Extrahepatic lymphoma
Mitochondriopathies (e.g. Navajo neurohepatopathy)
Early large bile-duct obstruction

Figure 5.1
The biliary tree.
The ramifying structures of the biliary system are shown schematically. The large segmental and area ducts have peribiliary glands (PGs). The finer branches are shown in an enlargement at upper left. Boxes at right show examples of biliary disease at the specific levels affected. PBC, primary biliary cirrhosis; PSC, primary sclerosing cholangitis.

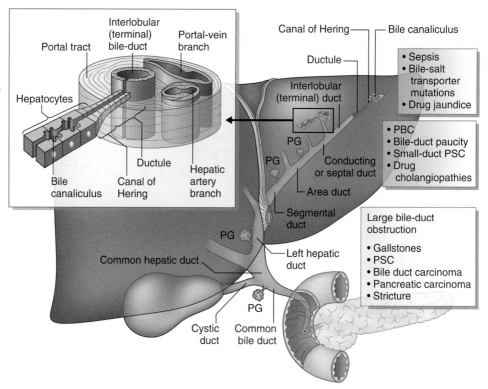

septicaemia[3] and cytokine release from extrahepatic lymphoma[4] are further examples of functional disorders of bile secretory physiology that may lead to intrahepatic cholestasis (discussed further in **Ch. 4**). The pathologist's first priority when cholestasis is present, nevertheless, is careful examination of the portal tracts for possible changes of mechanical large bile-duct obstruction, which are described below.

Large bile-duct obstruction

Biopsies from patients with large-duct obstruction are much less often seen than formerly because of improved imaging methods. However, the pathologist needs to be able to recognise the characteristic changes, especially following liver transplantation. From the first weeks of obstruction there is cholestasis in perivenular areas; that is to say, bile is visible under the microscope in the form of bile thrombi (bile plugs) in canaliculi and as yellow-brown pigment in hepatocytes and Kupffer cells (**Fig. 5.2**). The presence of canalicular bile thrombi distinguishes cholestasis from other pigmentations (**see Box 4.1**). Kupffer cells in cholestatic areas are enlarged and pigmented, containing both bile and diastase-resistant periodic acid–Schiff (PAS)-positive material. In recovering obstruction the Kupffer-cell changes persist while bile thrombi become smaller and less numerous. Finally, as in residual acute hepatitis, a few diastase–PAS-positive Kupffer cells may provide the only histological evidence of a recent episode of jaundice.

At first the hepatocytes in areas of cholestasis show little change, but with time they often become swollen. Their nuclei increase in size and number and a few apoptotic bodies and mitoses may be seen, indicating increased cell turnover. Individual hepatocytes or small groups of cells undergo **feathery degeneration**, characterised by rarefied and reticular cytoplasm (**Fig. 5.3**). The lesion is focal and the affected cells are typically surrounded

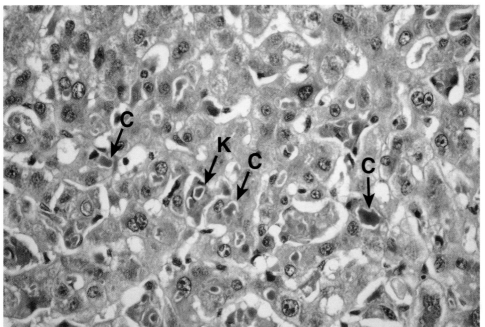

Figure 5.2
Cholestasis.
Bile is seen in the form of bile thrombi (bile plugs) in dilated canaliculi (C), as well as in Kupffer cells (K). (Needle biopsy, H&E.)

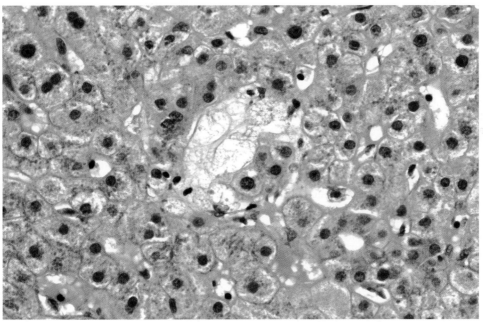

Figure 5.3
Cholestasis.
Small groups of swollen hepatocytes at centre have undergone feathery degeneration. Adjacent hepatocytes appear normal. (Wedge biopsy, H&E.)

by more or less normal hepatocytes. Feathery degeneration may be difficult to distinguish from the ballooning degeneration of hepatitis (**see Fig. 6.2**) or following liver transplantation, but in ballooning the cytoplasm is often granular rather than feathery and the lesion is more widespread in the lobule.

In a minority of patients with obstructed ducts **bile infarcts** form (**Fig. 5.4**). These are substantial areas of hepatocellular degeneration or death containing pale or bile-stained hepatocytes or discrete rounded cells that are difficult to distinguish from macrophages.

**Figure 5.4
Large bile-duct
obstruction with
bile infarct.**
A bile infarct is seen
at the centre of the
field near the portal
tract. Hepatocyte
nuclei are pyknotic
within the infarct.
Some of the pink
strands represent
fibrin. (Wedge
biopsy, H&E.)

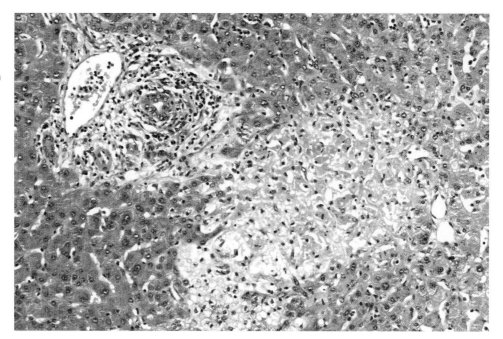

There are variable amounts of bile and fibrin, the latter often abundant. Reticulin fibres become progressively more difficult to demonstrate. Bile eventually leaches out of the infarct to leave a barely pigmented and scarcely stained lesion containing the ghosts of hepatocytes. Small bile infarcts may be found in severe cholestasis from any cause; larger infarcts such as the one shown in **Figure 5.4**, especially if adjacent to a portal tract, are highly suggestive of bile-duct obstruction. However, because such infarcts are seen in only a minority of patients with obstructed ducts, the diagnosis must usually be established by other criteria.

As a result of these various forms of hepatocellular damage in biliary obstruction, and indeed in cholestasis generally, a certain amount of inflammatory infiltration of the parenchyma is commonly seen after a period of some weeks. This infiltration is usually mild and restricted to the cholestatic areas, unlike the inflammation of an acute hepatitis. When cholestasis resulting from duct obstruction is prolonged, especially in older patients, inflammation and liver-cell damage are occasionally severe enough to raise the alternative possibility of an acute hepatitis. It is then helpful to note that in bile-duct obstruction the liver-cell plates remain for the most part intact, whereas in hepatitis they become irregular as a result of cell loss, swelling and regeneration. Central–portal (zone 3) bridging necrosis is not a feature of biliary obstruction.

Within a few days or weeks of the onset of duct obstruction a characteristic triad of portal changes develops,[5] consisting of portal oedema and swelling (**Fig. 5.5**), infiltration by inflammatory cells and increased numbers of bile-duct profiles at the margins of the portal tracts (**Figs 5.6 and 5.7**). These marginal bile-duct structures are the most consistent finding in the portal tracts and are rarely absent.[5] They may originate from canals of Hering, periportal stem cells or other sources[6] and are an early response to the increased portal tract pressure due to obstruction, circulating mediators[7] and expression of developmental proteins such as Notch receptors and Jagged proteins.[8] The term **ductular reaction** refers to these proliferated bile ductules accompanied by inflammation and stromal changes at the edges of the portal tracts.[9,10] Usage of 'ductular reaction' is now preferable to 'bile ductular proliferation' or 'typical' and 'atypical' bile ductules, which embody considerable imprecision.[6] The ductular structures may be of normal calibre or dilated, but

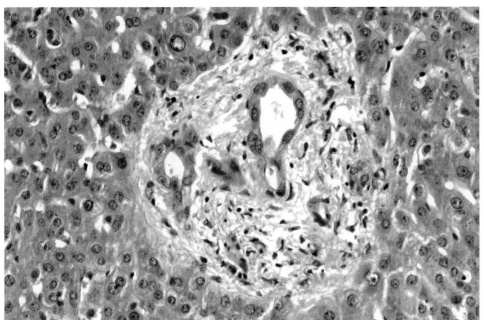

Figure 5.5
Large bile-duct obstruction.
The connective tissue of a small portal tract is oedematous. There is little inflammation in this example. (Wedge biopsy, H&E.)

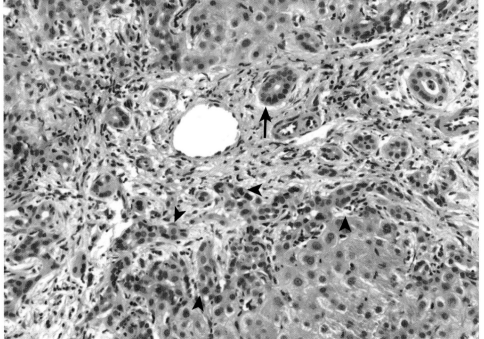

Figure 5.6
Large bile-duct obstruction.
A prominent ductular reaction (arrowheads) is present at the edge of an inflamed and oedematous portal tract. The original interlobular duct is marked by an arrow. (Needle biopsy, H&E.)

are often flattened with small or imperceptible lumens (**Fig. 5.7**) and variations in nuclear size, staining and location. These structures can be highlighted by immunostaining for cytokeratin 7 or 19 (**see Figs 5.24 and 5.25, below**). Surprisingly, bile is not usually seen within dilated ducts or ductules in uncomplicated obstruction; when it is present, sepsis should be suspected. The differentiation of the ductular reaction of biliary obstruction from that of chronic liver disease has already been discussed in **Chapter 4**.

Figure 5.7 Ductular reaction in large bile-duct obstruction.

The upper left-hand portion of **Figure 5.6** is shown at higher magnification. The irregular ductular structures at the edge of the portal tract show compressed, narrow lumens and an associated neutrophil infiltrate. (Needle biopsy, H&E.)

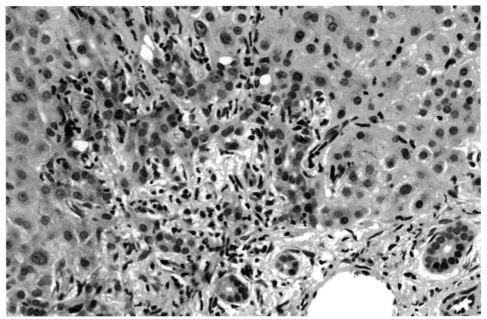

Within the oedematous, swollen portal tracts, especially around proliferated bile ducts, an inflammatory infiltrate develops, mediated by the complex interactions of cytokines and cellular adhesion molecules (some produced by biliary epithelium itself[11]) and proinflammatory agents such as endotoxin.[3] Neutrophils are prominent owing to the expression of the chemoattractant interleukin-8 by the ductular cells.[12] There may also be other cells, including lymphocytes and eosinophils. The presence of a few eosinophils is therefore not in itself sufficient evidence for a diagnosis of drug jaundice. As a result of the proliferative and inflammatory changes of bile-duct obstruction, the outlines of the portal tracts become irregular and the limiting plates of hepatocytes are disrupted to a variable extent. This disruption should be distinguished from interface hepatitis, in which the infiltrate is predominantly composed of lymphocytes and plasma cells, and in which the acute inflammatory changes of bile-duct obstruction are not seen.

In a few patients with bile-duct obstruction the portal changes are inconspicuous (**Fig. 5.5**) or even absent. Biliary obstruction should therefore be considered in the differential diagnosis of canalicular cholestasis without portal reaction (so-called 'pure' or 'bland' cholestasis). Conversely, portal changes resembling those of duct obstruction are occasionally found in severe acute hepatitis, when the parenchymal alterations make the diagnosis clear. Sometimes similar portal changes are seen without cholestasis near space-occupying lesions such as metastases,[13] usually together with sinusoidal dilatation. Portal inflammation without cholestasis is also found in patients with disease affecting one or other part of the biliary tree but without current obstruction of the segment biopsied. It is seen in chronic pancreatitis[14] and in patients with acute cholecystitis or choledocholithiasis.[15] Biopsies showing only an increased number of well-differentiated bile ductules at the portal interface, unaccompanied by inflammation or stromal changes, have been noted in patients with idiopathic **isolated ductular hyperplasia**[16] (**Fig. 5.8**). These patients have long-standing abnormalities in serum alanine aminotransferase and/or γ-glutamyl transferase, no proven biliary tract disease and an apparently good prognosis (although the cause of this reactive lesion is uncertain).

In a few instances of biliary obstruction, bile escapes from a duct into the connective tissue of a portal tract, giving rise to a *bile extravasate*. This leads to a phagocytic reaction,

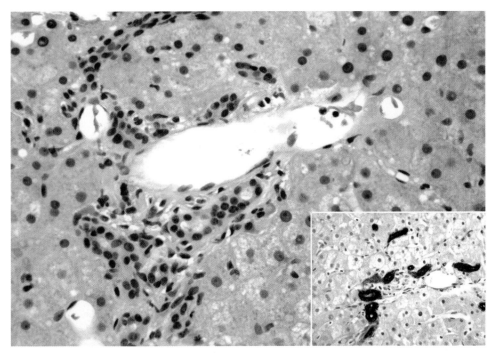

Figure 5.8 Isolated ductular hyperplasia.
Well-differentiated hyperplastic bile ductules are present in this biopsy from a patient with persistent liver function test abnormalities unrelated to viral hepatitis or demonstrable biliary disease. The absence of oedema and inflammation helps distinguish this lesion from large bile-duct obstruction. (Needle biopsy, H&E.) Inset: Immunostain for cytokeratin 7 on a deeper level highlights the bile ductules. (Needle biopsy, specific immunoperoxidase.) (Case kindly provided by Drs Bernard Traub and John B Herrington, III, Sleepy Hollow, New York, NY, USA.)

with or without foreign-body giant cells (**Fig. 5.9**). Bile extravasates, like large bile infarcts, are almost diagnostic of obstruction but are seen in only a minority of patients. If the extravasate extends beyond the confines of a portal tract into the adjacent parenchyma, the appearances at the periphery of the lesion are very like those of a bile infarct.

Chronic bile-duct obstruction and biliary cirrhosis

When bile-duct obstruction persists, the acute inflammatory reaction in the portal tracts is followed by increasing fibrosis. Production of fibrogenic cytokines by bile-duct epithelium contributes to this process.[17] Eventually the tracts are linked by broad fibrous septa. There is a variable degree of acute and chronic inflammatory infiltration; the chronic element is less striking than in PBC. In some patients the lesion appears to progress more by cholangitis than by obstruction, and cholestasis is therefore not always prominent or even present.

Interference with normal secretion of bile leads to several changes in hepatocytes adjacent to portal tracts and fibrous septa. The cells become swollen and separated by fibrous tissue, inflammatory cells and ductular structures (neocholangioles) derived from hepatocytes or bipotential stem cells.[18] Their cytoplasm is rarefied and may contain visible bile pigment, Mallory bodies, copper and copper-associated protein (**Fig. 5.10**). The last is seen in the form of fine red granules on haematoxylin and eosin (H&E) (**see Fig. 5.27** inset), staining variably with diastase–PAS and strongly with orcein or Victoria blue. The

Figure 5.9 Large bile-duct obstruction. Bile extravasate. Bile has escaped from a duct and has evoked a phagocytic reaction. (Needle biopsy, H&E.)

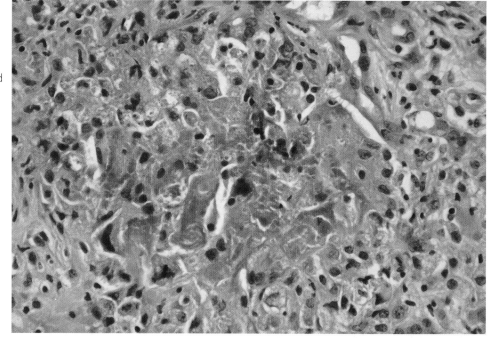

Figure 5.10 Chronic cholestasis. Hepatocytes near a portal tract (below) are swollen and pale-staining. Many contain Mallory bodies (lower arrow and triple arrow). Bile thrombi are also seen (top arrow). (Wedge biopsy, H&E.)

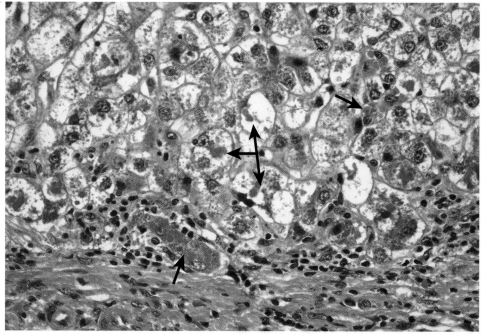

combination of all these changes is known as **chronic cholestasis** or **cholate stasis (pseudoxanthomatous change, precholestasis)** on the basis that some of the alterations probably result from the accumulation of toxic bile salts. Canalicular cholestasis is sometimes seen between the affected hepatocytes. The hepatocellular changes, ductular proliferation and associated fibrosis in the periportal or periseptal region in effect produce an irregular interface with the parenchyma.[19]

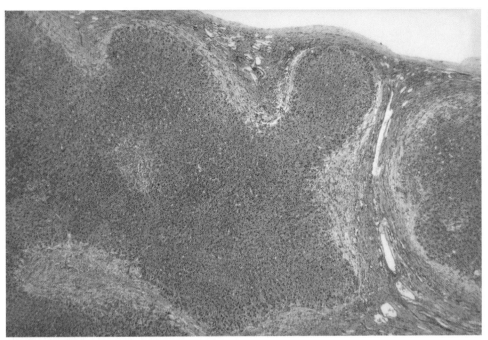

Figure 5.11
Secondary biliary cirrhosis.
Irregular nodules resemble pieces of a jigsaw puzzle. Note the narrow zone of oedema and ductular proliferation at the nodule margin. (Wedge biopsy, H&E.)

The fibrous septa which eventually form in chronic biliary tract disease surround and outline groups of classical hepatic lobules, leaving the normal vascular relationships essentially intact. Islands of parenchyma with characteristic protruding studs resemble the pieces of a jigsaw puzzle or land masses on a map (**Fig. 5.11**). Spherical nodules are sparse at first, in spite of evidence of liver-cell hyperplasia in the form of thickened liver-cell plates, seen particularly in patients with associated portal hypertension.[20] An occasional rounded parenchymal island may merely represent a tangential section of a complex parenchymal mass such as the one shown in **Figure 5.11**, rather than a true regeneration nodule of cirrhosis. This is especially common just deep to the liver capsule. A histological diagnosis of cirrhosis should therefore be made with caution, because at a fibrotic, precirrhotic stage considerable resolution can occasionally result if an obstruction is relieved.[21] Eventually, true **secondary biliary cirrhosis** develops, its biliary origin still evident from nodule shape and the regular, broad fibrous septa composed of loose collagen bundles with parallel arrangement (**Fig. 5.12**). A zone of oedema containing proliferated ductules is often diagnostically helpful and may be striking even at low magnification (the 'halo effect') (**Fig. 5.11**). Thus, many different structural characteristics make it possible to diagnose chronic biliary tract disease, even in the absence of cholestasis. Finally, however, an end-stage cirrhosis forms, no longer necessarily recognisable as biliary in origin.

Cholangitis: infection of the biliary tree

In biliary obstruction the inflammatory infiltrate around bile ducts in small portal tracts typically includes neutrophils. There is, therefore, cholangitis in a strictly histological sense, but this does not imply that there must be bacterial infection of the biliary tree or clinical ascending cholangitis. In the latter, neutrophils are more numerous and are found not only around ducts but also in their walls and lumens[22] (**Fig. 5.13**). Paradoxically, interlobular bile ducts are most affected, and larger ducts may appear histologically normal. The wall of a small duct may rupture, leading to abscess formation in the portal tract.

Figure 5.12
Secondary biliary cirrhosis.
Nodules are surrounded by loose bundles of parallel collagen fibres showing little compression. (Wedge biopsy, reticulin.)

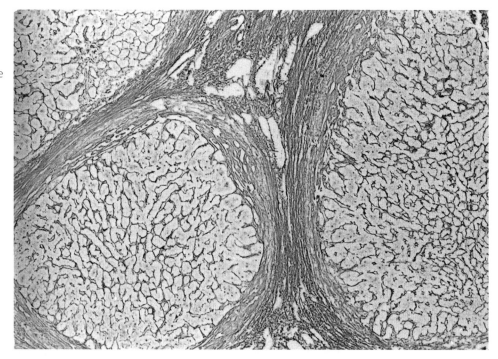

Figure 5.13
Acute cholangitis.
Many neutrophil leukocytes are seen in the walls and dilated lumens of the bile ducts, and in the surrounding connective tissue. (Wedge biopsy, H&E.)

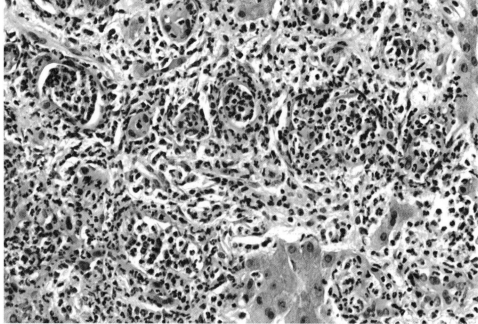

Neutrophils are seen in the sinusoids and abscesses may form in the acini. Associated lesions include fibrin thrombi in portal-vein branches, pyelophlebitis and various degrees of parenchymal necrosis,[23] the last probably related to hypoperfusion of the parenchyma. Cholestasis is more often absent than present. Causes of ascending cholangitis include cholecystitis and choledocholithiasis, strictures including those due to PSC, intrahepatic biliary stones,[24] AIDS cholangiopathy,[25,26] pancreatitis, neoplasia of the biliary tree and Caroli's disease. If cholangitis persists or recurs over a period of years, secondary biliary cirrhosis may develop. The histological features are then as described above in the section on bile-duct obstruction. Septicaemia uncommonly is associated with a particular form of histological cholangitis principally affecting the canals of Hering.[27] Affected ductules are dilated and filled with inspissated bile. Neutrophils accumulate around and sometimes within them. Larger ducts may be affected, as may the periportal parenchyma in which bile is seen in dilated bile canaliculi. These changes are easily confused with those of large bile-duct obstruction, but in obstruction the inspissated bile in the canals of Hering is not a feature unless there is concomitant sepsis. Sepsis more often gives rise to widespread canalicular cholestasis; the ductular cholestasis pattern (**see Fig. 15.12**) is seen in the minority of septic patients.[27] In toxic-shock syndrome the appearances of the small bile ducts can closely mimic ascending bacterial cholangitis.[28]

Primary sclerosing cholangitis

PSC is characterised by inflammation, strictures and saccular dilatations in the biliary tree. Typically found in adults with ulcerative colitis, it is also seen in neonates and children[29] and in the absence of inflammatory bowel disease. In a few cases the latter is Crohn's disease rather than ulcerative colitis.[30] Any part of the biliary tree may be affected, and involvement of the gallbladder[31] and pancreas[32] has been reported. The gallbladder shows intramural lymphoplasmacytic infiltrates and lymphoid aggregates.[33] Patients do not necessarily have symptoms referable to the liver or abnormal liver function tests.[34] The disease may recur after liver transplantation.[35] Lesions similar to those of PSC have been found in patients given arterial infusion of the anticancer drug fluorodeoxyuridine and other[36] chemotherapeutic agents.[37] Obliteration or narrowing of hepatic arteries and portal-vein branches suggests that, in drug-related cases at least, the bile-duct damage may have an ischaemic origin.[38] Systemic vasculitis, liver transplantation-related hepatic artery thrombosis or chronic rejection vasculopathy and, rarely, septic shock[39] are other causes of ischaemic bile-duct injury[40] (ischaemic cholangiopathy). Similar bile-duct injury occurs after lengthy hospitalisations in intensive care units or trauma (conditions likely to be associated with hypotension/hypoperfusion-hypoxia) in 'secondary sclerosing cholangitis in critically ill patients'.[41–43]

Final diagnosis of PSC normally rests on cholangiographic demonstration of the characteristic beading of bile ducts, but similar histological features, as described below, may be found in patients with normal cholangiograms. This can be explained on the basis of involvement of the smallest ducts, too small to be seen radiographically.[44] This **small-duct primary sclerosing cholangitis** corresponds approximately to the now obsolete label of 'pericholangitis', when applied to patients without cholangiographic abnormalities. Large- and small-duct forms of the disease frequently coexist. Progression of small-duct PSC to large-duct PSC occurs in approximately 20% of cases, usually over a decade.[45]

The features seen on liver biopsy depend in part on the location of strictures in relation to the biopsy site. If the biopsy is taken from a part of the liver unaffected by the primary disease but proximal to a stricture, then the changes, if any, will simply be those of bile-duct obstruction or cholangitis. The presence of chronic inflammation may lead to confusion with chronic hepatitis. If, on the other hand, the biopsy site is affected by the primary disease, there may be one or more features suggesting the diagnosis. These include periduct oedema and concentric fibrosis (**Fig. 5.14**), ductular proliferation, portal inflammation and atrophy or disappearance of the small ducts (**Fig. 5.15**). Loss of ducts is the most common finding in the smallest portal tracts, while periduct fibrosis is typical of medium-sized tracts.[46] Major bile ducts, as seen for example in explanted livers at transplantation, may be inflamed, ulcerated or dilated. They may also rupture, producing a perihilar **xanthogranulomatous cholangitis**.[47]

Figure 5.14 Primary sclerosing cholangitis. A bile duct is surrounded by a cuff of oedematous, inflamed fibrous tissue with an 'onion-skin' appearance. (Needle biopsy, H&E.)

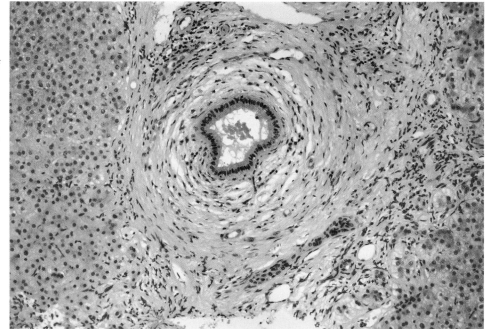

Figure 5.15 Primary sclerosing cholangitis. The inflamed portal tract lacks a bile duct. An aggregate of lymphocytes to the left of a small hepatic arteriole at the centre of the field is likely the former site of the duct. Inflammation extends into the adjacent parenchyma and there is interface hepatitis to the right of the portal tract. (Wedge biopsy, H&E.)

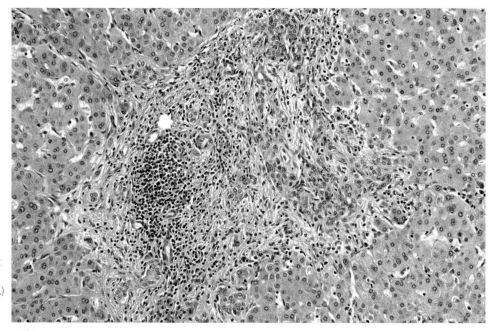

Loss of interlobular bile ducts from the smallest portal tracts can be assessed only in biopsy samples of adequate size, that is to say, containing several portal tracts. While interlobular ducts are not necessarily seen in all tracts because of the plane of section, arteries provide a useful guide: from 70–80%[48] to 92%[49] of arteries are normally accompanied by a duct lying near the centre of a portal tract. If there is doubt, for instance because ducts are difficult to identify in an inflammatory infiltrate, immunostaining of

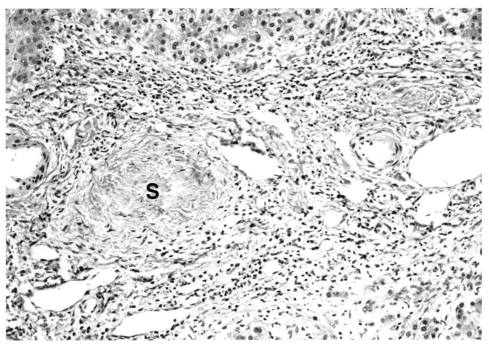

Figure 5.16
Primary sclerosing cholangitis.
The bile duct in a large portal tract has been replaced by a fibrous scar (S). (Wedge biopsy, H&E.)

duct-associated cytokeratins is helpful.[50] Suitable antibodies include AE-1 (Signet) and other antibodies against cytokeratins 7 and 19. In the presence of a ductular reaction, identification and counting of interlobular bile ducts are sometimes difficult.

The concentric fibrosis around medium-sized ducts is not entirely diagnostic, since it is occasionally found in other forms of biliary disease such as hepatolithiasis.[51] It is, however, a very helpful finding. The lamellar pattern of the fibrosis gives an 'onion-skin' appearance. The cuff of connective tissue around the duct may be oedematous and pale-staining or sclerotic, depending on the stage of the process. Inflammatory cells are seen in small numbers lying between the layers of collagen. The duct epithelium may show various degrees of atrophy, and sometimes disappears entirely, leaving a characteristic rounded fibro-obliterative scar[52] (**Fig. 5.16**). Staining with diastase–PAS often reveals irregular or regular thickening of the basement membrane material around both scarred and unscarred ducts.[53] In long-standing or severe cases, portal fibrosis gradually increases, fibrous septa form and secondary biliary cirrhosis may develop. In some patients, on the other hand, the lesions remain mild and clinically insignificant for many[30] years.[34] Portal tract fibrogenesis in sclerosing cholangitis and in PBC is in part attributed to an increased number of intrahepatic mast cells compared with other chronic liver diseases.[54] In fact, systemic mastocytosis has been associated with cholestasis[55] and a case of PSC.[56]

Parenchymal changes in PSC are usually less striking than the portal ones. Cholestasis may be seen as a result of large-duct obstruction or small-duct loss. In the later stages, the cholestasis is typically of the chronic type, with accumulation of copper and copper-associated protein. Extension of portal tract lymphoplasmacytic infiltrates into the periportal parenchyma (interface hepatitis) is common but not as a rule severe (**Fig. 5.15**). However, more severe interface hepatitis may be seen in patients with an unfavourable clinical course[30] or in an overlap syndrome with AIH. In children, the combination of AIH and PSC is well recognised.[57] Liver cells may undergo hyperplasia, indicated by thickening of cell plates.

Histological assessment of liver biopsies in patients with an established diagnosis of PSC is important for prognosis. Ludwig and colleagues[44,58,59] have proposed a histological

Figure 5.17 Cholangiocarcinoma in primary sclerosing cholangitis. Carcinoma has developed in the bile duct at left, still surrounded by periduct fibrosis (F). Invasive glands (arrows) are seen in the adjacent stroma. (Explanted liver, H&E.)

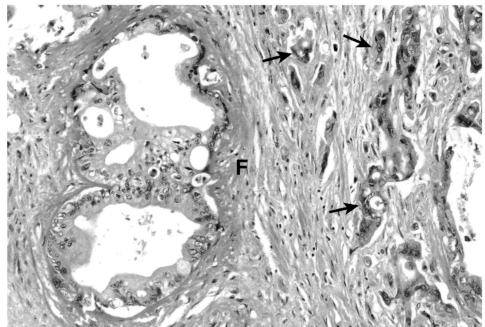

Figure 5.18 Bile-duct dysplasia in primary sclerosing cholangitis. The epithelium of the right portion of the bile duct is crowded and adenomatous and shows nuclear atypia. (Operative specimen, H&E.)

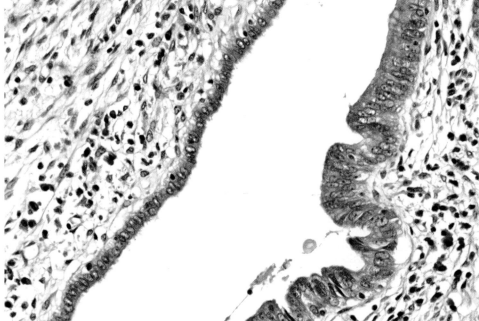

staging system based on essential and non-essential features. The stages correspond approximately to those of PBC: they are respectively designated portal, periportal, septal and cirrhotic.

There is an increased risk of carcinoma of the biliary tree in patients with sclerosing cholangitis[60] (**Fig. 5.17**) who may also have dysplasia of interlobular and septal bile ducts[61] (**Fig. 5.18**) and gallbladder,[62] including papillary bile-duct dysplastic lesions.[63] Cholangiocarcinoma-associated cytogenetic abnormalities such as polysomy (gains in chromosomes 3, 7 and 17) and loss of the CDKN2A gene for P16 at the 9p21 locus can be demonstrated in cytological and tissue specimens from bile ducts with dysplasia in PSC.[63a] The same risk of carcinoma does not appear to apply to the small-duct form of PSC.[64]

The main **differential diagnosis** of PSC is from chronic hepatitis, PBC and other forms of chronic biliary tract disease. In **chronic hepatitis** bile-duct numbers are normal, periduct fibrosis is not seen and cholestasis is very uncommon. Stains for copper and copper-associated protein are negative or near-negative unless cirrhosis has developed.[65] **PBC** closely resembles PSC in its later stages, and firm diagnosis usually requires cholangiography and testing for antimitochondrial antibodies (AMAs). However, the typical granulomatous cholangitis of PBC is not a feature of sclerosing cholangitis, although granulomas are very occasionally found in the liver.[66] Substantial chronic inflammation of portal tracts with or without lymphoid follicles favours PBC. Conversely, fibrous obliteration of ducts is much more characteristic of sclerosing cholangitis, and there is often dense portal fibrosis with relatively little inflammation. The main difference from **other chronic biliary diseases** is the loss of ducts and interface hepatitis. There is occasionally confusion between the focal duct dilatations of **Caroli's disease** and the cholangiectases which are typically seen in the large and medium-sized bile ducts in PSC.[52,67] **IgG4-associated cholangitis** (IAC), also termed **IgG4-related sclerosing cholangitis** (IRSC[68–71,71a]), a steroid-sensitive, autoimmune cholangiopathy, also needs consideration since it causes histological changes similar to PSC[72,73] and may raise the clinical question of cholangiocarcinoma.[73a] This condition is part of the spectrum of autoimmune diseases featuring IgG4+ plasma cells and sclerosis (IgG4-related disease[69]) which also includes autoimmune pancreatitis and certain cases of inflammatory pseudotumour.[74] Like PSC, the large ducts in IAC are surrounded by dense lymphoplasmacytic infiltrates (often with lymphoid aggregates and follicles), but in IAC the infiltrates extend deeply into the soft tissues surrounding the ducts with entrapment of nerves and obliterative phlebitis of large-calibre veins. In contrast to other chronic biliary diseases where IgG4+ plasma cells are absent or sparse, IAC shows numerous IgG4+ plasma cells on immunostaining (>25–30 per medium-power field[72]). A subgroup of more clinically aggressive PSC cases may also show such increased IgG4+ plasma cells.[75] Liver biopsies in IAC show portal tract infiltrates of lymphocytes, eosinophils and increased IgG4+ plasma cells (>5–10 per high-power field).[76,77] The inflammation is accentuated around portal vein branches and portal connective tissue is widened by storiform fibroinflammatory nodules.[77]

Primary biliary cirrhosis ♀ > ♂ 10x   AMA -- M2

PBC, generally regarded as an autoimmune disease, is characterised by a chronic non-suppurative destructive cholangitis, which can eventually lead to cirrhosis.[78] For much of its course the term 'cirrhosis' is not strictly applicable, but the name survives despite this inconsistency. PBC typically presents in middle life, but may also be found in the elderly, younger adults and uncommonly in adolescents.[79] Women are about 10 times more likely to be affected than men. In symptomatic patients the onset is insidious, with itching as the most common presenting symptom. Jaundice and histological cholestasis are usually absent in the early years of the disease. Characteristic findings on investigation of both symptomatic and asymptomatic patients include raised level serum alkaline phosphatase and the presence of AMAs. The antibodies are specifically the M2 type, directed against inner mitochondrial membrane autoantigens, which are members of the 2-oxo-acid dehydrogenase complex (2-OADC) of enzymes.[80] The most common of these antibodies reacts with the E2 subunit of the pyruvate dehydrogenase complex (PDC-E2). AMAs can be detected in more than 90% of patients. Serum IgM values are typically elevated.[81] Current hypotheses suggest that expression of 2-OADC antigens on bile-duct epithelium together with appropriate class II histocompatibility antigens, production of AMAs and T-lymphocyte response[82] mediate the bile-duct damage in PBC.[83] Cross-reactivity of human AMAs with bacterial antigens on *Escherichia coli* and other organisms that may infect patients with PBC has been suggested in the 'molecular mimicry' hypothesis.[84] Dysregulated interleukin-12 signaling[85] and increased circulating and intrahepatic T follicular helper cells (CD4+) involved in B cell activation[85a,85b] have also been described.

PBC is associated with a wide range of other conditions, many of them regarded as autoimmune in origin. The most common association is with the sicca complex of dry eyes and mouth.[86] Others include scleroderma, thyroiditis, rheumatoid arthritis, membranous glomerulonephritis and coeliac disease.

Liver biopsy plays an important part in diagnosis throughout the often long course of the disease. Four histological stages have been described[58,78,87] (**Box 5.2**). These are not always easy to determine in needle biopsies, partly because the lesions of PBC are unevenly distributed within the liver and partly because the stages overlap. For example, stage 1 bile-duct lesions and granulomas are sometimes seen in an established cirrhosis. From a practical point of view, however, the pathologist is usually able to decide whether the disease appears to be still in stage 1, with lesions more or less restricted to enlarged portal tracts, or whether it has extended to a significant degree into the adjacent parenchyma, with consequent alteration of acinar structure (the progressive lesion; stages 2, 3 or 4). This is of some clinical importance, because stage 1 often lasts for many years and the prognosis is therefore relatively favourable, especially in patients without symptoms referable to the liver. Having established in other patients that the disease has progressed beyond stage 1, the pathologist may also be able to determine with reasonable confidence that cirrhosis has developed. The patient is then at increased risk for hepatocellular carcinoma,[88,89] sometimes preceded by macroregenerative nodule formation.[90] However, other risk factors such as hepatitis C virus infection must be considered in patients with PBC who develop carcinoma.[91] Because different sets of differential diagnoses should be considered for the portal and the progressive lesion, these are considered separately in the following section.

Box 5.2 Stages of primary biliary cirrhosis

1. The florid duct lesion; portal hepatitis
2. Ductular reaction and periportal hepatitis
3. Scarring; bridging necrosis, septal fibrosis
4. Cirrhosis

The portal lesion of primary biliary cirrhosis

The bile-duct damage characteristic of early PBC mainly affects the septal and larger interlobular ducts, while the smaller interlobular ducts remain intact until later. The epithelium of the affected ducts becomes irregular and is infiltrated with lymphocytes. The basement membrane becomes disrupted, and the duct may rupture (**Fig. 5.19**). An inflammatory infiltrate is seen around or to one side of the duct. The denser parts of this infiltrate are mainly composed of lymphocytes, which may form aggregates or follicles with germinal centres (**Fig. 5.20**). Elsewhere there is a mixture of plasma cells (often abundant), eosinophils and neutrophils. The eosinophils contribute to bile-duct damage, granuloma formation and other aspects of the inflammatory response by releasing mediators which are located within their granules.[92] The biochemical and/or histological improvement seen in certain patients treated with ursodeoxycholic acid appears to be attributable in part to inhibition of eosinophil degranulation.[93] Of the various histological features of the disease, interface hepatitis appears to be the most resistant to improvement with ursodeoxycholic acid.[94]

In line with the presence of elevated serum IgM in individuals with PBC is the predominance of IgM-positive plasma cells in the portal tract plasmacytic infiltrates.[95] Specific IgM immunostaining can therefore be diagnostically useful (and contrasts with the IgG-predominant plasma cells seen in AIH[95,96]). CD1a-positive Langerhans cells may be increased within the predominantly lymphocytic intraepithelial bile-duct infiltrates.[97]

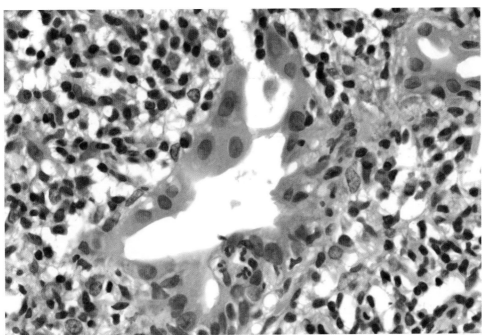

Figure 5.19
Primary biliary cirrhosis.
A damaged large interlobular bile duct shows an irregular configuration, partly attenuated epithelium and intraepithelial inflammatory cells. The surrounding infiltrate is rich in lymphocytes and plasma cells. (Wedge biopsy, H&E.)

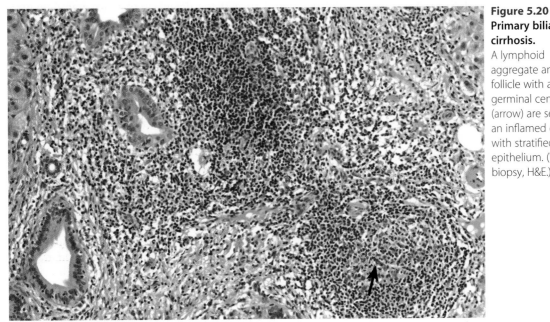

Figure 5.20
Primary biliary cirrhosis.
A lymphoid aggregate and a follicle with a germinal centre (arrow) are seen near an inflamed duct with stratified epithelium. (Wedge biopsy, H&E.)

Granulomas are present in many patients, although they are not necessarily seen in small biopsies; their absence does not therefore exclude the diagnosis. They take a variety of forms,[98] ranging from well-defined granulomas like those of sarcoidosis or tuberculosis (**Fig. 5.21**) to small focal collections of histiocytoid cells. Alternatively, there may be a substantial component of histiocytes or epithelioid cells within the inflammatory infiltrate, without formation of identifiable localised granulomas. A few intra-acinar granulomas may also be present (usually small intrasinusoidal clusters of histiocytes rather than well-formed

Figure 5.21
Primary biliary cirrhosis.
A well-formed epithelioid-cell granuloma (G) has formed near a damaged bile duct (arrow). The background infiltrate contains many lymphocytes, plasma cells and scattered eosinophils. (Needle biopsy, H&E.)

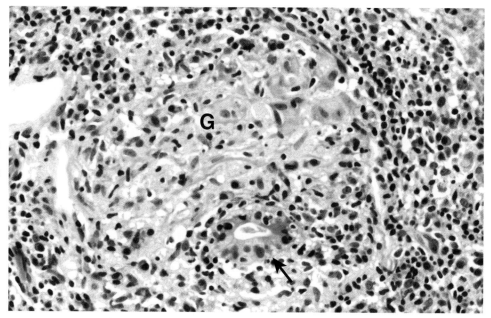

granulomas), but large numbers should suggest the diagnosis of other granulomatous diseases (**see Ch. 15**).

Not all liver biopsies from patients in this stage of the disease show the typical bile-duct lesions, so that a firm histological diagnosis cannot always be made. Small portal tracts may merely show 'non-specific' portal inflammation, in which case step sections may make the true diagnosis clear by revealing bile-duct lesions or granulomas. In a small number of patients with the **premature ductopenic variant** of PBC,[99] widespread bile-duct destruction and loss are accelerated at an early stage before the development of fibrosis or cirrhosis, with worse pruritus and clinical evidence of chronic cholestasis than would be anticipated.

Although in the first stage of PBC the lesions are by definition mainly portal, slight disruption of the limiting plate is common. Sinusoids may be infiltrated by lymphocytes, Kupffer cells are prominent and there may be focal necrosis[100] and thickening of liver-cell plates. Nodular regenerative hyperplasia, best recognised in reticulin preparations, is common even at this stage,[101,102] and together with portal vein narrowing[103] helps to explain the portal hypertension which frequently precedes the development of significant fibrosis or cirrhosis. Foci of small hepatocytes with basophilic cytoplasm and hyperchromatic nuclei (small-cell dysplasia) or hepatocytes with enlarged, pleomorphic nuclei (large-cell dysplasia) are occasionally found.[104]

Canalicular cholestasis is unusual in early PBC unless there is a complicating factor such as steroid-induced jaundice. Cholestasis of the chronic type (cholate stasis) does not develop until later, although small amounts of copper-associated protein are occasionally seen in periportal hepatocytes.

The **differential diagnosis of early PBC** includes other causes of portal inflammation and of bile-duct damage. The differentiation from **PSC** was discussed earlier. In PSC duct atrophy and fibrosis predominate and granulomas are seen only rarely.[66] **Drug injury** occasionally leads to bile-duct damage, but the ducts affected are smaller than those in early PBC; other parenchymal changes (fat, hepatocyte ballooning and apoptosis) are often present and the lesion is seen in the clinical context of an acutely jaundiced patient. Amoxicillin–clavulanic acid hepatotoxicity is an example of PBC-like, eosinophil-rich bile-duct damage.[105] Bile ducts are often abnormal in acute and chronic **viral hepatitis**, especially hepatitis C.[106] In hepatitis the epithelium of the affected ducts may be abnormal in only part of its circumference (**see Fig. 6.8**), and is typically stratified and vacuolated.[107] The surrounding infiltrate is almost entirely composed of lymphocytes, with few plasma cells or segmented leukocytes and no granulomas. Large numbers of eosinophils, sometimes seen in PBC,[108] are rare. In doubtful cases the clinical context and laboratory investigations usually make the diagnosis clear. Because in viral hepatitis the duct damage is focal and does not lead to extensive duct loss, the clinical and biochemical picture is not necessarily cholestatic. Other causes of bile-duct damage include **AIH**,[109] **bile-duct obstruction with suppuration**, **graft-versus-host disease** and **rejection of a grafted liver**. The last two situations are discussed in **Chapter 16**. Two rare causes of bile-duct damage associated with granulomas are **fascioliasis** and **sarcoidosis**, but in general this association strongly supports a diagnosis of PBC.

The progressive lesion of primary biliary cirrhosis

The disease now extends beyond the confines of the portal tracts and there is increasing fibrosis and alteration of acinar architecture. Bile-duct damage is less dramatic and granulomas are fewer, but there is a progressive fall in duct numbers. Duct numbers are best assessed in relation to arteries,[48] as already discussed in relation to PSC. The sites of former ducts are marked by aggregates of lymphocytes (**Fig. 5.22**). These sometimes show compression artefact, with rupture of lymphocyte nuclei. The inflammatory reaction may also obliterate periductal capillaries.[110]

The portal tracts expand progressively as the inflammatory process begins to extend from them into the adjacent parenchyma. At this time two apparently separate processes affect the future course of the disease. The first comprises a combination of biliary and cholestatic features, probably related to bile-duct loss, while the second closely resembles the interface hepatitis of chronic hepatitis.[19,111] The earliest and often most obvious biliary feature is a ductular reaction (**Fig. 5.23**). For a time this allows bile to drain from the parenchyma into the main ducts in spite of destruction of the medium-sized ducts.[112] It is

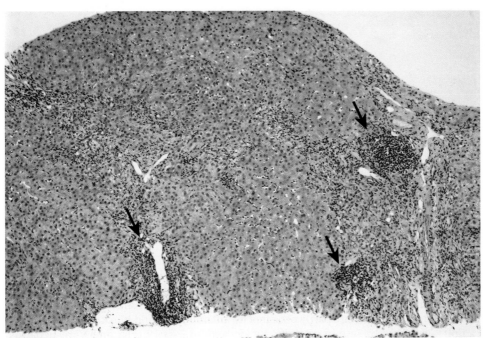

Figure 5.22 Primary biliary cirrhosis.
Aggregates of lymphocytes (arrows) mark the former sites of bile ducts in this inflamed, fibrotic liver. The picture is very typical of the progressive phase of the disease. (Needle biopsy, H&E.)

Figure 5.23 Primary biliary cirrhosis.
A widened portal tract shows chronic inflammation and a ductular reaction, but no native bile duct. The margins of the tract are blurred by fibrosis and interface hepatitis. (Wedge biopsy, H&E.)

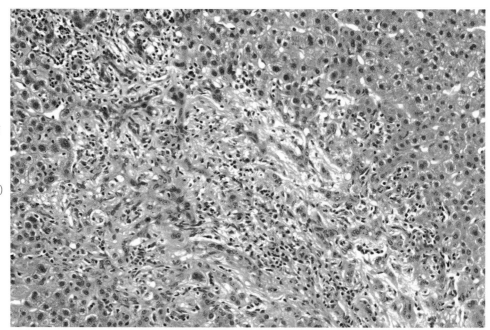

Figure 5.24 Stage 3 primary biliary cirrhosis.
The portal tract is chronically inflamed and fibrotic, without a readily identified bile duct. A ductular reaction is present, but obscured by the inflammation and fibrosis. Cholestasis is present at the periphery of the lobule (arrow). (Needle biopsy, H&E.)

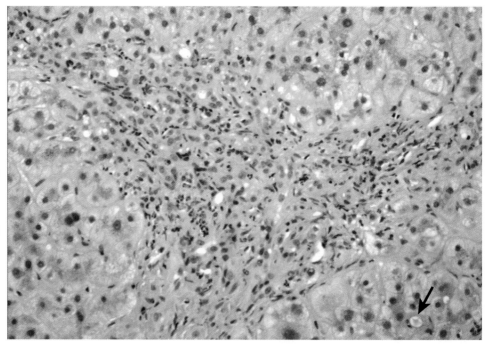

almost always associated with an infiltrate of neutrophils, so that it needs to be distinguished from the duct tortuosity and inflammation of mechanical bile-duct obstruction. The ductular reaction of PBC, and indeed of PSC, is often focal, representing a system of bypass channels in relation to a local interruption of bile flow through the duct system. If the ductular structures are partly obscured by inflammation and fibrosis (**Fig. 5.24**), they can be highlighted by immunostaining for cytokeratin 7 or 19 (**Fig. 5.25**).

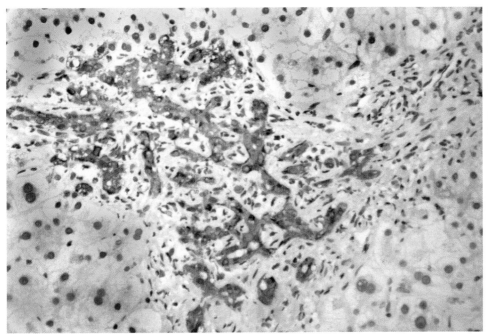

Figure 5.25 Stage 3 primary biliary cirrhosis.
The ductular reaction is highlighted by cytokeratin 7 immunostaining of a serial section of the same biopsy shown in **Figure 5.24**. (Needle biopsy, specific immunoperoxidase.)

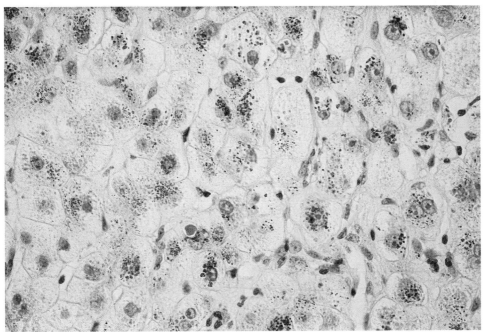

Figure 5.26 Primary biliary cirrhosis.
Heavy accumulation of copper-rich granules is seen in hepatocytes. Note the different colour of the canalicular bile thrombus slightly below centre. (Needle biopsy, rhodanine.)

Loss of bile ducts also leads to the chronic form of cholestasis marked by swelling of hepatocytes, bile staining, Mallory body formation and accumulation of copper (**Fig. 5.26**) and copper-associated protein (**Fig. 5.27**). Bile plugs are sometimes seen in canaliculi in the affected areas around portal tracts and septa, but more widespread canalicular cholestasis often reflects hepatocellular failure or associated sepsis. There may be many lipid-laden macrophages, forming diffuse or localised xanthomas.

Figure 5.27
Primary biliary cirrhosis.
Granular deposits of copper-associated protein have accumulated in hepatocytes near a fibrous septum (below) at a late stage of the disease. (Needle biopsy, Orcein.) Inset: Copper-associated protein in hepatocytes near the portal tract (PT) appears as fine red cytoplasmic granules. (Needle biopsy, H&E.)

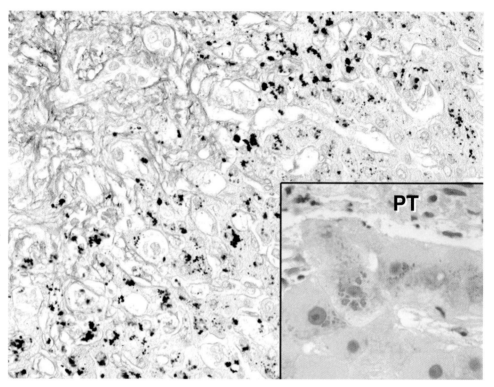

In addition to the cholestatic features described above, interface hepatitis of the classical, lymphoplasmacytic type is common in the progressive stage of PBC.[19] The infiltrate is rich in activated T cells.[111,113,114] Because this hepatocellular component is a regular feature of PBC, the finding of interface hepatitis together with the biliary features of PBC should not by itself lead to the diagnosis of an overlap syndrome (see below). Lymphocytes also form bridge-like extensions into the acini, and may be the forerunners of fibrous septa.[115] An increased number of intrahepatic mast cells is also present, which may have contributed to portal tract fibrosis.[54] Necrosis of perivenular hepatocytes has been noted.[100] There is therefore a histological resemblance to hepatitis. Hepatocellular dysplasia of small- or large-cell type may be present.[104]

The combination of cholestatic and hepatitic processes leads to increasing fibrosis. Portal inflammation diminishes, but lymphoid aggregates continue to mark the former sites of bile ducts (**Fig. 5.28**). Septa extend from the portal tracts and eventually come to link portal tracts to each other and to terminal hepatic venules.[115] In patients in whom the biliary and cholestatic features predominate, the cirrhosis which ultimately develops is generally of the biliary type. When hepatitic features predominate, the cirrhosis tends to be of posthepatitis type. All combinations of the two patterns may be seen.[116] Nodules often develop unevenly throughout the liver, so that nodular areas with the appearance of cirrhosis coexist with areas in which the acinar architecture remains preserved.

The **differential diagnosis of the progressive lesion** includes PSC and **other forms of chronic biliary disease**, on the one hand, and **chronic hepatitis** on the other.[117] The differentiation from primary PSC was discussed earlier; in the later stages of the two diseases it is often impossible to make the distinction histologically. With respect to other forms of chronic biliary obstruction and chronic hepatitis, the most important observation is that bile duct numbers remain normal in both, whereas they are characteristically reduced in PBC and in PSC (**Table 5.1**). Granulomas favour PBC over chronic hepatitis, as does chronic cholestasis, particularly when it is seen in the absence of cirrhosis.[65] There are also

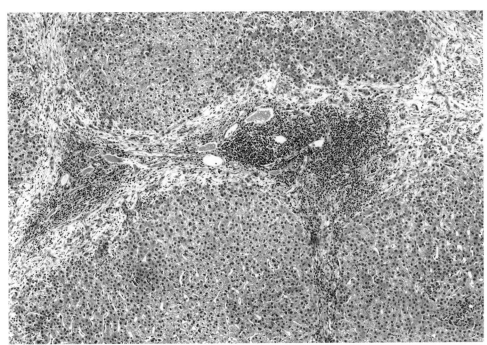

Figure 5.28
Primary biliary cirrhosis.
There is extensive scarring without nodule formation. Aggregates of lymphocytes mark the former sites of bile ducts, as in **Figure 5.22**. (Postmortem liver, H&E.)

rare cases of concomitant PBC and sarcoidosis with granulomas which may present the pathologist with unique diagnostic interpretive problems.[118] Difficulties remain even after these many factors are taken into account, especially if the biopsy specimen is small or fragmented. They can usually be resolved by consideration of the clinical context and laboratory investigations; a middle-aged woman with itching, high levels of serum alkaline phosphatase and AMAs is unlikely to be suffering from chronic viral hepatitis. There are, however, unusual cases which present as overlap syndromes, discussed briefly below.

Overlap syndromes, transitional diseases and autoimmune cholangitis

Establishing a clear-cut diagnosis of PBC or PSC is occasionally problematic when an unusually severe degree of lymphoplasmacytic interface hepatitis is superimposed on otherwise typical histopathological features of either disease (**Fig. 5.29**), raising the possibility of an **overlap syndrome**[119,120] with AIH. Such patients may show a mix of serum autoantibodies (some of which may be merely non-specific markers of immune disease), further clouding the diagnosis. In some instances there appears to be a genetic predilection for the hepatitic component, as in certain cases of PBC where a specific histocompatibility profile is present.[121] Rendering a diagnosis of either PBC/AIH or PSC/AIH overlap syndrome therefore requires close consultation between pathologist and clinician, taking into account and appropriately weighting the biopsy features, serological and biochemical data and cholangiographic findings.[57,119] The International Autoimmune Hepatitis Group recommends

Table 5.1 Causes of bile-duct damage and loss

Loss of ducts	Little or no loss
Primary sclerosing cholangitis	Bile-duct obstruction
Primary biliary cirrhosis	Viral hepatitis
Idiopathic ductopenia	Drug jaundice
Graft-versus-host disease	Parasitic duct disease
Chronic rejection of liver grafts	
Sarcoidosis	
Drug jaundice*	

*Note that, while many drugs produce bile duct injury without loss, there are also well-described cases where ductopenia and chronic cholestatic disease (sometimes requiring liver transplantation) are sequelae of drug hepatotoxicity.

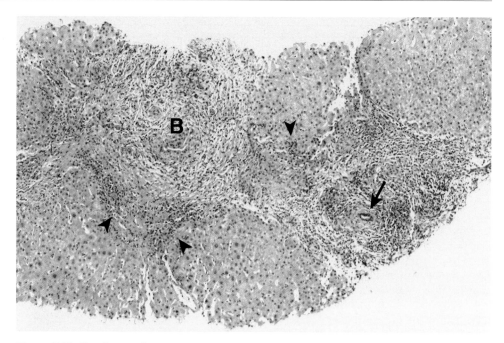

Figure 5.29 Overlap syndrome.
Biopsy from a young patient with ulcerative colitis, but clinicopathological and serological features suggesting primary sclerosing cholangitis–autoimmune hepatitis overlap syndrome. The biopsy features of biliary disease include abnormal bile-duct morphology (B), portal oedema and periduct fibrosis (arrow), while the extensive interface hepatitis (arrowheads) suggests an autoimmune component. (Needle biopsy, H&E.)

categorizing putative 'overlap' cases according to the predominating features as AIH, PBC or PSC/small duct PSC.[121a] Use of the clinicopathological scoring systems developed for AIH may be helpful in some cases,[122-124] although not devised for this purpose.[121a] The diagnostic dilemma of putative 'overlap' cases resides in the current imprecision in defining the individual outermost diagnostic borders of PBC, PSC and AIH,[125] insensitivity of tests used to detect serum mitochondrial antibodies,[81] non-specific generation of various autoantibodies and superimposition of histological features that may cloud the true diagnosis. A pathological diagnosis of overlap syndrome should therefore be made with due restraint whenever possible and only after careful examination of all the biopsy features, including bile-duct morphology, evidence of chronic cholestasis, lobular necroinflammatory changes and interface hepatitis. Paediatric liver biopsies from children with liver disease, serum autoantibodies and a clinical diagnosis suggestive of AIH require particularly careful microscopic evaluation for exclusion of overlap of AIH and PSC (**autoimmune sclerosing cholangitis** or **ASC**), an immune disorder which is significantly more common in children than adults.[126,127] Liver biopsy in ASC may demonstrate only the changes of chronic hepatitis without biliary features in a significant percentage of children with demonstrated biliary lesions on cholangiography.[127]

The interrelatedness of PBC, PSC and AIH as disorders of cellular immunity[128] is further highlighted by descriptions of clinical **transition** from one form to another. Such examples include cases of PBC progressing to AIH,[129,130] AIH progressing to PSC,[131] paediatric PSC patients with autoimmune serological and histopathological features,[132] and transplanted PBC patients who develop AIH in their allografts.[133]

A number of patients with typical biopsy features of PBC but no demonstrable serum AMAs have been described as cases of **autoimmune cholangitis** because of coexistent antinuclear or other autoantibodies, occasional corticosteroid responsiveness and other features that suggest an autoimmune clinical profile.[134] Such cases may reflect problems in the sensitivity of current mitochondrial antibody tests and are now usually considered to be examples of AMA-negative PBC.[81,119]

Other disorders with intrahepatic bile-duct loss

As indicated earlier, the loss of significant numbers of intrahepatic bile ducts (ductopenia) can be seen not only in PBC and PSC but also in several conditions listed in **Box 5.1**. In addition to these, there are patients in whom the pathogenesis of duct loss is poorly understood. Some of these may represent later stages of childhood **non-syndromatic paucity of intrahepatic bile ducts**.[135] In patients with **idiopathic adulthood ductopenia** – predominantly males with cholestatic biochemical profiles – duct loss could also be the end result of small-duct PSC or due to bile-duct damage associated with chronic hepatitis C[136] or autoimmune cholangitis.[137] Rarely, idiopathic adulthood ductopenia is familial.[138] Ductopenia due to the paraneoplastic effects of **Hodgkin's disease** was reported.[139] A group of asymptomatic patients with idiopathic ductopenia and elevated serum γ-glutamyl transferase activity has also been described.[140]

References

1 Jansen PLM, Sturm E. Genetic cholestasis, causes and consequences for hepatobiliary transport. Liver Int 2003;23:315–22.

2 Lee WS, Sokol RJ. Mitochondrial hepatopathies: advances in genetics and pathogenesis. Hepatology 2007;45:1555–65.

3 Crawford JM, Boyer JL. Clinicopathology conferences: inflammation-induced cholestasis. Hepatology 1998;28:253–60.

4 Turkish A, Levy J, Kato M, et al. Pancreatitis and paraneoplastic cholestasis as presenting manifestations of pancreatic lymphoma: evaluation, management, and clinical course in a child. J Pediatr Gastroenterol Nutr 2004;39:552–6.

5 Christoffersen P, Poulsen H. Histological changes in human liver biopsies following extrahepatic biliary obstruction. Acta Pathol Microbiol Scand 1970;212:150–7.

6 Roskams TA, Theise ND, Balabaud C, et al. Nomenclature of the finer branches of the biliary tree: canals, ductules, and ductular reactions in human livers. Hepatology 2004;39:1739–45.

7 LeSage G, Glaser S, Alpini G. Regulation of cholangiocyte proliferation. Liver 2001;21:73–80.

8 Nijjar SS, Wallace L, Crosby HA, et al. Altered Notch ligand expression in human liver disease. Further evidence for a role of the Notch signaling pathway in hepatic neovascularization and biliary ductular defects. Am J Pathol 2002;160:1695–703.

9 Gaya DR, Thorburn KA, Oien KA, et al. Hepatic granulomas: a 10 year single centre experience. J Clin Pathol 2003;56:850–3.

10 Gouw ASH, Clouston AD, Theise ND. Ductular reactions in human liver: diversity at the interface. Hepatology 2011;54:1853–63.

11 Liver transplantation database (LTD) investigators, Sakamoto T, Ezure T, et al. Interleukin-6, hepatocyte growth factor, and their receptors in biliary epithelial cells during a type I ductular reaction in mice: interactions between the periductal inflammatory and stromal cells and the biliary epithelium. Hepatology 1998;28:1260–8.

12 Isse K, Harada K, Nakanuma Y. IL-8 expression by biliary epithelial cells is associated with neutrophilic infiltration and reactive bile ductules. Liver Int 2007;27:672–80.

13 Gerber MA, Thung SN, Bodenheimer HC Jr, et al. Characteristic histologic triad in liver adjacent to metastatic neoplasm. Liver 1986;6:85–8.

14 Wilson C, Auld CD, Schlinkert R, et al. Hepatobiliary complications in chronic pancreatitis. Gut 1989;30:520–7.

15 Flinn WR, Olson DF, Oyasu R, et al. Biliary bacteria and hepatic histopathologic changes in gallstone disease. Ann Surg 1977;185:593–7.

16 Sonzogni A, Colloredo G, Fabris L, et al. Isolated idiopathic bile ductular hyperplasia in patients with persistently abnormal liver function tests. J Hepatol 2004;40:592–8.

17 Lewindon PJ, Pereira TN, Hoskins AC, et al. The role of hepatic stellate cells and transforming growth factor-beta-1 in cystic fibrosis liver disease. Am J Pathol 2002;160:1705–15.

18 Zhang L, Theise N, Chua M, et al. The stem cell niche of human livers: symmetry between development and regeneration. Hepatology 2008;48:1598–607.

19 Portmann B, Popper H, Neuberger J, et al. Sequential and diagnostic features in biliary cirrhosis based on serial histologic study in 209 patients. Gastroenterology 1985;88:1777–90.

20 Weinbren K, Hadjis NS, Blumgart LH. Structural aspects of the liver in patients with biliary disease and portal hypertension. J Clin Pathol 1985;38:1013–20.

21 Hammel P, Couvelard A, O'Toole D, et al. Regression of liver fibrosis after biliary drainage in patients with chronic

pancreatitis and stenosis of the common bile duct. N Engl J Med 2001;344:418–23.

22 Carpenter HA. Bacterial and parasitic cholangitis. Mayo Clin Proc 1998;73:473–8.

23 Shimada H, Nihmoto S, Matsuba A, et al. Acute cholangitis: a histopathologic study. J Clin Gastroenterol 1988;10:197–200.

24 Sasaki M, Nakanuma Y, Kim YS. Expression of apomucins in the intrahepatic biliary tree in hepatolithiasis differs from that in normal liver and extrahepatic biliary obstruction. Hepatology 1998;27:46–53.

25 Bouche H, Housset C, Dumont JL, et al. AIDS-related cholangitis: diagnostic features and course in 15 patients. J Hepatol 1993;17:34–9.

26 Pol S, Romana CA, Richard S, et al. Microsporidia infection in patients with the human immunodeficiency virus and unexplained cholangitis. N Engl J Med 1993;328:95–9.

27 Lefkowitch JH. Bile ductular cholestasis: an ominous histopathologic sign related to sepsis and 'cholangitis lenta.' Hum Pathol 1982;13:19–24.

28 Ishak KG, Rogers WA. Cryptogenic acute cholangitis – association with toxic shock syndrome. Am J Clin Pathol 1981;76:619–26.

29 Wilschanski M, Chait P, Wade JA, et al. Primary sclerosing cholangitis in 32 children: clinical, laboratory and radiographic features, with survival analysis. Hepatology 1995;22:1415–22.

30 Aadland E, Schrumpf E, Fausa O, et al. Primary sclerosing cholangitis: a long-term follow-up study. Scand J Gastroenterol 1987;22:655–64.

31 Jeffrey GP, Reed DW, Carrello S, et al. Histological and immunohistochemical study of the gall bladder lesion in primary sclerosing cholangitis. Gut 1991;32:424–9.

32 Kawaguchi K, Koike M, Tsuruta K, et al. Lymphoplasmacytic sclerosing pancreatitis with cholangitis: a variant of primary sclerosing cholangitis extensively involving pancreas. Hum Pathol 1991;22:387–95.

33 Abraham SC, Cruz-Correa M, Argani P, et al. Lymphoplasmacytic chronic cholecystitis and biliary tract disease in patients with lymphoplasmacytic sclerosing pancreatitis. Am J Surg Pathol 2003;27:441–51.

34 Broome U, Glaumann H, Hultcrantz R. Liver histology and follow up of 68 patients with ulcerative colitis and normal liver function tests. Gut 1990;31:468–72.

35 Graziadei IW, Wiesner RH, Batts KP, et al. Recurrence of primary sclerosing cholangitis following liver transplantation. Hepatology 1999;29:1050–6.

36 Kemeny MM, Battifora H, Blayney DW, et al. Sclerosing cholangitis after continuous hepatic artery infusion of FUDR. Ann Surg 1985;202:176–81.

37 Herrmann G, Lorenz M, Kirkowa-Reimann M, et al. Morphological changes after intra-arterial chemotherapy of the liver. Hepatogastroenterology 1987;34:5–9.

38 Ludwig J, Kim CH, Wiesner RH, et al. Floxuridine-induced sclerosing cholangitis: an ischemic cholangiopathy? Hepatology 1989;9:215–18.

39 Engler S, Elsing C, Flechtenmacher C, et al. Progressive sclerosing cholangitis after shock: a new variant of vanishing bile duct disorders. Gut 2003;52:688–93.

40 Deltenre P, Valla D-C. Ischemic cholangiopathy. J Hepatol 2006;44:806–17.

41 Gelbmann CM, Rümmele P, Wimmer M, et al. Ischemic-like cholangiopathy with secondary sclerosing cholangitis in critically ill patients. Am J Gastroenterol 2007;102:1221–9.

42 Voigtländer T, Negm AA, Schneider AS, et al. Secondary sclerosing cholangitis in critically ill patients: model of end-stage liver disease score and renal function predict outcome. Endoscopy 2012;44:1055–8.

43 Benninger J, Grobholz R, Oeztuerk Y, et al. Sclerosing cholangitis following severe trauma: description of a remarkable disease entity with emphasis on possible pathophysiologic mechanisms. World J Gastroenterol 2005;11:4199–205.

44 Ludwig J. Small-duct primary sclerosing cholangitis. Semin Liver Dis 1991;11:11–17.

45 Eaton JE, Talwalkar JA, Lazaridis KN, et al. Pathogenesis of primary sclerosing cholangitis and advances in diagnosis and management. Gastroenterology 2013;145:521–36.

46 Harrison RF, Hubscher SG. The spectrum of bile duct lesions in end-stage primary sclerosing cholangitis. Histopathology 1991;19:321–7.

47 Keaveny AP, Gordon FD, Goldar-Najafi A, et al. Native liver xanthogranulomatous cholangiopathy in primary sclerosing cholangitis: impact on posttransplant outcome. Liver Transpl 2004;10:115–22.

48 Nakanuma Y, Ohta G. Histometric and serial section observations of the intrahepatic bile ducts in primary biliary cirrhosis. Gastroenterology 1979;76:1326–32.

49 Crawford AR, Lin X-Z, Crawford JM. The normal adult human liver biopsy: a quantitative reference standard. Hepatology 1998;28:323–31.

50 Van Eyken P, Sciot R, Desmet VJ. A cytokeratin immunohistochemical study of cholestatic liver disease: evidence that hepatocytes can express 'bile duct-type' cytokeratins. Histopathology 1989;15:125–35.

51 Nakanuma Y, Yamaguchi K, Ohta G, et al. Pathological features of hepatolithiasis in Japan. Hum Pathol 1988;19:1181–6.

52 Ludwig J, MacCarty RL, LaRusso NF, et al. Intrahepatic cholangiectases and large-duct obliteration in primary sclerosing cholangitis. Hepatology 1986;6:560–8.

53 Fleming KA. Interlobular bile duct basement membrane thickening – a specific marker for primary sclerosing cholangitis (PSC)? J Pathol 1993;169(Suppl.): (abstract).

54 Farrell DJ, Hines JE, Walls AF, et al. Intrahepatic mast cells in chronic liver diseases. Hepatology 1995;22:1175–81.

55 Safyan EL, Veerabagu MP, Swerdlow SH, et al. Intrahepatic cholestasis due to systemic mastocytosis: a case report and review of literature. Am J Gastroenterol 1997;92:1197–200.

56 Baron TH, Koehler RE, Rodgers WH, et al. Mast cell cholangiopathy: another cause of sclerosing cholangitis. Gastroenterology 1995;109:1677–81.

57 Gregorio GV, Portmann B, Karani J, et al. Autoimmune hepatitis/sclerosing cholangitis overlap syndrome in childhood: a 16-year prospective study. Hepatology 2001;33:544–53.

58 Ludwig J, Dickson ER, McDonald GS. Staging of chronic nonsuppurative destructive cholangitis (syndrome of primary biliary cirrhosis). Virchows Arch Pathol Anat 1978;379:103–12.

59 Ludwig J, LaRusso NF, Wiesner RH. The syndrome of primary sclerosing cholangitis. In: Popper H, Shaffner F, editors. Progress in Liver Diseases, vol. IX. Philadelphia, PA: WB Saunders; 1990. p. 555–66.

60 Bergquist A, Ekbom A, Olsson R, et al. Hepatic and extrahepatic malignancies in primary sclerosing cholangitis. J Hepatol 2002;36:321–7.

61 Fleming KA, Boberg KM, Glaumann H, et al. Biliary dysplasia as a marker of cholangiocarcinoma in primary sclerosing cholangitis. J Hepatol 2001;34: 360–5.

62 Haworth AC, Manley PN, Groll A, et al. Bile duct carcinoma and biliary tract dysplasia in chronic ulcerative colitis. Arch Pathol Lab Med 1989;113:434–6.

63 Ludwig J, Wahlstrom HE, Batts KP, et al. Papillary bile duct dysplasia in primary sclerosing cholangitis. Gastroenterology 1992;102:2134–8.

63a Kerr SE, Fritcher EG, Campion MB, et al. Biliary dysplasia in primary sclerosing cholangitis harbors cytogenetic abnormalities similar to cholangiocarcinoma. Hum Pathol 2014;45:1797–804.

64 Björnsson E, Olsson R, Bergquist A, et al. The natural history of small-duct primary sclerosing cholangitis. Gastroenterology 2008;134:975–80.

65 Guarascio P, Yentis F, Cevikbas U, et al. Value of copper-associated protein in diagnostic assessment of liver biopsy. J Clin Pathol 1983;36:18–23.

66 Ludwig J, Colina F, Poterucha JJ. Granulomas in primary sclerosing cholangitis. Liver 1995;15:307–12.

67 Ludwig J. Surgical pathology of the syndrome of primary sclerosing cholangitis. Am J Surg Pathol 1989;13(Suppl. 1):43–9.

68 Stone JH. IgG4-related disease: nomenclature, clinical features, and treatment. Semin Diagn Pathol 2012;29:177–90.

69 Stone JH, Khosroshahi A, Deshpande V, et al. Recommendations for the nomenclature of IgG4-related disease and its individual organ system manifestations. Arthritis Rheum 2012;64:3061–7.

70 Nakazawa T, Naitoh I, Hayashi K, et al. Diagnosis of IgG4-related sclerosing cholangitis. World J Gastroenterol 2013;19:7661–70.

71 Okazaki K, Uchida K, Koyabu M, et al. IgG4 cholangiopathy – current concept, diagnosis, and pathogenesis. J Hepatol 2014.

71a Okazaki K, Uchida K, Koyabu M, et al. IgG4 cholangiopathy – current concept, diagnosis, and pathogenesis. J Hepatol 2014;61:690–5.

72 Björnsson E, Chari ST, Smyrk TC, et al. Immunoglobulin G4 associated cholangitis: description of an emerging clinical entity based on review of the literature. Hepatology 2007;45:1547–54.

73 Webster GJM, Pereira SP, Chapman RW. Autoimmune pancreatitis/IgG4-associated cholangitis – overlapping or separate diseases? J Hepatol 2009;51:398–402.

73a Graham RPD, Smyrk TC, Chari ST, et al. Isolated IgG4-related sclerosing cholangitis: a report of 9 cases. Hum Pathol 2014;45:1722–9.

74 Zen Y, Fujii T, Sato Y, et al. Pathological classification of hepatic inflammatory pseudotumor with respect to IgG4-related disease. Mod Pathol 2007;20:884–94.

75 Zhang L, Lewis JT, Abraham SC, et al. IgG4+ plasma cell infiltrates in liver explants with primary sclerosing cholangitis. Am J Surg Pathol 2010;34:88–94.

76 Umemura T, Zen Y, Hamano H, et al. Immunoglobulin G4-hepatopathy: association of immunoglobulin G4-bearing plasma cells in liver with autoimmune pancreatitis. Hepatology 2007;46:463–71.

77 Deshpande V, Sainani NI, Chung RT, et al. IgG4-associated cholangitis: a comparative histological and immunophenotypic study with primary sclerosing cholangitis on liver biopsy material. Mod Pathol 2009;22:1287–95.

78 Rubin E, Schaffner F, Popper H. Primary biliary cirrhosis. Chronic non-suppurative destructive cholangitis. Am J Pathol 1965;46:387–407.

79 Dahlan Y, Smith L, Simmonds D, et al. Pediatric-onset primary biliary cirrhosis. Gastroenterology 2003;125:1476–9.

80 Kaplan MM, Gershwin ME. Primary biliary cirrhosis. N Engl J Med 2005;353:1261–73.

81 Selmi C, Zuin M, Gershwin ME. The unfinished business of primary biliary cirrhosis. J Hepatol 2008;49:451–60.

82 Jones DEJ. Pathogenesis of primary biliary cirrhosis. J Hepatol 2003;39:639–48.

83 Leung PSC, Coppel RL, Ansari A, et al. Antimitochondrial antibodies in primary biliary cirrhosis. Semin Liver Dis 1997;17:61–9.

84 Neuberger J. Antibodies and primary biliary cirrhosis – piecing together the jigsaw. J Hepatol 2002;36:126–9.

85 Hirschfield GM, Liu X, Xu C, et al. Primary biliary cirrhosis associated with *HLA*, *IL12A*, and *IL12RB2* variants. N Engl J Med 2009;360:2544–55.

85a Wang L, Sun Y, Zhang Z, et al. CXCR5+ CD4+ T follicular helper cells participate in the pathogenesis of primary biliary cirrhosis. Hepatology 2015;61:627–38.

85b Webb GJ, Hirschfield GM. Follicles, germinal centers, and immune mechanisms in primary biliary cirrhosis. Hepatology 2015;61:424–7.

86 Culp KS, Fleming CR, Duffy J, et al. Autoimmune associations in primary biliary cirrhosis. Mayo Clin Proc 1982;57:365–70.

87 Scheuer P. Primary biliary cirrhosis. Proc R Soc Med 1967;60:1257–60.

88 Jones DEJ, Metcalf JV, Collier JD, et al. Hepatocellular carcinoma in primary biliary cirrhosis and its impact on outcomes. Hepatology 1997;26:1138–42.

89 Cavazza A, Caballeria L, Floreani A, et al. Incidence, risk factors, and survival of hepatocellular carcinoma in primary biliary cirrhosis: comparative analysis from two centers. Hepatology 2009;50:1162–8.

90 Terada T, Kurumaya H, Nakanuma Y, et al. Macroregenerative nodules of the liver in primary biliary cirrhosis: report of two autopsy cases. Am J Gastroenterol 1989;84:418–21.

91 Floreani A, Baragiotta A, Baldo V, et al. Hepatic and extrahepatic malignancies in primary biliary cirrhosis. Hepatology 1999;29:1425–8.

92 Neuberger J. Eosinophils and primary biliary cirrhosis – stoking the fire? Hepatology 1999;30:335–7.

93 Yamazaki K, Suzuki K, Nakamura A, et al. Ursodeoxycholic acid inhibits eosinophil degranulation in patients with primary biliary cirrhosis. Hepatology 1999;30:71–8.

94 Degott C, Zafrani ES, Callard P, et al. Histopathological study of primary biliary cirrhosis and the effect of ursodeoxycholic acid treatment on histology progression. Hepatology 1999;29:1007–12.

95 Daniels JA, Torbenson M, Anders RA, et al. Immunostaining of plasma cells in primary biliary cirrhosis. Am J Clin Pathol 2009;131:243–9.

96   Moreira RK, Revetta F, Koehler E, et al. Diagnostic utility of IgG and IgM immunohistochemistry in autoimmune liver disease. World J Gastroenterol 2010;16:453–7.

97   Graham RPD, Smyrk TC, Zhang L. Evaluation of Langerhans cell infiltrate by CD1a immunostain in liver biopsy for the diagnosis of primary biliary cirrhosis. Am J Surg Pathol 2012;36:732–6.

98   Nakanuma Y, Ohta G. Quantitation of hepatic granulomas and epithelioid cells in primary biliary cirrhosis. Hepatology 1983;3:423–7.

99   Vleggaar FP, van Buuren HR, Zondervan PE, et al. Jaundice in non-cirrhotic primary biliary cirrhosis: the premature ductopenic variant. Gut 2001;49:276–81.

100   Nakanuma Y. Necroinflammatory changes in hepatic lobules in primary biliary cirrhosis with less well-defined cholestatic changes. Hum Pathol 1993;24:378–83.

101   McMahon RF, Babbs C, Warnes TW. Nodular regenerative hyperplasia of the liver, CREST syndrome and primary biliary cirrhosis: an overlap syndrome? Gut 1989;30:1430–3.

102   Colina F, Pinedo F, Solís A, et al. Nodular regenerative hyperplasia of the liver in early histological stages of primary biliary cirrhosis. Gastroenterology 1992;102:1319–24.

103   Nakanuma Y, Ohta G, Kobayashi K, et al. Histological and histometric examination of the intrahepatic portal vein branches in primary biliary cirrhosis without regenerative nodules. Am J Gastroenterol 1982;77:405–13.

104   Nakanuma Y, Hirata K. Unusual hepatocellular lesions in primary biliary cirrhosis resembling but unrelated to hepatocellular neoplasms. Virchows Arch [A] 1993;422:17–23.

105   O'Donohue J, Oien KA, Donaldson P, et al. Co-amoxiclav jaundice: clinical and histological features and HLA class II association. Gut 2000;47:717–20.

106   Bach N, Thung SN, Schaffner F. The histological features of chronic hepatitis C and autoimmune chronic hepatitis: a comparative analysis. Hepatology 1992;15:572–7.

107   Christoffersen P, Poulsen H, Scheuer PJ. Abnormal bile duct epithelium in chronic aggressive hepatitis and primary biliary cirrhosis. Hum Pathol 1972;3:227–35.

108   Terasaki S, Nakanuma Y, Yamazaki M, et al. Eosinophilic infiltration of the liver in primary biliary cirrhosis: a morphological study. Hepatology 1993;17:206–12.

109   Czaja AJ, Carpenter HA. Autoimmune hepatitis with incidental histologic features of bile duct injury. Hepatology 2001;34:659–65.

110   Washington K, Clavien P-A, Killenberg P. Peribiliary vascular plexus in primary sclerosing cholangitis and primary biliary cirrhosis. Hum Pathol 1997;28:791–5.

111   Nakanuma Y, Saito K, Unoura M. Semiquantitative assessment of cholestasis and lymphocytic piecemeal necrosis in primary biliary cirrhosis: a histologic and immunohistochemical study. J Clin Gastroenterol 1990;12:357–62.

112   Yamada S, Howe S, Scheuer PJ. Three-dimensional reconstruction of biliary pathways in primary biliary cirrhosis: a computer-assisted study. J Pathol 1987;152:317–23.

113   Leon MP, Bassendine MF, Gibbs P, et al. Immunogenicity of biliary epithelium: study of the adhesive interaction with lymphocytes. Gastroenterology 1997;112:968–77.

114   Dienes HP, Lohse AW, Gerken G, et al. Bile duct epithelia as target cells in primary biliary cirrhosis and primary sclerosing cholangitis. Virchows Arch 1997;431:119–24.

115   Nakanuma Y. Pathology of septum formation in primary biliary cirrhosis: a histological study in the non-cirrhotic stage. Virchows Arch [A] 1991;419:381–7.

116   Scheuer PJ. Pathologic features and evolution of primary biliary cirrhosis and primary sclerosing cholangitis. Mayo Clin Proc 1998;73:179–83.

117   Williamson JM, Chalmers DM, Clayden AD, et al. Primary biliary cirrhosis and chronic active hepatitis: an examination of clinical, biochemical, and histopathological features in differential diagnosis. J Clin Pathol 1985;38:1007–12.

118   Stanca CM, Fiel MI, Allina J, et al. Liver failure in an antimitochondrial antibody-positive patient with sarcoidosis: primary biliary cirrhosis or hepatic sarcoidosis? Semin Liver Dis 2005;25:364–70.

119   Woodward J, Neuberger J. Autoimmune overlap syndromes. Hepatology 2001;33:994–1002.

120   Czaja AJ. Cholestatic phenotypes of autoimmune hepatitis. Clin Gastroenterol Hepatol 2014;12:1430–8.

121   Lohse AW, Meyer zum Büschenfelde K-H, Franz B, et al. Characterization of the overlap syndrome of primary biliary cirrhosis (PBC) and autoimmune hepatitis: evidence for it being a hepatitic form of PBC in genetically susceptible individuals. Hepatology 1999;29:1078–84.

121a Boberg KM, Chapman RW, Hirschfield GM, et al. Overlap syndromes: the International Autoimmune Hepatitis Group (IAIG) position statement on a controversial issue. J Hepatol 2011;54:374–85.

122   Hennes EM, Zeniya M, Czaja AJ, et al. Simplified criteria for the diagnosis of autoimmune hepatitis. Hepatology 2008;48:169–76.

123   Alvarez F, Berg PA, Biandin FB, et al. International Autoimmune Hepatitis Group report: review of criteria for diagnosis of autoimmune hepatitis. J Hepatol 1999;31:929–38.

124   Kaya M, Angulo P, Lindor KD. Overlap of autoimmune hepatitis and primary sclerosing cholangitis: an evaluation of a modified scoring system. J Hepatol 2000;33:537–42.

125   Czaja AJ. Overlap syndrome of primary biliary cirrhosis and autoimmune hepatitis: a foray across diagnostic boundaries. J Hepatol 2006;44:251–2.

126   Mieli-Vergani G, Vergani D. Paediatric autoimmune liver disease. Arch Dis Child 2013;98:1012–17.

127   Gregorio GV, Portmann B, Karani J, et al. Autoimmune hepatitis/sclerosing cholangitis overlap syndrome in childhood: a 16-year prospective study. Hepatology 2001;33:544–53.

128   Kita H, Mackay IR, Van de Water J, et al. The lymphoid liver: considerations on pathways to autoimmune injury. Gastroenterology 2001;120:1485–501.

129   Poupon R, Chazouilleres O, Corpechot C, et al. Development of autoimmune hepatitis in patients with typical primary biliary cirrhosis. Hepatology 2006;44:85–90.

130   Twaddell WS, Lefkowitch JH, Berk PD. Evolution from primary biliary cirrhosis to primary biliary cirrhosis/autoimmune hepatitis overlap syndrome. Semin Liver Dis 2008;28:128–34.

131   Abdo AA, Bain VG, Kichian K, et al. Evolution of autoimmune hepatitis to primary sclerosing cholangitis: a sequential syndrome. Hepatology 2002;36:1393–9.

132 Feldstein AE, Perrault J, El-Youssif M, et al. Primary sclerosing cholangitis in children: a long-term follow-up study. Hepatology 2003;38:210–17.

133 Jones DE, James OF, Portmann B, et al. Development of autoimmune hepatitis following liver transplantation for primary biliary cirrhosis. Hepatology 1999;30:53–7.

134 Brunner G, Klinge O. Ein der chronisch-destruierenden nicht-eitrigen Cholangitis ähnliches Krankheitsbild mit antinjukleären Antikörpern (Immuncholangitis). Dtsch Med Wochenschr 1987;112:1454–8.

135 Bruguera M, Llach J, Rodés J. Nonsyndromic paucity of intrahepatic bile ducts in infancy and idiopathic ductopenia in adulthood: the same syndrome? Hepatology 1992;15:830–4.

136 Dural AT, Genta RM, Goodman ZD, et al. Idiopathic adulthood ductopenia associated with hepatitis C virus. Dig Dis Sci 2002;47:1625–6.

137 Ludwig J. Idiopathic adulthood ductopenia: an update. Mayo Clin Proc 1998;73:285–91.

138 Burak KW, Pearson DC, Swain MG, et al. Familial idiopathic adulthood ductopenia: a report of five cases in three generations. J Hepatol 2000;32:159–63.

139 Crosbie OM, Crown JP, Nolan NPM, et al. Resolution of paraneoplastic bile duct paucity following successful treatment of Hodgkin's disease. Hepatology 1997;26:5–8.

140 Moreno A, Carreño CA, González C. Idiopathic biliary ductopenia in adults without symptoms of liver disease. N Engl J Med 1997;336:835–8.

General reading

Balistreri WF, Bezerra JA, Jansen P, et al. Intrahepatic cholestasis: summary of an AASLD single-topic conference. Hepatology 2005;42:222–35.

Bowlus CL, Gershwin ME. The diagnosis of primary biliary cirrhosis. Autoimmun Rev 2014;13:441–4.

Crawford JM. Development of the intrahepatic biliary tree. Semin Liver Dis 2002;22:213–26.

Czaja AJ, Bayraktar Y. Non-classical phenotypes of autoimmune hepatitis and advances in diagnosis and treatment. World J Gastroenterol 2009;15:2314–28.

Gouw ASH, Clouston AD, Theise ND. Ductular reactions in human liver: diversity at the interface. Hepatology 2011;54:1853–63.

Hirschfield GM, Gershwin ME. The immunobiology and pathophysiology of primary biliary cirrhosis. Annu Rev Pathol 2013;8:303–30.

Hirschfield GM, Karlsen TH, Lindor KD, et al. Primary sclerosing cholangitis. Lancet 2013;382:1587–99.

Kim WR, Ludwig J, Lindor KD. Variant forms of cholestatic diseases involving small bile ducts in adults. Am J Gastroenterol 2000;95:1130–8.

Li MK, Crawford JM. The pathology of cholestasis. Semin Liver Dis 2004;24:21–42.

Nakanuma Y, Zen Y, Portmann BC. Diseases of the bile ducts. In: Burt AD, Portmann BC, Ferrell LD, editors. MacSween's Pathology of the Liver. 6th ed. Edinburgh: Churchill Livingstone/Elsevier; 2012. p. 491–562.

Roberts SK, Ludwig J, LaRusso NF. The pathobiology of biliary epithelia. Gastroenterology 1997;112:269–79.

Roskams T, Desmet VJ. Ductular reaction and its diagnostic significance. Semin Diagn Pathol 1998;15:259–69.

Roskams TA, Theise ND, Balabaud C, et al. Nomenclature of the finer branches of the biliary tree: canals, ductules, and ductular reactions in human livers. Hepatology 2004;39:1739–45.

Stapelbroek JM, van Erpecum KJ, Klomp LWJ, et al. Liver disease associated with canalicular transport defects: current and future therapies. J Hepatol 2010;52:258–71.

Strazzabosco M, Fabris L. Development of the bile ducts: essentials for the clinical hepatologist. J Hepatol 2012;56:1159–70.

Wagner M, Zollner G, Trauner M. New molecular insights into the mechanisms of cholestasis. J Hepatol 2009;51:565–80.

Acute Viral Hepatitis

Introduction

Acute hepatitis is not usually an indication for liver biopsy. There are, however, at least three reasons why pathologists sometimes receive liver biopsy samples from patients with acute hepatitis. First, there may be doubt about the clinical diagnosis, or even a mistaken working diagnosis. Second, a diagnosis of hepatitis may be well established but the clinician needs information on the stage of the disease or its severity. Third, the patient may have received a liver transplant and the pathologist is being asked to help decide if symptoms or biochemical abnormalities are due to recurrent (or new) viral hepatitis or to some other cause such as rejection. For all these reasons, a knowledge of the pathology of acute hepatitis is essential. There is a further reason, no less important than the others: without a knowledge of acute hepatitis, the pathologist cannot hope to understand chronic hepatitis and cirrhosis, together the cause of most liver disease in the world. This chapter describes acute viral hepatitis and its immediate sequelae in the immunocompetent patient. The specific problems of diagnosing hepatitis in an immunosuppressed patient after transplantation are reviewed in **Chapter 16**.

The hepatitis viruses are listed in **Table 6.1**. While several other candidates have been extensively investigated in recent years, none has so far been established as a definite cause of viral hepatitis and most episodes of acute and chronic hepatitis can be attributed to one of the viruses listed, to autoimmune hepatitis (**Ch. 9**) or to a hepatotoxic agent (**Ch. 8**). An exception to this statement is fulminant hepatitis, the cause of which cannot currently be established in a substantial minority of patients,[1-3] including children.[4] Occasionally, a virus more often associated with infection of other organs, such as one of the herpesviruses[5-7] or an adenovirus,[8,9] gives rise to a severe hepatitis. These agents are further discussed in **Chapter 15**. Mild acute hepatitis has been reported in patients infected with the SARS virus (severe acute respiratory syndrome-associated coronavirus).[10,11]

Occasionally, mild serum liver test abnormalities and mild histological hepatitis ('bystander hepatitis') with apoptotic bodies, focal necrosis and lymphocytic inflammation are seen in systemic, non-hepatic viral infections such as pulmonary influenza and result from migration to the liver of, and collateral damage by, CD8 T lymphocytes.[12,13]

Pathological features

The essential components of the acute phase of hepatitis are inflammatory-cell infiltration and hepatocellular damage. Other features include cholestasis, Kupffer-cell activation, endotheliitis, bile-duct damage, the ductular reaction and hepatocellular regeneration.

Table 6.1 The hepatitis viruses

Virus	Type	Spread and disease
Hepatitis A (HAV)	RNA hepatovirus	Faecal–oral, acute
Hepatitis B (HBV)	DNA hepadnavirus	Parenteral, acute or chronic
Hepatitis C (HCV)	RNA hepacivirus	Parenteral or sporadic; acute, more often chronic
Hepatitis D (HDV)	RNA deltavirus, defective	Pathogenic when combined with HBV
Hepatitis E (HEV)	RNA virus	Faecal–oral, epidemic or sporadic acute disease

Figure 6.1 Acute viral hepatitis. Surviving hepatocytes in the perivenular area in the centre of the field are swollen and the area is infiltrated by inflammatory cells. (Needle biopsy, H&E.)

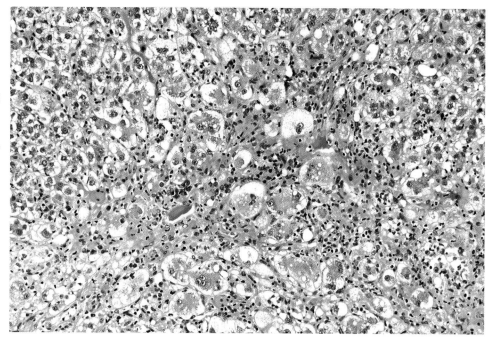

Hepatocellular damage

Changes seen under the light microscope range from minor degrees of cell swelling to cell death. They are accompanied by the inflammatory infiltration described below, reflecting the important role of cellular immunity in the pathogenesis of most forms of hepatitis. Both hepatocellular damage and inflammation are usually most severe in perivenular areas, giving rise to a characteristic histological pattern (**Fig. 6.1**). A periportal pattern of necrosis and inflammation, sometimes seen in hepatitis A, is less common.

The mildest and probably reversible change is cell swelling. The cytoplasm of affected cells is rarified, granular and sometimes finely vacuolated. The more severe degrees of cell swelling are called ballooning degeneration (**Fig. 6.2**). This differs from the feathery degeneration of cholestasis, in which the cytoplasm has a reticular pattern (**see Fig. 5.3**) and from the ballooning in steatohepatitis where the cytoplasm is less granular and more oedematous and 'clarifed' (**see Fig. 7.8**). Other hepatocytes undergo apoptosis, which is

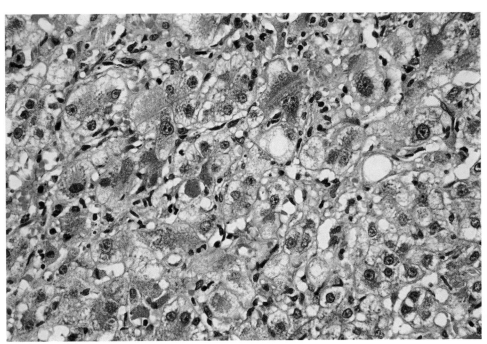

Figure 6.2 Acute viral hepatitis. Normal liver-cell plate structure is disrupted. Hepatocytes vary in size and some are ballooned and vacuolated. An apoptotic hepatocyte is seen left of centre. (Needle biopsy, H&E.)

an important method of cell death in hepatitis.[14] Shrinkage and increased staining of the cytoplasm, sometimes called acidophilic change or degeneration, is probably a precursor of apoptosis, in which the hepatocytes shrink further, become very dense and undergo fragmentation. The apoptotic bodies seen lying free in the sinusoids represent the largest fragments or entire unfragmented apoptotic cells (**Fig. 6.2**). They are also called acidophil bodies or Councilman bodies, Councilman having first described them in yellow fever[15,16] (**Fig. 6.3**). Apoptotic bodies sometimes contain pyknotic nuclear remnants and often appear to bulge beyond the plane of the section. Another form of hepatocellular damage in acute hepatitis is focal (spotty) necrosis, in which liver-cell plates are disrupted or replaced by small groups of lymphocytes and macrophages. Whether these mark a site of necrosis or of apoptosis is not clear; the damage to hepatocytes is deduced from their absence rather than seen. Whatever its mechanism, loss of hepatocytes or liver-cell drop-out, coupled with focal regeneration, leads to a characteristic irregularity of the liver-cell plates, which usually allows acute hepatitis to be distinguished from hepatocellular damage secondary to cholestasis. The loss of hepatocytes also leads to condensation of the extracellular matrix, best seen in reticulin preparations (**Fig. 6.4**).

Hepatocyte nuclei show prominent nucleoli and increased variation in size and may be multiple. When syncytial giant hepatocytes are very prominent, the term giant-cell hepatitis is appropriate.[17,18] This is only rarely of proven viral origin and is also more characteristic of acute hepatitis in neonates. In adults, autoimmune hepatitis and hepatitis C virus with or without human immunodeficiency virus co-infection are important associations.[19-23]

Cholestasis in the form of bile thrombi in canaliculi is common in acute hepatitis but rare in chronic hepatitis, which is diagnostically helpful. It is a result of damage to the bile-secretory apparatus of the hepatocytes, but may also result from interference with bile flow at the level of the portal tracts.[24] The term cholestatic hepatitis is best kept as a clinical description of patients with a prolonged cholestatic course. Mild hepatocellular siderosis or steatosis is occasionally seen.

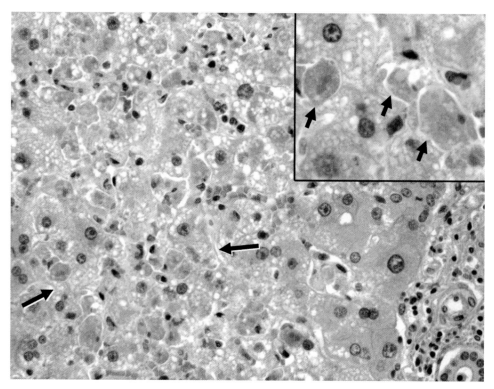

Figure 6.3 Acute yellow-fever hepatitis.
There is prominent mid-zonal necrosis (between arrows) with many apoptotic hepatocytes and scattered lymphocytes. The portal tract at lower right is mildly inflamed and there is relative preservation of periportal parenchyma. Inset: The numerous apoptotic (Councilman) bodies present (arrows) are characteristic of liver involvement in yellow fever. (Case kindly provided by Dr Matthias Szabolcs, New York, NY.)

The inflammatory infiltrate

Unlike classic acute inflammation, viral hepatitis is characterised by a mainly lymphocytic infiltrate within the parenchyma and portal tracts. In acute hepatitis, the most conspicuous inflammation is usually perivenular. The extent of portal inflammation is very variable and portal tracts may be either normal in size or expanded. The larger conducting tracts are often spared. The edges of small portal tracts may be well defined or blurred by outward extension of the infiltrate. This so-called spillover resembles the interface hepatitis of chronic hepatitis (**Ch. 9**) and may be difficult to distinguish from it. The parenchymal changes, clinical history and virological findings usually make the correct diagnosis clear.

While most of the infiltrating cells in acute hepatitis are small T lymphocytes,[25] plasma cells may also be prominent[26] and there are often a few neutrophils and eosinophils. The plasma cells do not necessarily indicate autoimmune hepatitis, nor do a few eosinophils prove a diagnosis of drug injury. Kupffer cells and other macrophages accumulate and enlarge, many of them forming discrete clumps together with lymphocytes. They may contain tan-brown ceroid pigment, staining with periodic acid–Schiff (PAS) agent after diastase digestion (**Fig. 6.5**). They may also contain stainable iron (**Fig. 6.6**), but this is less common.

Sinusoidal and venular endothelial cells also take part in the hepatitic process. Sinusoidal endothelial cells become swollen and may contain dense iron-positive granules[27]

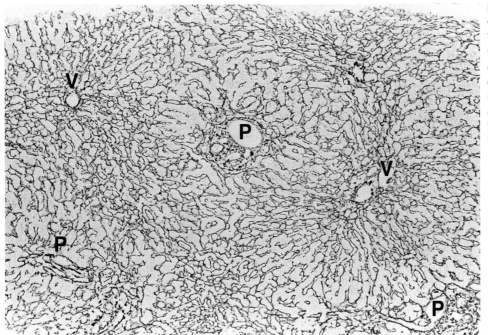

Figure 6.4 Acute viral hepatitis. The reticulin framework is condensed near the efferent venules (V), but not immediately around the portal tracts (P). (Needle biopsy, reticulin.)

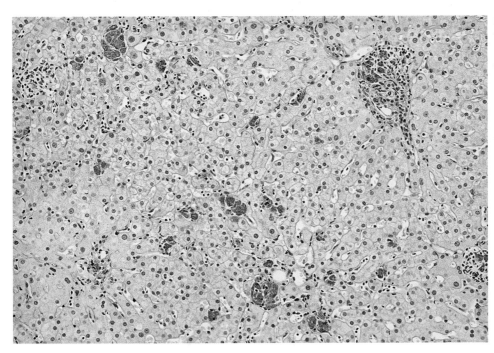

Figure 6.5 Acute viral hepatitis. Macrophages contain diastase periodic acid–Schiff (PAS)-positive material. (Needle biopsy, diastase–PAS.)

Figure 6.6 Acute viral hepatitis. Enlarged macrophages are strongly iron-positive. Some endothelial cells also contain dense Perls' stain-positive granules. (Section kindly provided by Dr Susan Davies, Cambridge, UK.) (Needle biopsy, Perls' stain.)

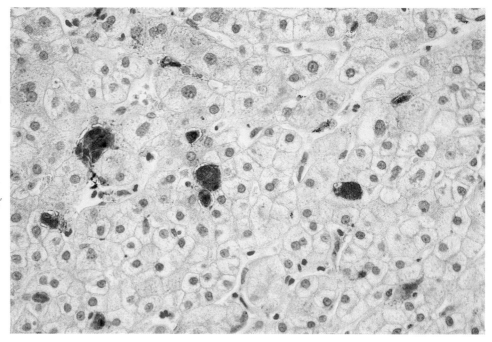

(**Fig. 6.6**). Terminal hepatic venules may show disruption of the endothelium and lymphocytic infiltration.

Portal changes

In contrast to chronic hepatitis, the parenchymal changes dominate the picture, but there is always some portal inflammation, affecting most or all of the small portal tracts (**Fig. 6.7**). The density of the infiltrate varies. Interlobular bile ducts may show abnormalities, including irregularity, crowding and stratification of the epithelium, cytoplasmic vacuolation and infiltration by lymphocytes (**Fig. 6.8**). These changes, together with formation of dense lymphoid structures (aggregates and follicles), are most often seen in hepatitis C. Bile-duct loss (ductopenia) is very rare.

Histological variants

The histological changes in acute hepatitis are infinitely variable, but a few patterns deserve special mention. These are confluent necrosis, bridging necrosis, necrosis of entire lobules and periportal necrosis.

Confluent necrosis signifies death of a substantial area of the parenchyma. Focal as opposed to zonal areas of confluent necrosis haphazardly distributed in relation to lobular zones are more likely to be due to causes other than acute viral hepatitis; possibilities to be considered include opportunistic infections with herpes simplex or zoster viruses and lymphoma. **Bridging necrosis (Figs 6.9, 6.10, and see Fig. 4.8)** is the term given to confluent necrosis linking terminal venules to portal tracts. A possible explanation for this location is that it represents the entire zone 3 of an acinus, a view supported by the curved shape of many bridges. Bridging necrosis is a manifestation of severe acute hepatitis but its distribution even within a single biopsy may be irregular. Necrosis and inflammation linking adjacent portal tracts without involvement of terminal venules should not strictly

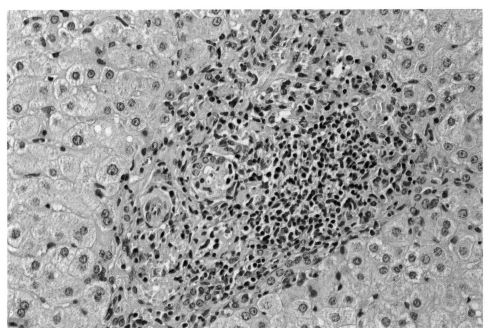

Figure 6.7 Acute viral hepatitis.
A portal tract is infiltrated by inflammatory cells, mainly lymphocytes. In places the infiltrate extends a short way into the adjacent parenchyma. (Needle biopsy, H&E.)

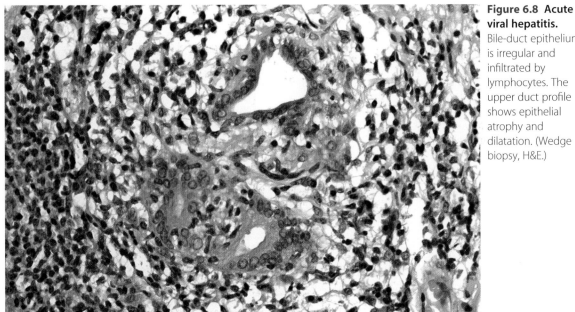

Figure 6.8 Acute viral hepatitis.
Bile-duct epithelium is irregular and infiltrated by lymphocytes. The upper duct profile shows epithelial atrophy and dilatation. (Wedge biopsy, H&E.)

be called bridging because it almost certainly has different pathogenetic significance; it results from widening of portal tracts, with or without periportal necrosis.

Bridges of confluent necrosis with subsequent collapse may be mistaken for the septa of chronic liver disease. In making the important distinction between them, the pathologist is often helped by stains for elastic tissue. Unlike stains for collagens, these normally give negative results in the parenchyma, but elastic tissue accumulates as septa age.[28] Recent collapse is therefore negative (**Fig. 6.11**), whereas old septa are positive. Substantial

Figure 6.9 Acute viral hepatitis: bridging necrosis. Two curved lines of collapse (arrows) extend from a portal tract (P). An efferent venule (V) is seen top centre. (Needle biopsy, H&E.)

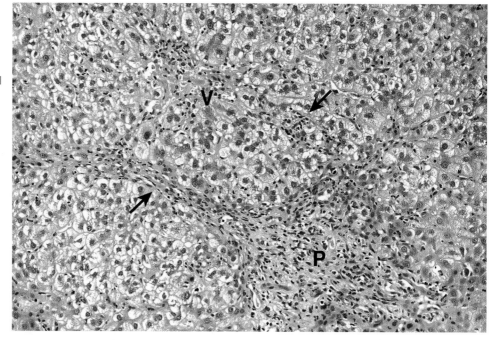

Figure 6.10 Acute viral hepatitis: bridging necrosis. Recent collapse following confluent necrosis is seen as condensation of reticulin, mimicking fibrosis. (Needle biopsy, reticulin.)

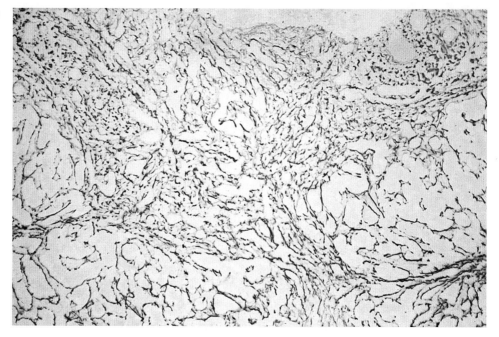

amounts of elastic tissue take months or years to accumulate, but small amounts can be detected by sensitive methods such as Victoria blue as early as 1 or 2 months after onset of hepatitis.[29]

In a minority of patients with acute viral hepatitis, confluent necrosis extends throughout entire lobules or acini (**panlobular** or **panacinar necrosis**) or several adjacent ones (**multilobular** or **multiacinar necrosis**). This is a common feature in patients with

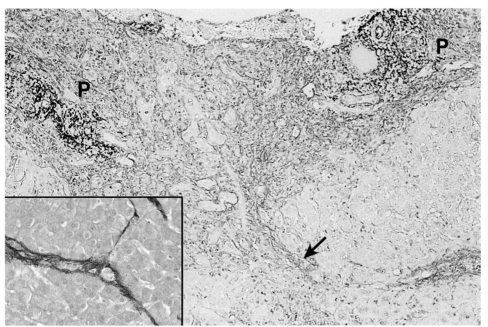

Figure 6.11 Acute hepatitis: bridging necrosis.
The field is the same as that shown in **Figure 6.9**. A stain for elastic fibres is positive in two portal tracts (P) but not in the intervening area of collapse. A necrotic bridge (arrow) is also negative. Inset: This contrasts with an elastic fibre-rich septum in chronic liver disease. (Needle biopsy, orcein.)

fulminant hepatitis. The term 'massive necrosis' is also sometimes used, but can be misleading in so far as a needle biopsy specimen may not be representative of the liver as a whole and can lead to over- or underestimation of the true extent of liver damage.[30] This throws doubt on the usefulness of liver biopsy as a means of assessing prognosis in severe acute hepatitis. Sometimes multilobular necrosis involves only the subcapsular zone, and a small needle specimen may then give a falsely pessimistic picture (**see Fig. 1.3**). In multilobular necrosis the parenchyma is replaced by collapsed stroma, inflammatory cells and activated macrophages (**Fig. 6.12**). Around the surviving portal tracts, there are prominent duct-like structures, some of which probably represent proliferation of pluripotential progenitor cells[31-33] (**see Fig. 4.13D**). Late-onset hepatic failure is a term used for patients developing encephalopathy between 8 and 24 weeks after onset of symptoms.[34] Study of liver biopsies and explanted livers from these patients has shown a consistent pattern of map-like necrosis together with areas of nodular regeneration.

Periportal necrosis rather than the more usual perivenular necrosis is a feature in some patients with hepatitis A (see below).

Individual causes of viral hepatitis

There are more similarities than differences between hepatitis types A, B, C, D and E, but certain patterns are more common in one type than another and are described here. They do not allow the pathologist to identify the cause of the hepatitis on histological appearance alone. The picture may be confused by the presence of more than one virus, or by additional damage resulting from alcohol abuse.

Hepatitis A

Two main patterns are described, occurring separately or together.[35-37] One is a histological picture of perivenular cholestasis with little liver-cell damage or inflammation,

Figure 6.12 Acute viral hepatitis: multilobular necrosis.
Portal tracts (P) can be identified but the parenchyma has been replaced by inflammatory cells, necrotic debris and duct-like structures. (Needle biopsy, H&E.)

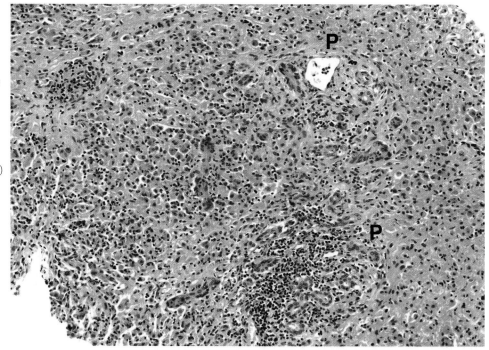

Figure 6.13 Hepatitis A.
Perivenular area showing irregularity of liver-cell plates and cholestasis, but only mild inflammatory infiltration. (Needle biopsy, H&E.)

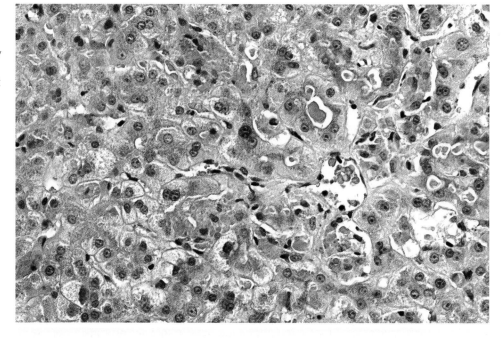

easily mistaken for other causes of cholestasis (**Fig. 6.13**). The second is a hepatitis with periportal necrosis and a dense portal infiltrate which includes abundant, often aggregated plasma cells (**Fig. 6.14**). These two patterns may be related, the cholestasis resulting from interruption of bile flow by the periportal necrosis.[23] Other patterns of hepatitis as described above are also found, but fulminant hepatitis with multilobular necrosis is rare. Extensive

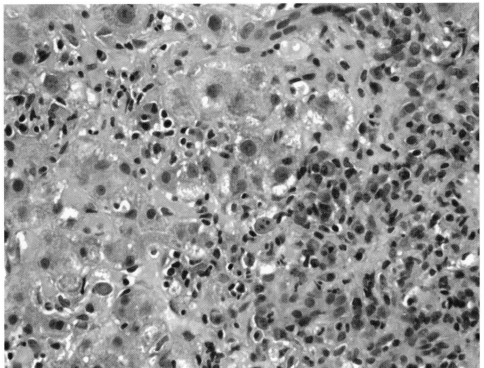

Figure 6.14
Hepatitis A.
The portal area at right is heavily infiltrated by lymphocytes and plasma cells, some of which extend into the adjacent parenchyma. The limiting plate is irregular. The picture resembles that of chronic hepatitis with interface hepatitis. (Needle biopsy, H&E.)

microvesicular change of hepatocytes, previously described in hepatitis D infection, has been seen also in severe acute hepatitis A (**Fig. 6.15**). Fibrin-ring granulomas have been reported.[38,39] A chronic course[40] is very rare.

Hepatitis B

The histological appearances are broadly similar to those of other forms of viral hepatitis. Some of the differences reported in the literature may well reflect patient selection rather than features specific for hepatitis B virus (HBV) infection. However, lymphocytes and macrophages sometimes lie in close contact with hepatocytes (peripolesis) or even invaginate them deeply (emperipolesis), which probably reflects the immunological nature of the cell damage. In a comparative study, periportal inflammation tended to be more severe in acute hepatitis B than in hepatitis C.[41] Liver cells and their nuclei may show a moderate degree of pleomorphism. In most cases of acute hepatitis, the hepatitis B core and surface antigens (HBcAg and HBsAg) are either not demonstrable or very sparse, but in one study of livers infected with an HBV mutant,[42] HBsAg could be demonstrated by immunostaining in over half of the patients and HBcAg in a minority. The presence of ground-glass hepatocytes (**Ch. 9**) or positive staining of surface material with Victoria blue or orcein indicates chronic disease. Recurrence of HBV infection after liver transplantation is an exception to this rule, both antigens being found in large amounts (**see Ch. 16**). In parenterally transmitted hepatitis, including types B and C, birefringent spicules of talc may be found in portal tracts as a result of intravenous drug abuse.[42]

Following clinical recovery of acute hepatitis B, occult infection and mild histological abnormalities including portal inflammation, focal necrosis, apoptosis and fibrosis may persist for at least a decade.[43]

**Figure 6.15
Hepatitis A.**
In this patient with a clinical picture of fulminant hepatitis, hepatocytes are swollen and microvesicular. There is cholestasis and a lymphocytic infiltrate. (Needle biopsy, H&E.)

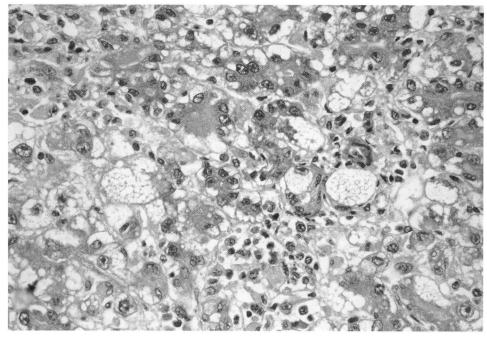

Reactivation of a previously occult or quiescent chronic hepatitis B infection may cause changes closely resembling acute hepatitis. In such instances the presence of: (1) portal tract lymphoid aggregates; (2) significant lymphoplasmacytic interface hepatitis; (3) any evidence of fibrosis on connective tissue stains; and (4) substantial positivity of HBsAg in hepatocytes on immunostaining points to the underlying chronicity of the process.

Hepatitis C

Usually the histological features of hepatitis C are those of any acute hepatitis, but two distinguishing features have been noted. First, there may be prominent infiltration of sinusoids by lymphocytes in the absence of severe liver-cell damage,[44] giving rise to a picture reminiscent of infectious mononucleosis (**Fig. 6.16**). Second, lymphoid follicles and bile-duct damage, features also associated with chronic hepatitis, may be seen within a few weeks or months of onset.[45] There may be cholestasis. The common finding of steatosis in hepatitis C is discussed in **Chapter 9**. Fulminant hepatitis C is very rare in the Western world,[3] but may be commoner in parts of Asia.[46]

Hepatitis D (delta hepatitis)

Co-infection or superinfection with the hepatitis D virus (HDV) alters the course of type B hepatitis. It encourages chronicity and enhances severity,[47–49] except after liver transplantation. The antigen, HDAg, can easily be demonstrated immunohistochemically in paraffin sections and is mainly found in hepatocyte nuclei (**Fig. 6.17**). These may have finely granular eosinophilic centres (so-called 'sanded' nuclei[50]). Cytoplasmic and membrane-associated staining is also sometimes seen.

Severe acute hepatitis in a patient with markers of HBV infection may be due to super-infection by HDV of a chronic HBV carrier.[51] In an outbreak of HDV infection among Venezuelan Indians, notable features included early small-droplet fatty change, sparse lymphocytes and abundant macrophages in the parenchyma and substantial portal

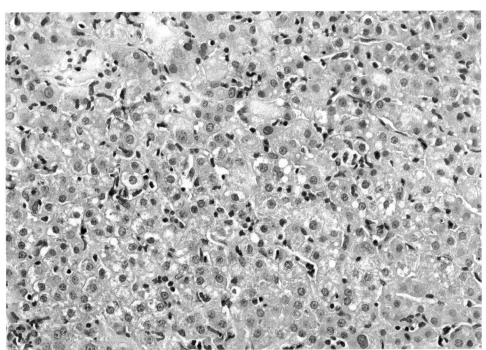

Figure 6.16
Acute hepatitis C.
In this example the main abnormality is infiltration of sinusoids by lymphocytes. (Needle biopsy, H&E.)

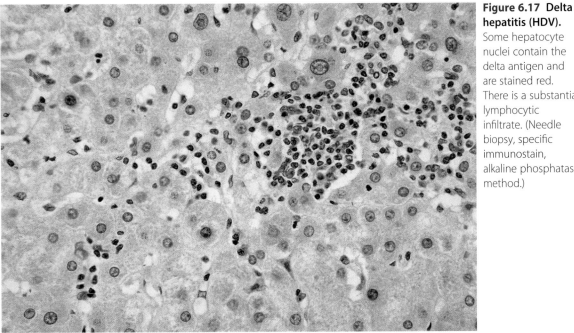

Figure 6.17 Delta hepatitis (HDV).
Some hepatocyte nuclei contain the delta antigen and are stained red. There is a substantial lymphocytic infiltrate. (Needle biopsy, specific immunostain, alkaline phosphatase method.)

infiltration.[52] Later in the attack, there was extensive necrosis and collapse. Microvesicular fatty change and acidophilic necrosis of hepatocytes have been reported from Colombia[53] and North America.[54] In non-immunosuppressed patients with current HDV infection, liver biopsy is likely to show substantial necrosis and inflammation. However, there are HDV-endemic regions where the virus produces little significant disease.[55] Following liver transplantation, on the other hand, HDV without HBV is sometimes demonstrable in the absence of hepatitic changes, indicating that HDV can survive in the absence of HBV. It does not then appear, however, to be capable of causing liver damage.[56]

Hepatitis E

Hepatitis E is the result of enteric infection by an RNA virus with four genotypes that infect humans.[57,58] The disease has caused epidemics in Asia and has also been found in Africa, North and South America and Europe. The epidemics are most often due to oral–faecal transmission of genotypes 1 and 2, which in 2005 resulted in an estimated >3 million symptomatic cases in endemic regions, according to a recent study.[59] Genotype 3, in contrast, infects humans and animals, including pigs, cattle, deer and rodents, and in North America and Europe can cause an acute hepatitis after ingestion of raw or undercooked contaminated meat.[57,60] Acute hepatitis E may also be mistaken as drug-induced liver injury.[61] HEV infection may cause severe decompensation of pre-existing chronic liver disease due to other causes.[62,63] Chronic hepatitis E has been described in organ transplant recipients[57,64–66] (**see Ch. 16**). Recent efforts to produce a vaccine have shown promise.[66a,66b]

There is little detailed information on the pathological changes of hepatitis E virus infection in humans (**Fig. 6.18**). In a small number of patients studied, the appearances were like those of hepatitis A, with prominent cholestasis and a predominantly portal and periportal inflammatory infiltrate.[67] Portal lymphoid aggregates and periportal ductular reaction with neutrophilia at the edges of portal tracts are also described.[60] Histological cholestasis has been described in an elderly patient with a prolonged cholestatic clinical course.[68] The liver of a pregnant woman with fatal hepatitis E showed little portal inflammation, much cholestasis and prominent phlebitis, and virus particles were seen in bile ductules by electron microscopy.[69]

**Figure 6.18
Hepatitis E.**
Hepatocytes are vacuolated and one to the left of centre is greatly enlarged and multinucleated. There is a mixed infiltrate and macrophages contain brown ceroid pigment. (Needle biopsy, H&E.)

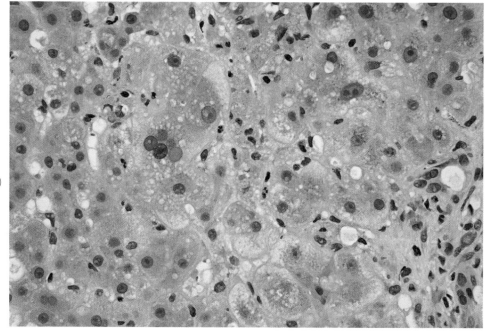

Differential diagnosis of acute viral hepatitis

The distinction of acute hepatitis from bile-duct obstruction rests mainly on the finding of typical hepatitic changes in the parenchyma. The portal tract oedema of duct obstruction is absent. Drug-related hepatitis may be indistinguishable from viral hepatitis and should always be suspected if the cause of the hepatitis is in doubt. Features more common in drug-induced than in viral hepatitis include sharply defined perivenular necrosis, granulomas, bile-duct damage, abundant neutrophils or eosinophils and a poorly developed portal inflammatory reaction. Cholestasis may overshadow the hepatitic features. Autoimmune hepatitis may have a clinically acute onset, histologically indistinguishable from viral hepatitis or alternatively with histological features of chronic disease. This is discussed more fully in **Chapter 9**. In steatohepatitis there is usually conspicuous fatty change. Mallory bodies may be present in ballooned hepatocytes and the infiltrate typically includes neutrophils. The key to the diagnosis is the presence of pericellular fibrosis in affected areas. The differentiation of acute from chronic hepatitis is briefly discussed under bridging necrosis in **Chapter 4**. While the parenchymal changes predominate in acute hepatitis, especially in perivenular areas, portal and periportal changes predominate in chronic disease. The distinction is sometimes difficult to make, especially when extensive lobular changes are found during an exacerbation of chronic hepatitis or in reactivated chronic hepatitis B, as described earlier.

Fate and morphological sequelae of acute viral hepatitis

Resolution

As far as can be deduced from the available evidence, most examples of hepatitis A, B and E are followed by complete or near-complete resolution and a return of the liver to normal. A chronic course is probably more common when hepatitis B is complicated by delta infection than otherwise, and in hepatitis C the risk of chronicity is high. Even in patients whose hepatitis resolves, some residual changes may persist for many months after clinical recovery (**Figs 6.19, 6.20**).

Scarring

Localised collapse, scarring and regeneration following severe hepatitis with bridging or panlobular necrosis sometimes produce a histological picture indistinguishable from cirrhosis.

Fatal outcome or need for liver transplantation

Necrosis is usually severe. Regenerative hyperplasia of surviving hepatocytes or progenitor cells may be seen.

Chronic hepatitis

Most individuals with hepatitis C virus infection develop chronic hepatitis. This has substantial impact on daily liver biopsy practice. Chronic hepatitis also develops in many patients with hepatitis B.

Figure 6.19 Acute viral hepatitis: residual changes. Short septa extend from the mildly inflamed portal tract to the left. Minimal inflammation and irregular liver-cell plates are seen around the efferent venule below right. (Needle biopsy, H&E.)

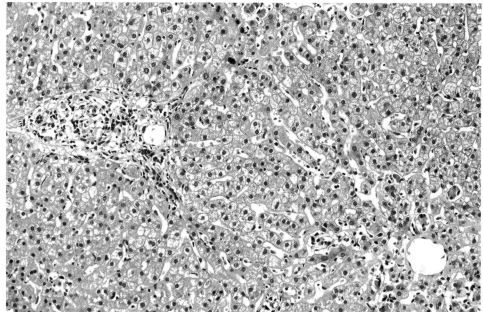

Figure 6.20 Acute viral hepatitis: residual changes. Slender septa link portal tracts (left and right), but the perivenular area (centre) is unaffected and architectural relationships are preserved. (Needle biopsy, reticulin.)

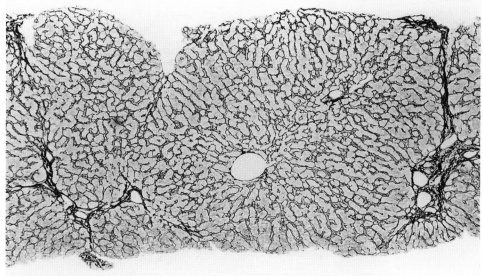

Cirrhosis

Cirrhosis resulting from infection with a hepatitis virus almost always follows a period of chronic hepatitis, with repeated or continuous hepatocellular necrosis and regeneration. Occasionally it may follow directly after a single episode of severe acute hepatitis.

Hepatocellular carcinoma

This may develop on the basis of cirrhosis in patients infected with HBV or hepatitis C virus. Occasionally, however, hepatocellular carcinoma is found in the absence of cirrhosis, usually after a prolonged period of chronic liver disease.[70]

References

1 Ben-Ari Z, Samuel D, Zemel R, et al. Fulminant non-A-G viral hepatitis leading to liver transplantation. Arch Intern Med 2000;160:388–92.

2 Petrovic LM, Arkadopoulos N, Demetriou AA. Activation of hepatic stellate cells in liver tissue of patients with fulminant liver failure after treatment with bioartificial liver. Hum Pathol 2001;32:1371–5.

3 Schiødt FV, Davern TJ, Shakil AO, et al. Viral hepatitis-related acute liver failure. Am J Gastroenterol 2003;98:448–53.

4 Kirsch R, Yap J, Roberts EA, et al. Clinicopathologic spectrum of massive and submassive hepatic necrosis in infants and children. Hum Pathol 2009;40:516–26.

5 Peters DJ, Greene WH, Ruggiero F, et al. Herpes simplex-induced fulminant hepatitis in adults: a call for empiric therapy. Dig Dis Sci 2000;45:2399–404.

6 Pinna AD, Rakela J, Demetris AJ, et al. Five cases of fulminant hepatitis due to herpes simplex virus in adults. Dig Dis Sci 2002;47:750–4.

7 Collin L, Moulin P, Jungers M, et al. Epstein–Barr virus (EBV)-induced liver failure in the absence of extensive liver-cell necrosis: a case for cytokine-induced liver dysfunction? J Hepatol 2004;41:174–5.

8 Wang WH, Wang HL. Fulminant adenovirus hepatitis following bone marrow transplantation. A case report and brief review of the literature. Arch Pathol Lab Med 2003;127:e246–8.

9 Longerich T, Haferkamp K, Tox U, et al. Acute liver failure in a renal transplant patient caused by adenoviral hepatitis superimposed on a fibrosing cholestatic hepatitis B. Hum Pathol 2004;35:894–7.

10 Chau TN, Lee KC, Yao H, et al. SARS-associated viral hepatitis caused by a novel coronavirus: report of three cases. Hepatology 2004;39:302–10.

11 Ng W-F, To K-F, Lam WWL, et al. The comparative pathology of severe acute respiratory syndrome and avian influenza A subtype H5N1: a review. Hum Pathol 2006;37:381–90.

12 Polakos NK, Cornejo JC, Murray DA, et al. Kupfer cell-dependent hepatitis occurs during influenza infection. Am J Pathol 2006;168:1169–78.

13 Adams DH, Hubscher SG. Systemic viral infections and collateral damage in the liver. Am J Pathol 2006;168:1057–9.

14 Lau JYN, Xie X, Lai MMC, et al. Apoptosis and viral hepatitis. Semin Liver Dis 1998;18:169–76.

15 Klotz O, Belt TH. The pathology of the liver in yellow fever. Am J Pathol 1930;6:663–89.

16 Dias LB Jr, Alves VAF, Kanamura C, et al. Fulminant hepatic failure in northern Brazil: morphological, immunohistochemical and pathogenic aspects of Lábrea hepatitis and yellow fever. Trans Roy Soc Trop Med Hyg 2007;101:831–9.

17 Phillips MJ, Blendis LM, Poucell S, et al. Syncytial giant-cell hepatitis. Sporadic hepatitis with distinctive pathological features, a severe clinical course and paramyxoviral features. N Engl J Med 1991;324:455–60.

18 Fimmel CJ, Guo L, Compans RW, et al. A case of syncytial giant cell hepatitis with features of a paramyxoviral infection. Am J Gastroenterol 1998;93:1931–7.

19 Devaney K, Goodman ZD, Ishak KG. Postinfantile giant-cell transformation in hepatitis. Hepatology 1992;16:327–33.

20 Lau JYN, Koukoulis G, Mieli-Vergani G, et al. Syncytial giant-cell hepatitis – a specific disease entity? J Hepatol 1992;15:216–19.

21 Protzer U, Dienes HP, Bianchi L, et al. Post-infantile giant cell hepatitis in patients with primary sclerosing cholangitis and autoimmune hepatitis. Liver 1996;16:274–82.

22 Ben-Ari Z, Broida E, Monselise Y, et al. Syncytial giant-cell hepatitis due to autoimmune hepatitis type II (LKM1+) presenting as subfulminant hepatitis. Am J Gastroenterol 2000;95:799–801.

23 Micchelli STL, Thomas D, Boitnott JK, et al. Hepatic giant cells in hepatitis C virus (HCV) mono-infection and HCV/HIV co-infection. J Clin Pathol 2008;61:1058–61.

24 Sciot R, Van Damme B, Desmet VJ. Cholestatic features in hepatitis A. J Hepatol 1986;3:172–81.

25 Volpes R, van den Oord JJ, Desmet VJ. Memory T cells represent the predominant lymphocyte subset in acute and chronic liver inflammation. Hepatology 1991;13:826–9.

26 Mietkiewski JM, Scheuer PJ. Immunoglobulin-containing plasma cells in acute hepatitis. Liver 1985;5:84–8.

27 Bardadin KA, Scheuer PJ. Endothelial cell changes in acute hepatitis. A light and electron microscopic study. J Pathol 1984;144:213–20.

28 Scheuer PJ, Maggi G. Hepatic fibrosis and collapse: histological distinction by orcein staining. Histopathology 1980;4:487–90.

29 Thung SN, Gerber MA. The formation of elastic fibers in livers with massive hepatic necrosis. Arch Pathol Lab Med 1982;106:468–9.

30 Hanau C, Munoz SJ, Rubin R. Histopathological heterogeneity in fulminant hepatic failure. Hepatology 1995;21:345–51.

31 Demetris AJ, Seaberg EC, Wennerberg A, et al. Ductular reaction after submassive necrosis in humans. Special emphasis on analysis of ductular hepatocytes. Am J Pathol 1996;149:439–48.

32 Roskams T, De Vos R, van Eyken P, et al. Hepatic OV-6 expression in human liver disease and rat experiments: evidence for hepatic progenitor cells in man. J Hepatol 1998;29:455–63.

33 Zhang L, Theise N, Chua M, et al. The stem cell niche of human livers: symmetry between development and regeneration. Hepatology 2008;48:1598–607.

34 Ellis AJ, Saleh M, Smith H, et al. Late-onset hepatic failure: clinical features, serology and outcome following transplantation. J Hepatol 1995;23:363–72.

35 Teixeira MR Jr, Weller IVD, Murray AM, et al. The pathology of hepatitis A in man. Liver 1982;2:53–60.

36 Abe H, Beninger PR, Ikejiri N, et al. Light microscopic findings of liver biopsy specimens from patients with hepatitis type A and comparison with type B. Gastroenterology 1982;82:938–47.

37 Okuno T, Sano A, Deguchi T, et al. Pathology of acute hepatitis A in humans. Comparison with acute hepatitis B. Am J Clin Pathol 1984;81:162–9.

38 Ponz E, Garcia-Pagan JC, Bruguera M, et al. Hepatic fibrin-ring granulomas in a patient with hepatitis A. Gastroenterology 1991;100:268–70.

39 Ruel M, Sevestre H, Henry-Biabaud E, et al. Fibrin ring granulomas in hepatitis A. Dig Dis Sci 1992;37:1915–17.

40 Inoue K, Yoshiba M, Yotsuyanagi H, et al. Chronic hepatitis A with persistent viral replication. J Med Virol 1996;50:322–4.

41 Chu CW, Hwang SJ, Luo JC, et al. Comparison of clinical, virologic and pathologic features in patients with acute hepatitis B and C. J Gastroenterol Hepatol 2001;16:209–14.

42 Uchida T, Shimojima S, Gotoh K, et al. Pathology of livers infected with 'silent' hepatitis B virus mutant. Liver 1994;14:251–6.

43 Yuki N, Nagaoka T, Yamashiro M, et al. Long-term histologic and virologic outcomes of acute self-limited hepatitis B. Hepatology 2003;37:1172–9.

44 Bamber M, Murray A, Arborgh BA, et al. Short incubation non-A, non-B hepatitis transmitted by factor VIII concentrates in patients with congenital coagulation disorders. Gut 1981;22:854–9.

45 Kobayashi K, Hashimoto E, Ludwig J, et al. Liver biopsy features of acute hepatitis C compared with hepatitis A, B and non-A, non-B, non-C. Liver 1993;13:69–73.

46 Chu CM, Sheen IS, Liaw YF. The role of hepatitis C virus in fulminant viral hepatitis in an area with endemic hepatitis A and B. Gastroenterology 1994;107:189–95.

47 Govindarajan S, De-Cock KM, Redeker AG. Natural course of delta superinfection in chronic hepatitis B virus-infected patients: histopathologic study with multiple liver biopsies. Hepatology 1986;6:640–4.

48 Verme G, Amoroso P, Lettieri G, et al. A histological study of hepatitis delta virus liver disease. Hepatology 1986;6:1303–7.

49 Lin H-H, Liaw Y-F, Chen T-J, et al. Natural course of patients with chronic type B hepatitis following acute hepatitis delta virus superinfection. Liver 1989;9:129–34.

50 Moreno A, Ramón Y, Cahal S, et al. Sanded nuclei in delta patients. Liver 1989;9:367–71.

51 Smedile A, Farci P, Verme G, et al. Influence of delta infection on severity of hepatitis B. Lancet 1982;ii:945–7.

52 Popper H, Thung SN, Gerber MA, et al. Histologic studies of severe delta agent infection in Venezuelan Indians. Hepatology 1983;3:906–12.

53 Buitrago B, Popper H, Hadler SC, et al. Specific histologic features of Santa Marta hepatitis: a severe form of hepatitis delta-virus infection in northern South America. Hepatology 1986;6:1285–91.

54 Lefkowitch JH, Goldstein H, Yatto R, et al. Cytopathic liver injury in acute delta virus hepatitis. Gastroenterology 1987;92:1262–6.

55 Rizzetto M. Hepatitis D: thirty years after. J Hepatol 2009;50:1043–50.

56 Davies SE, Lau JYN, O'Grady JG, et al. Evidence that hepatitis D virus needs hepatitis B virus to cause hepatocellular damage. Am J Clin Pathol 1992;98:554–8.

57 Wedemeyer H, Pischke S, Manns MP. Pathogenesis and treatment of hepatitis E virus infection. Gastroenterology 2012;142:1388–97.

58 Purcell RH, Emerson SU. Hepatitis E: an emerging awareness of an old disease. J Hepatol 2008;48:494–503.

59 Rein DB, Stevens GA, Theaker J, et al. The global burden of hepatitis E virus genotypes 1 and 2 in 2005. Hepatology 2012;55:988–97.

60 Malcolm P, Dalton H, Hussaini HS, et al. The histology of acute autochthonous hepatitis E virus infection. Histopathology 2007;51:190–4.

61 Chen EY, Baum K, Collins W, et al. Hepatitis E masquerading as drug-induced liver injury. Hepatology 2012;56:2420–3.

62 Hamid SS, Atiq M, Shehzad F, et al. Hepatitis E virus superinfection in patients with chronic liver disease. Hepatology 2002;36:474–8.

63 Ramachandran J, Eapen CE, Kang G, et al. Hepatitis E superinfection produces severe decompensation in patients with chronic liver disease. J Gastroenterol Hepatol 2004;19:134–8.

64 Kamar N, Selves J, Mansuy J-M, et al. Hepatitis E virus and chronic hepatitis in organ-transplant recipients. N Engl J Med 2008;358:811–17.

65 Kamar N, Mansuy J-M, Cointault O, et al. Hepatitis E virus-related cirrhosis in kidney- and kidney–pancreas-transplant recipients. Am J Transplant 2008;8:1744–8.

66 Aggarwal R. Hepatitis E: does it cause chronic hepatitis? Hepatology 2008;48:1328–30.

66a Zhang J, Zhang X-F, Huang S-J, et al. Long-term efficacy of a hepatitis E vaccine. N Engl J Med 2015;372:914–22.

66b Teshale E, Ward JW. Making hepatitis E a vaccine-preventible disease. N Engl J Med 2015;372:899–901.

67 Dienes HP, Hütteroth T, Bianchi L, et al. Hepatitis A-like non-A, non-B hepatitis: light and electron microscopic observations of three cases. Virchows Arch [A] 1986;409:657–67.

68 Mechnik L, Bergman N, Attali M, et al. Acute hepatitis E virus infection presenting as a prolonged cholestatic jaundice. J Clin Gastroenterol 2001;33:421–2.

69 Asher LVS, Innis BL, Shrestha MP, et al. Virus-like particles in the liver of a patient with fulminant hepatitis and antibody to hepatitis E virus. J Med Virol 1990;31:229–33.

70 Grando-Lemaire V, Guettier C, Chevret S, et al. Hepatocellular carcinoma without cirrhosis in the West: epidemiological factors and histopathology of the non-tumorous liver. Groupe d'Etude et de Traitement du Carcinome Hepatocellulaire. J Hepatol 1999;31:508–13.

General reading

Aggarwal R, Krawczynski K, Hepatitis E. An overview and recent advances in clinical and laboratory research. J Gastroenterol Hepatol 2000;15:9–20.

Jaeschke H, Gujral J, Bajt M. Apoptosis and necrosis in liver disease. Liver Int 2004;24:85–9.

Lavanchy D. Hepatitis B virus epidemiology, disease burden, treatment and current and emerging prevention and control measures. J Viral Hepat 2004;11:97–107.

Penin F, Dubuisson J, Rey FA, et al. Structural biology of hepatitis C virus. Hepatology 2004;39:5–19.

Purcell RH, Emerson SU. Hepatitis E: an emerging awareness of an old disease. J Hepatol 2008;48:494–503.

Schmid R. History of viral hepatitis: a tale of dogmas and misinterpretations. J Gastroenterol Hepatol 2001;16:718–22.

Theise ND, Bodenheimer HC, Ferrell LD Jr. Acute and chronic viral hepatitis. In: Burt AD, Portmann BC, Ferrell LD, editors. MacSween's Pathology of the Liver. 5th ed. Edinburgh: Churchill Livingstone/Elsevier; 2007. p. 399–442.

Steatosis, Steatohepatitis and Related Conditions

Steatosis

Steatosis (fatty change, fatty liver) is the accumulation of abnormal amounts of lipid in hepatocytes. Most steatosis is of the macrovesicular type, in which a single large fat vacuole or several smaller ones occupy the greater part of the cell, pushing the nucleus to the periphery (**Fig. 7.1**). The less common and often more serious type is microvesicular steatosis (**Fig. 7.2**). The fat in this type is finely divided and the nucleus remains central. The two types of steatosis are sometimes found together, though one type usually predominates.

Macrovesicular steatosis

Macrovesicular steatosis is common. It is frequently apparent by non-invasive imaging and may be accompanied by moderate abnormalities of serum aminotransferases, alkaline phosphatase and γ-glutamyl transpeptidase. Liver tests may be normal.[1] There are many causes of macrovesicular steatosis, of which the most common are listed in **Box 7.1**. It is usually not possible to determine the cause of uncomplicated large-droplet steatosis from histological examination alone.

The lipid in macrovesicular steatosis accumulates in hepatocytes because of increased triglyceride synthesis or decreased excretion.[2] Increased synthesis results from availability of excess free fatty acids and fatty acid precursors and from reduced fatty acid oxidation. Reduced excretion is a result of diminished apoprotein production, seen for example in protein malnutrition and alcohol abuse. Macrovesicular steatosis provides the background on which the important lesions of alcoholic and non-alcoholic steatohepatitis develop.[3] Moreover, macrovesicular steatosis is increasingly being recognised as a significant risk factor for hepatocellular carcinoma, even without preceding fibrosis or cirrhosis, particularly when widely prevalent risk factors for metabolic syndrome such as obesity and diabetes are present.[4-9] Most steatosis is **perivenular** (centrilobular regions/acinar zones 3). Alcohol use, adult obesity, diabetes and corticosteroid therapy typically show this location. Increasing amounts of steatosis extend to progressively involve mid-zonal and periportal regions

Box 7.1 Common causes of macrovesicular steatosis
Obesity and diabetes mellitus
Protein-calorie malnutrition
Total parenteral nutrition
Drugs and toxins (e.g. alcohol, corticosteroids)
Metabolic disorders (e.g. Wilson's disease)
Infections (e.g. hepatitis C)

**Figure 7.1
Macrovesicular
steatosis.**
There are large fat
vacuoles in
perivenular
hepatocytes,
displacing the nuclei
to the edges of the
cells. (Needle biopsy,
H&E.)

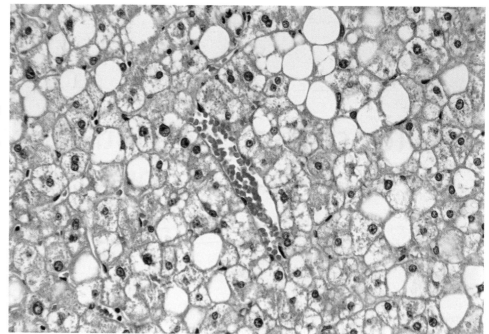

**Figure 7.2
Microvesicular
steatosis.**
Swollen hepatocytes
near an efferent
venule (right)
contain numerous
small vacuoles.
The nuclei have
maintained their
central position.
Some large fat
vacuoles are also
present. (Needle
biopsy, H&E.)

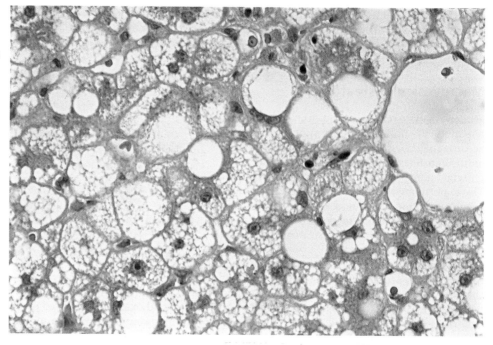

(acinar zones 2 and 1, respectively). With increasing amounts of macrovesicular fat there sometimes are interspersed clusters or patches of hepatocytes with microvesicular steatosis,[10] probably reflecting the evolution of large lipid vacuoles from progressive coalescence of small lipid droplets.[11,12] In contrast, **periportal steatosis** is more common in children with non-alcoholic fatty liver disease (discussed later), in patients on parenteral nutrition,

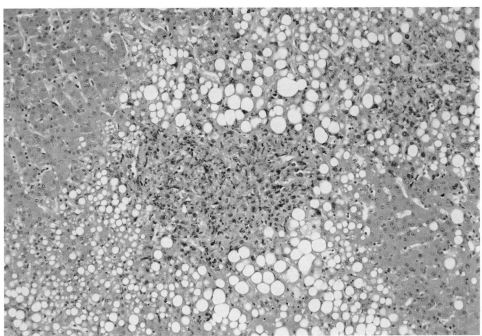

Figure 7.3
Periportal steatosis.
Liver biopsy from a patient with acquired immunodeficiency syndrome (AIDS) and portal tract infiltration by large-cell lymphoma. Periportal hepatocytes contain large fat vacuoles. (Needle biopsy, H&E.)

in kwashiorkor and protein-calorie malnutrition, and it is sometimes seen in acquired immunodeficiency syndrome (AIDS) (**Fig. 7.3**). In **focal fatty change**[13] more or less rounded foci of steatosis are seen in an otherwise normal liver and may be mistaken for neoplasms on imaging.

The histological **grade** of steatosis should be reported based on the percentage of hepatocytes which contain lipid vacuoles. One commonly used scoring system includes grades of minimal (<5%), mild (5–30%), moderate (30–60%) and marked (>60%). Provision of a numerical assessment to the nearest percentile is also recommended (e.g. 'marked macrovesicular steatosis is present involving approximately 90% of the parenchyma'). Periodic acid–Schiff and trichrome stains can be helpful in the assessment, providing contrast of the large lipid vacuoles against the more darkly stained background cytoplasm of hepatocytes. Digitised computer image analysis[14,15] is an alternative method of grading but from a practical standpoint is better suited to research settings.[16]

Occasionally lipid-laden hepatocytes rupture and the fat is then taken up by macrophages. The resulting lesion is a **lipogranuloma** (**Fig. 7.4**). Lipogranulomas are situated within the lobules, often near terminal venules. Serial sectioning may be needed to identify the fat in the centre of the lesion. Lipogranulomas may undergo fibrosis, but this does not appear to contribute to progressive liver disease and must be distinguished from the more important pericellular fibrosis characteristic of steatohepatitis (see below). Globules within portal tracts are usually the result of uptake of ingested or injected mineral oils by macrophages, rather than uptake of lipids[17] (**Fig. 7.5**). **Lipopeliosis** – the formation of large intrasinusoidal fat cysts following release of lipid from hepatocytes after transplantation – is described in **Chapter 16**.

The differential diagnosis of macrovesicular steatosis includes microvesicular steatosis. The presence of several fat vacuoles in one hepatocyte has to be distinguished from true microvesicular steatosis (below) in which vacuoles are generally less than 1 μm in diameter and may even be invisible in paraffin sections by light microscopy. The distinction is clinically important. The location of the nucleus helps to differentiate the two conditions. A

**Figure 7.4
Lipogranuloma.**
A lipogranuloma has formed near the terminal venule (V) in this moderately steatotic liver. Inset: The lipogranuloma contains large lipid vacuoles and aggregated Kupffer cells with scattered lymphocytes and a few eosinophils. (Needle biopsy, H&E.)

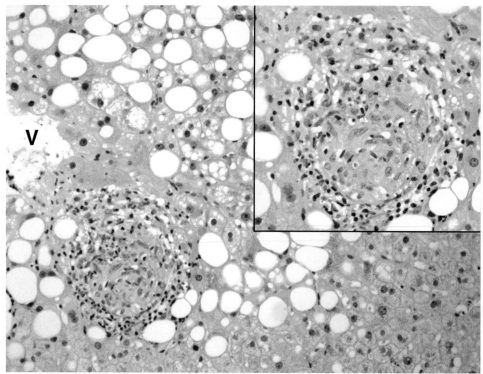

**Figure 7.5
Mineral oil globules.**
A row of vacuoles within macrophages is seen to the right of a portal venule. (Needle biopsy, H&E.)

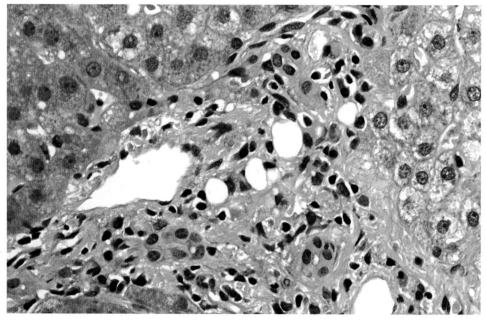

second differential diagnosis is from **stellate-cell hyperplasia (Fig. 7.6)**, in which the vacuoles are not in hepatocytes but in perisinusoidally located stellate cells.[18] Their nuclei are compressed into a crescentic shape by the vitamin A-rich globules. Stellate-cell hyperplasia may be unexplained, but should lead to investigation of possible overuse of vitamin A or other retinoids.

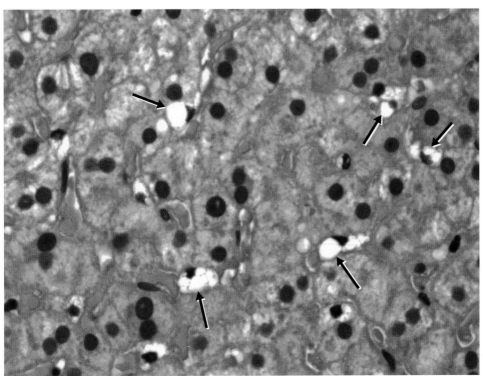

Figure 7.6 *HSC*
Stellate-cell hyperplasia. Stellate cells with single or multiple lipid vacuoles lie in the space of Disse between hepatocytes (arrows). Stellate-cell nuclei are small, intensely basophilic and indented by the cytoplasmic vacuoles. Hepatocyte nuclei are larger, less dense and rounded. (Needle biopsy, H&E.)

Microvesicular steatosis

In this serious and sometimes fatal condition, finely divided fat accumulates in hepatocyte cytoplasm as a result of mitochondrial damage leading to impaired β-oxidation.[19] Causes include acute fatty liver of pregnancy (**see Ch. 15**), hepatotoxic drugs such as valproate and nucleoside analogues (**see Ch. 8**), mitochondrial DNA depletion and deletion syndromes,[20] foamy degeneration in the alcoholic (see below) and total parenteral nutrition (**Box 7.2**). Another cause, Reye's syndrome, has declined sharply in incidence in recent years. In neonates and children, mitochondrial hepatopathies may need consideration.[20–22] Viral infections occasionally give rise to similar changes.[23]

Box 7.2 Main causes of microvesicular steatosis
Acute fatty liver of pregnancy
Alcoholic foamy degeneration
Drugs (e.g. nucleoside analogues, valproate)
Toxins (e.g. in Jamaican vomiting disease)
Total parenteral nutrition
Inborn errors of metabolism (e.g. urea cycle disorders)
Reye's syndrome
Infections

Histologically, the cytoplasmic lipid is seen to be very finely divided and is not always obvious in paraffin sections. It can be stained with oil red O in frozen sections. The affected hepatocytes are often swollen. Their nuclei remain central (**Fig. 7.2**).

The differential diagnosis is from macrovesicular steatosis and from conditions in which hepatocytes are swollen for other reasons, such as hepatitis. As discussed in **Chapter 13**, phospholipids and sphingolipids accumulate in various metabolic disorders. Cholesterol esters accumulate in hepatocytes in Wolman's disease and cholesterol ester storage disease, and glycogen accumulates in glycogen storage disease and diabetics with glycogenic hepatopathy (discussed later).

It bears noting that the terms 'macrovesicular steatosis' and 'microvesicular steatosis' are preferable for use (in lieu of the colloquial 'macrosteatosis' and 'microsteatosis').

Alcoholic and non-alcoholic fatty liver disease

The terms **alcoholic fatty liver disease** (AFLD) and **non-alcoholic fatty liver disease** (NAFLD) are used to describe the complete range of changes from uncomplicated macrovesicular steatosis to steatohepatitis and cirrhosis seen, respectively, in alcohol abuse and in obesity, diabetes, hyperlipidaemia and the metabolic syndrome. Insulin resistance, central (truncal) obesity, type 2 diabetes, hyperlipidaemia and systemic hypertension constitute the *metabolic syndrome*. NAFLD is considered the hepatic expression of the metabolic syndrome.[24,25] The wide prevalence of obesity and diabetes in industrialised countries and in other populations has brought NAFLD to increased attention in clinical and basic science. In the United States, NAFLD is currently the leading cause of abnormal serum aminotransferases and chronic liver disease.[26,27] A similar impact is likely in other Western countries and in other populations where the risk factors for NAFLD are prevalent. Emphasis on the histological evaluation of macrovesicular steatosis and related changes in liver biopsy, explant and postmortem specimens has consequently grown.

Systematic histological approach to macrovesicular fatty liver disease

Histological evaluation in AFLD and NAFLD should take into account not only the presence of large-droplet steatosis, but also evidence of hepatocellular damage, inflammation, fibrosis and siderosis which may also be present. The diagnosis of steatohepatitis should be rendered based on specific histological criteria (described in detail below). In AFLD and NAFLD there may be relatively inconspicuous *apoptotic bodies*.[28–30] *Focal lobular inflammation* (usually clusters of lymphocytes and activated Kupffer cells) may be seen (**Fig. 7.7**) but does not constitute steatohepatitis. *Hepatocyte ballooning, on the other hand, is a major feature of both early and of well-developed steatohepatitis* (**Figs 7.8** and **7.9**), for which careful inspection is warranted. Ballooned hepatocytes are often identifiable even at low magnification (**Fig. 7.8**). They show watery and oedematous, wispy, rarefied cytoplasm (**Fig. 7.9**). A variety of factors cause this type of ballooning, including perturbed metabolic pathways,[31] cytoskeletal damage[32] (particularly of keratins 8 and 18) and endoplasmic reticulum stress.[33] These ballooned hepatocytes appear to be moribund but yet 'undead', still capable of producing a variety of factors such as Sonic hedgehog which exerts both paracrine and autocrine effects.[33a,33b] Combination immunostaining for cytokeratins 8 and 18 (CK8/18) helps to demonstrate affected cells which show either absent or decreased cytoplasmic staining[32,34] (**Fig. 7.9, inset**). The most fully developed histopathological picture of steatohepatitis (**Fig. 7.10**) includes macrovesicular steatosis, hepatocyte ballooning, inflammation, intracellular Mallory–Denk bodies and perivenular fibrosis (discussed in detail below).

Uncomplicated steatosis in the majority of cases is not associated with significant portal tract inflammation. However, focal *minimal or mild portal lymphocytic infiltrates* are sometimes present in either steatosis or steatohepatitis.[35,36] More active cases of non-alcoholic steatohepatitis with advanced fibrosis sometimes present diagnostic difficulties because of substantial chronic portal inflammation (including lymphoid aggregates), which may raise the possibility of chronic hepatitis as an alternative diagnosis.[36] Any histological doubt on this issue should be resolved by discussion with the clinician and investigations to exclude causes of chronic hepatitis when necessary. Some adult and paediatric patients with NAFLD show positive serum *antinuclear and/or anti-smooth-muscle antibodies*,[37–39] raising a clinical suspicion of autoimmune hepatitis (AIH). However, these

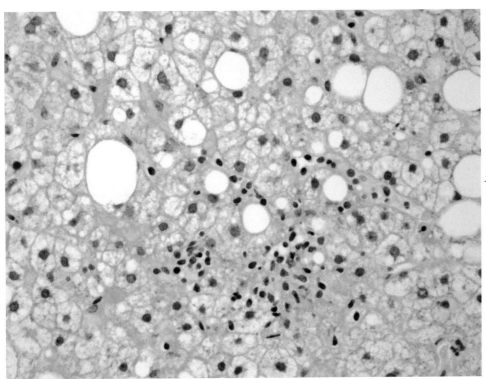

Figure 7.7
Macrovesicular steatosis with focal inflammation.
Scattered lymphocytes are present in this mildly fatty liver. This type of inflammation is relatively common, but does not constitute steatohepatitis. (Needle biopsy, H&E).

autoantibodies are usually low-titre and are considered non-specific. The characteristic portal lymphoplasmacytic inflammation, interface hepatitis and regenerative rosettes of AIH are typically absent in the majority of such cases. Rarely, antimitochondrial antibody may be positive.[40,41]

A connective tissue stain is important to evaluate the extent of any fibrosis and its distribution in the steatotic liver. When there is fibrosis in AFLD and NAFLD, it is usually present as a feature of steatohepatitis and is seen in centrilobular regions (acinar zone 3), as described below. Alternatively (and less frequently), there may be portal and periportal fibrosis accompanied by chronic inflammation (**Fig. 7.11**). This distribution is more common in paediatric NAFLD[42] and in morbidly obese individuals.[43–45]

An iron stain should also be reviewed for *siderosis*. Mild iron overload in Kupffer cells and/or hepatocytes may be seen in alcoholic patients because of altered intestinal iron absorption and in up to one-third of individuals with NAFLD due to **dysmetabolic iron overload syndrome (DIOS)**[46–51] (**Fig. 7.12**). Iron overload in this setting increases oxidative stress and hepatocyte apoptosis.[52] Significant hepatocellular siderosis should always prompt consideration of possible primary (genetic) iron overload.

Several systems exist to assess steatosis, inflammation and hepatocellular damage in NAFLD.[53–55] Matteoni and colleagues[54] characterised the spectrum of NAFLD according to four subtypes: NAFLD subtype 1 (simple steatosis); NAFLD subtype 2 (steatosis with inflammation); NAFLD subtype 3 (steatosis with hepatocellular ballooning degeneration – **Fig. 7.8**); and NAFLD subtype 4 (non-alcoholic steatohepatitis or NASH) (**Fig. 7.10**). (Subtypes 3 and 4 are now both considered NASH.)[53] Increased morbidity and mortality were associated with types 3 and 4. The NAFLD activity score[55] evaluates the unweighted sum of steatosis (scored 0–3), lobular inflammation (scored 0–2) and hepatocellular ballooning (scored 0–2) in order to determine the presence of NASH (values ≥5 are considered NASH, and <3 'not NASH'). A grading and staging system for NASH activity and fibrosis, respectively, is discussed later in the chapter (**see Table 7.1**). Similar scoring

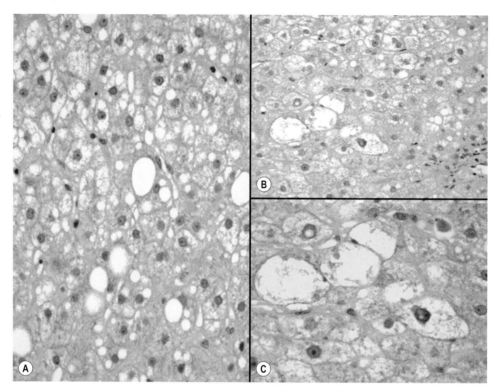

Figure 7.8 Hepatocyte ballooning in macrovesicular fatty liver disease.
A: This liver shows minimal steatosis but no hepatocyte ballooning. Note the uniform size of hepatocytes in this panel, some of which (at upper left) show pale, glycogen-containing cytoplasm, but no evidence of ballooning. **B:** A cluster of ballooned hepatocytes is evident at relatively low magnification. **C:** Ballooned hepatocytes are enlarged and show oedematous, wispy and rarefied cytoplasm. Ballooning of this type reflects significant hepatocellular damage, which is an important component of steatohepatitis, and the specimen should be examined carefully for frank steatohepatitis elsewhere. (Needle biopsy, H&E.)

systems have not been available for AFLD, although a recently proposed system utilises histological features (degree of fibrosis, degree of neutrophil infiltrates, type of cholestasis and presence of megamitochondria) to predict 90-day mortality.[56] Ultimately, the choice and use of a scoring system vary among pathologists and institutions and the system(s) used may be selected for specific clinical and research needs. At minimum, though, the pathologist needs to be able to determine when steatohepatitis is present and what degree of fibrosis, if any, has developed, since these features have impact on therapy and prognosis.[57]

Diabetes mellitus

In patients with diabetes mellitus, glycogen vacuolation of hepatocyte nuclei is common[58] (**Fig. 7.13**). These 'glycogen nuclei' are also seen in Wilson's disease (**see Ch. 14**), in non-alcoholic steatohepatitis and in biopsies from children and adolescents less than 14–15 years of age. Hepatomegaly in diabetics is not always attributable to steatosis: rarely, diabetics who are poorly controlled may develop Mauriac's syndrome,[58a] with abnormal serum liver tests and massive accumulation of glycogen in hepatocytes (**glycogenic**

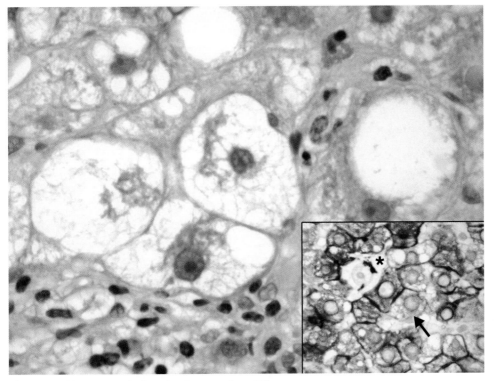

Figure 7.9 Hepatocyte ballooning in steatohepatitis.
The three conspicuously ballooned hepatocytes at the centre of this field have an oedematous, wispy and rarefied cytoplasm as well as clumped eosinophilic filamentous material (Mallory–Denk bodies). (Needle biopsy, H&E.) Inset: Combined immunohistochemical stain for cytokeratins 8 and 18 shows absent keratins in several hepatocytes at centre (arrow), one of which (*) contains several darkly stained Mallory–Denk bodies near the nucleus. (Needle biopsy, H&E. Inset: specific immunohistochemistry.)

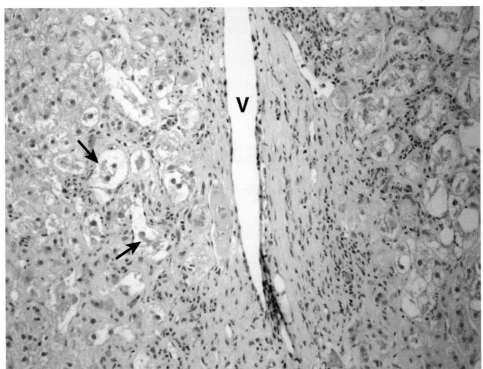

Figure 7.10 Non-alcoholic steatohepatitis (NASH).
The terminal venule (V) is surrounded by fibrosis and inflammation. Perivenular hepatocytes are swollen and show cytoplasmic Mallory–Denk bodies (arrows). (Needle biopsy, H&E.)

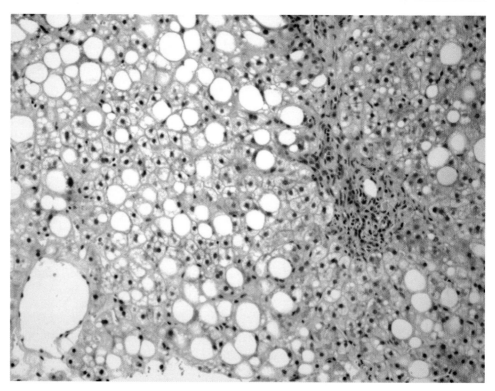

Figure 7.11
Steatosis with mild periportal fibrosis and chronic inflammation (non-alcoholic steatohepatitis (NASH) type 2).
This biopsy from an obese child shows large-droplet steatosis with mild periportal fibrosis and chronic inflammation (at right). This pattern in children with non-alcoholic fatty liver disease is referred to as NASH type 2. Note the absence of liver-cell ballooning, Mallory–Denk bodies, inflammation or fibrosis near the terminal venule at lower left. (Needle biopsy, H&E.)

hepatopathy[59]), giving rise to a picture closely resembling inherited glycogen storage disease (**Fig. 7.14**). Some diabetics with **diabetic hepatosclerosis**[60] (**Fig. 7.15**) show an increase in perisinusoidal type IV collagen[61] without a zonal predilection.

Steatohepatitis, alcoholic and non-alcoholic

In some patients with steatosis an inflammatory and fibrosing lesion, steatohepatitis, develops. This may then lead to cirrhosis. Some patients later develop hepatocellular carcinoma. Most patients with steatohepatitis are alcohol abusers or are overweight, diabetic or have a combination of attributes of the metabolic syndrome. The terms alcoholic steatohepatitis (ASH) and non-alcoholic steatohepatitis (NASH) are used accordingly. In a minority of patients NASH is associated with other factors, listed later in this chapter. The risk of developing steatohepatitis and cirrhosis in the alcoholic rises with the amount of alcohol consumed daily,[62] but genetic and other factors are also influential. Although simple steatosis in individuals with NAFLD has previously been considered a clinically benign and non-progressive condition, recent studies indicate the potential over time for progression to steatohepatitis, cirrhosis and hepatocellular carcinoma.[4–6]

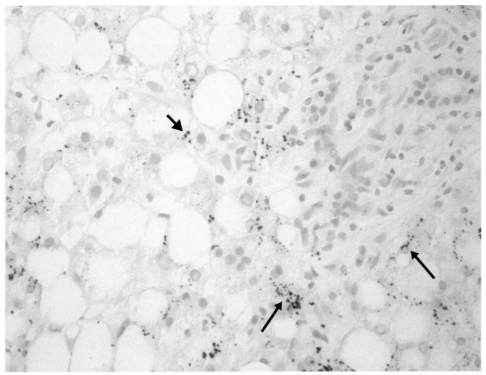

Figure 7.12 Dysmetabolic iron overload syndrome (DIOS).
This case of non-alcoholic fatty liver disease with marked steatosis is associated with mild siderosis of periportal hepatocytes (long arrows) and sinusoidal Kupffer cells (short arrow). (Needle biopsy, Prussian blue iron stain.)

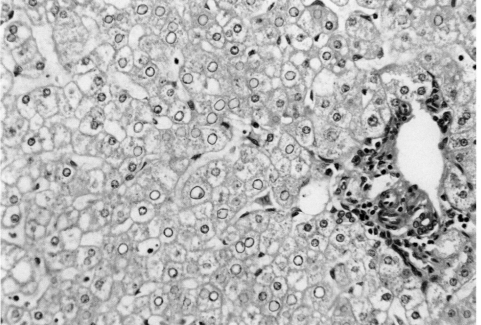

Figure 7.13 Diabetes mellitus. Glycogen vacuolation is seen in the nuclei of most periportal hepatocytes. (Needle biopsy, H&E.)

Figure 7.14
Mauriac syndrome with glycogenic hepatopathy.
Enlarged hepatocytes with abundant glycogen stores appear pale and have thickened cell membranes which resemble plant cell walls. The features are similar to those of glycogen storage disease. The subject was a poorly controlled diabetic with abnormal serum liver tests and hepatomegaly (note the diabetes-related 'glycogen nuclei' in periportal hepatocytes at upper left). (Needle biopsy, H&E.)

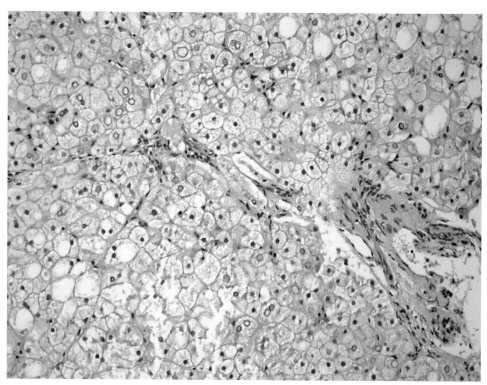

Figure 7.15
Diabetic hepatosclerosis.
A: Increased perisinusoidal collagen is evident (arrows). (H&E.)
B: The increased perisinusoidal collagen shows no zonal preference. (Trichrome stain.) (Photomicrographs kindly provided by Dr Elizabeth Brunt, St Louis, MO, USA.)

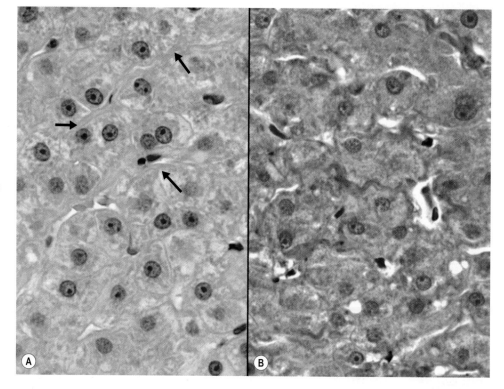

Pathological features of steatohepatitis

The changes in ASH and NASH are very similar, and the two conditions cannot usually be distinguished on histological grounds alone.[63] The main pathological features comprise hepatocellular damage, inflammation and fibrosis (**Box 7.3**). The following description is of the fully developed lesion.

Hepatocellular damage is generally most severe in, or even restricted to, perivenular areas (**Fig. 7.16**). It takes the form of cell swelling and clearing of the cytoplasm, together with the appearance of Mallory–Denk bodies (Mallory bodies, Mallory's hyalin[64]). The affected cells often do not contain obvious fat vacuoles, but these are visible in other parts of the parenchyma. The Mallory–Denk bodies consist of clumps and skeins of dense eosinophilic material, which sometimes forms a ring around the nucleus. When they are difficult to identify, positive immunostaining for p62 or ubiquitin is helpful[64,65] (**Fig. 7.17**). Swollen hepatocytes in steatohepatitis have reduced or absent filaments of keratins 8 and 18 (K8 and K18),[66] demonstrable by using specific K8 and K18 immunostains.[32,34] This feature can be used to distinguish steatohepatitic swelling from certain other causes of ballooning such as that seen in viral hepatitis where keratin 8/18 staining is preserved.[67] *Cams.2* This can be demonstrated with specific immunostains.[67] Hepatocytes may also contain megamitochondria, which are rounded or elongated eosinophilic bodies from 2 μm to 10 μm across (**Fig. 7.18**). These can be distinguished from Mallory–Denk bodies by their

Box 7.3 Main pathological features of steatohepatitis
Steatosis
Hepatocyte ballooning
Hepatocyte apoptosis
Mallory body formation
Inflammatory infiltration
Neutrophils
Lymphocytes
Sinusoidal cells
Fibrosis
Pericellular
Other

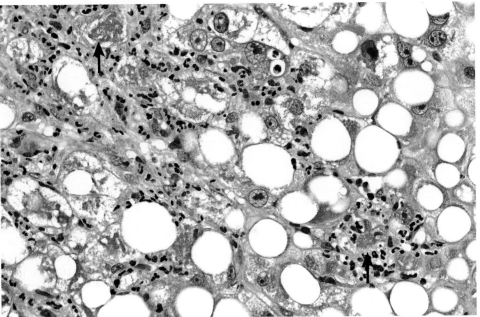

Figure 7.16 Alcoholic steatohepatitis. Inflammatory cells, mainly neutrophils, are clustered around and within hepatocytes, some of which contain densely stained Mallory bodies (arrows). Many hepatocytes contain large fat vacuoles. (Needle biopsy, H&E.)

**Figure 7.17
Mallory–Denk
bodies.**
The Mallory–Denk
bodies in this
example of
steatohepatitis stain
strongly for ubiquitin
(arrows). (Needle
biopsy, specific
immunostain for
ubiquitin.)

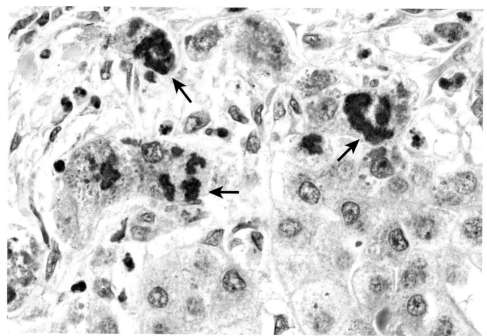

**Figure 7.18
Alcoholic
steatohepatitis.**
Two bright red giant
mitochondria are
marked with arrows.
Collagen fibres,
stained blue, are
seen around
ballooned
hepatocytes.
(Needle biopsy,
chromotrope–aniline
blue (CAB).)

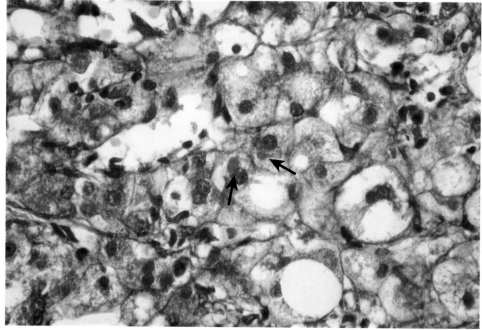

more definite outline and by red staining with chromotrope–aniline blue (CAB); Mallory–Denk bodies usually stain blue with the latter. Megamitochondria can be found in both ASH and NASH as well as in the livers of alcohol abusers in the absence of steatohepatitis.[68–71] Crystalline intramitochondrial inclusions can be seen on transmission electron microscopy in the giant mitochondria of NASH.[71]

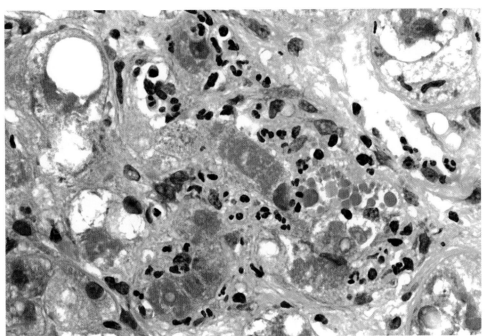

**Figure 7.19
Alcoholic
steatohepatitis.**
Hepatocytes contain
abundant Mallory–
Denk bodies and
neutrophils. (Needle
biopsy, H&E.)

The inflammatory infiltrate is characteristically rich in neutrophils but lymphocytes are also present. These are mainly T cells of CD4 and CD8 phenotype, and are found both in areas of steatohepatitis and in portal tracts.[72] Neutrophils surround or even infiltrate ballooned, Mallory–Denk body-containing hepatocytes (**Fig. 7.19**). Macrophages and other sinusoidal cells take part in the process. Kupffer cells may contain fat vacuoles.[72] Both macrophages and sinusoidal endothelial cells may contain stainable iron.[49]

Fibrosis is an integral part of the lesion of steatohepatitis. The most characteristic form of fibrosis is pericellular ('chicken-wire' fibrosis). Delicate or thicker strands of collagen surround ballooned hepatocytes to form a network which is well seen with trichrome stains (**Fig. 7.20**) and less easy to detect in reticulin preparations. The location corresponds to that of the cell damage and inflammation. In severe steatohepatitis, the fibrosis extends to the portal tracts as well as between perivenular areas, forming fibrous bridges often accompanied by a ductular reaction (**Fig. 7.21**). The evolution of such bridging fibrosis is similar to that seen in NASH.[73,74] Portal fibrosis is sometimes seen in the absence of the pericellular component.

These are the histological features of a classic, fully developed steatohepatitis. Like all pathological processes, however, steatohepatitis is an evolving lesion, which also varies in severity. For these reasons liver biopsy may show less obvious changes, not readily recognised as part of the spectrum. Mallory–Denk bodies may be absent or not demonstrable in the biopsy sample. The inflammatory infiltrate may be predominantly lymphocytic, and pericellular fibrosis may be slight or undetectable. In a small minority of patients the only indication of a probable steatohepatitis is finding a few swollen, Mallory–Denk body-containing hepatocytes without associated inflammation. This should always be reported and regarded as a sign that the patient may be at risk of progressive disease, which is more important from the point of view of patient management than the definition of minimal diagnostic criteria. The finding of pericellular fibrosis without any of the other changes of steatohepatitis may reflect past steatohepatitis.

Figure 7.20
Pericellular fibrosis.
Collagen fibres, stained blue, form a meshwork in this example of steatohepatitis.
(Needle biopsy, CAB.)

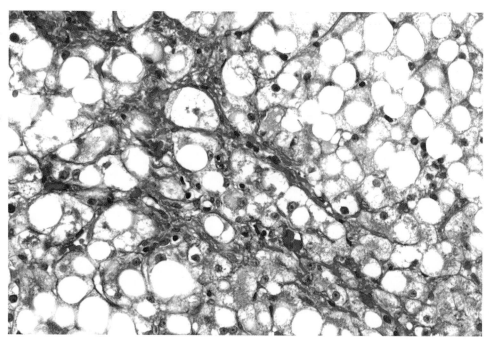

Figure 7.21
Fibrosis in alcoholic steatohepatitis.
Abundant collagen (C) has been laid down in a perivenular area, linked to a portal tract (P) by a fibrous bridge with ductular reaction (arrows). (Needle biopsy, Martius scarlet blue.)

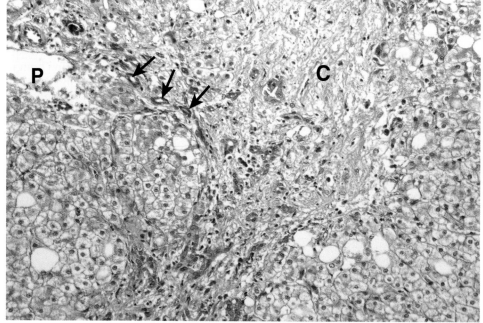

Non-alcoholic steatohepatitis

NASH has assumed increasing importance in recent years and the diagnosis is now a major clinical consideration when liver function tests are abnormal but viral markers are negative. The main clinical associations are listed in **Box 7.4**. It is important to note that, while obesity, diabetes and the metabolic syndrome are common associations with NASH, patients are not all obese,[75] and hyperlipidaemia and other disorders of lipid metabolism may need to be investigated. Certain drugs (amiodarone,[76] calcium channel blockers,[77] tamoxifen[78]) and toxins[79] and rare disorders such as Weber–Christian disease[80] (nodular panniculitis) are other possible causes. NASH can affect men, women, the elderly[81,82] and also children.[42] In **paediatric NASH**, a histological picture of steatosis, portal fibrosis with or without fibrous septa and a mainly lymphocytic infiltrate (**Fig. 7.12**) is more common than the typical perivenular lesion of adult NASH; in the paediatric population this is referred to as NASH type 2.[42] Normal or mildly elevated serum alanine aminotransferase does not exclude the presence of significant steatosis or fibrosis in this group.[83]

There is extensive literature on the pathogenesis of NASH, some of it cited under General reading at the end of this chapter. The exact mechanisms have not been fully elucidated, but many of the important factors involved have been defined. These include insulin resistance,[84] excess of free fatty acids in hepatocytes, lipid peroxidation[85] and oxidative stress.[86] Venous obstruction may be important in the progression to cirrhosis.[87] An element of genetic predisposition is likely[88,89] and NASH has been reported in kindreds.[90] Some of the above factors, such as excess of free fatty acids and oxidative stress, are common to NASH and ASH and help to explain their similarity.

The histological lesion in NASH (**Fig. 7.22**) is as described above under Pathological features of steatohepatitis, but may not be as severe as that in ASH. The presence of

Box 7.4 Main causes and associations of non-alcoholic steatohepatitis
Obesity
Diabetes mellitus
Metabolic syndrome
Hyperlipidaemia
Gastrointestinal surgery for obesity
Drugs and chemicals (e.g. amiodarone, tamoxifen, petrochemicals[79])

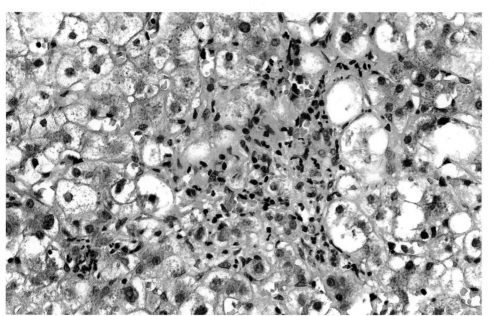

Figure 7.22 Non-alcoholic steatohepatitis. There is steatosis, hepatocellular ballooning and infiltration by neutrophils, as in the alcoholic counterpart. (Needle biopsy, H&E.)

abundant neutrophils and Mallory–Denk bodies should therefore lead to a suspicion of alcohol abuse. Glycogen vacuolation of nuclei is common in NASH.[63] Occasionally the lobular changes appear to be periportal rather than perivenular,[91] but this may reflect the difficulty of accurate localisation in two-dimensional sections. The pericellular fibrosis of NASH is very like that of ASH and is illustrated in **Figure 8.8**. It is associated with hepatocellular injury, as shown by ballooning degeneration and Mallory body formation.[92] As described earlier, in some patients fibrosis is confined to the portal areas.[43,93] Hepatocytes damaged by pathogenetic factors active in NASH may show impaired regeneration ('replicative senescence'), and such affected liver cells may display positive nuclear staining for the cell cycle inhibitor p21 on immunostaining.[73] In this setting, activation of periportal progenitor/stem cells to form a ductular reaction in tandem with fibrosis contributes to the bridging fibrosis and architectural obscuration seen in NASH as it progresses towards cirrhosis.[73] Even in later stages of ASH and NASH, some portal tracts may be spared and this can be a diagnostically helpful finding, further pointing to the centrilobular regions as the site of the initiating insult. The presence of spared portal tracts at the centres of cirrhotic nodules surrounded by fibrous septa bridging between central veins may render an appearance of 'reverse lobulation'.

Progression of the lesion to cirrhosis is variable but often slow.[94] Like other forms of cirrhosis it carries the risk of liver failure and hepatocellular carcinoma.[95–97] Clinical features associated with NASH are also common in patients who have received diagnoses of 'cryptogenic cirrhosis', many of whom represent the late stage of NASH[98–101] in which little or no histological evidence of steatosis or steatohepatitis remains (**Fig. 7.23**). Loss of steatosis has been linked to decreased hepatic delivery of insulin and fatty acids due to portal hypertension as well as abnormal serum adiponectin levels.[102,103] Such 'burnt-out' cases of NASH sometimes show sufficient portal and septal chronic inflammation as to suggest the endstage of a chronic hepatitis, or, alternatively, show bland fibrosis surrounding regenerative nodules. The periphery of nodules near fibrous septa and portal tracts should be carefully examined for residual evidence of hepatocyte ballooning and/or Mallory–Denk bodies (**Fig. 7.23, inset**). A scoring system for NASH has been devised, allowing semi-quantitative assessment and reporting of liver biopsy changes.[104–106] Separate scores are allotted for the severity of the hepatocyte damage and inflammation on the one hand, and for fibrosis and cirrhosis on the other (**Table 7.1**). As in the case of scoring in chronic viral hepatitis (**see Ch. 9**), the resulting numbers must be regarded as categories rather than measurements.

Histological differential diagnosis

The histological differential diagnosis of steatohepatitis includes other forms of hepatitis. In viral hepatitis and AIH the infiltrating cells are lymphocytes and plasma cells rather than neutrophils. In acute viral hepatitis there is collapse of the reticulin framework but the 'chicken-wire' pattern of pericellular fibrosis is not seen. There may be steatosis in patients with chronic hepatitis C, particularly genotype 3 infection[107] (**see Ch. 9**). Chronic hepatitis C accompanied by steatohepatitis is sometimes seen because of virus-related or co-morbid conditions associated with insulin resistance.[108] The fibrosis of venous outflow obstruction is usually linear and parasinusoidal rather than pericellular, but sometimes the hepatic fibrosis of long-standing cardiac disease can resemble that of steatohepatitis. The presence of congestion and absence of other features of steatohepatitis should make the diagnosis clear.

In chronic cholestasis with or without cirrhosis, hepatocytes near fibrous septa are typically ballooned and may contain Mallory–Denk bodies as well as bilirubin. Neutrophils are also seen. The correct diagnosis is made by attention to the location of the lesion, the general absence of steatosis, the presence of copper and copper-associated protein in the affected periportal hepatocytes, and to clinical circumstances. Amiodarone hepatotoxicity shows a similar periportal predilection of Mallory bodies and inflammation, often with

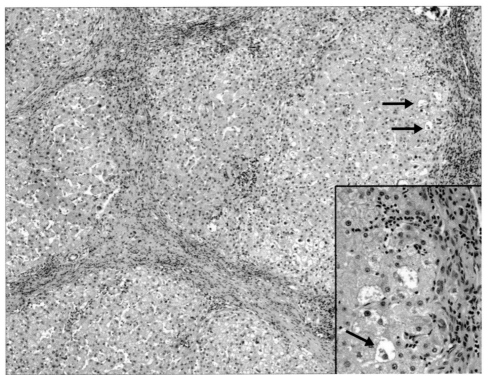

Figure 7.23 Late non-alcoholic steatohepatitis (NASH) presenting as 'cryptogenic cirrhosis'.
The non-descript cirrhotic nodules seen here are surrounded by fibrous septa with chronic
inflammatory cells. There is focal periseptal interface hepatitis at upper right (arrows) where residual
evidence of steatohepatitis is seen. Inset: Residual ballooning and intracellular Mallory–Denk bodies
(arrow) are the remaining histological features of preceding non-alcoholic fatty liver disease and
NASH. Note the absence of steatosis. (Explant liver, H&E.)

Table 7.1 A scoring system for steatohepatitis

Necroinflammatory grading	
Grade 1 (mild)	Steatosis (mainly macrovesicular) involving up to 66% of lobules; occasional ballooned perivenular hepatocytes; scattered neutrophils with or without lymphocytes; no or mild chronic portal inflammation
Grade 2 (moderate)	Steatosis of any degree; obvious ballooning (mainly perivenular); intralobular neutrophils, may be associated with perivenular pericellular fibrosis if evident; mild to moderate portal and intralobular chronic inflammation
Grade 3 (severe)	Panlobular steatosis; obvious perivenular ballooning and disarray; marked lobular inflammation; neutrophils may be concentrated in perivenular areas of ballooning and in areas of pericellular fibrosis if evident; portal inflammation mild or moderate
Fibrosis staging	
Stage 1	Pericellular fibrosis in perivenular areas, focal or extensive
Stage 2	As above, plus focal or extensive periportal fibrosis
Stage 3	Bridging fibrosis, focal or extensive
Stage 4	Cirrhosis

Adapted from Brunt et al.[104] with permission from Nature Publishing Group.

little or no steatosis.[109] Ballooning and Mallory–Denk bodies are also features of Wilson's disease; again, confusion with steatohepatitis is unlikely.

Because steatohepatitis is common in some populations, it is quite often found together with the changes of another liver disease in the same biopsy. Documented diseases coexisting with steatohepatitis include chronic hepatitis, primary biliary cirrhosis, iron storage disorders, drug-induced liver injury and metabolic disorders.[110] The pathologist should therefore consider whether all the changes seen in a biopsy can be explained by steatohepatitis alone.

Other alcohol-related liver lesions

Box 7.5 Liver lesions in the alcoholic
Steatosis
Macrovesicular
Microvesicular (foamy degeneration)
Steatohepatitis
Megamitochondria
Siderosis
Fibrosis
Pericellular
Perivenular
Portal
Cirrhosis
Hepatocellular carcinoma
Effects of non-hepatic alcohol-related diseases

The pathological features of ASH have been described earlier. A wide variety of other changes may be found in liver biopsies from drinkers (**Box 7.5**). In some alcohol abusers the liver is histologically normal or shows only mild macrovesicular steatosis. Portal tracts may contain lymphocytic infiltrates in the absence of other features of hepatitis.[111]

Alcoholic foamy degeneration

Alcoholic foamy degeneration[112] is a relatively rare, potentially life-threatening condition characterised by extensive microvesicular steatosis in perivenular areas. Macrovesicular fat may be seen elsewhere. There may be cholestasis, fine fibrosis and scanty Mallory bodies, but inflammation is minimal or absent and the condition is thus distinct from ASH. Biochemical and histological features of cholestasis have been described.[113]

Fibrosis

Fibrosis is occasionally seen in drinkers in the absence of severe steatosis or steatohepatitis. Perivenular fibrosis may be found with or without steatosis or steatohepatitis. Dense perivenular scarring with nearby Mallory–Denk bodies and steatohepatitis is occasionally seen with heavy alcohol use (**sclerosing hyaline necrosis**)[114,115] (**Fig. 7.24**). Pericellular fibrosis is an important component of steatohepatitis, as already noted, and should always be looked for with the help of a collagen stain. When it is found in the absence of the other features of steatohepatitis it may represent the remnant of a previous episode of this lesion. As such, it is a warning that the patient may be at risk of progressive disease if the cause is not removed. When the fibrosis is portal (**Fig. 7.25**), the possibility of associated biliary disease, alcoholic pancreatitis or coexisting viral hepatitis should be considered.

Fetal alcohol syndrome

In the fetal alcohol syndrome, children of mothers abusing alcohol during pregnancy have fatty livers together with perisinusoidal and portal fibrosis.[116]

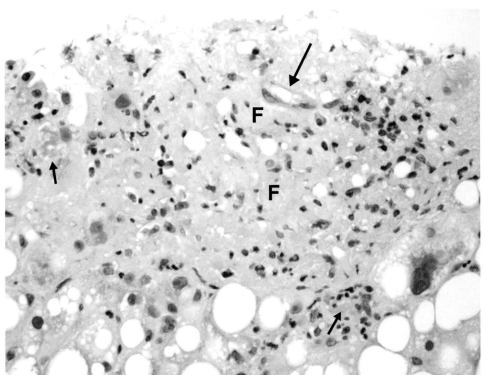

Figure 7.24
Sclerosing hyaline necrosis.
The efferent vein (long arrow) is surrounded by dense fibrosis (F) and inflammation in this alcohol-related lesion. Mallory–Denk bodies (short arrows) are present in the nearby swollen hepatocytes. (Needle biopsy, H&E.)

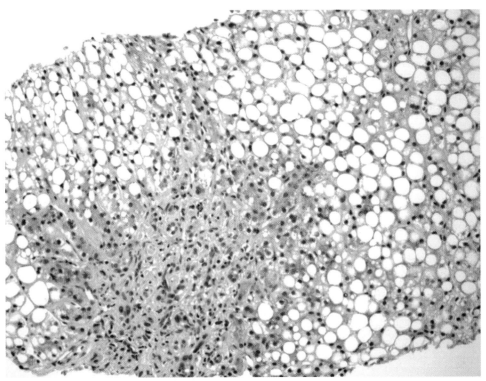

Figure 7.25
Portal fibrosis in an alcoholic.
A fibrotic portal tract with a stellate appearance is seen in this markedly fatty liver. Several bile ductular structures are evident within the fibrosis. The patient had a history of pancreatitis. (Needle biopsy, H&E.)

Cirrhosis

Cirrhosis in the alcoholic develops as a result of increasing fibrosis in steatohepatitis, together with nodular regeneration of the surviving parenchyma. There may also be other routes to cirrhosis, not involving steatohepatitis, but these are difficult to prove. Because steatohepatitis tends to involve all lobules, the cirrhosis is usually micronodular at first (**see Figs 10.12 and 10.13**). As the regeneration nodules enlarge, the cirrhosis remodels to a macronodular pattern and the original cause of the cirrhosis becomes more difficult or even impossible to establish on histological grounds. Venous occlusion is common,[117,118] and may be missed unless stains for collagen or elastic tissue are examined. Hepatocellular carcinoma may develop within the cirrhotic liver.

Other lesions

Alcohol-related lesions affecting organs other than the liver may cause liver changes. Chronic alcoholic pancreatitis has already been cited as a cause of portal fibrosis.[119] In patients with alcoholic cardiomyopathy the changes of right-sided heart failure may be found.

Finally, alcohol-related liver disease may coexist with other, non-alcohol-related liver diseases such as chronic hepatitis C. Alcohol consumption appears to accelerate the progression of fibrosis in hepatitis C.[120]

References

1 Fracanzani AL, Valenti L, Bugianesi E, et al. Risk of severe liver disease in nonalcoholic fatty liver disease with normal aminotransferase levels: a role for insulin resistance and diabetes. Hepatology 2008;48:792–8.

2 Burt AD, Mutton A, Day CP. Diagnosis and interpretation of steatosis and steatohepatitis. Semin Diagn Pathol 1998;15:246–58.

3 Day CP, James OFW. Steatohepatitis: a tale of two 'hits'? Gastroenterology 1998;114:842–5.

4 Sun B, Karini M. Obesity, inflammation, and liver cancer. J Hepatol 2012;56:704–13.

5 Baffy G, Brunt EM, Caldwell SH. Hepatocellular carcinoma in non-alcoholic fatty liver disease: an emerging menace. J Hepatol 2012;56:1384–91.

6 Guzman G, Brunt EM, Petrovic LM, et al. Does nonalcoholic fatty liver disease predispose patients to hepatocellular carcinoma in the absence of cirrhosis? Arch Pathol Lab Med 2008;132:1761–6.

7 Liu TC, Vachharajani N, Chapman WC, et al. Noncirrhotic hepatocellular carcinoma: derivation from hepatocellular adenoma? Clinicopathologic analysis. Mod Pathol 2014;27:420–32.

8 Paradis V, Albuquerque M, Mebarki M, et al. Cullin7: a new gene inivolved in liver carcinogenesis related to metabolic syndrome. Gut 2013;62:911–19.

9 Brunt EM. A novel genetic marker of liver disease aetiology in hepatocellular carcinoma: culling the metabolic syndrome. Gut 2013;62:808–9.

10 Tandra S, Yeh MM, Brunt EM, et al. Presence and significance of microvesicular steatosis in nonalcoholic fatty liver disease. J Hepatol 2011;55:654–9.

11 Martin S, Parton RG. Lipid droplets: a unified view of a dynamic organelle. Nat Rev Mol Cell Biol 2006;7:373–8.

12 Pawella LM, Hashani M, Eiteneuer E, et al. Perilipin discerns chronic from acute hepatocellular steatosis. J Hepatol 2014;60:633–42.

13 Wanless IR. Benign liver tumors. Clin Liver Dis 2002;6:513–26.

14 Franzén LE, Ekstedt M, Kechagias S, et al. Semiquantitative evaluation overestimates the degree of steatosis in liver biopsies: a comparison to stereological point counting. Mod Pathol 2005;18:912–16.

15 Hall AR, Dhillon AP, Green AC, et al. Hepatic steatosis estimated microscopically versus digital image analysis. Liver Int 2013;33:926–35.

16 Turlin B, Ramm GA, Purdie DM, et al. Assessment of hepatic steatosis: comparison of quantitative and semiquantitative methods in 108 liver biopsies. Liver Int 2009;29:530–5.

17 Wanless IR, Geddie WR. Mineral oil lipogranulomata in liver and spleen. A study of 465 autopsies. Arch Pathol Lab Med 1985;109:283–6.

18 Levine PH, Delgado Y, Theise ND, et al. Stellate-cell lipidosis in liver biopsy specimens. Recognition and significance. Am J Clin Pathol 2003;119:254–8.

19 Fromenty B, Berson A, Pessayre D. Microvesicular steatosis and steatohepatitis: role of mitochondrial dysfunction and lipid peroxidation. J Hepatol 1997;26(Suppl. 1):13–22.

20 Lee WS, Sokol RJ. Mitochondrial hepatopathies: advances in genetics and pathogenesis. Hepatology 2007;45:1555–65.

21 Lee WS, Sokol RJ. Mitochondrial hepatopathies: advances in genetics, therapeutic approaches, and outcomes. J Pediatr 2013;163:942–8.

22 Fellman V, Kotarsky H. Mitochondrial hepatopathies in the newborn period. Semin Fetal Neonatal Med 2011;16:222–8.

23 Aita K, Jin Y, Irie H, et al. Are there histopathologic characteristics particular to fulminant hepatic failure caused by human herpesvirus-6 infection? A case report and discussion. Hum Pathol 2001;32:887–9.

24 Marchesini G, Bugianesi E, Forlani G, et al. Nonalcoholic fatty liver, steatohepatitis, and the metabolic syndrome. Hepatology 2003;37:917–23.

25 Birkenfeld AI, Shulman GI. Nonalcoholic fatty liver disease, hepatic insulin resistance, and type 2 diabetes. Hepatology 2014;59:713–23.

26 Charlton M. Cirrhosis and liver failure in nonalcoholic fatty liver disease: molehill or mountain? Hepatology 2008;47:1431–3.

27 Ekstedt M, Franzen LE, Mathiesen UL, et al. Long-term follow-up of patients with NAFLD and elevated liver enzymes. Hepatology 2006;44:865–73.

28 Natori S, Rust C, Stadheim LM, et al. Hepatocyte apoptosis is a pathologic feature of human alcoholic hepatitis. J Hepatol 2001;34:248–53.

29 Ziol M, Tepper M, Lohez M, et al. Clinical and biological relevance of hepatocyte apoptosis in alcoholic hepatitis. J Hepatol 2001;34:254–60.

30 Feldstein AE, Canbay A, Angulo P, et al. Hepatocyte apoptosis and Fas expression are prominent features of human nonalcoholic steatohepatitis. Gastroenterology 2003;125:437–43.

31 Dumas M-E, Kinross J, Nicholson JK. Metabolic phenotyping and systems biology approaches to understanding metabolic syndrome and fatty liver disease. Gastroenterology 2014;46:46–62.

32 Lackner C, Gogg-Kamerer M, Zatloukal K, et al. Ballooned hepatocytes in steatohepatitis: the value of keratin immunohistochemistry for diagnosis. J Hepatol 2008;48:821–8.

33 Caldwell S, Ikura Y, Dias D, et al. Hepatocellular ballooning in NASH. J Hepatol 2010;53:719–23.

33a Guy CD, Suzuki A, Abdelmalek MF, et al. Treatment response in the PIVENS trial is associated with decreased hedgehog pathway activity. Hepatology 2015;61:98–107.

33b Hirsova P, Gores GJ. Ballooned hepatocytes, undead cells, Sonic hedgehog, and vitamin E: therapeutic implications for nonalcoholic steatohepatitis. Hepatology 2015;61:15–17.

34 Guy CD, Suzuki A, Burchette JL, et al. Costaining for keratins 8/18 plus ubiquitin improves detection of hepatocyte injury in nonalcoholic fatty liver disease. Hum Pathol 2012;43:790–800.

35 Colombat M, Charlotte F, Ratziu V, et al. Portal lymphocytic infiltrate in alcoholic liver disease. Hum Pathol 2002;33:1170–4.

36 Brunt EM, Kleiner DE, Wilson LA, et al. Portal chronic inflammation in nonalcoholic fatty liver disease (NAFLD): a histologic marker of advanced NAFLD – clinicopathologic correlations from the Nonalcoholic Steatohepatitis Clinical Research Network. Hepatology 2009;49:809–20.

37 Adams LA, Lindor KD, Angulo P. The prevalence of autoantibodies and autoimmune hepatitis in patients with nonalcoholic fatty liver disease. Am J Gastroenterol 2004;99:1316–20.

38 Cotler SJ, Kanji K, Keshavarzian A, et al. Prevalence and significance of autoantibodies in patients with non-alcoholic steatohepatitis. J Clin Gastroenterol 2004;38:801–4.

39 Patton HM, Lavine JE, Van Natta ML, et al. Clinical correlates of histopathology in pediatric nonalcoholic steatohepatitis. Gastroenterology 2008;135:1961–71.

40 Loria P, Lonardo A, Leonardi F, et al. Non-organ-specific autoantibodies in nonalcoholic fatty liver disease: prevalence and correlates. Dig Dis Sci 2003;48:2173–81.

41 Czaja AJ, Carpenter HA, Santrach PJ, et al. Genetic predisposition for immunologic features in chronic liver diseases other than autoimmune hepatitis. J Hepatol 1996;24:52–9.

42 Schwimmer JB, Behling C, Newbury R, et al. Histopathology of pediatric nonalcoholic fatty liver disease. Hepatology 2005;42:641–9.

43 Abrams GA, Kunde SS, Lazenby AJ, et al. Portal fibrosis and hepatic steatosis in morbidly obese subjects: a spectrum of nonalcoholic fatty liver disease. Hepatology 2004;40:475–83.

44 Skoien R, Richardson MM, Jonsson JR, et al. Heterogeneity of fibrosis patterns in non-alcoholic fatty liver disease supports the presence of multiple fibrogenic pathways. Liver Int 2013;33:624–32.

45 Kleiner DE, Berk PD, Hsu JY, et al. Hepatic pathology among patients without known liver disease undergoing bariatric surgery: observations and a perspective from the Longitudinal Assessment of Bariatric Surgery (LABS) Study. Semin Liver Dis 2014;34:98–107.

46 Deugnier Y, Brissot P, Loréal O. Iron and the liver: update 2008. J Hepatol 2008;48:S113–23.

47 Aigner E, Theurl I, Haufe H, et al. Copper availability contributes to iron perturbations in human nonalcoholic fatty liver disease. Gastroenterology 2008;135:680–8.

48 Nelson JE, Wilson L, Brunt EM, et al. Relationship between the pattern of hepatic iron deposition and histological severity in nonalcoholic fatty liver disease. Hepatology 2011;53:448–57.

49 Turlin B, Mendler MH, Moirand R, et al. Histologic features of the liver in insulin resistance-associated iron overload. A study of 139 patients. Am J Clin Pathol 2001;116:263–70.

50 Dongiovanni P, Fracanzani AL, Fargion S, et al. Iron in fatty liver and in the metabolic syndrome: a promising therapeutic target. J Hepatol 2011;55:920–32.

51 Nelson JE, Klintworth H, Kowdley KV. Iron metabolism in nonalcoholic fatty liver disease. Curr Gastroenterol Rep 2012;14:8–16.

52 Maliken BD, Nelson JE, Klintworth HM, et al. Hepatic reticuloendothelial system cell iron deposition is associated with increased apoptosis in nonalcoholic fatty liver disease. Hepatology 2013;57:1806–13.

53 Younossi ZM, Stepanova M, Rafiq N, et al. Pathologic criteria for nonalcoholic steatohepatitis: interprotocol agreement and ability to predict liver-related mortality. Hepatology 2011;53:1874–82.

54 Matteoni CA, Younossi ZM, Gramlich T, et al. Nonalcoholic fatty liver disease: a spectrum of clinical and pathological severity. Gastroenterology 1999;116:1413–19.

55 Kleiner DE, Brunt EM, Van Natta M, et al. Design and validation of a histological scoring system for nonalcoholic fatty liver disease. Hepatology 2005;41:1313–21.

56 Kleiner DE. The alcoholic hepatitis histologic score: structured prognostic biopsy evaluation comes to alcoholic hepatitis. Gastroenterology 2014;146:1156–8.

57 Angulo P. Diagnosing steatohepatitis and predicting liver-related mortality in patients with NAFLD: two distinct concepts. Hepatology 2011;53:1792–4.

58 Abraham S, Furth EE. Receiver operating characteristic analysis of glycogenated nuclei in liver biopsy specimens: quantitative evaluation of their relationship with diabetes and obesity. Hum Pathol 1994;25:1063–8.

58a Fitzpatrick E, Cotoi C, Quaglia A, et al. Hepatopathy of Mauriac syndrome: a retrospective review from a tertiary liver centre. Arch Dis Child 2014;99:354–7.

59 Torbenson M, Chen Y-Y, Brunt E, et al. Glycogenic hepatopathy. An underrecognized hepatic complication of diabetes mellitus. Am J Surg Pathol 2006;30:508–13.

60 Harrison SA, Brunt EM, Goodman ZD, et al. Diabetic hepatosclerosis: a novel entity or a rare form of nonalcoholic fatty liver disease? Arch Pathol Lab Med 2006;130:27–32.

61 Latry P, Bioulac-Sage P, Echinard E, et al. Perisinusoidal fibrosis and basement membrane-like material in the livers of diabetic patients. Hum Pathol 1987;18:775–80.

62 David K, Kowdley KV, Unalp A, et al. Quality of life in adults with nonalcoholic fatty liver disease: baseline data from the Nonalcoholic Steatohepatitis Clinical Research Network. Hepatology 2009;49:1904–12.

63 Itoh S, Yougel T, Kawagoe K. Comparison between nonalcoholic steatohepatitis and alcoholic hepatitis. Am J Gastroenterol 1987;82:650–4.

64 Zatloukal K, French SW, Stumptner C, et al. From Mallory to Mallory–Denk bodies: what, how and why? Exp Cell Res 2007;313:2033–49.

65 Banner BF, Savas L, Zivny J, et al. Ubiquitin as a marker of cell injury in nonalcoholic steatohepatitis. Am J Clin Pathol 2000;114:860–6.

66 Strnad P, Stumptner C, Zatloukal K, et al. Intermediate filament cytoskeleton of the liver in health and disease. Histochem Cell Biol 2008;129:735–49.

67 Lackner C, Gogg-Kamerer M, Zatloukal K, et al. Ballooned hepatocytes in steatohepatitis: the value of keratin immunohistochemistry for diagnosis. J Hepatol 2008;48:821–8.

68 Caldwell SH, Swerdlow RH, Khan EM, et al. Mitochondrial abnormalities in non-alcoholic steatohepatitis. J Hepatol 1999;31:430–4.

69 Sanyal AJ, Campbell-Sargent C, Mirshahi F, et al. Nonalcoholic steatohepatitis: association of insulin resistance and mitochondrial abnormalities. Gastroenterology 2001;120:1183–92.

70 Le TH, Caldwell SH, Redick JA, et al. The zonal distribution of megamitochondria with crystalline inclusions in nonalcoholic steatohepatitis. Hepatology 2004;39:1423–9.

71 Caldwell SH, de Freitas AR, Park SH, et al. Intramitochondrial crystalline inclusions in nonalcoholic steatohepatitis. Hepatology 2009;49:1888–95.

72 Lefkowitch JH, Haythe JH, Regent N. Kupffer cell aggregation and perivenular distribution in steatohepatitis. Mod Pathol 2002;15:699–704.

73 Richardson MM, Jonsson JR, Powell EE, et al. Progressive fibrosis in nonalcoholic steatohepatitis: association with altered regeneration and a ductular reaction. Gastroenterology 2007;133:80–90.

74 Gadd VL, Skoien R, Powell EE, et al. The portal inflammatory infiltrate and ductularreaction in human nonalcoholic fatty liver disease. Hepatology 2014;59:1393–405.

75 Bacon BR, Farahvash MJ, Janney CG, et al. Nonalcoholic steatohepatitis: an expanded clinical entity. Gastroenterology 1994;107:1103–9.

76 Simon JB, Manley PN, Brien JF, et al. Amiodarone hepatotoxicity simulating alcoholic liver disease. N Engl J Med 1984;311:167–72.

77 Babany G, Uzzan F, Larrey D, et al. Alcohol-like liver lesions induced by nifedipine. J Hepatol 1989;9:252–5.

78 Pinto HC, Baptista A, Camilo ME, et al. Tamoxifen-associated steatohepatitis – report of three cases. J Hepatol 1995;23:95–7.

79 Cotrium HP, De Freitas LAR, Freitas C, et al. Clinical and histopahological features of NASH in workers exposed to chemicals with or without associated metabolic conditions. Liver Int 2004;24:131–5.

80 Wasserman JM, Thung SN, Berman R, et al. Hepatic Weber–Christian disease. Semin Liver Dis 2001;21:115–18.

81 Noureddin M, Yates KP, Vaughn IA, et al. Clinical and histological determinants of nonalcoholic steatohepatitis and advanced fibrosis in elderly patients. Hepatology 2013;58:1644–54.

82 Koehler EM, Schouten JNL, Hansen BE, et al. Prevalence and risk factors of non-alcoholic fatty liver disease in the elderly: results from the Rotterdam study. J Hepatol 2012;57:1305–11.

83 Molleston JP, Schwimmer JB, Yates KP, et al. Histological abnormalities in children with nonalcoholic fatty liver disease and normal or mildly elevated alanine aminotransferase levels. J Pediatr 2014;164:707–13.

84 De Alwis NM, Day CP. Non-alcoholic fatty liver disease: the mist gradually clears. J Hepatol 2008;48:S104–12.

85 MacDonald GA, Bridle KR, Ward PJ, et al. Lipid peroxidation in hepatic steatosis in humans is associated with hepatic fibrosis and occurs predominantly in acinar zone 3. J Gastroenterol Hepatol 2001;16:599–606.

86 Seki S, Kitada T, Yamada T, et al. In situ detection of lipid peroxidation and oxidative DNA damage in non-alcoholic fatty liver diseases. J Hepatol 2002;37:56–62.

87 Wanless IR, Shiota K. The pathogenesis of nonalcoholic steatohepatitis and other fatty liver diseases: a four-step model including the role of lipid release and hepatic venular obstruction in the progression to cirrhosis. Semin Liver Dis 2004;24:99–106.

88 Valenti L, Fracanzani AL, Dongiovanni P, et al. Tumor necrosis factor alpha promoter polymorphisms and insulin resistance in nonalcoholic fatty liver disease. Gastroenterology 2002;122:274–80.

89 Namikawa C, Shu-Ping Z, Vyselaar JR, et al. Polymorphisms of microsomal triglyceride transfer protein gene and manganese superoxide dismutase gene in non-alcoholic steatohepatitis. J Hepatol 2004;40:781–6.

90 Struben VM, Hespenheide EE, Caldwell SH. Nonalcoholic steatohepatitis and cryptogenic cirrhosis within kindreds. Am J Med 2000;108:9–13.

91 Nagore N, Scheuer PJ. The pathology of diabetic hepatitis. J Pathol 1988;156:155–60.

92 Gramlich T, Kleiner DE, McCullough AJ, et al. Pathologic features associated with fibrosis in nonalcoholic fatty liver disease. Hum Pathol 2004;35:196–9.

93 Adler M, Schaffner F. Fatty liver hepatitis and cirrhosis in obese patients. Am J Med 1979;67:811–16.

94 Fassio E, Álvarez E, Domínguez N, et al. Natural history of nonalcoholic steatohepatitis: a longitudinal study of repeat liver biopsies. Hepatology 2004;40:820–6.

95 Shimada M, Hashimoto E, Taniai M, et al. Hepatocellular carcinoma in patients with non-alcoholic steatohepatitis. J Hepatol 2002;37:154–60.

96 Hui JM, Kench JG, Chitturi S, et al. Long-term outcomes of cirrhosis in nonalcoholic steatohepatitis compared with hepatitis C. Hepatology 2003;38:420–7.

97 Hashimoto E, Yatsuji S, Tobari M, et al. Hepatocellular carcinoma in patients with nonalcoholic steatohepatitis. J Gastroenterol 2009;44(Suppl. XIX):89–95.

98 Caldwell SH, Oelsner DH, Iezzoni JC, et al. Cryptogenic cirrhosis: clinical characterization and risk factors for underlying disease. Hepatology 1999;29:664–9.

99 Poonawala A, Nair SP, Thuluvath PJ. Prevalence of obesity and diabetes in patients with cryptogenic cirrhosis: a case–control study. Hepatology 2000;32:689–92.

100 Bugianesi E, Leone N, Vanni E, et al. Expanding the natural history of nonalcoholic steatohepatitis: from cryptogenic cirrhosis to hepatocellular carcinoma. Gastroenterology 2002;123:134–40.

101 Clark JM, Diehl AM. Nonalcoholic fatty liver disease: an underrecognized cause of cryptogenic cirrhosis. JAMA 2003;289:3000–4.

102 van der Poorten D, Samer CF, Ramezani-Moghadam M, et al. Hepatic fat loss in advanced nonalcoholic steatohepatitis: are alterations in serum adiponectin the cause? Hepatology 2013;57:2180–8.

103 Claudel T, Trauner M. Adiponectin, bile acids, and burnt-out nonalcoholic steatohepatitis: new light on an old paradox. Hepatology 2013;57:2106–9.

104 Brunt EM, Janney CG, Di Bisceglie AM, et al. Nonalcoholic steatohepatitis: a proposal for grading and staging the histological lesions. Am J Gastroenterol 1999;94:2467–74.

105 Yeh MM, Brunt EM. Pathology of nonalcoholic fatty liver disease. Am J Clin Pathol 2007;128:837–47.

106 Brunt EM, Neuschwander-Tetri BA, Kent DO, et al. Nonalcoholic steatohepatitis: histologic features and clinical correlations with 30 blinded biopsy specimens. Hum Pathol 2004;35:1070–82.

107 Negro F. Hepatitis C virus and liver steatosis: is it the virus? Yes it is, but not always. Hepatology 2002;36:1050–2.

108 Bedossa P, Moucari R, Chelbi E, et al. Evidence for a role of nonalcoholic steatohepatitis in hepatitis C: a prospective study. Hepatology 2007;46:380–7.

109 Lewis JH, Mullick F, Ishak KG, et al. Histopathologic analysis of suspected amiodarone hepatotoxicity. Hum Pathol 1990;21:59–67.

110 Brunt EM, Ramrakhiani S, Cordes BG, et al. Concurrence of histologic features of steatohepatitis with other forms of chronic liver disease. Mod Pathol 2003;16:49–56.

111 Engler S, Elsing C, Flechtenmacher C, et al. Progressive sclerosing cholangitis after shock: a new variant of vanishing bile duct disorders. Gut 2003;52:688–93.

112 Uchida T, Kao H, Quispe-Sjogren M, et al. Alcoholic foamy degeneration – a pattern of acute alcoholic injury of the liver. Gastroenterology 1983;84:683–92.

113 Suri S, Mitros FA, Ahluwalia JP. Alcoholic foamy degeneration and a markedly elevated GGT. A case report and literature review. Dig Dis Sci 2003;48:1142–6.

114 Edmondson HA, Peters RL, Reynolds TB, et al. Sclerosing hyaline necrosis of the liver in the chronic alcoholic. A recognizable clinical syndrome. Ann Intern Med 1963;59:646–73.

115 Wang J, Cornford ME, German J, et al. Sclerosing hyaline necrosis of the liver in Bloom syndrome. Arch Pathol Lab Med 1999;123:346–50.

116 Lefkowitch JH, Rushton AR, Feng-Chen KC. Hepatic fibrosis in fetal alcohol syndrome. Pathologic similarities to adult alcoholic liver disease. Gastroenterology 1983;85:951–7.

117 Goodman ZD, Ishak KG. Occlusive venous lesions in alcoholic liver disease. A study of 200 cases. Gastroenterology 1982;83:786–96.

118 Burt AD, MacSween RN. Hepatic vein lesions in alcoholic liver disease: retrospective biopsy and necropsy study. J Clin Pathol 1986;39:63–7.

119 Morgan MY, Sherlock S, Scheuer PJ. Portal fibrosis in the livers of alcoholic patients. Gut 1978;19:1015–21.

120 Siu L, Foont J, Wands JR. Hepatitis C virus and alcohol. Semin Liver Dis 2009;29:188–99.

General reading

Browning JD, Horton JD. Molecular mediators of hepatic steatosis and liver injury. J Clin Invest 2004;114: 147–52.

Brunt EM. Pathology of nonalcoholic fatty liver disease. Nat Rev Gastroenterol Hepatol 2010;7:195–203.

Brunt EM, Neuschwander-Tetri BA, Burt AD. Fatty liver disease: alcoholic and nonalcoholic. In: Burt AD, Portmann BC, Ferrell LD, editors. Macsween's Pathology of the Liver. 6th ed. Edinburgh: Churchill Livingstone/Elsevier; 2012. p. 293–360.

Brunt EM, Tiniakos DG. Histopathology of nonalcoholic fatty liver disease. World J Gastroenterol 2010;16: 5286–96.

Ekstedt M, Franzén LE, Mathiesen UL, et al. Long-term follow-up of patients with NAFLD and elevated liver enzymes. Hepatology 2006;44:865–73.

Kleiner DE, Brunt EM. Nonalcoholic fatty liver disease: pathologic patterns and biopsy evaluation in clinical research. Semin Liver Dis 2012;32:3–13.

Lucey MR, Mathurin P, Morgan TR. Medical progress: alcoholic hepatitis. N Engl J Med 2009;360:2758–69.

Mofrad P, Contos MJ, Haque M, et al. Clinical and histologic spectrum of nonalcoholic fatty liver disease associated with normal ALT values. Hepatology 2003;37:1286–92.

Reuben A. Pearls of pathology. Hepatology 2003;37:715–18.

Yeh MM, Brunt EM. Pathological features of fatty liver disease. Gastroenterology 2014;147:754–64.

Zafrani ES. Non-alcoholic fatty liver disease: an emerging pathological spectrum. Virchows Arch 2004;444:3–12.

Zatloukal K, French SW, Stumptner C, et al. From Mallory to Mallory–Denk bodies: what, how and why? Exp Cell Res 2007;313:2033–49.

Drugs and Toxins

Introduction

This chapter deals with the pathology of the important liver lesions attributed to drugs and toxins, with their recognition, and with their differential diagnosis. There are many hundreds of hepatotoxic drugs and other chemicals,[1] and new reports of adverse drug reactions appear regularly in the literature under the acronym DILI (drug-induced liver injury). Heightened awareness of DILI during the last two decades has resulted in the creation of multicentre networks and databases in the United States, the United Kingdom, Europe and Asia which serve as ongoing resources for reporting and evaluation of new cases, data retrieval and correlation, phenotype characterisation and standardisation of nomenclature.[2] The LiverTox website (http://livertox.nih.gov/index.html), developed by the Liver Disease Research Branch of the National Institute of Diabetes and Digestive and Kidney Diseases and the National Library of Medicine in the United States is a new and easily accessible source of information on some 650 different medications, herbal agents and supplements. Other search engines available on the internet, such as PubMed, are additional resources to consult when DILI is suspected. If a liver biopsy is obtained in order to determine the cause of hepatitis, jaundice, acute liver failure or other type of liver disease, the pathologist should bear in mind that a drug cannot be exonerated simply because an adverse reaction has not been reported; there is always a first time.

Chemical injury is not confined to drugs listed in pharmacopoeias. Herbal medicines and dietary supplements,[3–10] illicit drugs,[11–19] criminally administered poisons,[20] industrial chemicals,[21–24] vitamins[25,26] and foods[27,28] have all been held responsible for liver disease. Drugs used for the treatment of liver disease have themselves been suspected of causing liver damage.[29]

In his foreword to the second edition of Stricker's *Drug-Induced Hepatic Injury*,[30] Zimmerman wrote: 'virtually all known acute and chronic hepatic lesions can result from drug injury'. This important observation implies that drugs should be considered as a possible cause of any liver lesion found on biopsy, but some lesions are more often produced by drugs than others. Hepatocellular necrosis, hepatitis and cholestasis in particular should arouse a greater degree of suspicion, especially if no other cause has been found. Also, some groups of drugs are associated with particular kinds of injury; non-steroidal anti-inflammatory drugs (NSAIDs), for example, are often associated with hepatocellular injury, while neuroleptic drugs mostly cause cholestasis. However, these are generalisations and a drug which causes a dose-related hepatocellular necrosis in one patient may cause non-dose-related hepatitis, cholestasis or granulomas in another.[31,32]

The diagnostic pathologist should be aware of the potential of drugs and other substances to cause this wide variety of acute and chronic liver lesions and to know which lesions are most likely to be drug-induced. He or she should be familiar with their likely course and outcome, and the main points of similarity and difference from other, non-drug-related liver diseases. Finally, the pathologist should know where to look up the effects of individual drugs. The LiverTox site is found at http://livertox.nih.gov/php/searchchem.php.

Classification and mechanisms

Drugs may be regarded as producing liver injury in two main ways: *intrinsic* and *idiosyncratic* hepatotoxicity (**Table 8.1**). **Intrinsic (predictable) hepatotoxins** are those which predictably produce liver damage when taken in sufficient quantities. The type of damage is often characteristic of a particular drug; for example, the typical result of paracetamol (acetaminophen) overdose is hepatocellular necrosis and steatosis. Intrinsic hepatotoxicity can often be studied in laboratory animals. This type of hepatotoxicity is also frequently **zonal** in distribution; examples of this are the perivenular lesions of paracetamol and carbon tetrachloride and the periportal necrosis seen in phosphorus and ferrous sulfate toxicity. The mechanism of intrinsic hepatotoxicity can be **direct** or **indirect**; in the former, the chemical or its metabolites causes structural damage to cells and organelles, while in indirect intrinsic hepatotoxicity the chemical interferes with a specific metabolic pathway or cell component.

The more common kind of drug-related liver damage is **idiosyncratic (unpredictable)**. Only a small proportion of patients on a particular drug is affected, so that the adverse reaction is not detected in initial human trials. Antibiotics and psychoactive drugs are the most common cause of idiosyncratic DILI in Western countries.[30] Many different mechanisms for idiosyncratic hepatotoxicity have now been elucidated. They include individual genetic variation in the metabolism of drugs, and the development of immune reactions to a drug or its metabolites.[33] The immune reactions may be directed to neoantigens produced by the binding of reactive metabolites to hepatic drug-metabolising enzymes of the P450 system.[34,35] In some instances the distinction between an idiosyncratic and intrinsic

Table 8.1 Examples of liver lesions due to drugs and toxins

Lesion	Example of substance
Intrinsic hepatotoxicity	
Microvesicular steatosis	Valproate
Phospholipidosis	Amiodarone
Hepatocellular necrosis	Paracetamol (acetaminophen)
Fibrosis	Vitamin A
Cholestasis	Contraceptive steroids
Venous occlusion	Pyrrolizidine alkaloids
Angiosarcoma	Vinyl chloride
Idiosyncratic hepatotoxicity	
Hepatitis	Isoniazid
Cholestasis	Amoxicillin–clavulanic acid
Granuloma formation	Allopurinol

drug reaction is difficult to make. Typical idiosyncratic damage may follow a small dose of the offending drug, and cannot easily be studied in the laboratory. With the exception of a few drugs shown to cause liver damage in patients using a particular metabolic pathway, idiosyncratic drug injury is unpredictable in the sense that the susceptibility of individual patients cannot be tested before the drug is given.

Most intrinsic hepatotoxins produce liver damage within a few hours or days, whereas in the idiosyncratic type of injury there is often a latent period of many days, weeks or months[36] before liver disease becomes apparent. The latent period tends to shorten with repeated administration of the drug. Because of the latent period and the tendency for idiosyncratic injury to mimic non-drug-related liver diseases, clinicians and pathologists need to be alert to the possibility of idiosyncratic drug injury if diagnostic errors are to be avoided. The clinician may be helped by compiling specific data[37] and by using a causality scale.[38] The pathologist may be helped by finding a suspicious or characteristic pattern of injury.[39] Conclusive proof that a particular drug or combination of drugs is responsible is often impossible to obtain, although rechallenge (usually inadvertent) can provide strong circumstantial evidence. Liver injury may follow inadvertent rechallenge many years after a first episode.[40] Biochemical evidence of improvement after drug withdrawal is occasionally supported by a return to normal histology.[36]

Morphological categories

The categories described below represent the main changes attributed to drugs and toxins, apart from alcohol-related liver damage (**see Ch. 7**), neoplasms (**see Ch. 11**) and vascular lesions (**see Ch. 12**). A mixture of lesions may be found in the same liver: amiodarone, for example, produces both phospholipidosis and steatohepatitis, but by different mechanisms.[41] As already indicated, a single drug may give rise to different forms of hepatotoxicity in different patients. Phenylbutazone, for example, can cause necrosis, cholestasis, granuloma formation or combinations of these,[42] while the NSAIDs nimesulide and diclofenac can cause either severe hepatitis or cholestasis.[43,44]

Adaptation

Not all changes seen under the microscope necessarily represent liver damage. The increase in endoplasmic reticulum produced by long-term treatment with anticonvulsant drugs is commonly regarded as an adaptive phenomenon.[45,46] By light microscopy, this increase is seen as an abundance of pale-staining cytoplasm in hepatocytes (**see Figs 4.4 and 8.1**), which is difficult to distinguish from simple abundance of glycogen on a haematoxylin–eosin (H&E)-stained section.

Non-hepatitic liver-cell damage

One of the most common manifestations of intrinsic hepatotoxicity is **steatosis**. As discussed in **Chapter 7**, this may be macrovesicular or microvesicular. Macrovesicular steatosis, in which the nucleus of the hepatocyte is displaced by one or more fat vacuoles easily visible by light microscopy, is produced by chlorinated hydrocarbons and methotrexate, for example. It is common in patients on total parenteral nutrition,[47,48] although underlying disease may also contribute to the liver changes.[49] In patients treated with gold compounds for rheumatoid arthritis, intralobular lipogranulomas (focal accumulations of lipid-containing macrophages) have been found to contain gold pigment in the form of fine black or brown granules. These were also seen within portal lipid droplets.[50]

Causes of the more serious microvesicular steatosis[51] (**Fig. 8.2**) include treatment with the anticonvulsant drug valproate[52] and with the nucleoside analogue fialuridine.[53] An increased risk of acute liver failure with valproate use is seen in individuals with

Figure 8.1 Adaptation. Hepatocytes in this biopsy from a patient on antiepileptic drugs are enlarged and have abundant pale-staining cytoplasm. (Needle biopsy, H&E.)

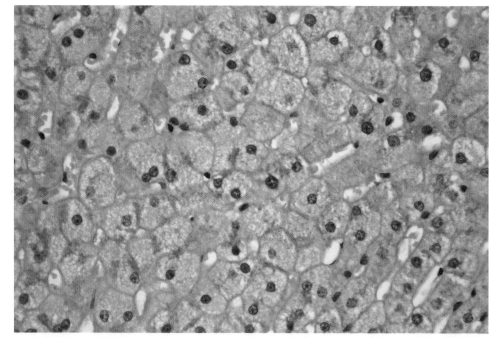

Figure 8.2 Microvesicular steatosis. In this example of valproate toxicity, the hepatocytes are swollen and finely vacuolated. (Recipient liver at transplantation, H&E.) (The section was kindly provided by Professor BC Portmann, London, UK.)

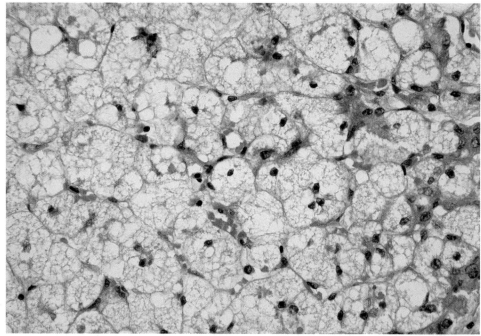

underlying mutations in the POLG1 gene for mitochondrial DNA polymerase gamma.[52a] This leads to the combination of microvesicular steatosis with mitochondrial abnormalities, found also in Reye's syndrome (**see Ch. 13**). Similar changes are reported after zidovudine,[54] didanosine (**Fig. 8.3**) and other nucleoside reverse transcriptase inhibitors in highly active antiretroviral therapy (HAART) for acquired immunodeficiency syndrome (AIDS).[55–58] In the microvesicular form of steatosis the fat within the hepatocytes is finely

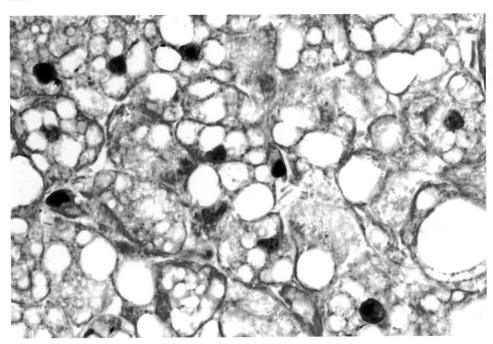

Figure 8.3 Didanosine-induced microvesicular steatosis. Small-droplet fat vacuoles are prominent in hepatocytes, most of which show nuclei maintained in a central position. (Needle biopsy, H&E.)

divided and is not always obvious with conventional stains. The hepatocyte nuclei remain in their normal central location, in contrast to macrovesicular steatosis. There is a variable degree of associated hepatocellular necrosis.

Several drugs, among them amiodarone[41] and trimethoprim-sulfamethoxazole (co-trimoxazole),[59] are causes of acquired **phospholipidosis**. Similar changes have been reported in patients receiving total parenteral nutrition.[60] Lamellar inclusions are seen within hepatocytes and other cells by electron microscopy (**see Fig. 17.3**). Light micros-copy of conventionally stained sections is not diagnostic.

In acute arsenic intoxication, a striking increase in hepatocyte mitoses has been reported, accompanied by ballooning, cholestasis and mild inflammation.[20] Markers of cell prolif-eration were also markedly increased.

An unusual form of cell injury is produced by cyanamide, used in alcohol aversion therapy.[61–63] Periportal hepatocytes contain large, pale-staining **cytoplasmic inclusion bodies**, giving the cells a superficial resemblance to the ground-glass cells of chronic type B hepatitis (**see Figs 4.4 and 9.13**). The inclusions are, however, orcein-negative and diastase–periodic acid–Schiff-positive.

Hepatocellular necrosis

Hepatocellular necrosis without the diffuse inflammatory lesion of hepatitis is usually a consequence of the intrinsic type of hepatotoxicity. A common example is suicidal or accidental overdose with the analgesic paracetamol.[64] Jaundice develops after an interval of days, during which available glutathione, which reacts with a toxic metabolite, is used up. The necrosis – like that of shock or heatstroke (**see Fig. 12.2**) – is most severe in perivenular regions (acinar zones 3) and is accompanied by little or no inflammation (**Fig. 8.4**). Kupffer cells contain brown ceroid pigment. Portal tracts usually remain normal. A few neutrophils and lymphocytes are sometimes also seen in necrotic regions, due to activation of innate immunity by damage-associated molecular pattern (DAMP) molecules such as high mobility group box-1 (HMGB1) and keratin 18 released from necrotic hepatocytes.[65–67] Complete recovery is possible. While most paracetamol-induced necrosis

**Figure 8.4
Hepatocellular
necrosis due to
paracetamol
(acetaminophen).**
Confluent necrosis
with little
inflammation is seen
in a perivenular area.
The surviving
parenchyma near
the portal tracts
(upper left and
upper right) shows
mild steatosis and
cholestasis. (Explant
liver, N, H&E.)

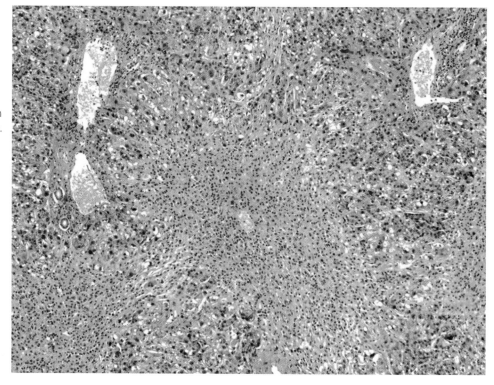

follows suicidal overdose, it is occasionally found in habitual drinkers taking large doses in the high therapeutic range.[68]

Hepatocellular necrosis, sometimes accompanied by steatosis, is also a feature of cocaine intoxication,[11,13,15] of glue sniffing and of solvent abuse.[16,69] In most instances the necrosis is perivenular and mid-zonal (in acinar zones 3 and 2), but periportal (zone 1) necrosis has been reported in a cocaine user.[70] 'Ecstasy' (3,4-methylenedioxymethamphetamine [MDMA]) can cause a hepatitic lesion of the kind described in the next section,[17,18,71] but there may also be confluent hepatocellular necrosis as a result of concurrent hyperthermia.[19] Other agents capable of causing confluent necrosis include industrial hydrochlorofluorocarbons.[21]

Acute drug-induced hepatitis

A large number of drugs of different chemical structure and with widely differing pharmacological actions occasionally give rise to acute hepatitis, and any drug should be regarded as a potential offender. Acute drug-induced hepatotoxicity is of the idiosyncratic type. The histological lesion is very like that of acute viral hepatitis, and often indistinguishable from it (**Figs 8.5 and 8.6**). Incriminated substances include antituberculous drugs,[72] NSAIDs, anaesthetics,[73,74] herbal remedies[4] and many others.

In the idiosyncratic injury of hepatitic type the latent period between exposure to the drug and clinically evident liver disease ranges from a few days to several months or longer, a long latent period sometimes making diagnosis difficult. However, correct diagnosis of idiosyncratic drug-induced hepatitis is most important, because inadvertent rechallenge may have serious consequences.

The hepatitis ranges in severity from a mild inflammatory lesion, sometimes combined with a cholestatic reaction (see under Steroid-induced cholestasis, below), to severe and

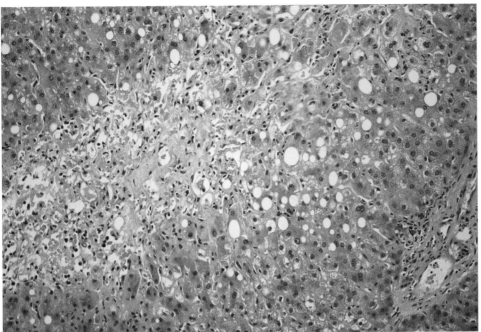

Figure 8.5 Drug-induced liver injury: hepatitic type.
In this acute hepatitis attributed to indometacin, necrosis in acinar zone 3 is well demarcated from the remaining parenchyma. The latter shows steatosis. Note the very mild portal inflammation (below right). (Needle biopsy, H&E.)

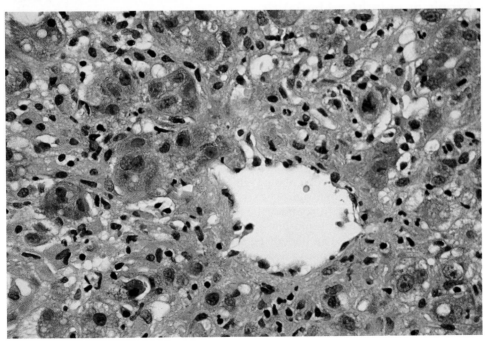

Figure 8.6 Drug-induced liver injury: hepatitic type.
There is a severe lobular hepatitis with disruption of liver-cell plates and apoptosis, attributed to ecstasy (3,4-methylenedi-oxymethamphetamine). The patient is the second of the two reported by Fidler and colleagues.[18] (Needle biopsy, H&E.)

even fatal disease.[75] In milder cases, removal of the drug usually leads to rapid improvement. Later uncommon outcomes also include cirrhosis and the development of autoimmune hepatitis (AIH).[76]

Differential diagnosis

Box 8.1 Features sometimes associated with drug-induced hepatitis
Demarcated perivenular (acinar zone 3) necrosis
Minimal hepatitis with canalicular cholestasis
Poorly developed portal inflammatory reaction
Abundant neutrophils
Abundant eosinophils
Epithelioid-cell granulomas

The possibility of drug idiosyncrasy should be considered in all patients with acute hepatitis, because in many cases the histological appearances are identical to those of viral hepatitis. A higher than usual degree of suspicion should be aroused when the hepatitis is histologically unusual (**Box 8.1**). Well-demarcated centrilobular confluent necrosis (**Fig. 8.5**) is common. There may be a very mild lobular hepatitis together with canalicular cholestasis. The portal inflammatory reaction may be poorly developed or even absent. Conversely, the portal infiltrate may be unusually rich in neutrophils or eosinophils, although the latter are neither proof of drug aetiology nor necessary for its diagnosis. The presence of epithelioid-cell granulomas increases the likelihood that drug idiosyncrasy is the correct diagnosis.

Chronic drug-induced hepatitis

Evolution of drug hepatotoxicity to chronic liver disease is relatively uncommon and usually requires prolonged or repeated exposure to the injurious agent.[77–79] The spectrum of histological changes includes chronic hepatitis, intrahepatic bile duct injury, ductopenia and chronic cholestasis, fibrosis and/or cirrhosis[39] A condition closely resembling AIH, with positive serum autoantibodies and active lymphoplasmacytic interface hepatitis on biopsy, may develop with certain drugs[80,81] (in the United States, most often due to nitrofurantoin[80,82] and minocycline[80,81,83]). Other drugs, herbal agents or dietary supplements have also been implicated, including methyldopa (**Fig. 8.7**), statins,[84,84a] diclofenac,[85] black cohosh and Ma huang.[81] The histological distinction between idiopathic AIH and DILI is often difficult.[86] Idiopathic AIH is favoured by the presence of more active interface hepatitis, portal, periportal and lobular plasma cells, rosettes, a higher stage of fibrosis and the presence of cirrhosis. Eosinophils may be seen in both AIH or DILI and therefore are not useful for discrimination.[86] In contrast, the presence of neutrophils in portal tracts and cholestasis within hepatocytes and bile canaliculi lends support for DILI.[86] Those cases where a drug has unmasked an underlying AIH often become clear when relapse occurs after withdrawal of immunosuppression.[85]

Differential diagnosis

Chronic viral hepatitis and AIH constitute the major histological differential diagnosis of chronic drug-induced hepatitis. Since some cases of acute hepatitis A virus (HAV) infection show abundant portal and periportal plasma cells with interface hepatitis on biopsy (therein resembling idiopathic AIH), acute HAV infection should be excluded by serum testing for IgM antibody to HAV.

Steatohepatitis

Steatohepatitis refers to a specific form of hepatic injury characterised by steatosis, hepatocellular ballooning, Mallory body formation, inflammation and pericellular fibrosis,

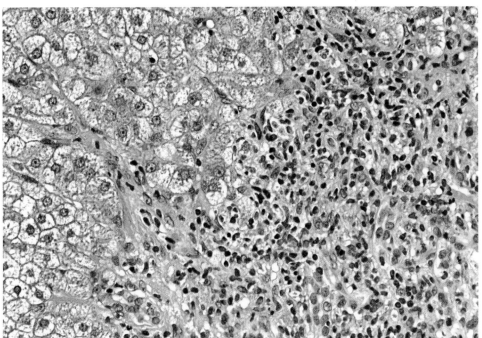

Figure 8.7 Drug-induced chronic hepatitis. Liver damage, here attributed to methyldopa, has taken the form of extensive interface hepatitis. There is a heavy lymphoplasmacytic infiltrate. (Needle biopsy, H&E.)

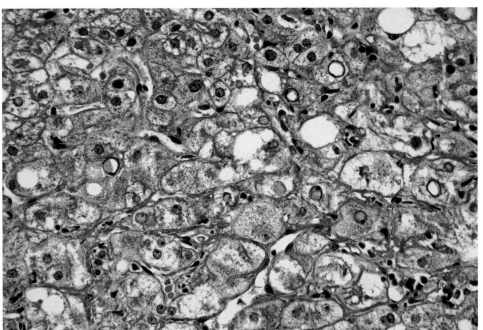

Figure 8.8 Steatohepatitis attributed to tamoxifen toxicity. Hepatocytes in the lower part of the field are swollen and surrounded by collagen, stained blue. There is also steatosis and nuclear vacuolation. (Needle biopsy, trichrome.) The patient is the third of the three reported by Pinto and colleagues.[91] (The biopsy was kindly provided by Professor Amelia Baptista, Lisbon, Portugal.)

sometimes progressing to cirrhosis. The most common cause is alcohol abuse (**see Ch. 7**). Drugs are among the causes of non-alcoholic steatohepatitis (NASH). Incriminated agents include synthetic oestrogens,[87] amiodarone[41,88] and tamoxifen[89–91] (**Fig. 8.8**). Similar changes are sometimes seen in patients on parenteral nutrition[47] and in industrial workers exposed to volatile petrochemical products.[22] In the case of amiodarone, steatosis itself

Figure 8.9 Hypervitaminosis A. Prominent, hypertrophied stellate cells with lipid vacuoles and peripheral dark, compressed nuclei are seen between hepatocytes, in perisinusoidal spaces (arrows). Some of the stellate cells are multivesicular (arrowheads). (Needle biopsy, H&E.)

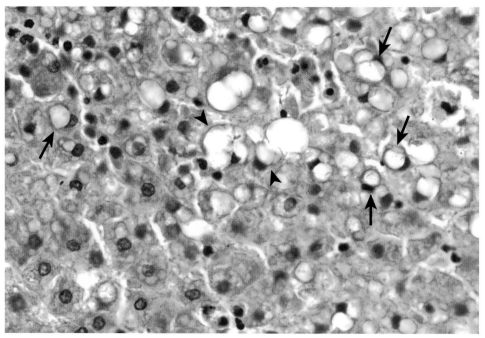

may be mild or absent,[92] but otherwise there is a close resemblance to other forms of NASH and to alcoholic steatohepatitis, including the potential for cirrhosis. However, amiodarone-related steatohepatitis has a periportal predilection, in contrast to the perivenular distribution seen with other causes of steatohepatitis. It is interesting to note that some patients with reported drug-related steatohepatitis were also obese,[91] which raises the possibility of an interaction between drug and other factors.

Fibrosis and cirrhosis

As already stated, cirrhosis may result from chronic drug-induced hepatitis. Progressive fibrosis and portal hypertension in a non-hepatitic setting are known complications of long-term exposure to arsenic or vinyl chloride. Excess intake of vitamin A (hypervitaminosis A) affects hepatic stellate cells which may appear unusually prominent[93] (**Fig. 8.9**). Perisinusoidal fibrosis, veno-occlusive disease and cirrhosis[26] are other consequences.

Pathologists are sometimes asked to report on liver biopsies from patients given or about to receive long-term methotrexate for psoriasis or rheumatoid arthritis. Although methotrexate was initially considered to be a potent hepatotoxin, doubt has more recently been thrown on its potential to cause serious liver disease in the absence of additional risk factors.[94] These include regular or heavy alcohol intake[95] and obesity.[96] Significant liver injury is reputedly less common in patients with rheumatoid arthritis than in those with psoriasis. Histological abnormalities attributed to methotrexate include steatosis, hepatocyte pleomorphism, portal fibrosis and inflammation, formation of fibrous septa extending from the portal tracts (**Fig. 8.10**) and cirrhosis. A grading system for methotrexate liver injury was developed by Roenigk and colleagues which scores the degree of fat, inflammation and fibrosis.[97] Minor changes such as focal necrosis and steatosis are common in baseline pretreatment biopsies, and are presumably related to the underlying disease (e.g. psoriasis) or to additional risk factors. Periportal septum formation is more likely to be due to methotrexate, whereas fibrosis mainly in perivenular regions should lead to suspicion of alcohol abuse or NASH.

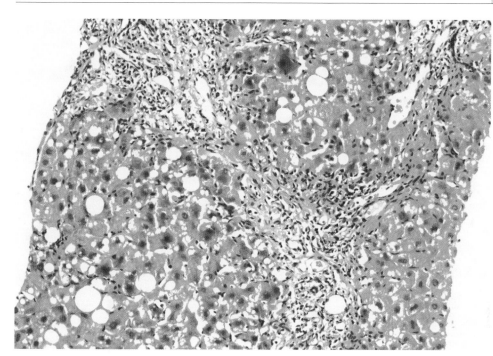

Figure 8.10 Liver damage attributed to methotrexate. Two portal tracts in this field show chronic inflammation and fibrosis extending outwards. The parenchyma shows steatosis. (Needle biopsy, H&E.)

Steroid-induced cholestasis

Steroid-induced cholestasis[98,99] lies on the borderline between intrinsic and idiosyncratic hepatotoxicity. On the one hand, it is reproducible in laboratory animals and some steroids cause biochemical abnormalities in humans in a predictable and dose-dependent manner. On the other hand, clinical liver disease cannot be predicted in the individual patient and is seen in only a small proportion of patients receiving anabolic or contraceptive steroids. Patients susceptible to contraceptive steroid-induced jaundice are also prone to develop cholestasis in late pregnancy.

The histological picture is one of canalicular cholestasis in perivenular areas, with little or no necrosis or inflammation beyond that attributable to the cholestasis itself (**Fig. 8.11**). Isolated hepatocytes may undergo feathery degeneration, and in prolonged cholestasis liver-cell rosettes are a common finding. Portal tracts usually remain normal but may be minimally inflamed. Because of the lack of necrosis and inflammation, this type of lesion is sometimes known as pure or bland cholestasis.

Differential diagnosis

The differential diagnosis is from other causes of bland cholestasis such as benign recurrent intrahepatic cholestasis, which is discussed in detail in **Chapter 5**.

Idiosyncratic drug-induced cholestasis

Idiosyncratic drug-induced cholestasis, typified by chlorpromazine jaundice[100] but also caused by many other drugs, differs from bland cholestasis in that some degree of portal inflammation is usually present (**Fig. 8.12**). There is sometimes inflammatory infiltration of the lobules and evidence of hepatocellular damage. Zimmerman and Ishak[101] therefore refer to this type of lesion as 'hepatocanalicular'. The portal infiltrate often includes eosinophils and these are occasionally abundant, but their absence does not exclude a

**Figure 8.11
Anabolic-
androgenic steroid
cholestasis.**
Bile canalicular
cholestasis is
prominent and
accentuated near
the efferent vein at
centre. (Needle
biopsy, H&E.)

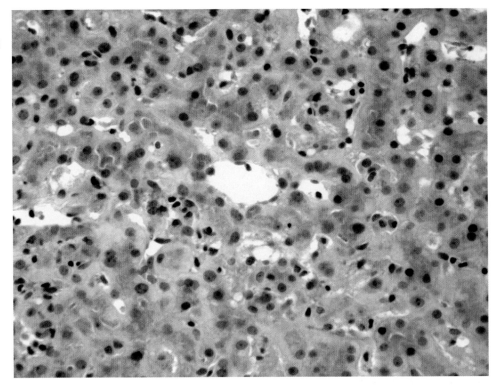

**Figure 8.12
Drug-induced
liver injury:
hepatocanalicular
type.**
In this patient with
jaundice following
chlorpromazine
therapy there is mild
inflammation of the
portal tract (lower
left) and swelling of
hepatocytes,
especially in the
perivenular area
(above, centre and
right). (Needle
biopsy, H&E.)

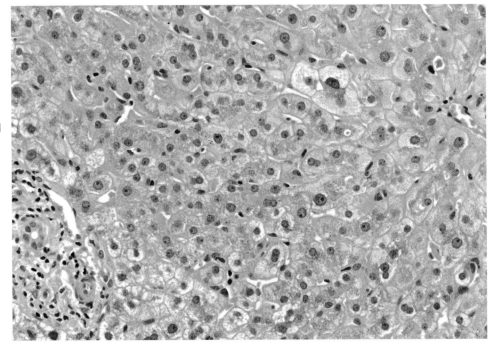

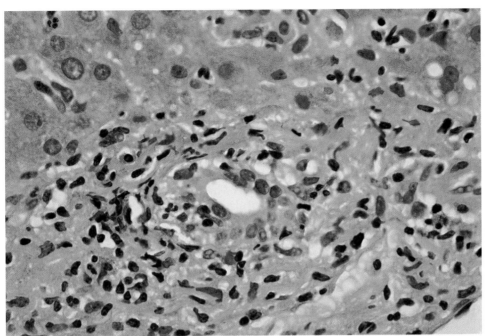

Figure 8.13 Drug-induced liver injury: hepatocanalicular type.
An inflamed portal tract from a patient with jaundice attributed to Augmentin (amoxicillin and clavulanic acid). The epithelium of an interlobular bile duct is irregular, vacuolated and infiltrated by lymphocytes. (Needle biopsy, H&E.) (Biopsy kindly provided by Dr Karin Oien, Glasgow, UK.)

diagnosis of drug-induced hepatocanalicular cholestasis. Small interlobular ducts often show abnormalities such as irregular distribution of epithelial cell nuclei, cytoplasmic vacuolation, variation in nuclear size and infiltration by lymphocytes. These changes are usually mild, but occasionally more severe (**Fig. 8.13**), even leading to ductopenia (see **vanishing bile duct syndrome**, below). The lobular changes (**Fig. 8.12**) are as in bland cholestasis, except for the additional element of inflammation and necrosis which is sometimes found, as mentioned above. There is therefore a spectrum of appearances in this type of cholestasis, from an almost bland cholestatic lesion to one resembling mild acute viral hepatitis. Even in the absence of necrosis and inflammation, hepatocellular changes are seen which possibly result from prolonged cholestasis itself, but which may also include an element of adaptive proliferation of the smooth endoplasmic reticulum. These changes include prominent hepatocellular swelling, abundant pale-staining cytoplasm and, commonly, multinucleation. Mitotic figures may be evident.[100]

Differential diagnosis

The differential diagnosis of idiosyncratic drug-induced cholestasis is from bile-duct obstruction, acute viral- or drug-induced hepatitis, and cholestasis of the bland type. Portal oedema, prominent neutrophils, marked ductular reaction and absence of lobular inflammation favour the first. In the absence of substantial portal inflammation the distinction between idiosyncratic drug jaundice and bland steroid-induced cholestasis becomes difficult to make and requires clinical information. In such circumstances bile-duct obstruction cannot be completely ruled out. The differential diagnosis also includes other causes of bland cholestasis, such as benign recurrent cholestasis (**see Ch. 4**). Severe liver-cell damage and inflammation favour viral hepatitis or the drug injury of hepatitic type, already discussed.

The clinical course of idiosyncratic drug jaundice varies. In most patients removal of the offending drug leads to rapid improvement. Occasionally the cholestasis is slow to improve but liver biopsy shows cholestasis only, with no fibrosis or other evidence of progressive disease. In rare instances true chronic disease develops on the basis of severe bile-duct damage and duct loss, with consequent fibrosis and other features of chronic biliary disease. The clinical picture resembles primary biliary cirrhosis. This **vanishing bile duct syndrome** has been reported after a number of drugs,[102,103] including chlorpromazine,[100] a combination of chlorpropamide with erythromycin ethylsuccinate,[104] prochlorperazine,[105] gold salts,[106] ciprofloxacin,[107] haloperidol,[108] ajmaline,[109] glycyrrhizin,[110] and amoxicillin and flucloxacillin,[111] among others. Augmentin (amoxicillin and clavulanic acid; **Fig. 8.13**) is a well-documented cause of cholestasis, with striking focal destruction of bile ducts in some biopsies.[112–115] This is occasionally associated with granuloma formation. Prolonged cholestasis may be the result of the duct damage and, in some patients, of duct loss.

More acute bile-duct injury is seen in poisoning with the herbicide paraquat.[116,117] Zimmerman and Ishak[101] designate this type of injury as ductal or cholangiodestructive, in contrast to canalicular and hepatocanalicular cholestasis.

Long-term parenteral nutrition, already noted in relation to steatosis and steatohepatitis in adults, may be associated in infants and children with a progressive form of liver injury, typified by cholestasis, hepatocellular damage, ductular reaction, fibrosis and even cirrhosis.[47,48,118] Whether the parenteral nutrition itself is responsible for all these changes is not proven.[48,49] The lesion may mimic bile-duct obstruction[119] (**see Fig. 13.18**).

Granulomas

Drugs are an important cause of otherwise unexplained granulomas. They are sometimes the only or main manifestation of a drug reaction, but can also form part of a cholestatic or hepatitic picture.[88] The granulomas may be portal (**Fig. 8.14**), parenchymal, or both. They usually show little or no necrosis, and are infiltrated by a variety of inflammatory cells, including plasma cells and eosinophils. Allopurinol has been reported to cause granulomas of the fibrin-ring type.[120] The list of drugs associated with hepatic granulomas

Figure 8.14 Drug-induced granuloma formation.

A portal tract contains a granuloma with many multinucleated giant cells. The patient became jaundiced after taking phenylbutazone. (Needle biopsy, H&E.)

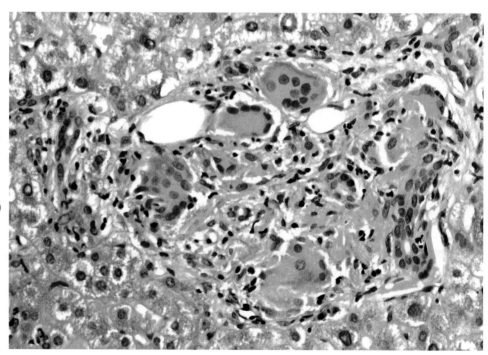

is small compared with the list of those causing hepatitis or cholestasis, but it is nevertheless substantial.[101,121,122]

Other lesions

Drugs may produce other hepatic lesions such as **nodular regenerative hyperplasia,**[123] as described with the combined chemotherapy agents 5-fluorouracil and oxaliplatin.[124]

Veno-occlusive disease, sinusoidal obstruction syndrome (**see Fig. 16.23**) and obliterative venopathy are other consequences of chemotherapy.[125]

References

1 Navarro VJ, Senior JR. Drug-related hepatotoxicity. N Engl J Med 2006;354:731–9.

2 Fontana RJ. Pathogenesis of idiosyncratic drug-induced liver injury and clinical perspectives. Gastroenterology 2014;46:914–28.

3 Stickel F, Patsenker E, Schuppan D. Herbal hepatotoxicity. J Hepatol 2005;43:901–10.

4 Fogden E, Neuberger J. Alternative medicines and the liver. Liver Int 2003;23:213–20.

5 Teschke R, Wolff A, Frenzel C, et al. Herbal hepatotoxicity: a tabular compilation of reported cases. Liver Int 2012;32:1543–56.

6 Navarro VJ, Seeff LB. Liver injury induced by herbal complementary and alternative medicine. Clin Liver Dis 2013;17:715–35.

7 Stickel F, Kessebohm K, Weimann R, et al. Review of liver injury associated with dietary supplements. Liver Int 2011;31:595–605.

8 Elinav E, Pinsker G, Safadi R, et al. Association between consumption of Herbalife® nutritional supplements and acute hepatotoxicity. J Hepatol 2007;47:514–20.

9 Schoepfer AM, Engel A, Fattinger K, et al. Herbal does not mean innocuous: ten cases of severe hepatotoxicity associated with dietary supplements from Herbalife® products.

10 Stickel F. Slimming at all costs: Herbalife-induced liver injury. J Hepatol 2007;47:444–6.

11 Kanel GC, Cassidy W, Shuster L, et al. Cocaine-induced liver cell injury: comparison of morphological features in man and in experimental models. Hepatology 1990;11:646–51.

12 Trigueiro de Araújo MS, Gerard F, Chossegros P, et al. Vascular hepatotoxicity related to heroin addiction. Virchows Arch [A] 1990;417:497–503.

13 Wanless IR, Dore S, Gopinath N, et al. Histopathology of cocaine hepatotoxicity. Report of four patients. Gastroenterology 1990;98:497–501.

14 Mallat A, Dhumeaux D. Cocaine and the liver. J Hepatol 1991;12:275–8.

15 Silva MO, Roth D, Reddy KR, et al. Hepatic dysfunction accompanying acute cocaine intoxication. J Hepatol 1991;12:312–15.

16 McIntyre AS, Long RG. Fatal fulminant hepatic failure in a 'solvent abuser'. Postgrad Med J 1992;68:29–30.

17 Ellis AJ, Wendon JA, Portmann B, et al. Acute liver damage and ecstasy ingestion. Gut 1996;38:454–8.

18 Fidler H, Dhillon A, Gertner D, et al. Chronic ecstasy (3,4-methylenedioxymethamphetamine) abuse: a recurrent and unpredictable cause of severe acute hepatitis. J Hepatol 1996;25:563–6.

19 Milroy CM, Clark JC, Forrest ARW. Pathology of deaths associated with 'ecstasy' and 'eve' misuse. J Clin Pathol 1996;49:149–53.

20 Brenard R, Laterre P-F, Reynaert M, et al. Increased hepatocyte mitotic activity as a diagnostic marker of acute arsenic intoxication. A report of two cases. J Hepatol 1996;25:218–20.

21 Hoet P, Graf MLM, Bourdi M, et al. Epidemic of liver disease caused by hydrochlorofluorocarbons used as ozone-sparing substitutes of chlorofluorocarbons. Lancet 1997;350:556–9.

22 Cotrim HP, Andrade ZA, Parana R, et al. Nonalcoholic steatohepatitis: a toxic liver disease in industrial workers. Liver 1999;19:299–304.

23 Kahl R. Toxic liver injury. In: Bircher J, Benhamou J-P, McIntyre N, et al., editors. Oxford Textbook of Clinical Hepatology. 2nd ed. Oxford: Oxford University Press; 1999. p. 1319 [chapter 18].

24 Cave M, Falkner KC, Ray M, et al. Toxicant-associated steatohepatitis in vinyl chloride workers. Hepatology 2010;51:474–81.

25 Bioulac-Sage P, Quinton A, Saric J, et al. Chance discovery of hepatic fibrosis in patient with asymptomatic hypervitaminosis A. Arch Pathol Lab Med 1988;112:505–9.

26 Jorens PG, Michielsen PP, Pelckmans PA, et al. Vitamin A abuse: development of cirrhosis despite cessation of vitamin A. A six-year clinical and histopathologic follow-up. Liver 1992;12:381–6.

27 Galler GW, Weisenberg E, Brasitus TA. Mushroom poisoning: the role of orthotopic liver transplantation. J Clin Gastroenterol 1992;15:229–32.

28 Nagai K, Hosaka H, Kubo S, et al. Vitamin A toxicity secondary to excessive intake of yellow-green vegetables, liver and laver. J Hepatol 1999;31:142–8.

29 Silva MO, Reddy KR, Jeffers LJ, et al. Interferon-induced chronic active hepatitis? Gastroenterology 1991;101:840–2.

30 Stricker GHC. Drug-Induced Hepatic Injury. 2nd ed. Amsterdam: Elsevier; 1992.

31 Lindgren A, Aldenborg F, Norkrans G, et al. Paracetamol-induced cholestatic and granulomatous liver injuries. J Int Med 1997;241:435–9.

32 Andrade RJ, Lucena MI, Garcia-Escaño MD, et al. Severe idiosyncratic acute hepatic injury caused by paracetamol (Letter). J Hepatol 1998;28:1078.

33 Kenna JG. Immunoallergic drug-induced hepatitis: lessons from halothane. J Hepatol 1997;26(Suppl. 1):5–12.

34 Robin M-A, Le Roy M, Descatoire V, et al. Plasma membrane cytochromes P450 as neoantigens and autoimmune targets in drug-induced hepatitis. J Hepatol 1997;26(Suppl. 1):23–30.

35 Eliasson E, Stål POA, Lytton S. Expression of autoantibodies to specific cytochromes P450 in a case of disulfiram hepatitis. J Hepatol 1998;29:819–25.

36 Grieco A, Vecchio FM, Greco AV, et al. Cholestatic hepatitis due to ticlopidine: clinical and histological recovery after drug withdrawal. Case report and review of the literature. J Hepatol 1998;10:713–15.

37 Agarwal VK, McHutcdhison J, Hoofnagle JH. Important elements for the diagnosis of drug-induced liver injury. Clin Gastroenterol Hepatol 2010;8:463–70.

38 Aithal GP, Watkins PB, Andrade RJ, et al. Case definition and phenotype standardization in drug-induced liver injury. Clin Pharmacol Ther 2011;89:806–15.

39 Kleiner DE, Chalasani NP, Lee WM, et al. Hepatic histological findings in suspected drug-induced liver injury: systemic evaluation and clinical associations. Hepatology 2014;59:661–70.

40 Paiva LA, Wright PJ, Koff RS. Long-term hepatic memory for hypersensitivity to nitrofurantoin. Am J Gastroenterol 1992;87:891–3.

41 Lewis JH, Mullick F, Ishak KG, et al. Histopathologic analysis of suspected amiodarone hepatotoxicity. Hum Pathol 1990;21:59–67.

42 Benjamin SB, Ishak KG, Zimmerman HJ, et al. Phenylbutzone liver injury: a clinical-pathologic survey of 23 cases and review of the literature. Hepatology 1981;1:255–63.

43 Banks AT, Zimmerman HJ, Ishak KG, et al. Diclofenac-associated hepatotoxicity: analysis of 180 cases reported to the Food and Drug Administration as adverse reactions. Hepatology 1995;22:820–7.

44 Van Steenbergen W, Peeters P, De Bondt J, et al. Nimesulide-induced acute hepatitis: evidence from six cases. J Hepatol 1998;29:135–41.

45 Jezequel AM, Librari ML, Mosca P, et al. Changes induced in human liver by long-term anticonvulsant therapy. Functional and ultrastructural data. Liver 1984;4:307–17.

46 Pamperl H, Gradner W, Fridrich L, et al. Influence of long-term anticonvulsant treatment on liver ultrastructure in man. Liver 1984;4:294–300.

47 Klein S, Nealon WH. Hepatobiliary abnormalities associated with total parenteral nutrition. Semin Liver Dis 1988;8:237–46.

48 Quigley EM, Marsh MN, Shaffer JL, et al. Hepatobiliary complications of total parenteral nutrition. Gastroenterology 1993;104:286–301.

49 Wolfe BM, Walker BK, Shaul DB, et al. Effect of total parenteral nutrition on hepatic histology. Arch Surg 1988;123:1084–90.

50 Landas SK, Mitros FA, Furst DE, et al. Lipogranulomas and gold in the liver in rheumatoid arthritis. Am J Surg Pathol 1992;16:171–4.

51 Fromenty B, Berson A, Pessayre D. Microvesicular steatosis and steatohepatitis: role of mitochondrial dysfunction and lipid peroxidation. J Hepatol 1997;26(Suppl. 1):13–22.

52 Zimmerman HJ, Ishak KG. Valproate-induced hepatic injury: analyses of 23 fatal cases. Hepatology 1982;2:591–7.

52a Hynynen J, Komulainen T, Tukiainen B, et al. Acute liver failure after valproate exposure in patients with *POLG1* mutations and the prognosis after liver transplantation. Liver Transplant 2014;20:1402–12.

53 Kleiner DE, Gaffey MJ, Sallie R, et al. Histopathologic changes associated with fialuridine hepatotoxicity. Mod Pathol 1997;10:192–9.

54 Chariot P, Drogou I, de Lacroix-Szmania I, et al. Zidovudine-induced mitochondrial disorder with massive liver steatosis, myopathy, lactic acidosis, and mitochondrial DNA depletion. J Hepatol 1999;30:156–60.

55 Van Huyen J-PD, Batisse D, Heudes D, et al. Alteration of cytochrome oxidase subunit I labeling is associated with severe mitochondriopathy in NRTI-related hepatotoxicity in HIV patients. Mod Pathol 2006;19:1277–88.

56 Spengler U, Lichterfeld M, Rockstroh JK. Antiretroviral drug toxicity – a challenge for the hepatologist? J Hepatol 2002;36:283–94.

57 Clark SJ, Creighton S, Portmann B, et al. Acute liver failure associated with antiretroviral treatment for HIV: a report of six cases. J Hepatol 2002;36:295–301.

58 Núñez M. Clinical syndromes and consequences of antiretroviral-related hepatotoxicity. Hepatology 2010;52:1143–55.

59 Muñoz SJ, Martinez-Hernandez A, Maddrey WC. Intrahepatic cholestasis and phospholipidosis associated with the use of trimethoprim–sulfamethoxazole. Hepatology 1990;12:342–7.

60 Degott C, Messing B, Moreau D, et al. Liver phospholipidosis induced by parenteral nutrition: histologic, biochemical, and ultrastructural investigations. Gastroenterology 1988;95:183–91.

61 Vazquez JJ, Guillen FJ, Zozaya J, et al. Cyanamide-induced liver injury. A predictable lesion. Liver 1983;3:225–30.

62 Bruguera M, Lamar C, Bernet M, et al. Hepatic disease associated with ground-glass inclusions in hepatocytes after cyanamide therapy. Arch Pathol Lab Med 1986;110:906–10.

63 Yokoyama A, Sato S, Maruyama K, et al. Cyanamide-associated alcoholic liver disease: a sequential histological evaluation. Alcohol Clin Exp Res 1995;19:1307–11.

64 Portmann B, Talbot IC, Day DW, et al. Histopathological changes in the liver following a paracetamol overdose: correlation with clinical and biochemical parameters. J Pathol 1975;117:169–81.

65 Antoine DJ, Dear JW, Lewis PS, et al. Mechanistic biomarkers provide early and sensitive detection of acetaminophen-induced acute liver injury at first presentation to hospital. Hepatology 2013;58: 777–87.

66 Ju C. Damage-associated molecular patterns: their iimpact on the liver and beyond during acetaminophen overdose. Hepatology 2012;56:1599–601.

67 Jaeschke H, Williams CD, Ramachandran A, et al. Acetaminophen hepatotoxicity and repair: the role of sterile inflammation and innate immunity. Liver Int 2012;32:8–20.

68 Maddrey WC. Hepatic effects of acetaminophen. Enhanced toxicity in alcoholics. J Clin Gastroenterol 1987;9:180–5.

69 Baerg RD, Kimberg DV. Centrilobular hepatic necrosis and acute renal failure in 'solvent sniffers. Ann Intern Med 1970;73:713–20.

70 Perino LE, Warren GH, Levine JS. Cocaine-induced hepatotoxicity in humans. Gastroenterology 1987;93:176–80.

71 Andreu V, Mas A, Bruguera M, et al. Ecstasy: a common cause of severe acute hepatotoxicity. J Hepatol 1998;29:394–7.

72 Mitchell I, Wendon J, Fitt S, et al. Antituberculous therapy and acute liver failure. Lancet 1995;345:555–6.

73 Neuberger J. Halothane hepatitis. Eur J Gastroentrol Hepatol 1998;10:631–3.

74 Lo SK, Wendon J, Mieli-Vergani G, et al. Halothane-induced acute liver failure: continuing occurrence and use of liver transplantation. Eur J Gastroenterol Hepatol 1998;10:635–9.

75 Paterson D, Kerlin P, Walker N, et al. Piroxicam induced submassive necrosis of the liver. Gut 1992;33:1436–8.

76 Björnsson E, Davidsdottir L. The long-term follow-up after idiosyncratic drug-induced liver injury with jaundice. J Hepatol 2009;50:511–17.

77 Aithal PG, Day CP. The natural history of histologically proved drug induced liver disease. Gut 1999;44:731–5.

78 Björnsson E, Davidsdottir L. The long-term follow-up after idiosyncratic drug-induced injury with jaundice. J Hepatol 2009;50:511–17.

79 Andrade RJ, Lucena MI, Kaplowitz N, et al. Outcome of acute idiosyncratic drug-induced liver injury: long-term follow-up in a hepatotoxicity registry. Hepatology 2006;44:1581–8.

80 Björnsson E, Talwalkar J, Treeprasertsuk S, et al. Drug-induced autoimmune hepatitis: clinical characteristics and prognosis. Hepatology 2010;51:2040–8.

81 Czaja AJ. Drug-induced autoimmune-like hepatitis. Dig Dis Sci 2011;56:958–76.

82 Sharp JR, Ishak KG, Zimmerman HJ. Chronic active hepatitis and severe hepatic necrosis associated with nitrofurantoin. Ann Intern Med 1980;92:14–19.

83 Gough A, Chapman S, Wagstaff K, et al. Minocycline induced autoimmune hepatitis and systemic lupus erythematosus-like syndrome. BMJ 1996;312:169–72.

84 Russo MW, Scobey M, Bonkovsky HL. Drug-induced liver injury associated with statins. Semin Liver Dis 2009;29:412–22.

84a Russo MW, Hoofnagle JH, Gu J, et al. Spectrum of statin hepatotoxicity: experience of the Drug-Induced Liver Injury Network. Hepatology 2014;60:679–86.

85 Scully LJ, Clarke D, Barr RJ. Diclofenac induced hepatitis. Three cases with features of autoimmune chronic active hepatitis. Dig Dis Sci 1993;38:744–51.

86 Suzuki A, Brunt EM, Kleiner DE, et al. The use of liver biopsy evaluation in discrimination of idiopathic autoimmune hepatitis versus drug-induced liver injury. Hepatology 2011;54:931–9.

87 Seki K, Minami Y, Nishikawa M, et al. 'Nonalcoholic steatohepatitis' induced by massive doses of synthetic estrogen. Gastroenterol Japon 1983;18:197–203.

88 Harrison RF, Elias E. Amiodarone-associated cirrhosis with hepatic and lymph node granulomas. Histopathology 1993;22:80–2.

89 Van Hoof M, Rahier J, Horsmans Y. Tamoxifen-induced steatohepatitis [letter]. Ann Intern Med 1996;124:855–6.

90 Cai Q, Bensen M, Greene R, et al. Tamoxifen-induced transient multifocal hepatic fatty infiltration. Am J Gastroenterol 2000;95:277–9.

91 Pinto HC, Baptista A, Camilo ME, et al. Tamoxifen-associated steatohepatitis – report of three cases. J Hepatol 1995;23:95–7.

92 Chang C-C, Petrelli M, Tomashefski JFJ, et al. Severe intrahepatic cholestasis caused by amiodarone toxicity after withdrawal of the drug. A case report and review of the literature. Arch Pathol Lab Med 1999;123:251–6.

93 Nollevaux M-C, Guiot Y, Horsmans Y, et al. Hypervitaminosis A-induced liver fibrosis: stellate cell activation and daily dose consumption. Liver Int 2006;26:182–6.

94 Tang H, Neuberger J. Review article: methotrexate in gastroenterology – dangerous villain or simply misunderstood? Aliment Pharmacol Ther 1996; 10:851–8.

95 Whiting OK, Fye KH, Sack KD. Methotrexate and histologic hepatic abnormalities: a meta-analysis. Am J Med 1991;90:711–16.

96 Newman M, Auerbach R, Feiner H, et al. The role of liver biopsies in psoriatic patients receiving long-term methotrexate treatment. Improvement in liver abnormalities after cessation of treatment. Arch Dermatol 1989;125:1218–24.

97 Roenigk HH Jr, Auerbach R, Maibach HI, et al. Methotrexate guidelines – revised. J Am Acad Dermatol 1982;6:145–55.

98 Sánchez-Osorio M, Duarte-Rojo A, Martinez-Benitez B, et al. Anabolic–androgenic steroids and liver injury. Liver Int 2008;28:278–82.

99 Ishak KG. Hepatic lesions caused by anabolic and contraceptive steroids. Semin Liver Dis 1981;1: 116–28.

100 Ishak KG, Irey NS. Hepatic injury associated with the phenothiazines. Clinicopathologic and follow-up study of 36 patients. Arch Pathol 1972;93:283–304.

101 Zimmerman HJ, Ishak KG. Hepatic injury due to drugs and toxins. In: MacSween RNM, Burt AD, Portmann BC, et al., editors. Pathology of the Liver. 4th ed. Edinburgh: Churchill Livingstone; 2002. p. 621 [chapter 14].

102 Degott C, Feldmann G, Larrey D, et al. Drug-induced prolonged cholestasis in adults: a histological semi-quantitative study demonstrating progressive ductopenia. Hepatology 1992;15:244–51.

103 Desmet VJ. Vanishing bile duct syndrome in drug-induced liver disease. J Hepatol 1997;26(Suppl. 1):31–5.

104 Geubel AP, Nakad A, Rahier J, et al. Prolonged cholestasis and disappearance of interlobular bile ducts following chlorpropamide and erythromycin ethylsuccinate. Case of drug interaction? Liver 1988;8:350–3.

105 Lok ASF, Ng IOL. Prochlorperazine-induced chronic cholestasis. J Hepatol 1988;6:369–73.

106 Basset C, Vadrot J, Denis J, et al. Prolonged cholestasis and ductopenia following gold salt therapy. Liver Int 2003;23:89–93.

107 Bataille L, Rahier J, Geubel A. Delayed and prolonged cholestatic hepatitis with ductopenia after long-term ciprofloxacin therapy for Crohn's disease. J Hepatol 2002;37:696–9.

108 Dincsoy HP, Saelinger DA. Haloperidol-induced chronic cholestatic liver disease. Gastroenterology 1982;83:694–700.

109 Larrey D, Pessayre D, Duhamel G, et al. Prolonged cholestasis after ajmaline-induced acute hepatitis. J Hepatol 1986;2:81–7.

110 Ishii M, Miyazaki M, Yamamoto T, et al. A case of drug-induced ductopenia resulting in fatal biliary cirrhosis. Liver 1993;13:227–31.

111 Davies MH, Harrison RF, Elias E, et al. Antibiotic-associated acute vanishing bile duct syndrome: a pattern associated with severe, prolonged, intrahepatic cholestasis. J Hepatol 1994;20:112–16.

112 Richardet J-P, Mallat A, Zafrani ES, et al. Prolonged cholestasis with ductopenia after administration of amoxicillin/clavulanic acid. Dig Dis Sci 1999;44:1997–2000.

113 O'Donohue J, Oien KA, Donaldson P, et al. Co-amoxiclav jaundice: clinical and histological features and HLA class II association. Gut 2000;47:717–20.

114 Hautekeete ML, Horsmans Y, Van Waeyenberge C, et al. HLA association of amoxicillin–clavulanate-induced hepatitis. Gastroenterology 1999;117:1181–6.

115 Ryley NG, Fleming KA, Chapman RWG. Focal destructive cholangiopathy associated with amoxicillin/clavulinic acid (Augmentin). J Hepatol 1995;23:278–82.

116 Mullick FG, Ishak KG, Mahabir R, et al. Hepatic injury associated with paraquat toxicity in humans. Liver 1981;1:209–21.

117 Yang C-J, Lin J-L, Lin-Tan D-T, et al. Spectrum of toxic hepatitis following intentional paraquat ingestion: analysis of 187 cases. Liver Int 2012;32:1400–6.

118 Baker AL, Rosenberg IH. Hepatic complications of total parenteral nutrition. Am J Med 1987;82:489–97.

119 Body JJ, Bleiberg H, Bron D, et al. Total parenteral nutrition-induced cholestasis mimicking large bile duct obstruction. Histopathology 1982;6:787–92.

120 Vanderstigel M, Zafrani ES, Lejonc JL, et al. Allopurinol hypersensitivity syndrome as a cause of hepatic fibrin-ring granulomas. Gastroenterology 1986;90:188–90.

121 Ishak KG, Zimmerman HJ. Drug-induced and toxic granulomatous hepatitis. Baillières Clin Gastroenterol 1988;2:463–80.

122 Lewis JH, Kleiner DE. Hepatic injury due to drugs, chemicals and toxins. In: Burt AD, Portmann BC, Ferrell LD, editors. MacSween's Pathology of the Liver. 5th ed. Edinburgh: Churchill Livingstone/Elsevier; 2007. p. 649–760.

123 Reshamwala PA, Kleiner DE, Heller T. Nodular regenerative hyperplasia: not all nodules are created equal. Hepatology 2006;44:7–14.

124 Hubert C, Sempoux C, Horsmans Y, et al. Nodular regenerative hyperplasia: a deleterious consequence of chemotherapy for colorectal liver metastases? Liver Int 2007;27:938–43.

125 De Bruyne R, Portmann B, Samyn M, et al. Chronic liver disease related to 6-thioguanine in children with acute lymphoblastic leukaemia. J Hepatol 2006;44:407–10.

General reading

Aithal PG, Day CP. The natural history of histologically proved drug induced liver disease. Gut 1999;44:731–5.

deLemos AS, Foureau DM, Jacobs C, et al. Drug-induced liver injury with autoimmune features. Semin Liver Dis 2014;34:194–204.

Goodman ZD. Drug hepatotoxicity. Clin Liver Dis 2002;6:381–98.

Hoofnagle JH, Serrano J, Knoben JE, et al. LiverTox: a website on drug-induced liver injury. Hepatology 2013;57:873–4.

Kaplowitz N, DeLeve LD. Drug-Induced Liver Disease. 3rd ed. Waltham, MA: Academic Press; 2013.

Kleiner DE, Chalasani NP, Lee WM, et al. Hepatic histological findings in suspected drug-induced liver injury: systemic evaluation and clinical associations. Hepatology 2014;59:661–70.

Larrey D. Drug-induced liver diseases. J Hepatol 2000;32(Suppl. 1):77–88.

Leise MD, Poterucha JJ, Talwalkar JA. Drug-induced liver injury. Mayo Clin Proc 2014;89:95–106.

Lewis JH, Kleiner DE. Hepatic injury due to drugs, herbal compounds, chemicals and toxins. In: Burt AD, Portmann BC, Ferrell LD, editors. MacSween's Pathology of the Liver. 6th ed. Edinburgh: Churchill Livingstone/Elsevier; 2012. p. 645–760.

Navarro VJ, Senior JR. Drug-related hepatotoxicity. N Engl J Med 2006;354:731–9.

Ramachandran R, Kakar S. Histological patterns in drug-induced liver disease. J Clin Pathol 2009;62:481–92.

Stricker GHC. Drug-Induced Hepatic Injury. 2nd ed. Amsterdam: Elsevier; 1992.

Watkins PB, Seeff LB. Drug-induced liver injury: summary of a single topic clinical research conference. Hepatology 2006;43:618–31.

Zimmerman HJ. Hepatotoxicity: The Adverse Effects of Drugs and Other Chemicals on The Liver. Philadelphia, PA: Lippincott Williams & Wilkins; 1999.

Chronic Hepatitis

Definition and causes

Chronic hepatitis is a common reason for persistently abnormal liver function tests[1] and forms the background for the development of much cirrhosis[2] and hepatocellular carcinoma. It is defined as persistence of liver injury with raised aminotransferase levels or viral markers for more than 6 months.[3] This definition, though artificial, helps to establish a borderline in studies of acute and chronic hepatitis. In practice, however, this borderline is not always easy to draw, because acute self-limiting hepatitis is sometimes prolonged beyond 6 months and chronic hepatitis may have an acute or indefinable onset. Many chronic liver diseases have an inflammatory component, but the term chronic hepatitis is often restricted to a limited number of causes (**Box 9.1**). The pathology of chronic hepatitis in the majority is fairly characteristic: the basic lesion is portal tract-based chronic inflammation, sometimes with variable degrees of periportal interface hepatitis and/or lobular necroinflammation. Features such as interface hepatitis and lymphocytic infiltration are sometimes seen in other conditions such as primary biliary cirrhosis and primary sclerosing cholangitis, as discussed in **Chapter 5**. For the sake of clarity, a diagnosis of chronic hepatitis should therefore include the probable cause whenever possible.

Box 9.1 Classic causes of chronic hepatitis
Hepatitis B, with or without hepatitis D virus infection
Hepatitis C
Autoimmune hepatitis
Drug-induced hepatitis
Wilson's disease
Alpha-1-antitrypsin deficiency

Classification and nomenclature

The current classification is three-tiered and includes designation of the *aetiology*, the *grade* of necroinflammation and the *stage* of fibrosis/cirrhosis. This classification replaces the obsolete terms 'chronic persistent hepatitis', 'chronic active hepatitis' and 'chronic lobular hepatitis'.[4,5] The primacy of aetiology in this classification is conceptually important, since the appearances on a given liver biopsy at any one time in chronic hepatitis reflect differing pathobiologic pathways such as viral kinetics or activity (or quiescence) of the immune system. This classification system is easily used in biopsy reporting in the form of single-line diagnosis, an example being '*Chronic hepatitis B with mild activity and mild periportal fibrosis (Grade 2, Stage 2)'*. The several systems available for semi-quantitative scoring of the grade and stage are discussed in detail at the end of the chapter.

Use of liver biopsy in chronic hepatitis

Box 9.2 Uses of liver biopsy in chronic hepatitis
Establishment of the diagnosis
Diagnosis of incidental lesions
Assessment of histological activity (grading)
Evaluation of types of necrosis
Evaluation of structural changes (staging)
Clues to aetiology and possible superinfection
Immunohistochemical assessment of viral antigens
Monitoring of therapy

Liver biopsy continues to play an important role in the diagnosis and management of patients with chronic hepatitis.[6–9] Biopsy may guide decisions on when to initiate or when to stop treatment[10] and, in patients with multiple aetiological agents, may help to establish their relative importance. Examples of the latter include the patient with chronic hepatitis C who has co-morbid risk factors for non-alcoholic fatty liver disease, or the patient with thalassaemia and viral hepatitis. Large-cell and small-cell change (dysplasia), possible predictors of hepatocellular carcinoma, are sometimes found before cirrhosis develops but will be discussed with the latter, in **Chapter 10**.

Box 9.2 lists the possible reasons for liver biopsy in chronic hepatitis.

Histological features of chronic hepatitis

Portal changes

Box 9.3 Histological features of chronic type C hepatitis
Difficult to distinguish from acute hepatitis C
Often mild, but cirrhosis commonly develops
Lymphoid follicles in portal tracts
Damaged interlobular bile ducts
Lobular activity, including acidophil bodies
Large-droplet steatosis
Lymphocytes in sinusoids
Granulomas

Most small portal tracts are infiltrated to a variable extent by lymphocytes together with smaller numbers of plasma cells and occasional segmented leukocytes (**Box 9.3**). A few eosinophils are often present. Lymphoid aggregates and lymphoid follicles with germinal centres are common in, but not exclusive to, hepatitis C. Larger conducting tracts are less affected than small terminal tracts and this has to be taken into account in assessing the severity of a hepatitis.

In the mildest forms of chronic hepatitis, the infiltrate is confined to portal tracts (**Fig. 9.1**) and the margins of the tracts remain regular. In the more severe forms, infiltration extends into the adjacent parenchyma, as described below. In mild chronic hepatitis, the tracts are often enlarged and short fibrous spurs may be seen extending from them (**Fig. 9.2**). These and other structural changes are most easily evaluated in reticulin or collagen stains. Interlobular bile ducts may be damaged, as shown by irregularity of the epithelial wall, vacuolation and infiltration by lymphocytes.

Parenchymal changes
The periportal lesion: interface hepatitis

In all but the mildest forms of chronic hepatitis, the inflammatory infiltrate extends from the portal tracts into the adjacent parenchyma and there is destruction of hepatocytes

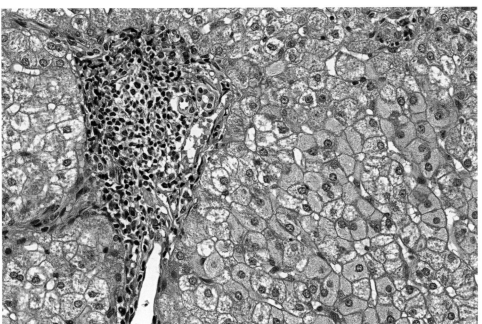

Figure 9.1 Chronic hepatitis B, mild. The portal tract is heavily infiltrated with lymphocytes. These do not extend beyond the margins of the tract, the limiting plate of hepatocytes is intact and interface hepatitis is absent. Some hepatocytes have a ground-glass appearance. (Needle biopsy, H&E.)

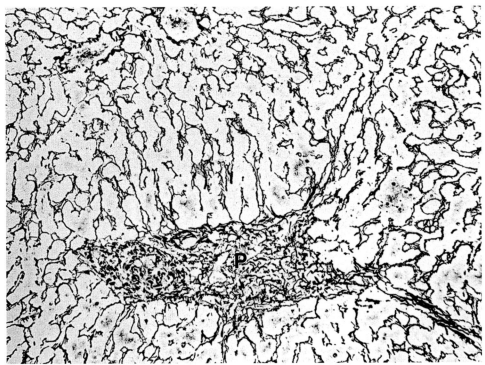

Figure 9.2 Chronic hepatitis. Short septa extend from the slightly enlarged portal tract (P) but normal architectural relationships are preserved. (Needle biopsy, reticulin.)

**Figure 9.3
Interface hepatitis.**
In contrast to the upper margin of this portal tract, the edges of the lower margin are blurred by inflammatory infiltration and hepatocyte loss. (Needle biopsy, H&E.)

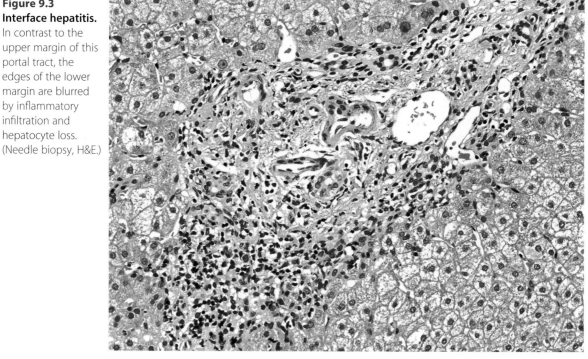

**Figure 9.4
Interface hepatitis.**
At a higher magnification than **Fig. 9.3**, lymphocytes are seen infiltrating between surviving hepatocytes. The interface between inflamed portal tract and parenchyma is irregular. (Needle biopsy, H&E.)

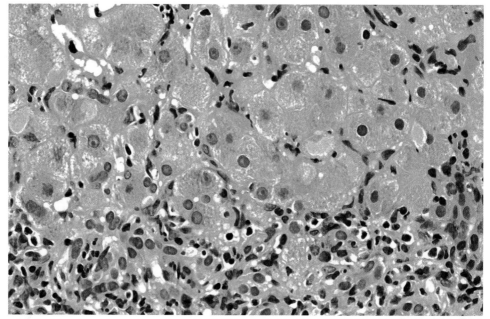

(**Figs 9.3, 9.4**). This process of interface hepatitis or piecemeal necrosis is most easily identified by the irregularity of the limiting plates of hepatocytes around the portal tracts. The term 'interface hepatitis' is now often preferred to the older term 'piecemeal necrosis' because there is evidence to suggest that apoptosis rather than necrosis may be involved.[11,12] However, the relative roles played by apoptosis and necrosis in viral hepatitis are not yet entirely clear, because the two processes share several characteristics.[13]

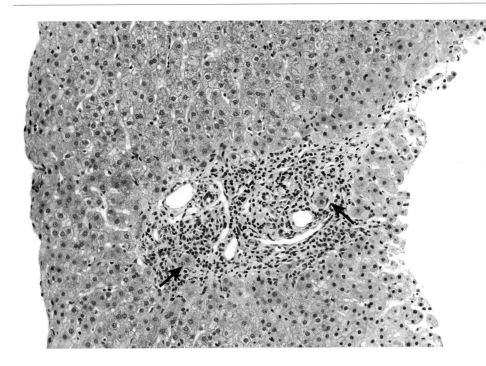

Figure 9.5
Chronic hepatitis,
mild to moderate.
The lower edge of
the portal tract
shows interface
hepatitis, with
trapping of
hepatocytes in the
infiltrate (arrows).
(Needle biopsy, H&E.)

Interface hepatitis at its mildest is recognised by lymphocytes in the periportal paren-chyma, in association with hepatocellular damage. In more severe examples, trapped surviving hepatocytes may be seen within the inflammatory infiltrate (**Fig. 9.5**) and fibrous septa extend from the portal tract (**Fig. 9.6**). In cirrhotic livers the process is seen at the edges of nodules and septa rather than immediately around portal tracts (**see Fig. 10.19**); in either case, however, the hepatitic process involves the interface between connective tissue and parenchyma.

Interface hepatitis varies not only in severity, but also in the extent of involvement of the interface, whatever its exact location. This is taken into consideration in some grading systems. With more severe interface hepatitis and liver-cell damage, periportal progenitor cells may become activated to produce a ductular reaction (proliferated bile ductules).[14] The blurring of the margins of the portal tracts in such instances then results from the combination of periportal chronic inflammatory cells and the ductular structures (**Fig. 9.7**). The presence of scattered neutrophils near the ductules should not be confused with biliary obstruction, cholangitis or a presumed drug reaction; they are normal con-stituents of the ductular reaction, mediated by cytokines expressed by the ductular cells.[15]

The lobular lesion

Deeper within the parenchyma there are varying degrees of hepatocellular damage and inflammation, sometimes called the lobular component or lobular hepatitis. Most commonly, this takes the form of focal necrosis, but confluent and bridging necrosis may also be seen. Panlobular necrosis is rare in chronic hepatitis. Also uncommon is the finding of severe lobular hepatitis in the absence of substantial portal and periportal inflammation.[16] The severity of lobular hepatitis correlates with the accumulation of pro-genitor cells.[17]

Focal (spotty) necrosis is seen as areas of hepatocyte loss with infiltration by lym-phocytes, macrophages and other cells. Each area covers the space normally occupied by up to about four or five hepatocytes (**Fig. 9.8**). Larger areas of hepatocyte loss are referred

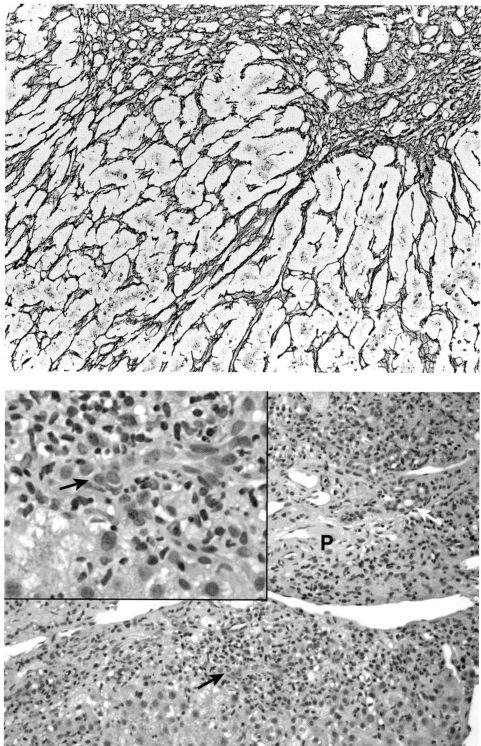

**Figure 9.6
Chronic hepatitis
with fibrosis.**
Fibrosis extends from
the portal tract
above into the
parenchyma. (Needle
biopsy, reticulin.)

Figure 9.7 Ductular reaction in chronic hepatitis with marked activity.
The margins of the portal tract (P) above and below are expanded and effaced by marked interface
hepatitis. The white arrow marks the native bile duct. Within the irregular border of interface hepatitis
at bottom are bile ductular structures (ductular reaction), one of which (arrow) is enlarged in the
inset. Inset: Scattered neutrophils surround and partially infiltrate the flattened ductule (arrow) in this
area of lymphoplasmacytic interface hepatitis. (Needle biopsy, H&E.)

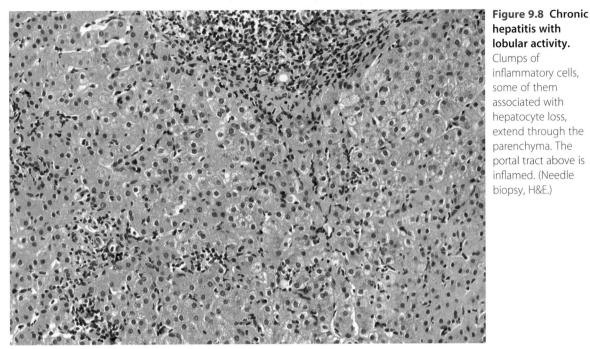

Figure 9.8 Chronic hepatitis with lobular activity. Clumps of inflammatory cells, some of them associated with hepatocyte loss, extend through the parenchyma. The portal tract above is inflamed. (Needle biopsy, H&E.)

to as confluent necrosis (**see Ch. 4**). As in acute hepatitis, bridging necrosis refers to confluent necrosis and collapse linking vascular structures and is usually restricted to bridges linking portal tracts to terminal hepatic venules.

Severe lobular hepatitis is often accompanied by the formation of small rounded or ovoid gland-like clusters of surviving hepatocytes, so-called hepatitic rosettes (**Fig. 9.9**). Unlike cholestatic rosettes (**see Ch. 4**), these are embedded in connective tissue and probably form as a result of hyperplasia of hepatocytes trapped in a collapsed and inflamed area of parenchyma.

In a minority of patients with chronic hepatitis some of the hepatocytes fuse to form multinucleated giant cells like those of neonatal hepatitis (**Fig. 9.10**). In adults this is termed *postinfantile giant-cell transformation*; it is an occasional feature of autoimmune hepatitis (AIH) and of chronic hepatitis C (with or without human immunodeficiency virus (HIV) co-infection),[18,19] typically present only in perivenular regions.

Other hepatocyte changes seen in chronic hepatitis include steatosis, iron deposition and oncocytic change. Steatosis is most common in chronic hepatitis C and is further discussed under that heading below, as is siderosis. Iron deposits are sometimes focal.[20] Substantial hepatocellular siderosis should always lead to consideration of possible hereditary haemochromatosis, but siderosis is not necessarily related to an *HFE* gene mutation.[21] Oncocytic change results from the accumulation of large numbers of closely packed mitochondria in hepatocytes, giving them a granular, densely eosinophilic appearance[22,23] (**Fig. 9.11**). These cells are most common within hepatitic rosettes. Mitochondrial hyperplasia in these cells appears to be a compensatory response to mitochondrial DNA dysfunction.[24] Finally, the appearance of bile thrombi in dilated canaliculi is most unusual in chronic hepatitis. While this type of cholestasis could result from an acute exacerbation of chronic disease, alternative explanations such as drug hepatotoxicity should be considered.

In some patients with chronic viral or AIH, distinctive eosinophilic and diastase periodic acid–Schiff (PAS)-positive inclusions are seen in sinusoidal endothelial cells[25] (**Fig. 9.12**). The inclusions have been shown to contain immunoglobulins.[26]

Figure 9.9 Chronic hepatitis, severe, with rosette formation. Parenchymal architecture has been completely disrupted. Surviving hepatocytes have formed gland-like rosettes, which are separated by bridges of collapse and inflammation. (Needle biopsy, H&E.)

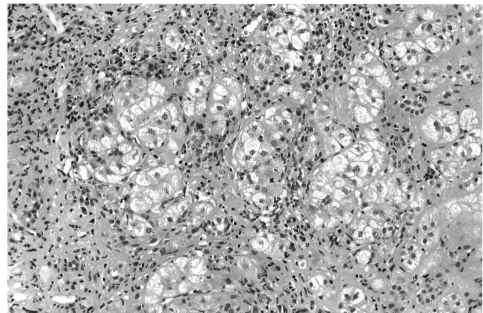

Figure 9.10 Postinfantile giant-cell transformation in chronic hepatitis. The affected perivenular hepatocytes are enlarged and pale with multiple nuclei (arrows). In adults this may be seen in autoimmune hepatitis or in chronic hepatitis C with or without human immunodeficiency virus (HIV) co-infection. (Needle biopsy, H&E.)

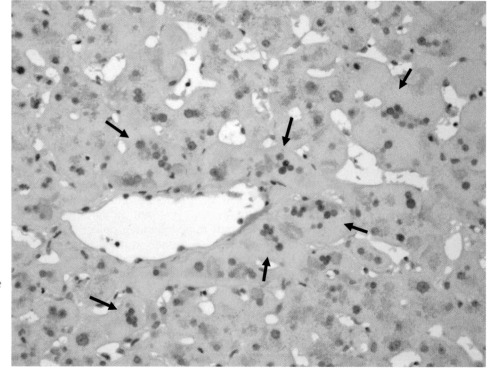

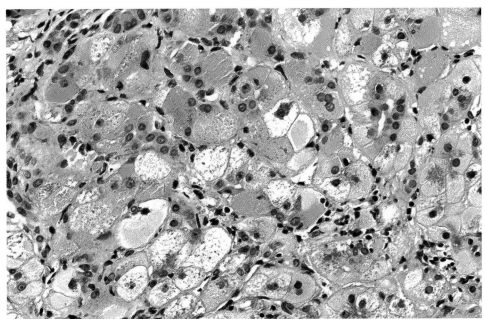

Figure 9.11 Oncocyte formation in chronic hepatitis. Some of the hepatocytes in this severe chronic hepatitis have intensely eosinophilic granular cytoplasm. Others have a ground-glass appearance. (Needle biopsy, H&E.)

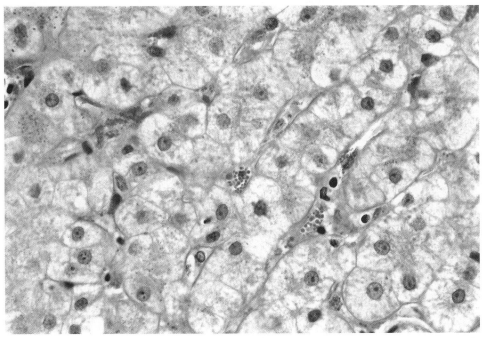

Figure 9.12 Sinusoidal inclusion-containing endothelial cells. In this example of chronic hepatitis C, multiple small granular inclusions are seen in the endothelium. (Needle biopsy, diastase–PAS.)

Individual causes of chronic hepatitis

Chronic hepatitis B and D

Chronic hepatitis B infection in both adults and children[27,28] goes through a series of phases marked by different serological, histological and immunocytochemical findings.[29] It begins with a period of immune tolerance, in which there are high levels of hepatitis B virus (HBV)-DNA in serum. Hepatitis B e-antigen (HBeAg) is positive and anti-HBe negative. Histological activity varies, and both interface hepatitis and lobular hepatitis may be seen on liver biopsy. However, low levels of activity are more common. The surface antigen, HBsAg, is most abundant in the characteristic **ground-glass hepatocytes (Fig. 9.13)**. The ground-glass cells are typically scattered singly throughout the parenchyma at this stage of infection. Their name derives from the finely granular appearance of the central part of the cytoplasm, which is rich in endoplasmic reticulum and hepatitis B surface material. Other organelles are located at the cell periphery and often appear to be separated from the ground-glass area by a pale halo. HBsAg can be demonstrated immunohistochemically **(Fig. 9.14)** and with orcein or Victoria blue methods. It is most abundant in the ground-glass hepatocytes, but can also be seen in a membranous or submembranous location in hepatocytes without a ground-glass pattern. The differential diagnosis of ground-glass hepatocytes is from the oncocytic cells described in the previous section, from drug-induced hypertrophy of the endoplasmic reticulum **(see Fig. 8.1)** and from inclusion-containing hepatocytes in cyanamide toxicity **(see Ch. 8)**, Lafora's disease, immunosuppressed transplant patients **(see Fig. 4.4C and Ch. 16)** and fibrinogen storage disease.[30] Clinical circumstances together with immunostaining for HBsAg make confusion unlikely.

The core antigen, HBcAg, is also demonstrable by immunostaining **(Fig. 9.14)**. It is mainly located in hepatocyte nuclei, but also in cytoplasm when necroinflammatory activity is high. Positive nuclear staining correlates with viral load.[31] Nuclei which contain large amounts of core protein sometimes have a pale, homogeneous appearance on haematoxylin and eosin (H&E)-stained sections and have been described as 'sanded'[32] **(Fig. 9.15)**.

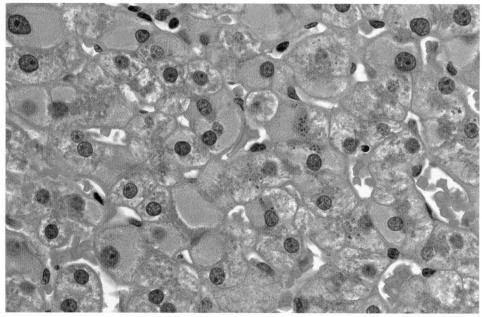

Figure 9.13
Chronic hepatitis B with ground-glass hepatocytes.
In many hepatocytes the central part of the cytoplasm has a homogeneous ground-glass appearance. A paler-staining halo is seen around the ground-glass areas in some cells. (Needle biopsy, H&E.)

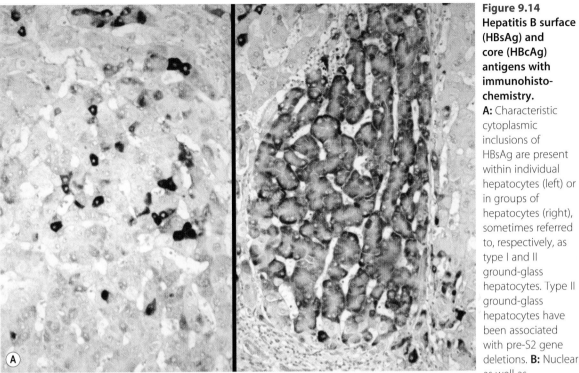

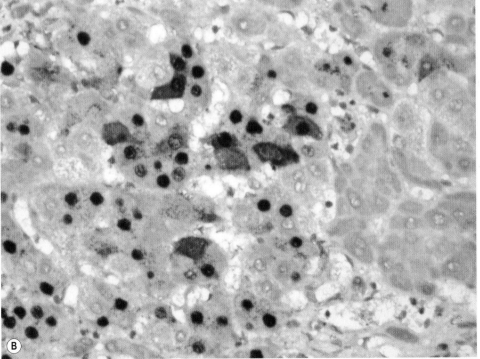

Figure 9.14
Hepatitis B surface (HBsAg) and core (HBcAg) antigens with immunohisto-chemistry.
A: Characteristic cytoplasmic inclusions of HBsAg are present within individual hepatocytes (left) or in groups of hepatocytes (right), sometimes referred to, respectively, as type I and II ground-glass hepatocytes. Type II ground-glass hepatocytes have been associated with pre-S2 gene deletions. **B:** Nuclear as well as cytoplasmic staining of HBcAg is present in this case, consistent with active viral replication. (Explant liver, specific immunoperoxidase stains.)

**Figure 9.15
'Sanded' nuclei
with hepatitis B
core antigen.**
In this case of
chronic hepatitis B
the pale
homogeneous
appearance of the
affected hepatocyte
nuclei (long arrows)
reflects the presence
of many intranuclear
core particles.
Several normal-
appearing nuclei are
in the field (short
arrows). Many
hepatocytes have
ground-glass
inclusions. (Needle
biopsy, H&E.)

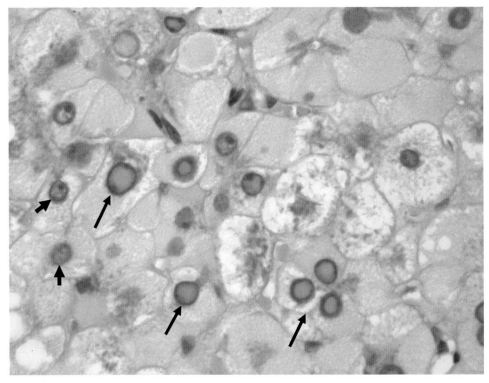

The immunotolerant phase of chronic HBV infection is followed by immune clearance and seroconversion to a non-replicative phase in which HBeAg disappears from serum to be replaced by anti-HBe. During the phase of immune clearance, of very variable length, histological activity is typically high.

In the third, non-replicative phase, histological activity is usually considered to be low, as are markers of viral replication. However, in a large study of liver biopsies from patients in this phase, about one-third showed varying degrees of interface hepatitis, sometimes in the presence of normal aminotransferase levels.[33] Lobular activity was not necessarily accompanied by portal and periportal inflammation. Ground-glass hepatocytes may be clustered in focal accumulations in the late replicative or non-replicative phases. These clusters show dense marginal and/or submembranous HBsAg on immunostain (**Fig. 9.14A**), reflecting the presence of pre-S2 mutant forms of HBV with deletions in the gene encoding the pre-S2 envelope protein.[34,35] These deletions appear to confer protection from immunological attack as well as enhanced cell proliferative capacity favouring hepatocellular carcinoma.

Reactivation of virus replication and histological activity are common and may develop when chemotherapy[35a] or immunomodulatory agents are administered, or in association with the emergence of viral mutants. In some of these mutants, expression of HBeAg is defective and histological activity is unexpectedly high, in spite of the negative HBeAg and presence of anti-HBe.

Finally, in a minority of patients with chronic HBV infection, HBsAg becomes negative and anti-HBs appears in the serum. HBV-DNA may still be detectable in small amounts in serum and liver.

This complex evolution, not always as orderly as the above simplified description might suggest, is marked by a very variable degree of fibrosis, depending on the severity and timing of the hepatitic process. Cirrhosis may develop at any stage, especially in patients whose HBV infection is complicated by infection with other viruses such as hepatitis C virus (HCV) and hepatitis delta virus (HDV).[36]

Apart from the presence of ground-glass hepatocytes and HBV antigens, there are other features which characterise chronic hepatitis B. Marked variation in the size and appearance of hepatocyte nuclei has been described,[37] as has close contact between hepatocytes and lymphocytes,[38] in keeping with the immunological nature of the hepatitis. The lymphocytes are usually of CD8+ type, in contrast to the portal infiltrate, which is rich in CD4+ lymphocytes, B lymphocytes and dendritic cells.[39] Lymphoid follicles are occasionally found in portal tracts but are less common and less prominent than in hepatitis C.[40]

Infection with HDV modifies infection with HBV, as already noted in **Chapter 6**. Its presence is associated with relatively high histological activity except after liver transplantation. Inflammation is rarely restricted to portal tracts, and there is likely to be substantial inflammation in periportal areas as well as deeper within the lobules. Positive immunostaining for HDV (**see Fig. 6.17**) denotes active infection. A 'sanded' appearance similar to that produced by hepatitis core protein may be seen when there is abundant HDV in hepatocyte nuclei.[41] In the presence of HDV infection there is a greater risk of chronicity than with HBV alone, and liver-associated mortality is increased.[42] Once cirrhosis has developed in patients with hepatitis B, HDV infection confers a greater risk of developing hepatocellular carcinoma and a higher mortality.[43] The prevalence of HDV infection has declined since the 1970s and 1980s as a result of measures to eradicate HBV infection.[44]

Chronic hepatitis C

Chronic hepatitis C affects more than 170 million persons worldwide.[45] It is not usually life-threatening until cirrhosis develops, typically several decades after onset of the hepatitis. Factors associated with faster progression to cirrhosis include older age,[46] male sex, fibrosis on initial biopsy,[47] high necroinflammatory activity on initial biopsy,[48] iron deposition (see Pathological features, below), alcohol consumption, previous HBV infection[49] and HIV infection.[50] There are six different genotypes of the virus,[51] affecting disease severity and response to specific treatment[52]; patients with genotypes 2 and 3 respond best to specific therapy.

The use of liver biopsy in the management of patients with HCV infection has been the subject of extensive discussion. There are serious efforts to replace biopsy to some extent with formulae based on biochemical findings,[53,54] but these fail to predict histological findings accurately.[8,9] Repeatedly normal or near-normal serum aminotransferases suggest mild histological changes,[55] yet a substantial proportion of such patients has been found to have serious liver damage and even cirrhosis.[56,57] The consensus view appears to be that liver biopsy currently continues to provide useful information not obtainable in other ways.[7,58,59]

Pathological features

The histological features of chronic hepatitis C, although not completely diagnostic in themselves, are very characteristic[40,60] (**Box 9.4**). The portal infiltrate is rich in lymphocytes which often form aggregates or follicles, some of them with prominent germinal centres (**Fig. 9.16**). These follicles are easily identified in reticulin preparations (**Fig. 9.17**). Follicles are not restricted to hepatitis C and can also be found in hepatitis B, AIH, primary biliary

---

Box 9.4 Conditions sometimes associated with features of autoimmune hepatitis

Drug hepatotoxicity (e.g. minocycline, nitrofurantoin)

Chronic hepatitis C

HIV disease with immune reconstitution

Transition from other autoimmune diseases (e.g. PBC)

Overlap syndromes (autoimmune hepatitis/PBC; autoimmune hepatitis/PSC)

After liver transplantation

Recurrent chronic hepatitis C
Recurrent chronic hepatitis C treated with interferon
De novo autoimmune hepatitis
Alloimmune late rejection

HIV, human immunodeficiency virus; PBC, primary biliary cirrhosis; PSC, primary sclerosing cholangitis.

Figure 9.16
Chronic hepatitis C.
The portal tract (top left) is heavily infiltrated by lymphocytes, which extend irregularly into the adjacent tissue. A lymphoid follicle with germinal centre has formed. (Needle biopsy, H&E.) (Reproduced from Scheuer PJ, Ashrafzadeh P, Sherlock S, et al. The pathology of hepatitis C. *Hepatology* 1992; **15**: 567–571.)

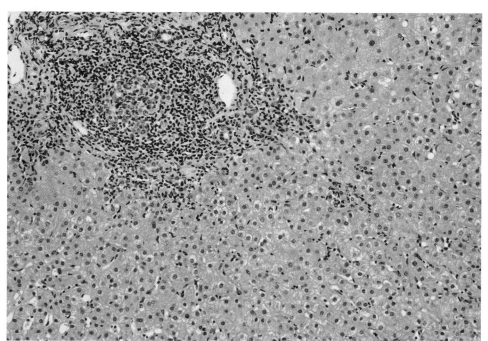

Figure 9.17
Chronic hepatitis C.
The prominent pale area in the portal tract is the site of a lymphoid follicle. (Needle biopsy, reticulin.)

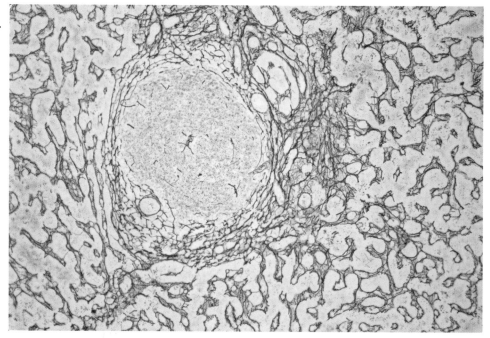

cirrhosis and primary sclerosing cholangitis, but in hepatitis C they are particularly common and prominent. Within, or to one side of, the lymphoid infiltrates, damaged interlobular bile ducts may be seen, as in acute hepatitis. The damage takes the form of vacuolation, stratification and crowding of epithelial cells, and infiltration by lymphocytes.[61] The virus has been demonstrated in bile-duct epithelium and in bile.[62] Bile-duct damage is occasionally, but by no means always, associated with a clinically cholestatic course, and rare ductopenia has been reported.[63,64]

The intralobular changes typically include acidophilic degeneration of hepatocytes and formation of acidophil bodies, already described in **Chapter 6**. Confluent necrosis is uncommon. Sinusoids are focally or diffusely infiltrated by lymphocytes, giving rise in some biopsies to a striking beaded appearance reminiscent of infectious mononucleosis. Epithelioid-cell granulomas and lipogranulomas are occasionally found in lobules or portal tracts[65,66,66a] and clumped material somewhat like Mallory-Denk bodies has been reported in periportal hepatocytes.[67] The presence of talc crystals in liver tissue, seen by polarised light microscopy, is a specific but insensitive marker of intravenous drug abuse.[68]

Iron deposition is common even in the absence of the frequently found *HFE* mutations of hereditary haemochromatosis and may influence progression of the disease.[69,70] Iron is seen not only in hepatocytes, but also in macrophages, endothelial cells and portal tracts.[71,72]

There is an extensive recent literature on the significance of steatosis in chronic hepatitis C. As already noted, steatosis is more common in hepatitis C than in other forms of chronic hepatitis and may be quite severe. It is a risk factor for progression,[73,74] and can interfere with therapy. The steatosis is often associated with obesity, diabetes or alcohol consumption.[65-78] However, in infection with HCV genotype 3[79,80] and very occasionally other genotypes,[81] the virus appears to have a direct effect and the steatosis improves after successful treatment.[82,83] The mechanism for the steatosis may be interference by the viral core protein with lipoprotein assembly and secretion.[84] In addition to steatosis, features of steatohepatitis such as pericellular fibrosis have been reported.[85] Polyarteritis nodosa is a rare complication of chronic hepatitis C.[85a]

The development of reliable and clinically useful methods for detecting viral proteins by immunohistochemistry has been hampered by the small amounts of virus present in each cell, at least in immunocompetent patients. Although results using a monoclonal antibody against HCV envelope protein have been reported,[86] an immunostain for the identification of HCV in routine practice currently remains unavailable.

In biopsies taken early in the course of the disease, the hepatitis is often mild, with little interface hepatitis or fibrosis. With time, fibrous septa extend from expanded portal tracts and link vascular structures. Fibrosis linking portal tracts has the appearance of web-like membranes on three-dimensional reconstruction.[87] A pericellular pattern of fibrosis in perivenular areas has been reported in children.[88] Spontaneous clearance of virus[89,89a] or specific treatment of the infection[90] may bring about dramatic improvement of the fibrosis and structural changes. Drug hepatotoxicity has recently been reported with administration of direct-acting antiviral HCV agents, resulting in an acute hepatitis characterized by focal lobular necrosis, portal and periportal eosinophils, lymphocyes and plasma cells.[90a]

Autoimmune hepatitis

AIH is diagnosed mainly on the basis of serum autoantibodies and absence of evidence for other causes of chronic hepatitis. The autoantibody profile is the basis for subclassification into different types.[91] The commonly assayed autoantibodies include anti-nuclear and anti-smooth-muscle antibodies (ANA, ASMA) and liver–kidney microsomal (LKM) antibodies. Other non-standard antibodies which may be present include soluble liver antigen (SLA), atypical peripheral antineutrophil cytoplasmic antibodies (atypical pANCA) and anti-liver cytosol antibodies.[92-94] Antimitochondrial antibodies (AMAs) may be present in up to 35% of patients with otherwise typical AIH; they may persist for many years without clinical impact or evidence of primary biliary cirrhosis.[95] Histological evidence is important not only for confirming the diagnosis, but also as a means of detecting other conditions with which AIH may be confused. Histology is therefore one component of scoring systems which can be utilised in clinical practice.[96,97]

While there are no pathognomonic histological features of AIH, there is a characteristic picture in many patients before treatment. Biopsy shows active disease, with much hepatocellular damage and a heavy infiltrate of lymphocytes and plasma cells in portal tracts, at the interface and deep within the parenchyma (**Figs 9.18, 9.19**). Plasma cells in clusters in interface regions are often striking. Eosinophils may also be present.[98] Lymphoid follicles are less

Figure 9.18 Autoimmune hepatitis with rosette formation.
Rounded hepatitic rosettes, some with a visible lumen (arrow), are surrounded by compressed sinusoids, fibrous tissue and inflammatory cells. (Needle biopsy, H&E.)

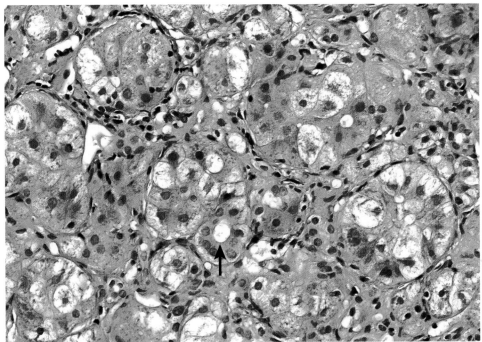

Figure 9.19 Autoimmune hepatitis.
Inflammatory cells including plasma cells extend from the portal tract (left) into the parenchyma as part of the process of interface hepatitis. (Needle biopsy, H&E.)

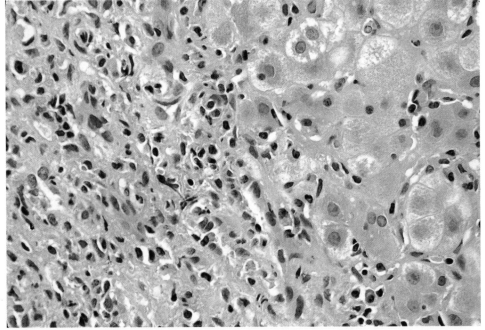

prominent than in hepatitis C. Bridging necrosis is common and surviving hepatocytes often form hepatitic rosettes (**Fig. 9.14**). Prominent syncytial giant hepatocytes in an adult hepatitis (**Fig. 9.10**), while not diagnostic, should always raise the possibility of AIH.[99,100]

This classic histological picture is not, however, the only one seen in AIH, and communication between pathologist and clinician is important to ensure a correct diagnosis.[101]

Plasma cells are not always present in large numbers. In some patients the hepatitis is much milder, and in some there may be cholestasis, bile-duct damage or even ductopenia.[102,103] In adults, this has to be distinguished from the bile-duct lesions of primary biliary cirrhosis and the relatively uncommon overlap syndromes (**see Ch. 5**). In children, AIH is often associated with an autoimmune form of sclerosing cholangitis.[104,105]

AIH is regarded as a chronic disease in all patients, but the clinical onset is sometimes acute. In a study of 26 patients biopsied within 6 months of onset,[106] most showed evidence of chronicity and a few had cirrhosis. However, careful analysis of connective tissue septa with the help of several connective tissue stains (**see Ch. 6**) sometimes suggests recent onset with rapid development of nodules. Furthermore there is a small subgroup of patients with a variant histological form of AIH characterised by centrilobular necrosis and inflammation, as in an acute hepatitis[107-110] (**Fig. 9.20**). The lesion is seen in perivenular regions where there are foci of hepatocyte drop-out and/or apoptosis, collections of lymphocytes with or without plasma cells, and, typically, intrasinusoidal ceroid-laden Kupffer cells. The centrilobular necroinflammatory lesion may be the only histological manifestation of AIH, or it may be accompanied by the portal and periportal lymphoplasmacytic inflammation more typical of AIH. Some studies have suggested that the centrilobular necroinflammatory lesion is the early histological form of AIH which eventually progresses to a more classical chronic form of AIH based in portal and periportal regions.

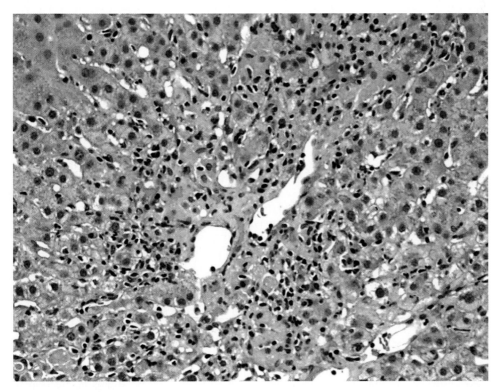

Figure 9.20 **Autoimmune hepatitis: histological variant form with centrilobular necrosis and inflammation.**
The liver parenchyma around the efferent vein (centre) shows hepatocyte drop-out and numerous inflammatory cells, including lymphocytes, plasma cells and clusters of tan ceroid-laden Kupffer cells. This type of centrilobular necroinflammation may be the only histological manifestation of autoimmune hepatitis, or may be present in combination with classical portal inflammation with interface hepatitis. (Needle biopsy, H&E.)

Exacerbation of disease severity may favour the development of confluence of the two patterns, resulting in central-to-portal bridging necrosis or even multilobular and massive necrosis.

Patients with AIH usually respond rapidly to corticosteroid therapy. Biopsy following treatment shows varying degrees of resolution of the necroinflammatory process and sometimes dramatic improvement in fibrosis and structural changes.[111,112] Liver biopsy helps to determine when corticosteroid treatment can safely be withdrawn.[10] The degree of plasma-cell infiltration is a predictor of relapse,[113] and worsening histological activity appears to correlate with progression of fibrosis.[114] Biopsy therefore continues to play an important role in patient management.

Other conditions with features of autoimmune hepatitis

Histological changes closely resembling AIH may occur in other settings (**Box 9.4**), sometimes accompanied by positive serum autoantibodies and elevated γ-globulin levels. The microscopic changes and generation of autoantibodies may be triggered by viral infection (chronic hepatitis C with autoimmune features[115]), drugs with idiosyncratic effects (nitrofurantoin and minocycline,[116,117] statins,[118,119] diclofenac,[119] black cohosh[120]) or medication-related immunomodulatory changes in an immunosuppressed individual (immune reconstitution after antiretroviral therapy in HIV disease[121]; after liver transplantation – **see Ch. 16**). In such cases, the interpretation of AIH-like features merits clinical discussion along with review of current or recently changed medications. The type and titre of autoantibodies, γ-globulin level and the biopsy findings need to be factored into specific changes in management.

The potential for AIH to 'overlap' with other liver diseases of autoimmune nature, such as primary biliary cirrhosis and primary sclerosing cholangitis,[121a] was discussed in **Chapter 5**. Infrequently, one autoimmune disease may transition over time to another, such as primary biliary cirrhosis evolving to AIH. The transition may be evident as heightened necroinflammation, including interface hepatitis and bridging necrosis.[122,123]

Differential diagnosis of chronic hepatitis

In biopsies with inflammation confined to portal tracts, other possibilities to be considered include **resolving acute hepatitis, non-specific inflammation near a focal lesion, primary biliary cirrhosis** and **lymphoma**. The nature of the infiltrate and involvement of most or all portal tracts in chronic hepatitis should resolve the issue in most cases, but clinical information is also needed.

More severe chronic hepatitis needs to be distinguished from **acute hepatitis**, which is sometimes difficult. As discussed in **Chapter 6**, staining for elastic fibres may enable recently formed bridges to be distinguished from old fibrous septa. Canalicular cholestasis, common in acute hepatitis, is not often found in chronic hepatitis. In HBV infection in an immunocompetent patient the presence of HBsAg-containing ground-glass hepatocytes indicates chronic disease.

Other diseases to be considered in the more severe forms include **chronic biliary diseases**, especially primary biliary cirrhosis and primary sclerosing cholangitis, α_1-**antitrypsin deficiency, Wilson's disease, lymphoma** and **drug injury**. Loss of bile ducts and periportal accumulation of copper-associated protein suggest biliary disease rather than chronic hepatitis. α_1-Antitrypsin deficiency can be diagnosed by appropriate staining (**see Ch. 13**), while Wilson's disease (**see Ch. 14**) should be established principally by clinical features and biochemical findings. The infiltrates of various lymphomas are usually extensive and irregular and may undergo necrosis. Drugs sometimes cause a liver disease closely resembling AIH, or may act as a trigger, unmasking latent autoimmunity, as discussed above. As in all liver diseases, correlation of clinical and histological findings reduces the risk of diagnostic error.

Semi-quantitative scoring: grading and staging

Scoring is now widely used to evaluate liver biopsies before treatment, to monitor the effects of treatment and to assess the effects of new therapies in clinical trials. It consists of two components, their names borrowed from oncology: **grading** and **staging**. Grading refers to the scoring of the necroinflammatory lesion of a hepatitis, including the various types and degrees of hepatocellular damage and the location and extent of the inflammatory process. Staging records the extent of fibrosis and of changes in structure, including the development of cirrhosis. In many scoring systems, grading is subdivided into categories such as portal inflammation, interface hepatitis and lobular hepatitis, whereas staging is expressed as a single scale.

Assessment of fibrosis can also be carried out using morphometric measurement of collagen.[124,125] This gives an accurate measurement of the amount of fibrous tissue per unit area, but does not take structural changes such as nodule formation into account. Staging and morphometry should therefore be viewed as complementary to each other and not as alternatives.

Scoring is semi-quantitative rather than quantitative, in the sense that, while scores are usually expressed as numbers, they do not represent measurements. Scoring involves subjective assessment of the various relevant histological features in a biopsy, and the scores allotted will inevitably vary somewhat from observer to observer depending on experience and personal bias. For this reason, scores allotted at different times or by different observers cannot be directly compared. This limits the usefulness of scoring as a routine reporting procedure.

Before embarking on scoring, the pathologist should consider carefully why the scores are required. This will help to determine the most suitable system for the particular purpose or project. For example, if what is needed is a decision as to whether the chronic hepatitis in a particular patient is mild, moderate or severe, a simple system will suffice, and will usually have the advantage over more complex systems in so far as the latter tend to be associated with greater intra- and interobserver variation and are also more time-consuming. If, on the other hand, the purpose is to evaluate a group of biopsies in a clinical trial of a new treatment regime, then a complex system is more appropriate. A complex system would allow analysis not only of the overall severity of the changes, but also of individual features such as interface hepatitis and lobular activity. Examples of two simple systems are given in **Box 9.5**.[126,127] The simple staging system proposed by the METAVIR group[128] is given in **Box 9.6** and **Table 9.1**, and the more complex and widely used Ishak system,[128] derived from the earlier Knodell Histology Activity Index,[129] in **Table 9.2**. Examples of grading and staging are shown in **Figures 9.21** and **9.22**.

The results of a particular study can be compared in a general way with those of another, but, because of the subjective nature of scoring, the numbers themselves cannot be directly compared or combined. Each study therefore stands on its own to some extent and the observers are free to modify a published scoring system to suit a particular purpose. For instance, a scoring range for steatosis, siderosis or bile-duct damage could be devised and added if required.

Reproducibility of scoring is improved when it is performed by more than one observer.[130] There should then be an initial discussion using a multi-headed microscope in order to ensure that all observers agree on the criteria used to score each feature. At the end of a study, discrepancies between observers can be resolved by joint discussion at the microscope. In a clinical trial, it may be helpful to reassess a proportion of biopsies in order to test intraobserver variation. The scoring should be performed by the same observer or observers throughout, and is usually done without knowledge of clinical data.

Box 9.5 A simple scoring system for chronic hepatitis

Grade

Portal inflammation and interface hepatitis

0 Absent or minimal
1 Portal inflammation only
2 Mild or localised interface hepatitis
3 Moderate or more extensive interface hepatitis
4 Severe and widespread interface hepatitis

Lobular activity

0 None
1 Inflammatory cells but no hepatocellular damage
2 Focal necrosis or apoptosis
3 Severe hepatocellular damage
4 Damage includes bridging confluent necrosis

Stage

0 No fibrosis
1 Fibrosis confined to portal tracts
2 Periportal or portal–portal septa but intact vascular relationships
3 Fibrosis with distorted structure but no obvious cirrhosis
4 Probable or definite cirrhosis

Modified from Scheuer PJ. Classification of chronic viral hepatitis: a need for reassessment. *J Hepatol* 1991; **13**: 372–374.

Interpretation of the results of scoring

Box 9.6 The METAVIR staging system

F0 No fibrosis
F1 Stellate enlargement of portal tracts but without septum formation
F2 Enlargement of portal tracts with rare septum formation
F3 Numerous septa without cirrhosis
F4 Cirrhosis

Modified from Bedossa P, Bioulac-Sage P, Callard P, et al. Intraobserver and interobserver variations in liver biopsy interpretation in patients with chronic hepatitis C. *Hepatology* 1994; **20**: 15–20.

When the scores from a group of biopsies are assessed, the statistical methods used to evaluate the results must be appropriate for categorical data. An example of a suitable method is that used by Lagging et al.[131] Some grading systems are divided into several categories. In the case of the Ishak score, these are interface hepatitis, confluent necrosis, lobular activity and portal inflammation. For each of these four categories the scale from 0 to 4 or 0 to 6 is not exactly linear, and it is therefore not acceptable to add the four scores together and then to manipulate the result as if it were a true mathematical sum. To put the matter another way, a score of 2 for any particular feature does not denote exactly twice 1 or precisely half of 4, but simply a score somewhere between 1 and 3. Nevertheless, total grading scores are often used and published. In routine practice a total grading score gives an approximate indication of the severity of a patient's hepatitis, but no information on the relative contribution of each category. In clinical trials of new therapies, total grading scores are potentially misleading and the effect of the therapy on each individual grading category should be examined.

Table 9.1 The METAVIR algorithm

Interface hepatitis* (piecemeal necrosis)		Lobular necrosis†		Overall histological activity‡
0	+	0	=	0
0	+	1	=	1
0	+	2	=	2
1	+	0	=	1
1	+	1	=	1
1	+	2	=	2
2	+	0	=	2
2	+	1	=	2
2	+	2	=	3
3	+	0	=	3
3	+	1	=	3
3	+	2	=	3

*Interface hepatitis scored 0 (none), 1 (mild), 2 (moderate), 3 (severe).
†Lobular necrosis scored 0 (none or mild), 1 (moderate), 2 (severe).
‡Histological activity scored 0 (none), 1 (mild), 2 (moderate), 3 (severe).
Modified from Bedossa P, Poynard T, the METAVIR cooperative study group. An algorithm for the grading of activity in chronic hepatitis C. *Hepatology* 1996; **24**: 289–293.

Table 9.2 The Ishak scoring system

Category	Score
Grading	
Periportal or periseptal interface hepatitis	
Absent	0
Mild (focal, few portal areas)	1
Mild/moderate (focal, most portal areas)	2
Moderate (continuous around <50% of tracts or septa)	3
Severe (continuous around >50% of tracts or septa)	4

Table 9.2 Continued

Category	Score
Confluent necrosis	
Absent	0
Focal	1
Zone 3 necrosis in some areas	2
Zone 3 necrosis in most areas	3
Zone 3 necrosis + occasional portal–central bridging	4
Zone 3 necrosis + multiple portal–central bridging	5
Panacinar or multiacinar necrosis	6
Focal (spotty) lytic necrosis, apoptosis and focal inflammation*	
Absent	0
<2 foci per 10 × objective	1
2–4 foci per 10 × objective	2
5–10 foci per 10 × objective	3
>10 foci per 10 × objective	4
Portal inflammation	
None	0
Mild, some or all portal areas	1
Moderate, some or all portal areas	2
Moderate/marked, all portal areas	3
Marked, all portal areas	4
Staging	
No fibrosis	0
Fibrous expansion of some portal areas, with or without short fibrous septa	1
Fibrous expansion of most portal areas, with or without short fibrous septa	2
Fibrous expansion of most portal areas with occasional portal–portal bridging	3
Fibrous expansion of portal areas with marked bridging (portal–portal and portal–central)	4
Marked bridging (portal–portal and/or portal–central) with occasional nodules (incomplete cirrhosis)	5
Cirrhosis, probable or definite	6

*Does not include diffuse sinusoidal infiltration by inflammatory cells.
Adapted from Ishak K, Baptista A, Bianchi L, et al. Histological grading and staging of chronic hepatitis. *J Hepatol* 1995; **22**: 696–699.

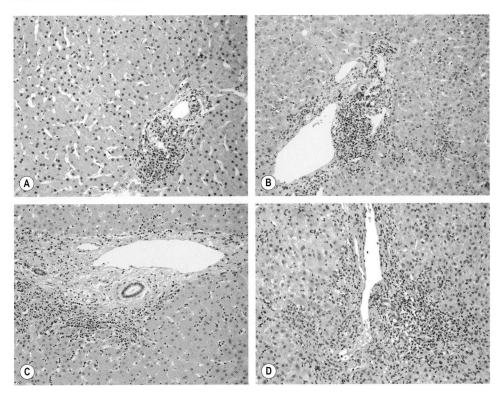

Figure 9.21 Grading of chronic hepatitis.
The examples of grading shown in these four panels emphasise the portal/periportal necroinflammatory component of chronic hepatitis; lobular activity also should be taken into account, but is frequently less prominent. **A:** Minimal activity (grade 1). Inflammation is confined to the portal tracts and there is no interface hepatitis. The lobular parenchyma is quiescent. **B:** Mild activity (grade 2). Focal interface hepatitis is now present (right periportal region) in addition to portal tract inflammation. A few lobular necroinflammatory foci are also seen at right. **C:** Moderate activity (grade 3). More extensive interface hepatitis is present than in grade 2, but involving <50% of the circumference of most portal tracts. In this example, the portal tract edges above and to the right show relative sparing. **D:** Marked activity (grade 4). The portal tract is diffusely inflamed and shows extensive circumferential interface hepatitis. Similar changes affect virtually all portal tracts with this grade of activity, often with considerable lobular activity. (Needle biopsies, H&E.)

The possibility or indeed likelihood of sampling variation must also be kept in mind.[132] In chronic hepatitis C, there are differences between the findings in the left and the right lobe of the liver.[133] More importantly, small-needle biopsy samples may be misleading. Recent studies have thrown light on this particular issue. In one study using image analysis to assess fibrosis, the ability of the image analysis to predict a METAVIR fibrosis score diminished progressively in specimens less than 25 mm long.[124] In another study, reducing the sample size optically led to underestimation of disease severity in samples less than 20 mm long and 1.4 mm wide.[134] According to this study, samples obtained with fine needles were considered unsatisfactory for scoring. Another group recommended that the use of fine needles in diffuse HCV-related liver disease should be restricted to early non-fibrotic lesions.[135] While not all investigators agree that fine-needle specimens are inadequate for grading and staging,[136] specimen size is clearly a critical issue.

Figure 9.22 Staging of chronic hepatitis.
A: Minimal fibrosis (stage 1). This type of modest fibrosis sometimes takes the form of rounded fibrous expansion of some portal tracts (shown at left). In other cases, minimal fibrosis consists of occasional short fibrous scars at the edges of some, but not all, portal tracts (shown at arrows in right panel). **B:** Mild fibrosis (stage 2). Most portal tracts have a stellate contour due to periportal fibrosis, as shown here.

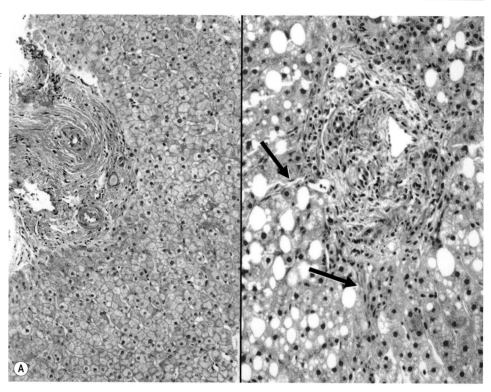

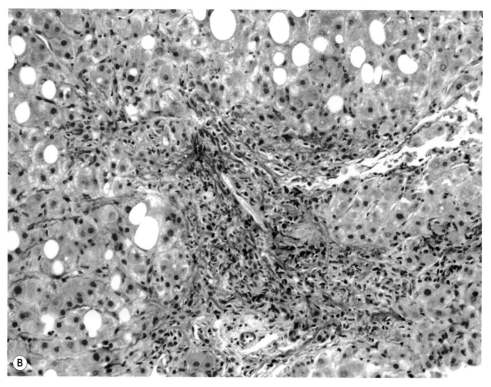

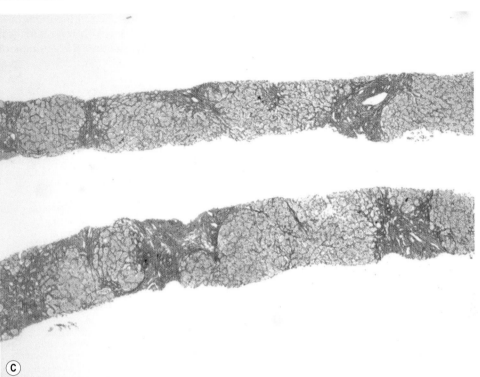

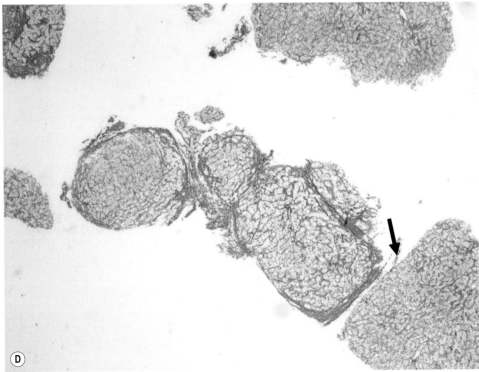

Figure 9.22, cont'd
C: Extensive bridging fibrosis with nodularity, but without cirrhosis (stage 3). This biopsy specimen consisted of several cores of liver tissue. Portal-to-portal bridging fibrosis is prominent in the left-hand portions of both cores, while more architecturally preserved parenchyma with stellate scarring of portal tracts is evident at right. Developing parenchymal nodules are also seen at left. Fully established cirrhosis is not demonstrated. **D:** Cirrhosis (stage 4). Architecturally abnormal regenerative nodules are evident and are circumscribed by diffuse fibrosis. Needle biopsy samples sometimes contain fragments of cirrhotic nodules (at arrow) which have been shelled out and separated from the adjacent fibrous septa. Such regenerative fragments frequently have a 'squared-off' or 'flat-top' appearance at their edges. (**A, B,** needle biopsies: trichrome stain; **C, D,** needle biopsies: reticulin stain.)

In conclusion, many factors limit the accuracy of semi-quantitative scoring in chronic hepatitis.[137] Awareness of these factors, careful attempts to minimise observer variation and appropriate interpretation of the results should ensure the continued usefulness of grading and staging in clinical practice and research.

References

1 Berasain C, Betes M, Panizo A, et al. Pathological and virological findings in patients with persistent hypertransaminasaemia of unknown aetiology. Gut 2000;47:429–35.

2 Hano H, Takasaki S. Three-dimensional observations on the alterations of lobular architecture in chronic hepatitis with special reference to its angioarchitecture for a better understanding of the formal pathogenesis of liver cirrhosis. Virchows Arch 2003;443:655–63.

3 Burt AD. Diseases of the Liver and Biliary Tract. Standardization of Nomenclature, Diagnostic Criteria, and Prognosis. New York: Raven Press; 1994.

4 Desmet VJ, Gerber M, Hoofnagle JH, et al. Classification of chronic hepatitis: diagnosis, grading and staging. Hepatology 1994;19:1513–20.

5 International Working Party. Terminology of chronic hepatitis, hepatic allograft rejection, and nodular lesions of the liver: summary of recommendations developed by an international working party, supported by the World Congresses of Gastroenterology, Los Angeles 1994. Am J Gastroenterol 1994;89:S177–81.

6 Andriulli A, Festa V, Leandro G, et al. Usefulness of a liver biopsy in the evaluation of patients with elevated ALT values and serological markers of hepatitis viral infection: an AIGO study. Dig Dis Sci 2001;46:1409–15.

7 European Association for the Study of the Liver. EASL Clinical Practice Guidelines: management of chronic hepatitis B virus infection. J Hepatol 2012;57:167–85.

8 European Association for the Study of the Liver. EASL Clinical Practice Guidelines: management of hepatitis C virus infection. J Hepatol 2014;60:392–420.

9 Manns MP, Czaja AJ, Gorham JD, et al. AASLD Practice Guidelines. Diagnosis and management of autoimmune hepatitis. Hepatology 2010;51:2193–213.

10 Czaja AJ, Carpenter HA. Histological features associated with relapse after corticosteroid withdrawal in type 1 autoimmune hepatitis. Liver Int 2003;23:116–23.

11 Lau JYN, Xie X, Lai MMC, et al. Apoptosis and viral hepatitis. Semin Liver Dis 1998;18:169–76.

12 Oksuz M, Akkiz H, Isiksal F, et al. Expression of Fas antigen in liver tissue of patients with chronic hepatitis B and C. Eur J Gastroenterol Hepatol 2004;16:341–5.

13 Jaeschke H, Gujral J, Bajt M. Apoptosis and necrosis in liver disease. Liver Int 2004;24:85–9.

14 Eleazar JA, Memeo L, Jhang JS, et al. Progenitor cell expansion: an important source of hepatocyte regeneration in chronic hepatitis. J Hepatol 2004;39:552–6.

15 Isse K, Harada K, Nakanuma Y. IL-8 expressed by biliary epithelial cells is associated with neutrophilic infiltration and reactive bile ductules. Liver Int 2007;27:672–80.

16 Liaw YF, Chu CM, Chen TJ, et al. Chronic lobular hepatitis: a clinicopathological and prognostic study. Hepatology 1982;2:258–62.

17 Libbrecht L, Desmet V, Van Damme B, et al. Deep intralobular extension of human hepatic 'progenitor cells' correlates with parenchymal inflammation in chronic viral hepatitis: can 'progenitor cells' migrate? J Pathol 2000;192:373–8.

18 Protzer U, Dienes HP, Bianchi L, et al. Post-infantile giant cell hepatitis in patients with primary sclerosing cholangitis and autoimmune hepatitis. Liver 1996;16:274–82.

19 Micchelli STL, Thomas D, Boitnott JK, et al. Hepatic giant cells in hepatitis C virus (HCV) mono-infection and HCV/HIV co-infection. J Clin Pathol 2008;61:1058–61.

20 Lefkowitch JH, Yee HT, Sweeting J, et al. Iron-rich foci in chronic viral hepatitis. Hum Pathol 1998;29:116–18.

21 Martinelli AL, Filho AB, Franco RF, et al. Liver iron deposits in hepatitis B patients: association with severity of liver disease but not with hemochromatosis gene mutations. Gastroenterol Hepatol 2004;19:1036–41.

22 Lefkowitch JH, Arborgh BA, Scheuer PJ. Oxyphilic granular hepatocytes. Mitochondrion-rich liver cells in hepatic disease. Am J Clin Pathol 1980;74:432–41.

23 Gerber MA, Thung SN. Hepatic oncocytes. Incidence, staining characteristics, and ultrastructural features. Am J Clin Pathol 1981;75:498–503.

24 Tanji K, Bhagat G, Vu TH, et al. Mitochondrial DNA dysfunction in oncocytic hepatocytes. Liver Int 2003;23:397–403.

25 Iwamura S, Enzan H, Saibara T, et al. Appearance of sinusoidal inclusion-containing endothelial cells in liver disease. Hepatology 1994;20:604–10.

26 Iwamura S, Enzan H, Saibara T, et al. Hepatic sinusoidal endothelial cells can store and metabolize serum immunoglobulin. Hepatology 1995;22:1456–61.

27 Broderick AL, Jonas MM. Hepatitis B in children. Semin Liver Dis 2003;23:59–68.

28 Boxall E, Sira J, Standish RA, et al. The natural history of hepatitis B in perinatally infected carriers. Arch Dis Child Fetal Neonatal Ed 2004;89:F456–60.

29 Fattovich G. Natural history and prognosis of hepatitis B. Semin Liver Dis 2003;23:47–58.

30 Callea F, De Vos R, Togni R, et al. Fibrinogen inclusions in liver cells: a new type of ground-glass hepatocyte. Immune light and electron microscopic characterization. Histopathology 1986;10:65–73.

31 Serinoz E, Varli M, Erden E, et al. Nuclear localization of hepatitis B core antigen and its relations to liver injury, hepatocyte proliferation, and viral load. J Clin Gastroenterol 2003;36:269–72.

32 Bianchi L, Gudat F. Sanded nuclei in hepatitis B: eosinophilic inclusions in liver cell nuclei due to excess in hepatitis B core antigen formation. Lab Invest 1976;35:1–5.

33 Ter Borg F, ten Kate FJ, Cuypers HT, et al. A survey of liver pathology in needle biopsies from HBsAg and anti-HBe positive individuals. J Clin Pathol 2000;53:541–8.

34 Wang H-C, Wu H-C, Chen C-F, et al. Different types of ground glass hepatocytes in chronic hepatitis B virus infection contain specific pre-S mutants that may induce endoplasmic reticulum stress. Am J Pathol 2003;163:2441–9.

35 Mathai AM, Alexander J, Kuo F-Y, et al. Type II ground-glass hepatocytes as a marker of hepatocellular carcinoma in chronic hepatitis B. Hum Pathol 2013;44:1665–71.

35a Hsu C, Tsou H-H, Lin S-J, et al. Chemotherapy-induced hepatitis B reactivation in lymphoma patients with resolved HBV infection: a prospective study. Hepatoloy 2014;59:2092–100.

36 Mathurin P, Thibault V, Kadidja K, et al. Replication status and histological features of patients with triple (B, C, D) and dual (B, C) hepatic infections. J Viral Hepat 2000;7:15–22.

37 Bianchi L, Gudat F. Chronic hepatitis. In: MacSween RNM, Anthony PP, Scheuer PJ, et al., editors. Pathology of the Liver. 3rd ed. Edinburgh: Churchill Livingstone; 1994. p. 349–96.

38 Dienes HP, Popper H, Arnold W, et al. Histologic observations in human hepatitis non-A, non-B. Hepatology 1982;2:562–71.

39 van den Oord JJ, De Vos R, Facchetti F, et al. Distribution of non-lymphoid, inflammatory cells in chronic HBV infection. J Pathol 1990;160:223–30.

40 Scheuer PJ, Ashrafzadeh P, Sherlock S, et al. The pathology of hepatitis C. Hepatology 1992;15:567–71.

41 Moreno A, Ramón y Cahal S, Marazuela M, et al. Sanded nuclei in delta patients. Liver 1989;9:367–71.

42 Abiad H, Ramani R, Currie JB, et al. The natural history of hepatitis D virus infection in Illinois state facilities for the developmentally disabled. Am J Gastroenterol 2001;96:534–40.

43 Fattovich G, Giustina G, Christensen E, et al. Influence of hepatitis delta virus infection on morbidity and mortality in compensated cirrhosis type B. The European Concerted Action on Viral Hepatitis (Eurohep). Gut 2000;46: 420–6.

44 Rizzetto M. Hepatitis D: thirty years after. J Hepatol 2009;50:1043–50.

45 Poynard T, Ratziu V, Benhamou Y, et al. Natural history of HCV infection. Best Pract Res Clin Gastroenterol 2000;14:211–28.

46 Ghany MG, Kleiner DE, Alter H, et al. Progression of fibrosis in chronic hepatitis C. Gastroenterology 2003;124:97–104.

47 Ryder SD. Progression of hepatic fibrosis in patients with hepatitis C: a prospective repeat liver biopsy study. Gut 2004;53:451–5.

48 Fontaine H, Nalpas B, Poulet B, et al. Hepatitis activity index is a key factor in determining the natural history of chronic hepatitis C. Hum Pathol 2001;32:904–9.

49 Giannini E, Ceppa P, Botta F, et al. Previous hepatitis B virus infection is associated with worse disease stage and occult hepatitis B virus infection has low prevalence and pathogenicity in hepatitis C virus-positive patients. Liver Int 2003;23:12–18.

50 Poynard T, Mathurin P, Lai CL, et al. A comparison of fibrosis progression in chronic liver diseases. J Hepatol 2003;38:257–65.

51 Webster G, Barnes E, Brown D, et al. HCV genotypes – role in pathogenesis of disease and response to therapy. Best Pract Res Clin Gastroenterol 2000;14:229–40.

52 Roffi L, Redaelli A, Colloredo G, et al. Outcome of liver disease in a large cohort of histologically proven chronic hepatitis C: influence of HCV genotype. Eur J Gastroenterol Hepatol 2001;13:501–6.

53 Imbert-Bismut F, Ratziu V, Pieroni L, et al. Biochemical markers of liver fibrosis in patients with hepatitis C virus infection: a prospective study. Lancet 2001;357:1069–75.

54 Afdhal NH. Diagnosing fibrosis in hepatitis C: is the pendulum swinging from biopsy to blood tests? Hepatology 2003;37:972–4.

55 Persico M, Persico E, Suozzo R, et al. Natural history of hepatitis C virus carriers with persistently normal aminotransferase levels. Gastroenterology 2000;118:760–4.

56 Nutt AK, Hassan HA, Lindsey J, et al. Liver biopsy in the evaluation of patients with chronic hepatitis C who have repeatedly normal or near-normal alanine aminotransferase levels. Am J Med 2000;109:62–4.

57 Kyrlagkitsis I, Portmann B, Smith H, et al. Liver histology and progression of fibrosis in individuals with chronic hepatitis C and persistently normal ALT. Am J Gastroenterol 2003;98:1588–93.

58 Dienstag JL. The role of liver biopsy in chronic hepatitis C. Hepatology 2002;36:S152–60.

59 Rockey DC, Caldwell SH, Goodman ZD, et al. Liver biopsy. Hepatology 2009;49:1017–44.

60 Bach N, Thung SN, Schaffner F. The histological features of chronic hepatitis C and autoimmune chronic hepatitis: a comparative analysis. Hepatology 1992;15:572–7.

61 Kaji K, Nakanuma Y, Sasaki M, et al. Hepatitic bile duct injuries in chronic hepatitis C: histopathologic and immunohistochemical studies. Mod Pathol 1994;7:937–45.

62 Haruna Y, Kanda T, Honda M, et al. Detection of hepatitis C virus in the bile and bile duct epithelial cells of hepatitis C virus-infected patients. Hepatology 2001;33:977–80.

63 Delladetsima JK, Makris F, Psichogiou M, et al. Cholestatic syndrome with bile duct damage and loss in renal transplant recipients with HCV infection. Liver 2001;21:81–8.

64 Kumar KS, Saboorian MH, Lee WM. Cholestatic presentation of chronic hepatitis C: a clinical and histological study with a review of the literature. Dig Dis Sci 2001;46:2066–73.

65 Gaya DR, Thorburn D, Oien KA, et al. Hepatic granulomas: a 10 year single centre experience. J Clin Pathol 2003;56:850–3.

66 Ozaras R, Tahan V, Mert A, et al. The prevalence of hepatic granulomas in chronic hepatitis C. J Clin Gastroenterol 2004;38:449–52.

66a Zhu H, Bodenheimer HC, Clain DJ, et al. Hepatic lipogranulomas in patients with chronic liver disease: association with hepatitis C and fatty liver disease. World J Gastroenterol 2010;16:5065–9.

67 Lefkowitch JH, Schiff ER, Davis GL, et al. Pathological diagnosis of chronic hepatitis C: a multicenter comparative study with chronic hepatitis B. Gastroenterology 1993;104:595–603.

68 Sherman KE, Lewey SM, Goodman ZD. Talc in the liver of patients with chronic hepatitis C infection. Am J Gastroenterol 1995;90:2164–6.

69   Bonkovsky HL, Troy N, McNeal K, et al. Iron and HFE or TfR1 mutations as comorbid factors for development and progression of chronic hepatitis C. J Hepatol 2002;37:848–54.

70   Martinelli AL, Ramalho LN, Zucoloto S. Hepatic stellate cells in hepatitis C patients: relationship with liver iron deposits and severity of liver disease. J Gastroenterol Hepatol 2004;19:91–8.

71   Pirisi M, Scott CA, Avellini C, et al. Iron deposition and progression of disease in chronic hepatitis C. Role of interface hepatitis, portal inflammation, and HFE missense mutations. Am J Clin Pathol 2000;113: 546–54.

72   Metwally MA, Zein CO, Zein NN. Clinical significance of hepatic iron deposition and serum iron values in patients with chronic hepatitis C infection. Am J Gastroenterol 2004;99:286–91.

73   Wyatt J, Baker H, Prasad P, et al. Steatosis and fibrosis in patients with chronic hepatitis C. J Clin Pathol 2004;57:402–6.

74   Fartoux L, Chazouillères O, Wendum D, et al. Impact of steatosis on progression of fibrosis in patients with mild hepatitis C. Hepatology 2005;41:82–7.

75   Adinolfi LE, Gambardella M, Andreana A, et al. Steatosis accelerates the progression of liver damage of chronic hepatitis C patients and correlates with specific HCV genotype and visceral obesity. Hepatology 2001;33:1358–64.

76   Monto A, Alonzo J, Watson JJ, et al. Steatosis in chronic hepatitis C: relative contributions of obesity, diabetes mellitus, and alcohol. Hepatology 2002;36:729–36.

77   Sheikh MY, Choi J, Qadri I, et al. Hepatitis C virus infection: molecular pathways to metabolic syndrome. Hepatology 2008;47:2127–33.

78   Hu KQ, Kyulo NL, Esrailian E, et al. Overweight and obesity, hepatic steatosis, and progression of chronic hepatitis C: a retrospective study on a large cohort of patients in the United States. J Hepatol 2004;40:147–54.

79   Rubbia-Brandt L, Quadri R, Abid K, et al. Hepatocyte steatosis is a cytopathic effect of hepatitis C virus genotype 3. J Hepatol 2000;33:106–15.

80   Serfaty L, Andreani T, Giral P, et al. Hepatitis C virus induced hypobetalipoproteinemia: a possible mechanism for steatosis in chronic hepatitis C. J Hepatol 2001;34:428–34.

81   Colloredo G, Sonzogni A, Rubbia-Brandt L, et al. Hepatitis C virus genotype 1 associated with massive steatosis of the liver and hypo-β-lipoproteinemia. J Hepatol 2004;40:562–3.

82   Hofer H, Bankl HC, Wrba F, et al. Hepatocellular fat accumulation and low serum cholesterol in patients infected with HCV-3a. Am J Gastroenterol 2002;97:2880–5.

83   Kumar D, Farrell GC, Fung C, et al. Hepatitis C virus genotype 3 is cytopathic to hepatocytes: reversal of hepatic steatosis after sustained therapeutic response. Hepatology 2002;36:1266–72.

84   Lonardo A, Adinolfi LE, Loria P, et al. Steatosis and hepatitis C virus: mechanisms and significance for hepatic and extrahepatic disease. Gastroenterology 2004;126:586–97.

85   Clouston AD, Jonsson JR, Purdie DM, et al. Steatosis and chronic hepatitis C: analysis of fibrosis and stellate cell activation. J Hepatol 2001;34:314–20.

85a Saadoun D, Terrier B, Semoun O, et al. Hepatitis C virus-associated polyarteritis nodosa. Arthritis Care Res (Hoboken) 2011;63:427–35.

86   Verslype C, Nevens F, Sinelli N, et al. Hepatic immunohistochemical staining with a monoclonal antibody against HCV-E2 to evaluate antiviral therapy and reinfection of liver grafts in hepatitis C viral infection. J Hepatol 2003;38:208–14.

87   Hoofring A, Boitnott J, Torbenson M. Three-dimensional reconstruction of hepatic bridging fibrosis in chronic hepatitis C viral infection. J Hepatol 2003;39:738–41.

88   Badizadegan K, Jonas MM, Ott MJ, et al. Histopathology of the liver in children with chronic hepatitis C infection. Hepatology 1998;28:1416–23.

89   Sugiyasu Y, Yuki N, Nagaoka T, et al. Histological improvement of chronic liver disease after spontaneous serum hepatitis C virus clearance. J Med Virol 2003;69:41–9.

89a Stenkvist J, Nystrom J, Falconer K, et al. Occasional spontaneous clearance of chronic hepatitis C virus in HIV-infected individuals. J Hepatol 2014;61:957–61.

90   Pol S, Carnot F, Nalpas B, et al. Reversibility of hepatitis C virus-related cirrhosis. Hum Pathol 2004;35:107–12.

90a Fujii Y, Uchida Y, Mochida S. Drug-induced immunoallergic hepatitis during combination therapy with daclatasvir and asunaprevir. Hepatology 2015;61:400–1.

91   Al Khalidi JA, Czaja AJ. Current concepts in the diagnosis, pathogenesis, and treatment of autoimmune hepatitis. Mayo Clin Proc 2001;76:1237–52.

92   Krawitt EL. Autoimmune hepatitis. N Engl J Med 2006;354:54–66.

93   Heneghan MA, McFarlane IG. Of mice and women: toward a mouse model of autoimmune hepatitis. Hepatology 2005;42:17–20.

94   Czaja AJ, Bayraktar Y. Non-classical phenotypes of autoimmune hepatitis and advances in diagnosis and treatment. World J Gastroenterol 2009;15:2314–28.

95   O'Brien C, Joshi S, Feld JJ, et al. Long-term follow-up of antimitochondrial antibody-positive autoimmune hepatitis. Hepatology 2008;48:550–6.

96   Alvarez F, Berg PA, Biandin FB, et al. International Autoimmune Hepatitis Group report: review of criteria for diagnosis of autoimmune hepatitis. J Hepatol 1999;31:929–38.

97   Hennes EM, Zeniya M, Czaja AJ, et al. Simplified criteria for the diagnosis of autoimmune hepatitis. Hepatology 2008;48:169–76.

98   Goldstein NS, Soman A, Gordon SC. Portal tract eosinophils and hepatocyte cytokeratin 7 immunoreactivity helps distinguish early-stage, mildly active primary biliary cirrhosis and autoimmune hepatitis. Am J Clin Pathol 2001;116:846–53.

99   Devaney K, Goodman ZD, Ishak KG. Postinfantile giant-cell transformation in hepatitis. Hepatology 1992;16:327–33.

100 Lau JYN, Koukoulis G, Mieli-Vergani G, et al. Syncytial giant-cell hepatitis – a specific disease entity? J Hepatol 1992;15:216–19.

101 Carpenter HA, Czaja AJ. The role of histologic evaluation in the diagnosis and management of autoimmune hepatitis and its variants. Clin Liver Dis 2002;6: 397–417.

102   Czaja AJ, Carpenter HA. Autoimmune hepatitis with incidental histologic features of bile duct injury. Hepatology 2001;34:659–65.

103   Zolfino T, Heneghan MA, Norris S, et al. Characteristics of autoimmune hepatitis in patients who are not of European Caucasoid ethnic origin. Gut 2002;50:713–17.

104   Gregorio GV, Portmann B, Karani J, et al. Autoimmune hepatitis/sclerosing cholangitis overlap syndrome in childhood: a 16-year prospective study. Hepatology 2001;33:544–53.

105   Mieli-Vergani G, Vergani D. Autoimmune hepatitis in children. Clin Liver Dis 2002;6:335–46.

106   Burgart LJ, Batts KP, Ludwig J, et al. Recent-onset autoimmune hepatitis. Biopsy findings and clinical correlations. Am J Surg Pathol 1995;19:699–708.

107   Pratt DS, Fawaz KA, Rabson A, et al. A novel histological lesion in glucocorticoid-responsive chronic hepatitis. Gastroenterology 1997;113:664–8.

108   Te HS, Koukoulis G, Ganger DR. Autoimmune hepatitis: a histological variant associated with prominent centrilobular necrosis. Gut 1997;41:269–71.

109   Singh R, Nair S, Farr G, et al. Acute autoimmune hepatitis presenting with centrizonal liver disease: case report and review of the literature. Am J Gastroenterol 2002;97:2670–3.

110   Misdraji J, Thiim M, Graeme-Cook FM. Autoimmune hepatitis with centrilobular necrosis. Am J Surg Pathol 2004;28:471–8.

111   Cotler SJ, Jakate S, Jensen DM. Resolution of cirrhosis in autoimmune hepatitis with corticosteroid therapy. J Clin Gastroenterol 2001;32:428–30.

112   Czaja AJ, Carpenter HA. Decreased fibrosis during corticosteroid therapy of autoimmune hepatitis. J Hepatol 2004;40:646–52.

113   Verma S, Gunuwan B, Mendler M, et al. Factors predicting relapse and poor outcome in type I autoimmune hepatitis: role of cirrhosis development, patterns of transaminases during remission and plasma cell activity in the liver biopsy. Am J Gastroenterol 2004;99:1510–16.

114   Czaja AJ, Carpenter HA. Progressive fibrosis during corticosteroid therapy of autoimmune hepatitis. Hepatology 2004;39:1631–8.

115   Czaja AJ, Carpenter HA. Histological findings in chronic hepatitis C with autoimmune features. Hepatology 1997;26:459–66.

116   Goldstein NS, Bayati N, Silverman AL, et al. Minocycline as a cause of drug-induced autoimmune hepatitis. Report of four cases and comparison with autoimmune hepatitis. Am J Clin Pathol 2000;114:591–8.

117   Björnsson E, Talwalkar J, Treeprasertsuk S, et al. Drug-induced autoimmune hepatitis: clinical characteristics and prognosis. Hepatology 2010;51:2040–8.

118   Alla V, Abraham J, Siddiqui J, et al. Autoimmune hepatitis triggered by statins. J Clin Gastroenterol 2006;40:757–61.

119   deLemos AS, Foureau DM, Jacobs C, et al. Drug-induced liver injury with autoimmune features. Semin Liver Dis 2014;34:194–204.

120   Lynch CR, Folkers ME, Hutson WR. Fulminant hepatic failure associated with the use of black cohosh: a case report. Liver Transpl 2006;12:989–92.

121   O'Leary JG, Zachary K, Misdraji J, et al. De novo autoimmune hepatitis during immune reconstitution in an HIV-infected patient receiving highly active antiretroviral therapy. Clin Infect Dis 2008;46:e12–14.

121a. Czaja AJ. Cholestatic phenotypes of autoimmune hepatitis. Clin Gastroenterol Hepatol 2014;12:1430–8.

122   Poupon R, Chazouillieres O, Corpechot C, et al. Development of autoimmune hepatitis in patients with typical primary biliary cirrhosis. Hepatology 2006;44:85–90.

123   Twaddell WS, Lefkowitch J, Berk PD. Evolution from primary biliary cirrhosis to primary biliary cirrhosis/autoimmune hepatitis overlap syndrome. Semin Liver Dis 2008;28:128–34.

124   Bedossa P, Dargere D, Paradis V. Sampling variability of liver fibrosis in chronic hepatitis C. Hepatology 2003;38:1449–57.

125   Wright M, Thursz M, Pullen R, et al. Quantitative versus morphological assessment of liver fibrosis: semi-quantitative scores are more robust than digital image fibrosis area estimation. Liver Int 2003;23:28–34.

126   Scheuer PJ. Classification of chronic viral hepatitis: a need for reassessment. J Hepatol 1991;13:372–4.

127   Bedossa P, Poynard T, the METAVIR cooperative study group. An algorithm for the grading of activity in chronic hepatitis C. Hepatology 1996;24:289–93.

128   Bedossa P, Bioulac-Sage P, Callard P, et al. Intraobserver and interobserver variations in liver biopsy interpretation in patients with chronic hepatitis C. Hepatology 1994;20:15–20.

129   Ishak K, Baptista A, Bianchi L, et al. Histological grading and staging of chronic hepatitis. J Hepatol 1995;22:696–9.

130   Knodell RG, Ishak KG, Black WC, et al. Formulation and application of a numerical scoring system for assessing histological activity in asymptomatic chronic active hepatitis. Hepatology 1981;1:431–5.

131   Lagging LM, Westin J, Svensson E, et al. Progression of fibrosis in untreated patients with hepatitis C virus infection. Liver 2002;22:136–44.

132   Guido M, Rugge M. Liver biopsy sampling in chronic viral hepatitis. Semin Liver Dis 2004;24:89–97.

133   Regev A, Berho M, Jeffers LJ, et al. Sampling error and intraobserver variation in liver biopsy in patients with chronic HCV infection. Am J Gastroenterol 2002;97:2614–18.

134   Colloredo G, Guido M, Sonzogni A, et al. Impact of liver biopsy size on histological evaluation of chronic viral hepatitis: the smaller the sample, the milder the disease. J Hepatol 2003;39:239–44.

135   Brunetti E, Silini E, Pistorio A, et al. Coarse vs. fine needle aspiration biopsy for the assessment of diffuse liver disease from hepatitis C virus-related chronic hepatitis. J Hepatol 2004;40:501–6.

136   Petz D, Klauck S, Rohl FW, et al. Feasibility of histological grading and staging of chronic viral hepatitis using specimens obtained by thin-needle biopsy. Virchows Arch 2003;442:238–44.

137   Rousselet M-C, Michalak S, Dupré F, et al. Sources of variability in histological scoring of chronic hepatitis. Hepatology 2005;41:257–64.

General reading

Carpenter HA, Czaja AJ. The role of histologic evaluation in the diagnosis and management of autoimmune hepatitis and its variants. Clin Liver Dis 2002;6:397–417.

Czaja AJ. Autoimmune liver disease. Curr Opin Gastroenterol 2003;19:232–42.

De Vos R, Verslype C, Depla E, et al. Ultrastructural visualization of hepatitis C virus components in human and primate liver biopsies. J Hepatol 2002;37:370–9.

Fattovich G, Bortolotti F, Donato F. Natural history of chronic hepatitis B: special emphasis on disease progression and prognostic factors. J Hepatol 2008;48:335–52.

Ganem D, Prince AM. Hepatitis B virus infection – natural history and clinical consequences. N Engl J Med 2004;350:1118–29.

Goodman ZD. Grading and staging systems for inflammation and fibrosis in chronic liver diseases. J Hepatol 2007;47:598–607.

Ishak KG. Pathologic features of chronic hepatitis. A review and update. Am J Clin Pathol 2000;113:40–55.

Lai CL, Ratziu V, Yuen MF, et al. Viral hepatitis B. Lancet 2003;362:2089–94.

Mani H, Kleiner DE. Liver biopsy findings in chronic hepatitis B. Hepatology 2009;49:S61–71.

McFarlane IG. Definition and classification of autoimmune hepatitis. Semin Liver Dis 2002;22:317–24.

Penin F, Dubuisson J, Rey FA, et al. Structural biology of hepatitis C virus. Hepatology 2004;39:5–19.

Ramadori G, Saile B. Portal tract fibrogenesis in the liver. Lab Invest 2004;84:153–9.

Scheuer PJ, Standish RA, Dhillon AP. Scoring of chronic hepatitis. Clin Liver Dis 2002;6:335–47.

Seeff LB. Natural history of chronic hepatitis C. Hepatology 2004;36:S35–46.

Theise ND, Bodenheimer HC Jr, Ferrell LD. Acute and chronic viral hepatitis. In: Burt AD, Portmann BC, Ferrell LD, editors. MacSween's Pathology of the Liver. 6th ed. Edinburgh: Churchill Livingstone/Elsevier; 2012. p. 361–402.

Washington MK. Autoimmune liver disease: overlap and outliers. Mod Pathol 2007;20:S15–30.

Cirrhosis

Introduction

Cirrhosis is a diffuse process in which the normal lobules are replaced by architecturally abnormal nodules separated by fibrous tissue.[1,2] The nodules, which are most commonly the result of regenerative hyperplasia following hepatocellular injury, are functionally less efficient than normal hepatic parenchyma and there is a profound disturbance of vascular relationships.

Several different kinds of information can be obtained about the cirrhotic liver by means of liver biopsy (**Box 10.1**). The most important functions of biopsy are to establish a diagnosis, to assess the cause of the cirrhosis as far as possible and to detect hepatocellular carcinoma (HCC).

Box 10.1 Main information from liver biopsy in cirrhosis
Diagnosis of cirrhosis
Assessment of cause
Stage of development
Histological activity
Detection of hepatocellular carcinoma

Diagnosis of cirrhosis by liver biopsy

The ease with which the pathologist can diagnose cirrhosis from a biopsy specimen depends on the sample as well as on the criteria used. The sample may be sufficiently big, and the nodules sufficiently small, to make the diagnosis obvious. On the other hand a slender core from within a large cirrhotic nodule can be difficult to identify as such (**see Fig. 1.4**). There are occasions when the pathologist can do no more than hint at the possible diagnosis.

The type of biopsy needle used also influences the ease of diagnosis. Very narrow needles may be adequate to obtain tumour samples, but may be inadequate for the accurate diagnosis of medical conditions. For example, in staging chronic hepatitis thin-needle biopsies obtained under computed tomographic guidance may underdiagnose cirrhosis for advanced bridging fibrosis.[3] Some clinicians prefer to use the TruCut type of needle when cirrhosis is suspected in order to lessen the risk of fragmentation,[4,5] but suitable samples can usually be obtained with needles of the aspiration type.[6,7] Transjugular biopsy is used when there is a risk of haemorrhage by other routes. The combination of biopsy with laparoscopy has been advocated.[8,9] Operative wedge biopsies of cirrhotic liver give an accurate idea of the relative proportions of parenchyma and stroma in the liver as a whole.[10]

Box 10.2 Cirrhosis: diagnostic criteria

Fundamental

Nodularity

Fibrosis

Relative

Fragmentation

Abnormal structure

Hepatocellular changes

Regenerative hyperplasia

Pleomorphism

Large-cell dysplasia (large-cell change)

Small-cell dysplasia (small-cell change)

Excess copper-associated protein

The histological criteria for a diagnosis of cirrhosis are outlined in **Box 10.2**. The two fundamental criteria, nodularity and fibrosis, reflect the definition of cirrhosis. When there are well-defined, rounded nodules surrounded by fibrous septa the diagnosis is easily established. Underestimating the stage of fibrosis because of specimen fragmentation (see below) is a concern, particularly when scoring biopsies in chronic hepatitis.[11] Correlation with clinical and laboratory data helps surmount this problem. Occasionally, a nodular appearance just deep to the liver capsule is not representative of the whole liver but has resulted from transection of a tongue or peninsula extending from the main bulk of the parenchyma.

In many patients the relative criteria listed in **Box 10.2** are equally important. They allow a tentative diagnosis of cirrhosis to be reached, readily converted to a firm diagnosis when correlated with other data. A diagnosis of cirrhosis therefore requires communication between pathologist and clinician, and cannot be exactly equated with a histological stage.[12]

Fragmentation

Fragmentation of the specimen, either at the time of biopsy or during processing in the laboratory, should itself suggest the possibility of cirrhosis (**Fig. 10.1**). The specimen is more likely to break into fragments when needles of the aspiration type (e.g. Menghini) are used. Other biopsy specimens that are likely to fragment are metastatic tumours surrounded by reactive fibrous tissue, and HCC.

Figure 10.1 Cirrhosis: fragmented sample.

A specimen obtained by the aspiration biopsy method has broken into rounded fragments peripherally circumscribed by fibrosis. (Needle biopsy, reticulin.)

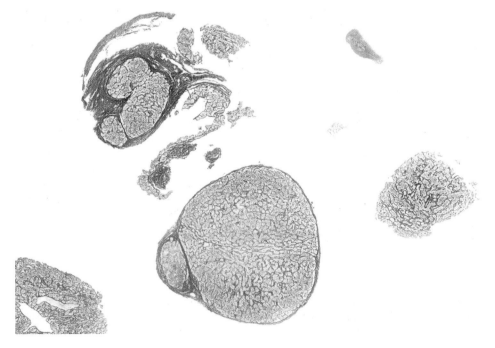

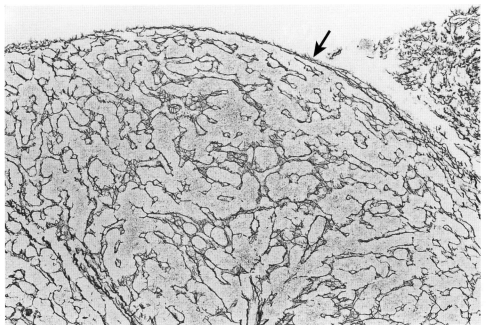

Figure 10.2
Cirrhosis: selective
sampling.
A nodule has been
cored out of the
connective tissue
by the biopsy
procedure, but a thin
layer of connective
tissue (arrow) has
adhered to the
nodule margin.
(Needle biopsy,
reticulin.)

Abnormal structure

Structural changes should be assessed by means of a reticulin preparation, preferably not counterstained. This may show two features not readily seen with other stains. First, although nodules are readily cored out of the dense fibrous stroma of a cirrhotic liver during aspiration biopsy, a thin layer of connective tissue tends to adhere to the nodules over much of their surface (**Fig. 10.2**). This layer may be difficult to see even with the help of collagen stains, and is easily missed in haematoxylin and eosin (H&E)-stained sections (**Fig. 10.3**). Second, minor alterations of structure become apparent even in those nodules which closely mimic normal liver. Such alterations include abnormal orientation of reticulin fibres resulting from different patterns and rates of growth in different areas (**Fig. 10.4**) and approximation of portal tracts and terminal venules. The number of venules may be abnormally large in relation to the number of portal tracts (**Fig. 10.5**), and the latter are sometimes abnormally small and poorly formed (**see Fig. 1.4**). A more obvious structural abnormality in cirrhosis is the presence of septa linking central veins (terminal hepatic venules) to portal tracts. These septa must be distinguished from recently formed necrotic bridges.

In wedge biopsies, excess fibrous tissue in and near the capsule and crowding of vessels must be distinguished from the changes of cirrhosis. The latter extend through the specimen, whereas the former is confined to the capsular and immediately subcapsular area.[13] Very occasionally a wedge biopsy of part of a large, well-differentiated regeneration nodule fails to show the histological features of cirrhosis.

Hepatocellular changes

In some biopsies from cirrhotic livers the hepatocytes are normal in appearance and arrangement, so that diagnosis rests on the structural changes discussed above. In others there are more or less obvious abnormalities of growth.

**Figure 10.3
Cirrhosis: selective
sampling.**
Same field as in
Fig. 10.2. In a
haematoxylin and
eosin preparation
the thin layer of
connective tissue is
not easily seen.
(Needle biopsy, H&E.)

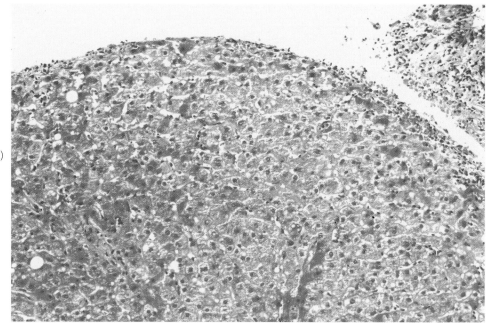

**Figure 10.4
Cirrhosis: distorted
reticulin pattern.**
The distortion has
resulted from
abnormal and
irregular hepatocyte
growth patterns.
(Needle biopsy,
reticulin.)

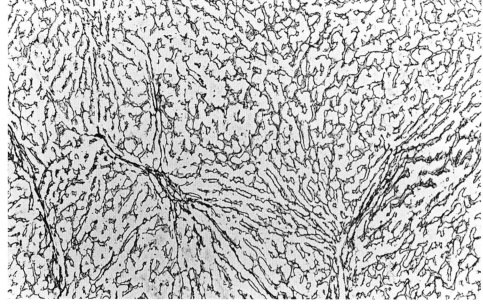

Regeneration is suggested by thickening of the liver-cell plates (**Fig. 10.6**). In any liver an oblique plane of sectioning will cause a few plates to appear more than one cell thick, but widespread double-cell plates are seen when there is active growth. Hepatocytes in hyperplastic areas contain little or no lipofuscin pigment, even near terminal venules. Regeneration is not always evident in cirrhosis because it is not a continuous process. Its absence does not therefore exclude the diagnosis. Conversely, its presence does not prove cirrhosis, because it is found also in other circumstances, for example after an acute hepatitis and in the precirrhotic stages of chronic biliary diseases.

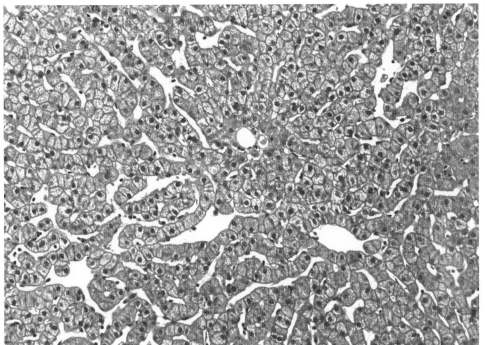

**Figure 10.5
Cirrhosis: abnormal vascular relationships.**
Several venous channels are seen near to each other.
(Wedge biopsy, H&E.)

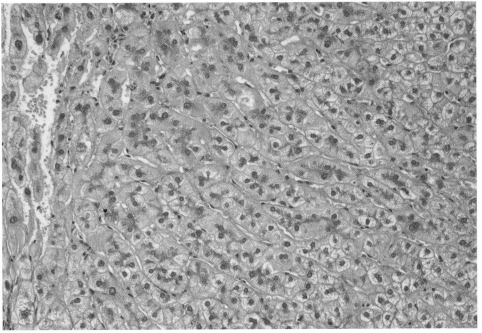

**Figure 10.6
Cirrhosis: hepatocellular regeneration.**
Liver-cell plates are two or more cells thick, indicating active growth.
(Needle biopsy, H&E.)

A very characteristic feature of cirrhosis is the presence of adjacent populations of hepatocytes growing at different rates and having different cell and nuclear characteristics (**Fig. 10.7**). This **pleomorphism** gives rise to the abnormalities of reticulin pattern already mentioned, notably a tendency for reticulin fibres in the different growth areas to lie in different directions.

**Figure 10.7
Cirrhosis: different
cell populations.**
The parenchymal
cells in area A are
smaller than those in
area B, which also
show a rounded and
nodular growth
pattern. (Wedge
biopsy, H&E.)

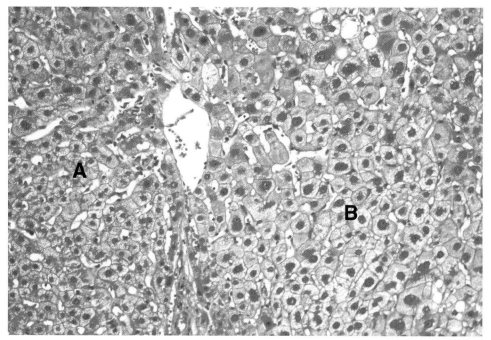

In a minority of cirrhotic livers the hepatocytes show structural atypia of a degree sufficient to warrant a label of **dysplasia**, an appearance further discussed in **Chapter 11**. Two types have been described: large-cell dysplasia[14] and small-cell dysplasia.[15] Because of the controversial status of either type as a precursor of malignant change,[16] some authors prefer to call them large-cell change and small-cell change.[16,17] In the large-cell form, the cells are enlarged and their nuclei are hyperchromatic and irregular in shape, with prominent nucleoli (**Fig. 10.8**). Nuclear–cytoplasmic ratio is normal or only moderately increased.[18] This type of dysplasia was first described in an African population with a high incidence of HCC and hepatitis B virus (HBV) infection.[14] It is most often seen in patients with HBV and HCV infection but may also be evident in other chronic liver diseases.[19] There is evidence of an association of large-cell dysplasia with an increased risk of development of HCC independently of other risk factors.[20,21] Decreased expression of cell cycle checkpoint markers, presence of cytoplasmic DNA micronuclei and shortened telomeres in large-cell change are evidence favouring a disposition to HCC.[22] Demonstration of an increased hepatocyte proliferation rate as a risk for carcinoma is also important.[23] Care should be taken not to interpret the nuclear atypia which may be associated with cholestasis as large-cell dysplasia.[17]

In small-cell dysplasia the nuclear–cytoplasmic ratio is increased but the overall size of the affected cells is less than normal (**Fig. 10.9**). Zones of dysplastic hepatocytes of either type support a diagnosis of cirrhosis, and are regarded by some clinicians as an indication for increased monitoring for HCC. A finding of dysplasia of either type should therefore be specifically mentioned in liver biopsy reports.

Differential diagnosis

When there is nodularity and evidence of regeneration but little or no fibrosis, **nodular regenerative hyperplasia** should be considered. In **congenital hepatic fibrosis** the acinar architecture remains intact and the ductal plate malformation is seen. In **chronic hepatitis** with fibrosis and structural abnormalities, the differential diagnosis is between active

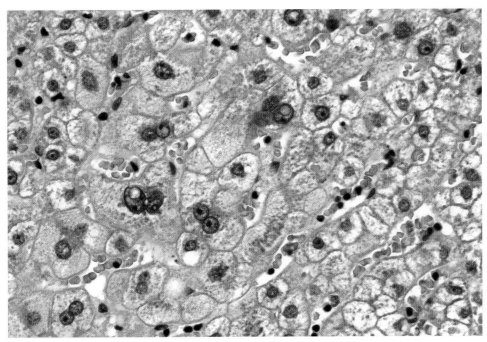

Figure 10.8
Cirrhosis: large-cell dysplasia (large-cell change).
The nuclei of the enlarged hepatocytes at centre and left are irregular in shape and vary greatly in size and staining intensity. Several of these cells are multinucleated. Compare with the normal hepatocytes at right and in the upper left-hand corner. (Wedge biopsy, H&E.)

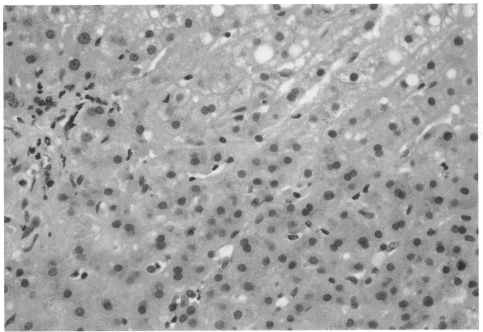

Figure 10.9
Cirrhosis: small-cell dysplasia (small-cell change).
The hepatocytes below and to the right have normal-sized nuclei, but their overall size is reduced. Nuclear–cytoplasmic ratios are therefore increased. (Needle biopsy, H&E.)

cirrhosis and chronic hepatitis that has not yet reached the stage of cirrhosis. This problem cannot always be resolved on the basis of a liver biopsy. Similar doubt may arise in steatohepatitis. The presence of substantial quantities of copper and copper-associated protein in non-cholestatic chronic liver disease supports a diagnosis of cirrhosis.[24] Cirrhotic nodules can usually be distinguished from well-differentiated **HCC**. In the latter the cell plate architecture is more abnormal, reticulin may be scanty or absent and the cells have malignant cytological characteristics. Also, hepatocellular siderosis is often present secondarily in cirrhosis of varied aetiology (**see Ch. 14**) but is typically absent in tumour cells of HCC.

Assessment of cause

Box 10.3 Main causes of cirrhosis

Viral hepatitis (B, C, D)

Alcohol abuse

Obesity, insulin resistance/metabolic syndrome

Biliary disease

Metabolic disorders

Haemochromatosis

Wilson's disease

α_1-Antitrypsin deficiency, etc.

Venous outflow obstruction

Drugs and toxins

Autoimmune disease

Box 10.4 Cirrhosis: assessment of cause

Pattern of nodules and fibrosis

Bile ducts

Blood vessels

Steatohepatitis

Evidence of viral infection

Abnormal deposits

Iron

Copper, copper-associated protein

α_1-Antitrypsin globules

Biopsy may help to establish the cause of a cirrhosis. In some of the categories listed in **Box 10.3** the histological appearances are diagnostic. The term 'cryptogenic' should only be applied when full clinical and laboratory investigations have been completed and the features listed in **Box 10.4** have been assessed. This can be achieved by means of a small range of routine stains. There is evidence to suggest that many examples of cryptogenic cirrhosis result from non-alcoholic steatohepatitis (NASH), not evident histologically at the time of diagnosis.[25] Some cases of cirrhosis are due to mutations in genes for specific cellular keratins[26] or for bile canalicular transporter proteins.[27]

Pattern of nodules and fibrosis

Irregularly shaped nodules suggest the possibility of a biliary cause, especially if there is perinodular oedema, ductular reaction and chronic cholestasis. In a precirrhotic stage of venous outflow obstruction there is regular fibrosis in perivenular regions (acinar zones 3). Sinusoids are dilated. Portal tracts show little or no abnormality or sometimes have changes mimicking biliary tract obstruction.[28] Certain features are indicative of earlier chronic hepatitis that evolved to cirrhosis. Irregular, slender fibrous septa emanating from portal tracts, lymphoplasmacytic infiltrates, lymphoid aggregates or follicles and foci of interface hepatitis should prompt consideration of the several causes of chronic hepatitis.

Confluent fibrosis which replaces multiple adjacent lobules is a common feature in several types of cirrhosis, particularly following steatohepatitis and chronic hepatitis of viral or autoimmune aetiology. It is also seen in the less common 'postnecrotic' cirrhosis which develops rapidly, within a few months of a severe viral or drug-induced acute hepatitis. Needle biopsy samples in such cases may show entire cores, portions of cores and especially the subcapsular region occupied by fibrous tissue, residual portal tracts and many ductular structures (**see Fig. 4.13C**), mild chronic inflammatory cell infiltrates, entrapped regenerative liver-cell rosettes and collections of small neovessels (see Blood vessels, below).

Bile ducts

Assessment of bile-duct numbers in cirrhosis is very important. The number of ducts should approximately equal the number of arteries of similar size and location, but the pathologist must bear in mind that not every portal tract will necessarily contain a bile duct in the plane of section. Definite duct loss should prompt consideration of primary biliary cirrhosis or primary sclerosing cholangitis. In some cases ductopenia is drug-related or is associated with other conditions,[29] so the clinical history is important. In children or young adults, other ductopenic syndromes should also be considered. Typical bile-duct lesions of primary biliary cirrhosis, with or without granulomas, are still sometimes found at a stage of cirrhosis.

Periductal fibrosis may be very prominent in primary sclerosing cholangitis. Ductular reaction is a non-specific finding, but when severe and focal it often reflects biliary disease. Following extensive hepatocellular damage in cirrhosis – for example, after variceal haemorrhage – there is sometimes a very extensive ductular reaction which can be mistaken for cholangiocarcinoma.

Blood vessels

Occluded, narrowed or recanalised veins suggest that the cirrhosis may be the result of venous outflow block, but they are also found in cirrhosis from other causes.[30,31] Portal and hepatic venous thrombosis has indeed been implicated in the progression of cirrhosis in general.[32] Recognition of venous lesions is often difficult without the help of stains for collagen or elastic fibres. Neovascularisation of fibrotic portal tracts, areas of confluent fibrosis and bridging fibrous septa in cirrhosis produce numerous lymphatic and capillary channels, particularly in chronic hepatitis B and C.[33]

Steatohepatitis

This is found in alcohol abusers and in individuals at risk for non-alcoholic fatty liver disease, as a manifestation of drug toxicity, or for no obvious underlying reason (**see Ch. 7**). In amiodarone toxicity the fatty change is usually absent. Steatohepatitis must be distinguished from chronic cholestasis, in which there are also swollen hepatocytes containing Mallory bodies (**see Ch. 5**).

Evidence of viral infection

Features of chronic hepatitis, particularly interface hepatitis and lymphocytic infiltration, are often but by no means always due to infection with one of the hepatitis viruses. Liver-cell dysplasia also favours a viral cause. Ground-glass hepatocytes, Victoria blue or orcein stains (**Fig. 10.10**) and immunostains for viral antigens (**see Fig. 9.14**) help in the diagnosis of HBV infection, but tissue evidence of HBV antigens is not always present or detectable. Lymphoid aggregates or follicles should suggest the possibility of hepatitis C (**Fig. 10.11**). More than one virus or other causal agent may be responsible for a patient's cirrhosis. Abundant plasma cells raise the possibility of autoimmune hepatitis but are also sometimes found in viral hepatitis.

Abnormal deposits

Severe parenchymal siderosis should always raise the possibility of hereditary haemochromatosis, even when another cause is also evident. However, stainable iron often accumulates in cirrhosis from any cause.[34,35] Lack of significant haemosiderin in the connective tissue of portal tracts or fibrous septa in a cirrhosis points to a cause other than hereditary haemochromatosis (**see Fig. 14.12**). In hereditary haemochromatosis the nodules are sometimes irregular, as in biliary cirrhosis.

Copper and copper-associated protein can often be detected in cirrhosis, whatever its cause.[24] Large amounts at the edges of the nodules suggest biliary disease. Staining of entire

**Figure 10.10
Hepatitis B surface
antigen in hepatitis
B virus (HBV)-
related cirrhosis.**
Many hepatocytes
show positive
cytoplasmic staining
for HBV surface
antigen. This staining
method also
demonstrates elastic
tissue fibres in the
fibrous tissue.
(Recipient liver from
transplantation,
Victoria blue.)

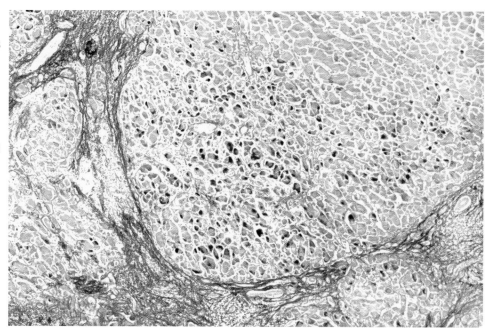

**Figure 10.11
Cirrhosis following
hepatitis C virus
infection.**
Lymphoid
aggregates are still
visible. The patient
was also infected
with GBV-C (the
so-called hepatitis G
virus). (Recipient liver
from transplantation,
H&E.)

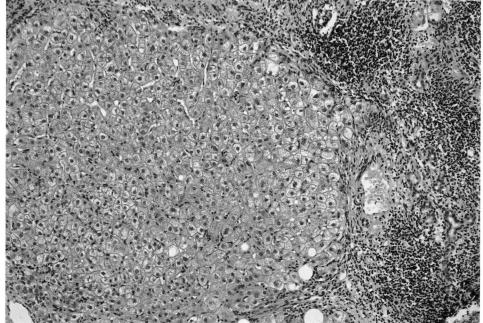

nodules is seen in Wilson's disease, but other nodules may be negative. In some stages of
the disease the copper is not histochemically demonstrable, so that negative staining does
not exclude the diagnosis. Abundant copper and Mallory bodies are also features of Indian
childhood cirrhosis and other forms of copper toxicosis.[36,37]

α_1-Antitrypsin bodies should always be looked for in cirrhosis. Immunocytochemical
staining is more sensitive than diastase–periodic acid–Schiff.

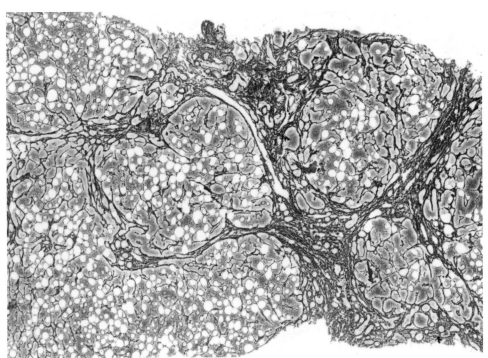

**Figure 10.12
Cirrhosis:
micronodular
pattern.**
Nodules are of
lobular size or
smaller. (Needle
biopsy, reticulin.)

Anatomical type

Because of possible sampling error, the pathologist cannot confidently assess nodule size in the rest of the liver on the basis of a biopsy specimen. This is usually of little consequence to the patient, though one biopsy study has suggested a significant correlation of the hepatic venous pressure gradient in portal hypertension with small nodule size.[38] Nevertheless, primary classification of cirrhosis by nodule size is no longer appropriate, because aetiology is clinically much more important.

However, nodule size does influence the ease of histological diagnosis. When nodules are of the size order of the lobules from which they are derived, several nodules are usually seen in one biopsy and diagnosis is easy (**Figs 10.12, 10.13**). When nodules are larger (**Fig. 10.14**), more subtle diagnostic criteria need to be considered. The most difficult anatomical type to recognise is **incomplete septal cirrhosis**. This is characterised by indistinct nodularity, slender septa, some of which end blindly, poorly formed small portal tracts and abnormal relationships between portal tracts and efferent venules[39] (**Fig. 10.15**). There is evidence of hepatocytic hyperplasia, giving rise to crowding of reticulin fibres in adjacent areas. Sinusoidal dilatation is common, while inflammation and necrosis are generally modest or absent. A reticulin preparation is important for diagnosis because the slender septa are easily missed (**Figs 10.15, 10.16**). The diagnosis is more easily made in wedge biopsies than in needle specimens. A relationship to various forms of non-cirrhotic portal hypertension has been demonstrated,[39-42] but it has also been postulated that incomplete septal cirrhosis can represent a burnt-out form of macronodular cirrhosis.[43] The incomplete septa could also reflect resorption of fibrous tissue, a type of 'regressed cirrhosis'.

**Figure 10.13
Cirrhosis:
micronodular
pattern.**
Similar field as in
Fig. 10.12. There is
steatosis. (Needle
biopsy, H&E.)

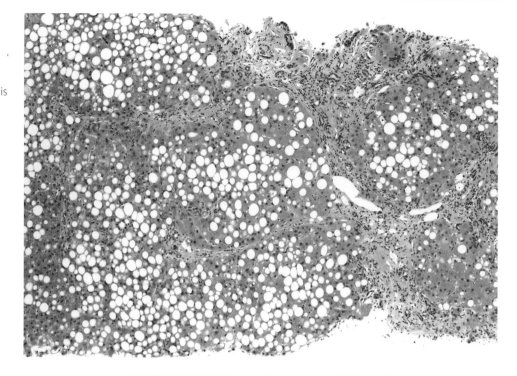

**Figure 10.14
Cirrhosis:
macronodular
pattern.**
Nodules are
larger than in
Figs 10.12, 10.13.
The magnification is
slightly smaller.
(Needle biopsy,
reticulin.)

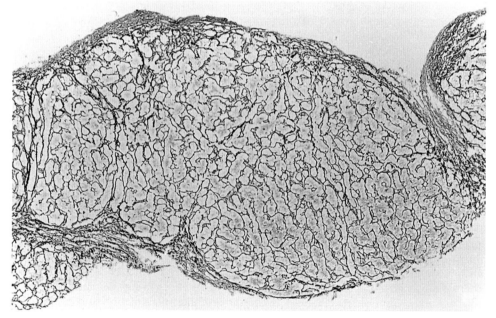

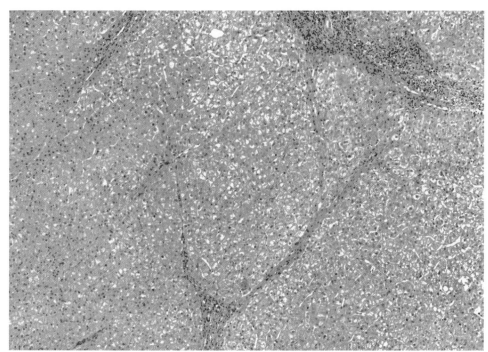

**Figure 10.15
Cirrhosis:
incomplete septal
pattern.**
The parenchyma is
nodular but only
partially surrounded
by fibrous septa.
Note the
incompleted fibrous
septum emerging
vertically from the
portal tract at
bottom. (Wedge
biopsy, H&E.)

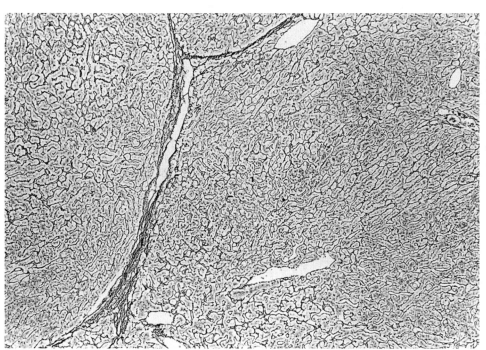

**Figure 10.16
Cirrhosis:
incomplete septal
pattern.**
Slender septa and
vessels are present.
There is a small
portal tract on the
right, towards the
top of the figure.
(Wedge biopsy,
reticulin.)

Figure 10.17 Early (developing) cirrhosis. There is extensive fibrosis and architectural distortion in this biopsy from an alcohol abuser. Nodules are beginning to form but are not yet clearly defined. (Needle biopsy, reticulin.)

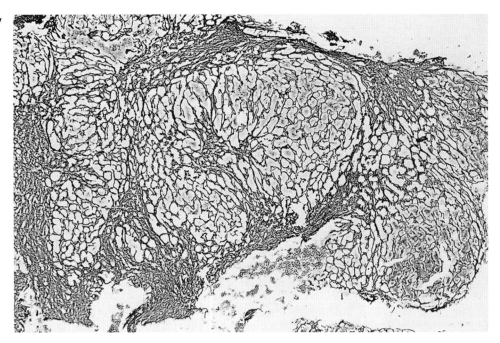

Stage of development

In some patients, cirrhosis is obvious and appears mature, in the sense that the well-demarcated nodules and dense fibrosis give an impression of long-standing disease. In others there is doubt as to whether there is cirrhosis or merely fibrosis. An impression may be gained that cirrhosis is incipient or at an early stage of development (**Fig. 10.17**). When doubt is unresolved, a report of 'developing cirrhosis' or 'incomplete cirrhosis' is sometimes appropriate. The concept of incomplete cirrhosis is recognised in the staging system of Ishak et al.[44] Once cirrhosis is fully established, reversion to a normal lobular pattern is unlikely. Indeed, reversibility of cirrhosis is a controversial subject[45] and the pathologist should consider this prospect cautiously, taking into account the type of biopsy sample, the underlying disease process and the possibility of sampling error. Diminished fibrosis following therapy does not automatically confer a return to normal liver-cell plate structure and vascular relationships.[2] Despite these caveats, reports of regression of cirrhosis of varied aetiologies[46,47] deserve attention.

Paradoxically, there may be confusion between mild chronic hepatitis and an inactive, well-established cirrhosis. This reflects difficulty in diagnosing some examples of late cirrhosis by needle biopsy, because of a tendency for nodule size to increase with time.

Histological activity

Activity is a convenient term to describe the rate of progression of the cirrhosis. It is usually taken to mean the various forms of liver-cell damage and inflammation typical of chronic viral hepatitis. In cirrhosis following steatohepatitis, however, the severity of the latter should also be taken into account.

In an inactive cirrhosis the interface between septa and nodules is sharply defined (**Fig. 10.18**). Cellular infiltration is mild and may be confined to the septa. There is little or no focal necrosis or intranodular inflammation. In an active, rapidly progressive cirrhosis

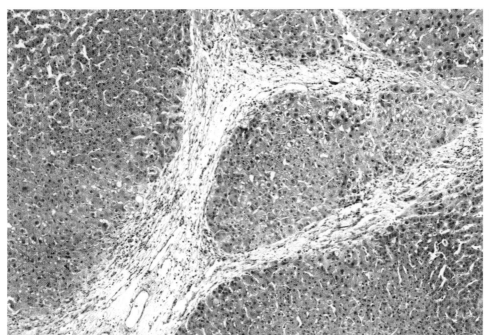

Figure 10.18
Inactive cirrhosis.
Nodules are sharply outlined and inflammatory cells are scanty. (Wedge biopsy, H&E.)

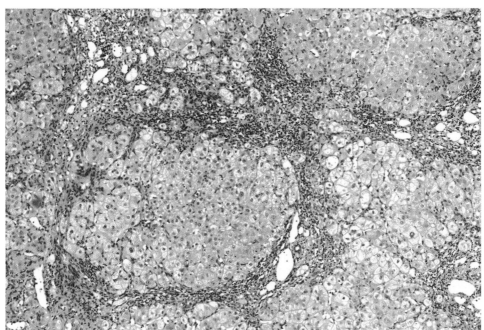

Figure 10.19
Active cirrhosis.
The outline of the nodule is blurred by interface hepatitis and there is a heavy inflammatory infiltrate. (Wedge biopsy, H&E.)

on the other hand, the interface is blurred by hepatocellular damage and inflammation (**Fig. 10.19**). Isolated hepatocytes or groups of cells may be seen within the inflamed septa. There is hepatocellular damage and inflammation deep within the nodules.

Histological activity often varies in severity from one part of the liver to another. Comparison of activity in multiple biopsies from an individual patient should therefore be made with caution and with reference to clinical and biochemical data.

Complications

Hypoperfusion leads to coagulative necrosis involving whole nodules or their centres.[31] This is sometimes referred to as **nodular infarction**.

In recent years, advances in imaging and examination of explanted cirrhotic livers after transplantation have led to extensive discussion of the pathology and nomenclature of nodules different in appearance from the rest, and usually larger in diameter. The relationship of these nodules to HCC has been debated, and is further discussed in **Chapter 11**. An international working party[48] has recommended that the old term adenomatous hyperplasia should no longer be used, and that the nodules should be subdivided into **large regenerative nodules (macroregenerative nodules)** and **dysplastic nodules**. The latter are further subclassified as low-grade and high-grade. The dysplastic nodules differ from macroregenerative nodules in their content of dysplastic (atypical) hepatocytes and their more expansile growth pattern. However, the distinction between macroregenerative nodules and low-grade dysplastic nodules is often difficult, as is the distinction between high-grade dysplastic nodules and well-differentiated **HCC**, a very important complication of cirrhosis. In addition to the three large nodule types described by the working party, the group also defined **dysplastic foci**, clusters of dysplastic hepatocytes less than 1 mm in diameter.[49] In making a microscopic diagnosis and differentiating between these various possibly preneoplastic nodules, the pathologist must bear in mind that needle biopsy samples of a nodule may not be representative of the entire nodule, and that HCC may have arisen in a part not sampled by the needle.

References

1 Anthony PP, Ishak KG, Nayak NC, et al. The morphology of cirrhosis: definition, nomenclature, and classification. Bull World Health Org 1977;55:521–40.

2 Desmet VJ, Roskams T. Cirrhosis reversal: a duel between dogma and myth. J Hepatol 2004;40:860–7.

3 Petz D, Klauck S, Röhl FW, et al. Feasibility of histological grading and staging of chronic viral hepatitis using specimens obtained by thin-needle biopsy. Virchows Arch 2003;442:238–44.

4 Rockey DC, Caldwell SH, Goodman ZD, et al. Liver biopsy. Hepatology 2009;49:1017–44.

5 Colombo M, Del Ninno E, de Francis R, et al. Ultrasound-assisted percutaneous liver biopsy: superiority of the Tru-Cut over the Menghini needle for diagnosis of cirrhosis. Gastroenterology 1988;95:487–9.

6 Bateson MC, Hopwood D, Duguid HL, et al. A comparative trial of liver biopsy needles. J Clin Pathol 1980;33:131–3.

7 Littlewood ER, Gilmore IT, Murray-Lyon IM, et al. Comparison of the Trucut and Surecut liver biopsy needles. J Clin Pathol 1982;35:761–3.

8 Orlando R, Lirussi F, Okolicsanyi L. Laparoscopy and liver biopsy: further evidence that the two procedures improve the diagnosis of liver cirrhosis. A retrospective study of 1,003 consecutive examinations. J Clin Gastroenterol 1990;12:47–52.

9 Jalan R, Harrison DJ, Dillon JF, et al. Laparoscopy and histology in the diagnosis of chronic liver disease. Q J Med 1995;88:559–64.

10 Imamura H, Kawasaki S, Bandai Y, et al. Comparison between wedge and needle biopsies for evaluating the degree of cirrhosis. J Hepatol 1993;17:215–19.

11 Everhart JE, Wright EC, Goodman ZD, et al. Prognostic value of Ishak fibrosis stage: findings from the Hepatitis C Antiviral Long-Term Treatment Against Cirrhosis trial. Hepatology 2010;51:585–94.

12 Desmet VJ, Roskams T. Reversal of cirrhosis: evidence-based medicine? Gastroenterology 2003;125:629–30.

13 Petrelli M, Scheuer PJ. Variation in subcapsular liver structure and its significance in the interpretation of wedge biopsies. J Clin Pathol 1967;20:743–8.

14 Anthony PP, Vogel CL, Barker LF. Liver cell dysplasia: a premalignant condition. J Clin Pathol 1973;26:217–23.

15 Watanabe S, Okita K, Harada T, et al. Morphologic studies of the liver cell dysplasia. Cancer 1983;51:2197–205.

16 Lee RG, Tsamandas AC, Demetris AJ. Large cell change (liver cell dysplasia) and hepatocellular carcinoma in cirrhosis: matched case–control study, pathological analysis, and pathogenetic hypothesis. Hepatology 1997;26:1415–22.

17 Natarajan S, Theise ND, Thung SN, et al. Large-cell change of hepatocytes in cirrhosis may represent a reaction to prolonged cholestasis. Am J Surg Pathol 1997;21:312–18.

18 Roncalli M, Borzio M, Tombesi MV, et al. A morphometric study of liver cell dysplasia. Hum Pathol 1988;19:471–4.

19 Hodges TR, Millward-Sadler GH, Barbatis C, et al. Heterozygous MZ alpha-1-antitrypsin deficiency in adults with chronic active hepatitis and cryptogenic cirrhosis. N Engl J Med 1981;304:557–60.

20 Libbrecht L, Craninx M, Nevens F, et al. Predictive value of liver cell dysplasia for development of hepatocellular carcinoma in patients with non-cirrhotic and cirrhotic chronic viral hepatitis. Histopathology 2001;39:66–71.

21 Borzio M, Bruno S, Roncalli M, et al. Liver cell dysplasia is a major risk factor for hepatocellular carcinoma in cirrhosis: a prospective study. Gastroenterology 1995;108:812–17.

22 Kim H, Oh B-K, Roncalli M, et al. Large liver cell change in hepatitis B virus-related liver cirrhosis. Hepatology 2009;50:752–62.

23 Borzio M, Trerè D, Borzio F, et al. Hepatocyte proliferation rate is a powerful parameter for predicting hepatocellular carcinoma development in liver cirrhosis. J Clin Pathol Mol Pathol 1998;51:96–101.

24 Guarascio P, Yentis F, Cevikbas U, et al. Value of copper-associated protein in diagnostic assessment of liver biopsy. J Clin Pathol 1983;36:18–23.

25 Caldwell SH, Oelsner DH, Iezzoni JC, et al. Cryptogenic cirrhosis: clinical characterization and risk factors for underlying disease. Hepatology 1999;29:664–9.

26 Ku N-O, Gish R, Wright TL, et al. Keratin 8 mutations in patients with cryptogenic liver disease. N Engl J Med 2001;344:1580–7.

27 Gotthardt D, Runz H, Keitel V, et al. A mutation in the canalicular phospholipid transporter gene, ABCB4, is associated with cholestasis, ductopenia, and cirrhosis in adults. Hepatology 2008;48:1157–66.

28 Kakar S, Batts KP, Poterucha JJ, et al. Histologic changes mimicking biliary disease in liver biopsies with venous outflow impairment. Mod Pathol 2004;17:874–8.

29 Kim WR, Ludwig J, Lindor KD. Variant forms of cholestatic diseases involving small bile ducts in adults. Am J Gastroenterol 2000;95:1130–8.

30 Burt AD, MacSween RN. Hepatic vein lesions in alcoholic liver disease: retrospective biopsy and necropsy study. J Clin Pathol 1986;39:63–7.

31 Nakanuma Y, Ohta G, Doishita K. Quantitation and serial section observations of focal venocclusive lesions of hepatic veins in liver cirrhosis. Virchows Arch [A] 1985;405:429–38.

32 Wanless IR, Wong F, Blendis LM, et al. Hepatic and portal vein thrombosis in cirrhosis: possible role in development of parenchymal extinction and portal hypertension. Hepatology 1995;21:1238–47.

33 Yamauchi Y, Michitaka K, Onji M. Morphometric analysis of lymphatic and blood vessels in human chronic viral liver diseases. Am J Pathol 1998;153:1131–7.

34 Deugnier Y, Turlin B, Le Quilleuc D, et al. A reappraisal of hepatic siderosis in patients with end-stage cirrhosis: practical implications for the diagnosis of hemochromatosis. Am J Surg Pathol 1997;21:669–75.

35 McGuinness PH, Bishop GA, Painter DM, et al. Intrahepatic hepatitis C RNA levels do not correlate with degree of liver injury in patients with chronic hepatitis C. Hepatology 1996;23:676–87.

36 Mehrotra R, Pandey RK, Nath P. Hepatic copper in Indian childhood cirrhosis. Histopathology 1981;5:659–65.

37 Müller T, Langner C, Fuchsbichler A, et al. Immunohistochemical analysis of Mallory bodies in Wilsonian and non-Wilsonian hepatic copper toxicosis. Hepatology 2004;39:963–9.

38 Nagula S, Jain D, Groszmann RJ, et al. Histological-hemodynamic correlation in cirrhosis – a histological classification of the severity of cirrhosis. J Hepatol 2006;44:111–17.

39 Sciot R, Staessen D, Van Damme B, et al. Incomplete septal cirrhosis: histopathologic aspects. Histopathology 1988;13:593–603.

40 Lopez JI. Does incomplete septal cirrhosis link non-cirrhotic nodulations with cirrhosis? Histopathology 1989;15:318–20.

41 Bernard P-H, Le Bail B, Cransac M, et al. Progression from idiopathic portal hypertension to incomplete septal cirrhosis with liver failure requiring liver transplantation. J Hepatol 2004;22:495–9.

42 Nakanuma Y, Hoso M, Sasaki M, et al. Histopathology of the liver in non-cirrhotic portal hypertension of unknown etiology. Histopathology 1996;28:195–204.

43 Nevens F, Staessen D, Sciot R, et al. Clinical aspects of incomplete septal cirrhosis in comparison with macronodular cirrhosis. Gastroenterology 1994;106:459–63.

44 Ishak K, Baptista A, Bianchi L, et al. Histological grading and staging of chronic hepatitis. J Hepatol 1995;22:696–9.

45 Friedman SL. Liver fibrosis – from bench to bedside. J Hepatol 2003;38:S38–53.

46 Serpaggi J, Carnot F, Nalpas B, et al. Direct and indirect evidence for the reversibility of cirrhosis. Hum Pathol 2006;37:1519–26.

47 Ellis EL, Mann DA. Clinical evidence for the regression of liver fibrosis. J Hepatol 2012;56:1171–80.

48 International Working Party. Terminology of nodular hepatocellular lesions. Hepatology 1995;22:983–93.

49 International Consensus Group for Hepatocellular Neoplasia. Pathologic diagnosis of early hepatocellular carcinoma: a report of the international consensus group for hepatocellular neoplasia. Hepatology 2009;49:658–64.

General reading

Crawford JM. Liver cirrhosis. In: MacSween RNM, Burt AD, Portmann BC, et al., editors. Pathology of the Liver. 4th ed. Edinburgh: Churchill Livingstone/Elsevier; 2002. p. 575–620.

Desmet VJ, Roskams T. Cirrhosis reversal: a duel between dogma and myth. J Hepatol 2004;40:860–7.

International Consensus Group for Hepatocellular Neoplasia. Pathologic diagnosis of early hepatocellular carcinoma: a report of the International Consensus Group for Hepatocellular Neoplasia. Hepatology 2009;49:658–64.

Neoplasms and Nodules

Introduction

This chapter is intended to provide a working overview of the tumours and tumour-like nodular lesions that the pathologist will encounter with some frequency in everyday practice. The majority of these can be classified according to the putative cells of origin (hepatocytes, bile-duct epithelium and endothelium) from which they arise (**Table 11.1**) and immunohistochemistry can often be used effectively to distinguish histogenesis. Neoplastic and nodular lesions of adults are covered first, followed by lesions in children and a section on cytopathological diagnosis. The reader is encouraged to consult the references and general reading list for additional details and coverage of some of the rarer tumours.

Neoplasms and nodules in adults

Benign lesions

Hepatocellular (liver-cell) adenoma

Hepatocellular adenomas are solitary or occasionally multiple tumours composed of hepatocytes. Macroscopically they are well defined but often not encapsulated. The cells of the tumour closely resemble normal hepatocytes (**Fig. 11.1**). Nuclei are small and regular and mitoses are almost never seen. These features are evident in fine-needle aspiration biopsies (FNABs).[1] The cells are arranged in normal or thickened trabeculae interspersed with prominent arteries and thin-walled blood vessels. In adenomas, reticulin is normal or sometimes reduced, but extensive loss is in most cases confined to areas of necrosis or haemorrhage. The latter are characteristically found in adenomas in oral contraceptive users, and are responsible for pain and for the serious complication of haemoperitoneum. They probably also explain the fibrous scars which are sometimes found in the lesions. Regular septa, portal tracts and bile ducts are, however, absent; this distinguishes hepatocellular adenomas both from non-neoplastic liver and from macroregenerative nodules (MRNs: large regenerative nodules) in cirrhosis as well as focal nodular hyperplasia (FNH). Exceptions to this rule may occur in patients with multiple adenomas (adenomatosis[2]) where bile ducts can become entrapped within the lesions[3] and in the inflammatory adenoma where focal ductular reaction is sometimes present (see below).

Table 11.1 Classification of liver tumours and nodular lesions

Putative cell of origin	Benign	Malignant
Hepatocyte	Liver cell adenoma MRN FNH NRH PNT	Hepatocellular carcinoma Fibrolamellar carcinoma Hepatoblastoma
Bile-duct epithelium	Bile-duct adenoma Cystadenoma Adenofibroma	Cholangiocarcinoma Cystadenocarcinoma
Mixed liver cell and bile-duct cell	Mesenchymal hamartoma	Combined hepatocellular cholangiocarcinoma
Endothelial cell	Haemangioma Infantile haemangioendothelioma*	Angiosarcoma Epithelioid haemangioendothelioma

MRN, macroregenerative nodule; FNH, focal nodular hyperplasia; NRH, nodular regenerative hyperplasia; PNT, partial nodular transformation.
*Some cases may behave more aggressively and are capable of metastasis.

**Figure 11.1
Hepatocellular
adenoma, steatotic
type.**
Liver cells appear
normal or contain fat
vacuoles. Isolated
blood vessels (upper
left) or vessels within
small amounts of
connective tissue,
but without
accompanying bile
ducts ('pseudo-portal
tracts') (upper right)
are seen within the
lesion. (Operative
specimen, H&E.)

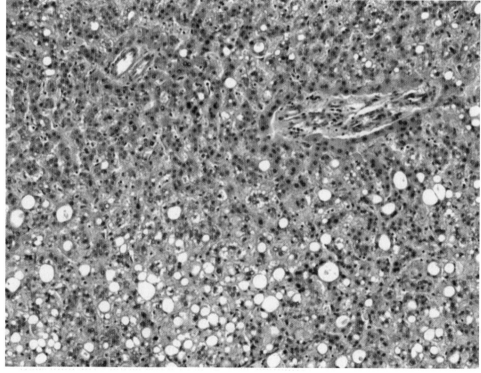

Table 11.2 Diagnostic distinctions between hepatocellular adenoma (HCA) and focal nodular hyperplasia (FNH)

Lesion	Routine diagnostic features	Key immunohistochemical stain(s)
HCA	Benign-appearing hepatocytes Thickened cords and trabeculae Interspersed venules and arterioles Absence of bile ducts	
HCA Subtype (%)		
(Gene mutation)		
Steatotic (30–40%) (*HNF-1A* inactivating mutation)	Macrovesicular steatosis No cytological atypia	**LFABP:** absent (compared to positive in normal liver)
β-catenin (10–15%) (*β-catenin* activating mutation)	Nuclear atypia Acini	**β-Catenin:** nuclear and/or cytoplasmic positivity **GS:** diffuse, strong positivity
Inflammatory (40–50%) (*activating mutations in IL6ST [codes for gp130], STAT3 and GNAS*)	Inflammation in pseudo-portal tracts Sinusoidal dilatation/ectasia may be present Focal ductular reaction may be present Steatosis sometimes present	**SAA:** cytoplasmic positivity **CRP:** cytoplasmic positivity
Unclassified (10%)	No distinctive features	None identified
FNH	Central stellate scar Thick-walled artery within scar Ductular reaction at edge of scar Cirrhosis-like nodular parenchyma	**GS:** Map-like broad fields of cytoplasmic positivity

LFABP: liver-type fatty acid protein; SAA: serum amyloid A; CRP: C-reactive protein; IL6ST: interleukin 6 signal transducer; STAT3: signal transducer and activator of transcription 3; GNAS: guanine nucleotide binding protein (G Protein), alpha stimulating activity polypeptide.

Adenomas may contain Dubin–Johnson-like pigment[4] or show steatohepatitis with Mallory–Denk bodies.[5] Non-necrotising granulomas within adenomas are also described.[6,7]

Genetic–histological correlations have allowed subclassification of adenomas into several subtypes with distinctive immunohistochemical signatures (**Table 11.2**).[8–14] Approximately 30–40% of adenomas show *HNF-1α* inactivating mutations and these typically contain fat but show no cytological atypia[10–15] (**Fig. 11.1**). Activating β-catenin gene mutations are seen in some 10–15% of adenomas with cytological atypia and acini[16] and these tumours are more likely to show transformation to hepatocellular carcinoma (HCC) and the chromosome gains and losses seen in HCC.[17] Transformation is more common in men and metabolic syndrome appears to be a risk factor.[18] The third subtype of adenoma is the inflammatory adenoma (**Fig. 11.2**), which shows small amounts of connective tissue ("pseudo-portal tracts") containing chronic inflammatory cell infiltrates (occasionally with adjacent ductular reaction) and/or sinusoidal dilatation. This subtype has been linked to *IL6ST, STAT3* and *GNAS*-activating gene mutations[16] and increased

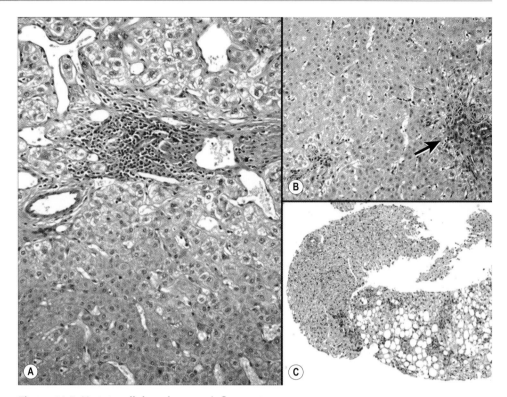

Figure 11.2 Hepatocellular adenoma, inflammatory type.
The histological hallmark of this type of hepatocellular adenoma is the presence of scattered lymphocytic inflammation. **A:** The pseudo-portal tract contains a mild lymphocytic infiltrate and abnormal blood vessels, but no bile ducts. **B:** In contrast to most hepatocellular adenomas, a few foci of ductular reaction (arrow) may be seen in this type of adenoma, usually near or within pseudo-portal tracts. **C:** Inflammatory adenomas sometimes show large-droplet fat vacuoles, as in this needle biopsy. Note the focality of the steatosis as well as the many abnormal blood vessels. (**A, B,** operative specimen, H&E; **C,** needle biopsy, H&E.)

interleukin-6 signalling[19] and represents some 40–50% of adenomas. The last hepatocellular adenoma subtype accounts for 10% of adenomas, shows no unique histological or immunohistochemical features and is as yet genomically unclassified. The percentage of each adenoma subtype may vary depending on the population studied.[20]

Distinguishing adenoma from either FNH or well-differentiated HCC can be diagnostically challenging. Targeted use of immunohistochemical stains may be necessary for such distinctions (**Table 11.2**).[21] In the case of adenoma vs HCC, loss of reticulin, nuclear atypia and mitotic activity and the presence of many acinar structures favour carcinoma. Immunohistochemical demonstration of nuclear and/or cytoplasmic β-catenin overexpression is often helpful evidence of transition to carcinoma, but is not invariably present.[22]

Most hepatocellular adenomas arise in women of child-bearing age, usually after prolonged use of oral contraceptives.[23] Use of anabolic/androgenic steroids is a risk factor for both adenoma and HCC,[24] particularly in Fanconi's anaemia.[25,26] **Adenomatosis**,[27,28] in which multiple tumours are seen throughout the liver, is much less common, is associated with *HNF-1α* mutations and shows female predominance.[2] A subgroup of these cases is familial and associated with diabetes.[2,28–30] Adenomatosis is also seen in patients taking anabolic/androgenic steroids[31] or in patients without risk factors.[32] Hepatocellular adenomas may also arise in patients with diabetes[33] or type I glycogen storage disease[34] (usually the inflammatory subtype[35]) and in children or young adults (see Neoplasms and nodules in children, below). In older and elderly men, metabolic syndrome is of growing concern for the development of adenomas and possible evolution to HCC.[36]

Focal nodular hyperplasia

FNH is a fairly common lesion, seen in either sex and at any age. FNH is a reactive, hyperplastic response of polyclonal[37] hepatocytes, fibrous stroma and bile ductules due to a putative pre-existing arterial malformation.[38–41] FNH, unlike liver-cell adenoma, does not appear to be caused by oral contraceptives. Although oral contraceptives may cause an increase in size and vascularity,[42] they do not appear to influence the number or size of these lesions.[43] Bleeding and rupture are rare, as is recurrence after resection.[44] Features of FNH and adenoma are only very occasionally seen in the same tumour, and the occurrence of the two lesions in the same liver may be coincidental.[45] There may be multiple FNHs in the same patient, and such individuals often have other lesions, including vascular anomalies (hepatic haemangioma, telangiectasis of the brain, berry aneurysm, dysplastic systemic arteries, portal-vein atresia), central nervous system neoplasms (meningioma, astrocytoma)[46,47] and hemihypertrophy.[48]

Macroscopically, the nodules are well demarcated from the normal hepatic parenchyma. They are usually pale, and are dissected by fibrous septa into nodules, giving them an appearance very like that of cirrhosis. There may be a prominent central fibrous scar (**Fig. 11.3**) with closely associated smooth-muscle actin immunostain-positive activated stellate cells.[49] Histologically, the appearance is also very like that of inactive cirrhosis. The dense fibrous septa contain large thick-walled and sometimes narrowed arteries, as well as bile-duct-like structures probably derived from metaplastic liver-cell plates[50] or from progenitor cells.[40] Cytokeratin 7 immunostain highlights the bile ductular structures (**Fig. 11.4**) and helps distinguish FNH from adenoma.[51] The presence of bile-duct cells in fine-needle aspiration cytology of FNH is helpful in distinguishing this lesion from HCC.[52] In radiologically guided needle biopsies, the pathologist should be made aware that a mass

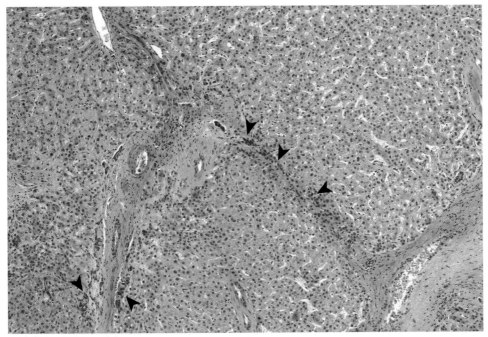

Figure 11.3 Focal nodular hyperplasia. Part of a central scar with abnormal arterioles has been sampled. Radiating fibrous septa show small bile-duct-like structures at their edges (arrowheads). The parenchyma is nodular. (Operative specimen, H&E.)

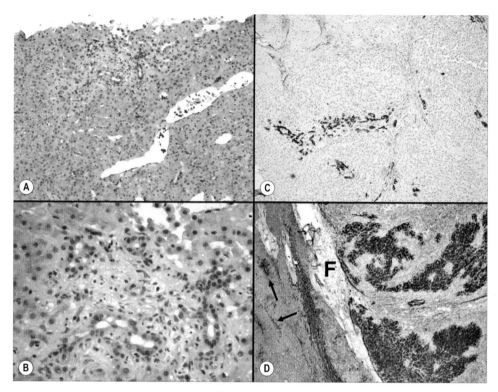

Figure 11.4 Focal nodular hyperplasia (FNH).
Needle biopsies of FNH are sometimes diagnostic problems due to the region sampled.
A, B: A needle biopsy of FNH taken from near the fibrous scar and its associated ductular reaction could be mistaken for biliary obstruction. These fields highlight the oedematous stroma and ductular structures. **C:** Immunostain for cytokeratin 7 helps confirm the presence of ductular reaction as an important component of FNH. **D:** Immunostain for glutamine synthetase demonstrates the characteristic 'geographic' or 'map-like' pattern in the lesional parenchyma. Compare to the normal limited staining of centrilobular hepatocytes outside the lesion (arrows). F = central fibrous scar. (**A, B,** Needle biopsy, H&E. **C,** Operative specimen, specific immunohistochemistry. **D,** Operative specimen, specific immunohistochemistry.)

lesion is being sampled, since the proliferated bile-duct-like structures and reactive stroma may otherwise suggest the diagnosis of mechanical bile-duct obstruction[53] (**Fig. 11.4**).

Lesions that grossly resemble FNH are also occasionally seen in Budd–Chiari syndrome.[54] Microscopically, these masses show hyperplastic, regenerative nodules in combination with other features, including central scars and multiple arterial structures. Some vary histologically so as to suggest crossover lesions between large regenerative nodules, FNH and liver-cell adenoma.[55] They appear to result from hyperarterialisation of regions of decreased hepatic venous blood flow.[55,56] FNH is also seen after liver transplantation in allografts with vascular perfusion abnormalities.[57]

FNH and adenoma are sometimes difficult to distinguish because of certain shared histological features, including the presence of isolated arterioles, thickened and nodular hepatocellular parenchyma, fibrosis and (in the inflammatory adenoma) inflammation and ductular reaction. The map-like staining pattern of broad islands of parenchyma in FNH seen with glutamine synthetase (GS) immunostain is helpful in confirming FNH (**Fig. 11.5**).[58]

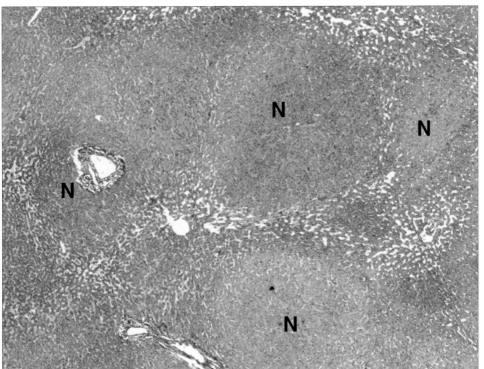

Figure 11.5 Nodular regenerative hyperplasia. This abnormal, nodular growth pattern is not accompanied by fibrosis and therefore differs from cirrhosis. The parenchymal nodules (N) are often adjacent to (nodule at bottom) or surrounding portal tracts (nodule at left of centre). The intervening liver shows flattened and compressed liver-cell plates and sinusoidal dilatation. (Wedge biopsy, H&E.)

Nodular regenerative hyperplasia

In nodular regenerative hyperplasia (NRH) multiple hyperplastic parenchymal nodules with thickened liver-cell plates are seen but fibrosis is absent or slight[59] (**Fig. 11.3**). This distinguishes the lesion from cirrhosis. In some cases perisinusoidal fibrosis is found in the compressed liver tissue between nodules. Portal tracts may be found at the centres of the nodules but this is not invariable. Diagnosis is often difficult in needle-biopsy specimens. The nodularity may be more clearly seen in reticulin preparations (**Fig. 11.6**). A wedge liver biopsy may be required to establish the diagnosis and to exclude an important differential: incomplete septal cirrhosis (**see Ch. 10**).

NRH is associated with a wide range of conditions, mainly rheumatic diseases, myeloproliferative disorders and chronic venous congestion.[60–62] Patients with NRH may have received therapeutic drugs, including corticosteroids, anabolic steroids, oral contraceptives, antineoplastics,[63] anticonvulsants and immunosuppressive agents.[60,64,65] NRH has also been associated with the toxic-oil syndrome,[66] Behçet's disease,[67] early histological stages of primary biliary cirrhosis,[68] coeliac disease with anticardiolipin antibodies,[69] livers containing metastatic neuroendocrine tumours[70] and non-cirrhotic livers in which HCC has developed.[71] Some patients with NRH have portal hypertension. Serum alkaline phosphatase and γ-glutamyl transpeptidase levels may be elevated.[62,68]

Wanless and co-workers[72] have postulated that the basic lesion is portal venous thrombosis, leading to atrophy and compensatory hyperplasia. Arterial lesions, particularly arteriosclerosis of ageing, may also contribute to these changes.[62] Portal venous thrombosis has also been invoked in the pathogenesis of the rare **partial nodular transformation**, in which somewhat larger nodules are found, often localised to the perihilar region, where they may cause portal hypertension.[73,74] NRH, FNH and partial nodular transformation share the common feature of liver-cell hyperplastic growth in the form of nodules; they

**Figure 11.6
Nodular
regenerative
hyperplasia.**
Reticulin stain of a
field which
highlights the
regenerative nodules
and the absence of
fibrosis. (Postmortem
liver, reticulin.)

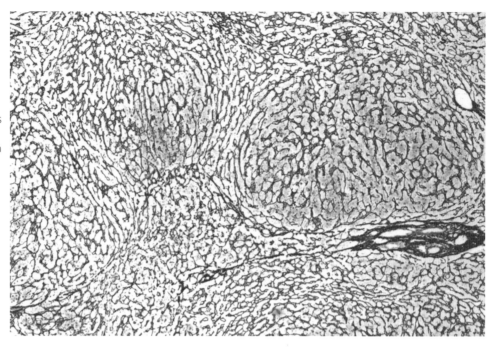

have accordingly been grouped under the umbrella heading of 'nodular transformation'
by Wanless.[75]

Bile-duct adenoma

Bile-duct adenomas are small, grey-white, usually subcapsular nodules measuring from 1
to 20 mm in diameter,[76] which may represent hamartomatous peribiliary glands or reactive
biliary lesions with features of foregut pyloric metaplasia, rather than a neoplasm.[77,78] They
are more often solitary than multiple. Histologically, they are composed of small, well-
formed ducts embedded in a stroma of mature fibrous tissue which may contain chronic
inflammatory cells, often densely aggregated at the periphery of the lesion[76,79,80] (**Fig. 11.7**).
Their chief importance is that they may be mistaken for metastatic carcinoma, both macroscopically and microscopically. They differ from microhamartomas (von Meyenburg
complexes) in that the ducts are smaller and more numerous, are usually not dilated and
do not contain bile.[76,81] Periodic acid–Schiff (PAS)-positive, diastase-resistant globules of
α_1-antitrypsin within the bile-duct epithelium of multiple adenomas were described in a
patient with heterozygous α_1-antitrypsin deficiency.[82] The bile-duct adenoma should also
be distinguished from the rare **biliary adenofibroma**, a much larger tumour composed of
tubulocystic bile-duct structures with apocrine metaplasia and intraluminal bile embedded
in fibrous stroma, resembling fibroadenoma of the breast.[83]

Biliary cystadenoma

Biliary cystadenoma is a multilocular tumour, the cystic spaces of which contain mucoid
fluid and are lined by columnar, mucin-secreting epithelium which may form papillary
projections. A variant with subepithelial **mesenchymal stroma** containing myofibroblasts
occurs in women.[84,85] Malignant change is common.[86]

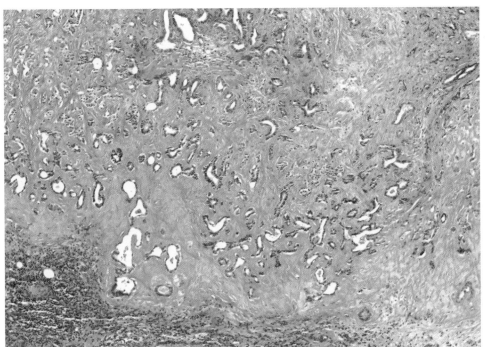

Figure 11.7
Bile-duct adenoma.
This subcapsular tumour consists of closely packed bile ducts set in a dense fibrous stroma. A dense collection of lymphocytes is seen at the edge of the lesion (bottom). (Operative specimen, H&E.)

Haemangioma

The cavernous haemangioma is the most common benign tumour of the liver, found incidentally at autopsy or operation and occasionally seen in biopsy material.[87] A few reach a large and clinically significant size. As in other sites, the lesions are composed of endothelium-lined channels supported by a fibrous stroma (**Fig. 11.8**). Lesional tissue sometimes extends irregularly into adjacent liver.[88] Complications include thrombosis, sclerosis and calcification.[89] Spontaneous rupture is recorded but uncommon. A distinction should be made between cavernous haemangiomas and peliosis (**see Ch. 12**); the latter lacks the complete endothelial layer and fibrous trabeculae. **Lymphangioma** of the liver has been reported as part of multiorgan lymphangiomatosis or as a solitary hepatic lesion,[90] but is very rare. The endothelium-lined channels of this neoplasm are empty or contain lymph with occasional leukocytes. It should not be mistaken for mesenchymal hamartoma (see Neoplasms and nodules in children, below).

Mesenchymal and neural tumours

Connective-tissue elements, adipocytes and smooth muscle of the liver, nerve sheaths of intrahepatic nerves and other mesenchymal cells may give rise to rare tumours, including lipomas, myelolipomas, angiomyelolipomas,[91,92] schwannomas and neurofibromas,[93-95] solitary fibrous tumours[96] and chondromas.[97] **Angiomyolipomas** resemble their more common renal counterparts, and contain blood vessels, smooth muscle (myoid cells) and fat.[98] These components allow subcategorisation into mixed, lipomatous, myomatous and angiomatous types, in decreasing order of frequency.[99,100] Multiple tumours may be present.[101,102] Muscle cells may be partly of epithelioid type, with finely granular eosinophilic cytoplasm and pleomorphic nuclei[103-106] (**Fig. 11.9**). These may be mistaken for hepatocytes or malignant cells, particularly in cases where the component of fat is minimal. Megakaryocytes and other bone marrow elements are commonly present. Positive HMB-45 immunostaining of the myoid cells is a major diagnostic feature.[99,106] **Pseudolipomas**[107]

**Figure 11.8
Haemangioma.**
Blood-filled spaces
are separated by
fibrous septa. A thick
capsule is seen at
right. (Operative
specimen, H&E.)

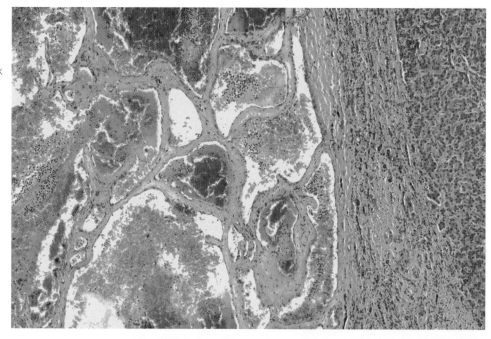

**Figure 11.9
Angiomyolipoma.**
The tumour shows
myoid cells with
ample granular
cytoplasm
resembling
hepatocytes. Fat
vacuoles, seen at
right, were variably
scattered through
the tumour, as were
small blood vessels.
(Operative specimen,
H&E.)

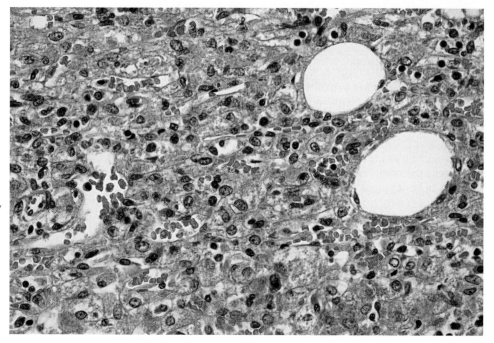

probably represent separated nodules of peritoneal fat which become embedded in the liver capsule.

Inflammatory pseudotumour

Lesions of inflammatory pseudotumour may be solitary or multiple and usually occur in young, male patients with constitutional symptoms, fever and weight loss. They may

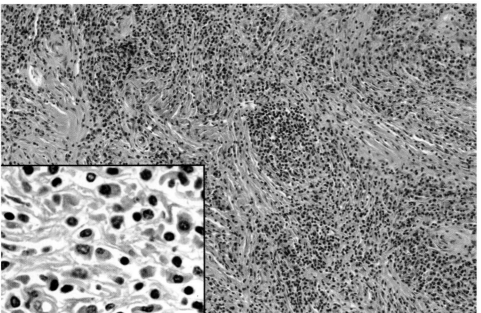

Figure 11.10
Inflammatory
pseudotumour.
Dense infiltrates of
plasma cells,
lymphocytes and
histiocytes with
interwoven bundles
of collagen are seen.
Inset: Plasma cells
are unusually
prominent.
(Operative specimen,
H&E.)

sometimes involve structures near the porta hepatis with resultant biliary problems or portal hypertension, or may mimic HCC.[108] Surgical resection is the treatment of choice, when possible. The microscopic hallmark of inflammatory pseudotumour is the extensive poly-clonal plasma-cell infiltrates which are intermixed with lymphocytes, eosinophils, foamy histiocytes and variable degrees of stromal proliferation, including spindle cells in bundles and whorls with associated fibrosis[109] (**Fig. 11.10**). Granulomas and partly obliterated blood vessels may be present. The lesion falls within a diagnostically controversial spectrum ranging from an inflammatory–reparative process (possibly infectious in aetiology) to a low-grade stromal malignancy termed inflammatory myofibroblastic tumour.[110,111] Some have been thought to be follicular dendritic cell tumours related to Epstein–Barr virus infec-tion.[112] Immunostains are helpful to characterise individual cases. Among these, smooth-muscle actin will highlight the extent of the myofibroblastic component and activin-like kinase 1 expression in the spindle cells favours a diagnosis of inflammatory myofibroblastic tumour.[110,111] Infrequently, such lesions are part of the spectrum of IgG4-related disease[113–115] and show abundant IgG4-positive plasma cells with IgG4 immunostain.

Malignant lesions

Precursors of hepatocellular carcinoma

A number of hepatocellular changes and nodular lesions have been considered premalig-nant or precursors[116] of HCC, and these are discussed below. Despite refinements in the terminology of these lesions provided by panels of hepatic pathologists,[117–119] the precise sequence of histological and molecular changes in the presumed multistep pathogenesis of HCC in humans has not been established. The importance of recognition of these worrisome lesions is based on the need for close patient surveillance and possible surgical resection (or liver transplantation) once they are identified pathologically. The presence of one or more of these lesions should be clearly stated in the pathologist's report.

Non-neoplastic liver tissue may show varying degrees of **liver-cell dysplasia (LCD)** of either large- or small-cell type (**see Figs 10.8, 10.9**). **Large-cell LCD (large-cell change)** is the type most often observed and features cell and nuclear enlargement, nuclear pleomorphism, multinucleation and multiple nucleoli and increased nuclear staining[120] (**see Figs 10.8, 11.38**). Its distribution is random within lobules or cirrhotic nodules and should be distinguished from the variations in nuclear morphology seen in perivenular hepatocytes with ageing, in the presence of cholestasis or in methotrexate therapy. This type of dysplasia was first associated with hepatitis B virus infection, cirrhosis and HCC[121,122] and subsequently with a four- to fivefold increased risk of HCC in several studies.[123,124] Affected cells are usually aneuploid[125] and may have attendant chromosomal abnormalities.[126] However, it has been considered merely an effect of cholestasis[127] or a derangement in normal liver-cell polyploidisation[128] and has not been proven to be a direct pathogenetic precursor lesion of HCC. Nevertheless, it is a strong independent risk factor for the development of HCC[129,130] and thereby identifies patients requiring more diligent surveillance.

Small-cell LCD (small-cell change) is characterised by enlarged, hyperchromatic nuclei within small hepatocytes (increased nuclear–cytoplasmic ratio) arranged in crowded clusters[131] (**see Figs 10.9, 11.39**). These foci show high cellular proliferation rates[132] and an overall cytological resemblance to HCC, and may originate from progenitor cells.[129] These features have lent support to small-cell LCD as a true precursor lesion that is subject to the later cellular events leading to the development of HCC.[133]

Other cellular changes cited as indicators of premalignancy include intracytoplasmic Mallory bodies,[134] irregular areas of regeneration showing hepatocyte glycogenosis, oncocytic change (**see Ch. 9**) or bulging nodularity,[135] iron-negative foci in siderotic MRNs[136] and 'iron-free foci' in livers of patients with hereditary haemochromatosis[137]; the last may show large-cell LCD.[137] Clusters of large-cell or small-cell dysplastic hepatocytes less than 1 mm in diameter have been termed **dysplastic foci** by an international working party.[118]

The **MRN** is an unusually large regenerative nodule measuring 0.8 cm or more in diameter which develops in cirrhosis or other chronic liver disease[138] (**Fig. 11.11**). MRNs are particularly common in macronodular cirrhosis.[139] They may be paler or more bile-stained than the surrounding liver.[118] The cirrhotic liver may harbour several MRNs, which may coexist with HCC elsewhere in the liver or may contain foci of carcinoma. Cirrhotic explant livers should be carefully examined for these lesions[117,140] and for LCD.[141]

The MRN histologically shows hyperplastic liver parenchyma arranged in plates two or three cells thick, which is typical of cirrhosis. The nodule contains portal tracts and fibrous septa with bile ducts, hepatic arteries and portal-vein branches, and shows no cellular atypia or disorder in the liver-cell plate arrangement. Steatosis, haemosiderin, bile plugs and Mallory bodies may be present.[138,142] The terms 'adenomatous hyperplasia', a former synonym of MRN, as well as subdivisions into MRN types I and II,[139] are not currently advocated for use.[118]

The **dysplastic nodule (borderline nodule)** shows atypical architectural and/or cytological features that are not acceptable for a benign MRN, but which fall diagnostically short of frank HCC.[118,143] Dysplastic nodules may show varying degrees of large- and small-cell LCD, increased cellularity and foci where the liver cords are less cohesive, focal loss of reticulin fibres or pseudoacini[117,118,140,143] (**Fig. 11.12**).

The major diagnostic concern is to distinguish MRNs and dysplastic nodules from HCC. Certain features seen in these nodules are associated with high risk of progression to carcinoma, including an increased ratio of nuclear density, clear-cell change, small-cell dysplasia and fatty change.[144] Increased mitotic activity, loss of reticulin fibres, formation of broad trabeculae and an infiltrative margin are helpful evidence of carcinoma.[117,140,145,146] Demonstration of clonality and loss of heterozygosity[147] and increased cell proliferative indices[148] are further supportive evidence of HCC.

Hepatocellular carcinoma

HCC ranks fifth among malignant tumours worldwide.[122] Epidemiological and other studies of HCC have defined geographical variations in the incidence and prevalence of

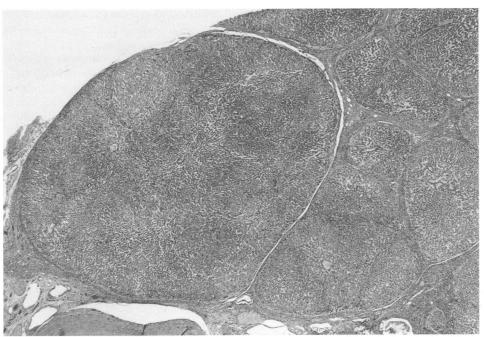

Figure 11.11
Macroregenerative nodule.
This low-magnification view demonstrates the increased size of the nodule at right compared with the cirrhotic nodules at left. (Operative specimen, H&E.) (Illustration kindly provided by Dr Kamal Ishak, Washington, DC, USA.)

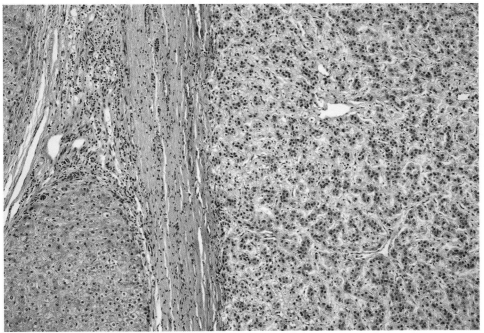

Figure 11.12
Dysplastic nodule.
The dysplastic nodule at right shows hepatocytes arranged in pseudoacini, with a less cohesive growth pattern centrally. A cirrhotic nodule is present at lower left. The patient had an inactive cirrhosis due to tyrosinaemia. (Explant liver, H&E.)

this tumour, as well as a multifactorial aetiology.[149] Chronic necrosis and inflammation of the liver are important driving forces in the multistep process of hepatocarcinogenesis[150,151] in the context of underlying risk factors such as hepatitis B and C viral infections,[122] iron overload,[152] aflatoxin exposure[153] and the presence of fatty liver disease.[154–156] At the molecular level, identification of genetic changes that control cell cycling and apoptosis,[157] as well as oncogene expression,[158] gene deletions and amplifications,[159] mutation of tumour suppressor genes such as *p53*,[160] expression of vascular and cellular growth factors[161–166] and proliferation of hepatic stem cells or their progeny[167–169] constitute a large and growing literature on this subject.

The majority of HCCs develop in cirrhotic liver.[170] The cause of the cirrhosis is usually known, even in many cases labelled as 'cryptogenic' where risk factors for non-alcoholic fatty liver disease (**see Ch. 7**) become apparent.[155] The non-cirrhotic setting accounts for a substantial number of cases from North America[171] and elsewhere[172] and can be seen in hepatitis B virus carriers[173,174] or in those with suspected occult hepatitis B[172] in individuals infected with hepatitis C virus,[175] and, increasingly, in non-alcoholic fatty liver disease with large-droplet fatty liver.[176] In older and elderly non-cirrhotic men with metabolic syndrome and without cirrhosis, hepatocellular adenoma may precede the development of HCC.[36] HCC may even develop within ectopic liver.[177] The cirrhosis associated with carcinoma is often macronodular in pattern, except for the micronodular cirrhosis seen in genetic haemochromatosis and chronic hepatitis C. The cirrhosis is usually inactive, although inflammation and necrosis may be seen near the tumour itself. Tumours may be multifocal.[178] Intrahepatic tumour spread is both portal (via portal-vein branches) and lobular.[179] Rarely, HCC may spontaneously regress.[122,180,181] Following transplantation, cirrhotic explant livers require careful examination for small carcinomas and precursor lesions which are clinically undetected.[182] Pathology reports on explants or partial resections with HCC should specify the number of lesions and their sizes, as well as the histological grade and evidence of vascular invasion,[183] since these factors affect TNM staging and other prognostic classifications.[184]

The outstanding histological features of HCC are the resemblance of the tumour cells to normal hepatocytes, and of their arrangement to the trabeculae of normal liver (**Fig. 11.13**). However, the trabeculae are for the most part thicker and reticulin is often scanty or even absent (**Fig. 11.14**). This paucireticulin pattern is even helpful in FNABs (see Cytopathological diagnosis, below). In exceptional cases where there may be an increase in reticulin, other histological features and/or the clinical behaviour of the tumour must be used as diagnostic criteria of malignancy. Rarely, the trabecular pattern and even

Figure 11.13 Hepatocellular carcinoma.

Note the trabecular–sinusoidal structure and resemblance of the tumour cells to normal hepatocytes. (Needle biopsy, H&E.)

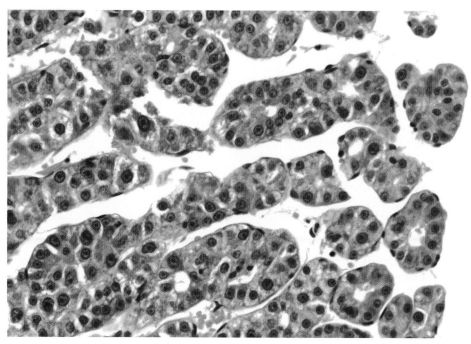

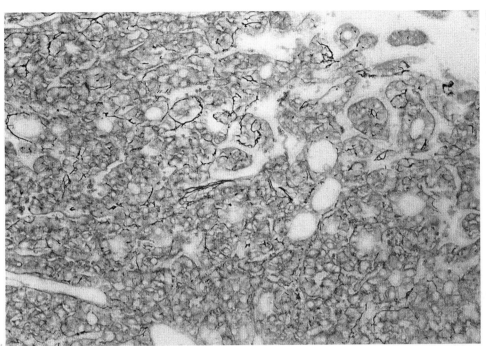

**Figure 11.14
Hepatocellular
carcinoma.**
Reticulin is scanty in
this example.
(Needle biopsy,
reticulin.)

bile production is mimicked by primary tumours ('hepatoid carcinomas') of the stomach, ovary and other sites[185,186] (see section on Metastatic tumour, below). Between the tumour trabeculae in HCC there is a network of vascular channels lined by endothelium which is positive with immunostains for CD34,[161,162] factor VIII-related antigen and *Ulex europaeus* lectin.[187] The endothelial lining of these channels is a particularly helpful diagnostic feature in fine-needle aspirates. The absence of portal tracts and a cohesive connective tissue framework in the tumour results in a characteristic fragmentation of needle biopsy specimens with separation of tumour trabeculae that is readily observed at low magnification (**see Ch. 4**, **Fig. 4.1**). Although connective tissue stroma is uncommon except in **fibrolamellar carcinoma** (described below), focal areas of fibrosis may follow tumour necrosis. In addition, a small percentage of HCCs are **scirrhous HCCs** and must be distinguished from fibrolamellar HCC, cholangiocarcinoma and metastatic carcinoma. The risk factors for this variant include chronic hepatitis B and C, steatosis and steatohepatitis (with or without cirrhosis).[188] In this setting, the hepatocellular origin of the tumour can be confirmed with the combination of glypican-3 (GPC-3) and arginase-1 immunostains[188] (see further discussion of immunohistochemistry below). The so-called **sclerosing carcinoma**[189] has been associated with hypercalcaemia but represents a poorly defined category in which some tumours may be of cholangiocyte origin. The **adenoid (acinar)** variant of HCC (**Fig. 11.15**) should not be confused with adenocarcinoma of the biliary tree. Bile-duct carcinomas are usually scirrhous, mucin-secreting tumours, whereas the characteristic secretion of HCCs is bile, seen in a minority of tumours in spaces homologous with normal bile canaliculi. The large repertoire of histological features of HCC also includes the 'steatohepatitic-HCC' (SH-HCC) variant which recapitulates many of the features seen in benign steatohepatitis[190] (**Fig. 11.16A**), the 'lymphoepithelioma-like' HCC (**Fig. 11.16B**) with admixed lymphocytes (predominantly T-lymphocytes with fewer B cells) and variable association with Epstein–Barr virus[191–194] (**Fig. 11.16**) and the 'chromophobe HCC with abrupt anaplasia' variant.[195] Mixed or combined tumours designated **combined hepatocellular–cholangiocarcinoma** are also well described, with special stains and

Figure 11.15 Hepatocellular carcinoma. Adenoid pattern. Other areas of this tumour showed a more typical trabecular structure. (Postmortem liver, H&E.)

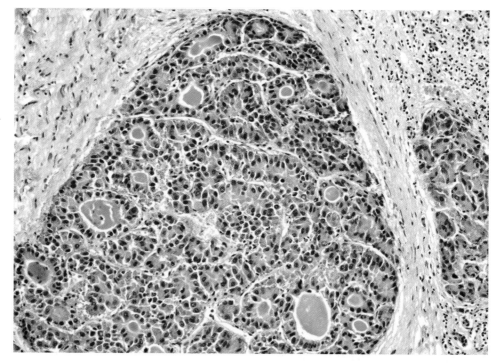

Figure 11.16 Hepatocellular carcinoma (HCC).
A: Steatohepatitic variant of HCC (SH-HCC). The neoplastic cells are ballooned and show oedematous and rarefied cytoplasm, focal intratumour inflammation and numerous Mallory–Denk bodies.
B: Lymphoepithelioma variant of HCC. This tumour elicits prominent lymphocytic infiltrates, chiefly T cells. (Operative specimens, H&E.)

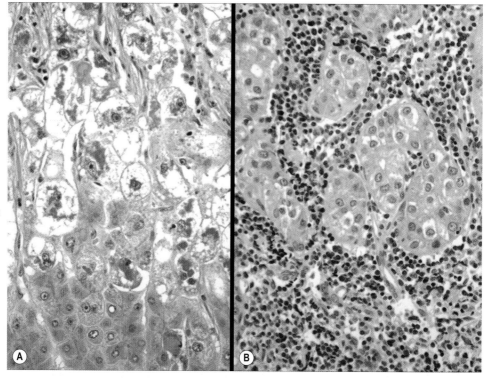

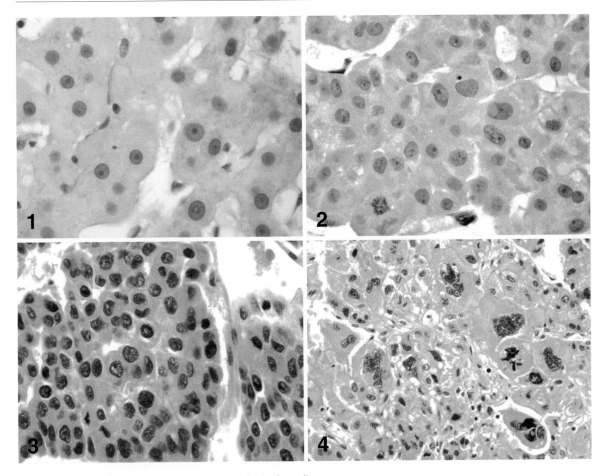

Figure 11.17 Hepatocellular carcinoma: cytological grading.
Grades 1–4 are illustrated in the respective panels. Grade 1 (well-differentiated) tumours have small, round nuclei similar to those of normal and cirrhotic liver. Grades 2 and upwards show progressive alterations in nuclear contour, chromatin coarseness and chromaticity. Grade 4 shows marked anaplasia with giant, multinucleated tumour cells and atypical mitotic figures. (Needle biopsies, H&E.)

immunohistochemical features representative of both hepatocellular and bile-duct epithelial derivation.[196] Progenitor/stem-cell constituents are sometimes present[197] (discussed below).

At a cellular level variants include giant-cell forms with multinucleated tumour cells (a bad prognostic sign[198]) (**Fig. 11.17**), spindle-cell or sarcomatoid tumours[199,200] and clear-cell carcinomas. The last must be distinguished from metastatic renal adenocarcinoma and PAX-8 immunostain nuclear positivity is helpful evidence of the latter.[201,202] Fine-needle aspiration yields diagnostic material in a high proportion of patients.[203–206] Histological grading of HCC from 1 to 4 is based on nuclear features, with grade 1 HCC resembling normal hepatocytes and grade 2 showing prominent nucleoli, hyperchromatism and nuclear membrane irregularities.[207] Grades 3 and 4 show progressively greater nuclear pleomorphism, the latter featuring anaplastic and giant tumour cells (**Fig. 11.17**).

When there is doubt about the hepatocellular origin of a carcinoma, further evidence can sometimes be gained from the characteristics of the tumour cells. In HCC these often contain fat and glycogen, and may also contain α_1-antitrypsin globules, even in patients without genetic α_1-antitrypsin deficiency. Mallory–Denk bodies may be found in the cytoplasm of the tumour cells,[208] particularly in the SH-HCC variant.[190] Evidence of hepatocellular origin is also provided when immunohistochemical stains of paraffin sections are positive for albumin, fibrinogen, liver-cell cytokeratins (8 and 18), α_1-antitrypsin or α_1-antichymotrypsin.[209–213]

There are several possible immunohistochemical strategies for confirming the diagnosis of HCC (**Fig. 11.18** and **Table 11.3**). One established approach is to begin with the quartet of cytokeratin 7, cytokeratin 20, Hep Par 1 ('hepatocyte') and polyclonal carcinoembryonic antigen (pCEA). HCC typically is negative for both cytokeratin 7 and cytokeratin 20,[214] while Hep Par 1 stains normal and malignant hepatocytes (and, rarely, several extrahepatic tumours[215]). Hep Par 1 staining may be only patchy in needle biopsies of HCC or negative with more poorly differentiated tumours, liabilities which can be surmounted using other immunostains. pCEA provides positive staining of the carbohydrate moiety of biliary glycoprotein on the apical surfaces or canalicular structures of the HCC cells (**Fig. 11.19**) and on bile canaliculi in non-neoplastic liver tissue. CD10 shows similar results to pCEA but is less sensitive.[216] α-Fetoprotein is an unreliable immunostain for HCC,[217] in contrast to hepatoblastoma, where most cases stain positively. Arginase-1 immunostain shows excellent sensitivity for HCC.[218] The immunostain for thyroid transcription factor-1, often used in the diagnosis of lung carcinomas, showed positive cytoplasmic (not nuclear) staining in the majority of HCCs in one study,[219] which may be helpful in specific diagnostic settings.

The trio of GPC-3, GS and heat shock protein 70 immunostains is proving to be an exceptionally robust combination for the diagnosis of HCC, particularly when any two of the three are positive.[220] GPC-3, a cell-surface heparan sulphate proteoglycan, usually shows cytoplasmic positivity in the tumour cells, but may also be membranous or canalicular. It has particular value in staining poorly differentiated HCCs that are negative with Hep Par 1 and is also applicable to fine-needle aspiration specimens.[221] However, cirrhotic nodules and hepatocytes in chronic hepatitis C with high-grade necroinflammatory activity may also show strong GPC-3 positivity.[222,223] Positive GPC-3 staining may also be seen in certain germ cell tumours,[224] ovarian clear-cell carcinoma,[225] squamous cell carcinoma of the lung,[226] some gastrointestinal tract carcinomas and acinar pancreatic carcinoma.[227] GS staining in non-neoplastic liver is restricted to the cytoplasm of perivenular hepatocytes, while HCC shows diffuse strong lesional staining.[119,220] Heat shock protein 70 shows focal nucleocytoplasmic positivity in HCC.[119] This panel of three immunostains also helps distinguish dysplastic lesions from HCC.[220]

Certain tumours wiith partial histological and immunohistochemical features of HCC but other admixed elements (such as partial glandular differentiation or less well-differentiated regions) that suggest the presence of 'stemness' or progenitor/stem-cell features can be further evaluated with hepatic progenitor/stem-cell immunhistochemical markers, including neural cell adhesion molecule (NCAM), epithelial cell adhesion molecule (EpCAM), cytokeratin 7 and CK19, c-KIT (CD 117) and CD133.[228–230] CK19 positivity has been associated with HCC invasiveness.[231]

Fibrolamellar carcinoma

This tumour usually develops in non-cirrhotic liver in older children and adults and carries a better prognosis (because of its resectability[232] and absence of cirrhosis[233]) than typical HCC.[234–239] The lesions are solitary or multiple and occasionally resemble FNH macroscopically in having a central fibrous scar.[240] The unique histological features distinguish this tumour from routine HCC. Fibrous lamellae are arranged in parallel separate groups of large, densely eosinophilic tumour cells[236,241] which produce transforming growth factor-β[242] (**Fig. 11.20**). The eosinophilia is due to the presence of abundant mitochondria.[235,243] Tumour cells commonly contain eosinophilic, diastase–PAS-negative globules which stain immunohistochemically for C-reactive protein, fibrinogen and α_1-antitrypsin,

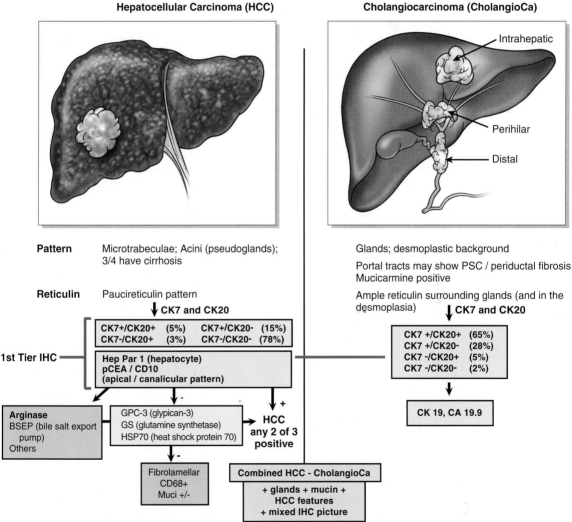

Metastasis

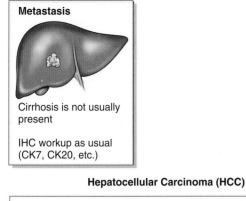

Cirrhosis is not usually present

IHC workup as usual (CK7, CK20, etc.)

Hepatocellular Carcinoma (HCC)

Cholangiocarcinoma (CholangioCa)

Intrahepatic

Perihilar

Distal

Pattern	Microtrabeculae; Acini (pseudoglands); 3/4 have cirrhosis	Glands; desmoplastic background
		Portal tracts may show PSC / periductal fibrosis Mucicarmine positive
Reticulin	Paucireticulin pattern	Ample reticulin surrounding glands (and in the desmoplasia)

↓ CK7 and CK20

↓ CK7 and CK20

1st Tier IHC

CK7+/CK20+	(5%)	CK7+/CK20-	(15%)
CK7-/CK20+	(3%)	CK7-/CK20-	(78%)

Hep Par 1 (hepatocyte)
pCEA / CD10
(apical / canalicular pattern)

CK7 +/CK20+	(65%)
CK7 +/CK20-	(28%)
CK7 -/CK20+	(5%)
CK7 -/CK20-	(2%)

CK 19, CA 19.9

Arginase
BSEP (bile salt export pump)
Others

GPC-3 (glypican-3)
GS (glutamine synthetase)
HSP70 (heat shock protein 70)

+ → **HCC any 2 of 3 positive**

-

Fibrolamellar
CD68+
Muci +/-

Combined HCC - CholangioCa
+ glands + mucin +
HCC features
+ mixed IHC picture

Figure 11.18 Immunohistochemical work-up of primary malignant liver tumours.
The standard diagnostic work-up (in yellow) of these primary hepatic malignancies utilises cytokeratins 7 and 20, hep par 1 (hepatocyte or hepatocyte-specific antigen) and polyclonal carcinoembryonic antigen (pCEA). Other second- and third-tier immunostains (in lavender) may be necessary for less-than-well-differentiated tumours, for histological variants, and for tumours with mixed features. Percentages for CK7 and CK20 are cited in Reference 214.

Table 11.3 Immunohistochemical stains in the evaluation of hepatic tumours

Tumour	Recommended immunostain(s)
Heptatocellular carcinoma	Hep Par 1 (hepatocyte) Polyclonal carcinoembryonic antigen* Cytokeratin 7/20 pair (−/− staining)[†] GPC-3/GS/HSP70 trio[‡]
Hepatoblastoma	α-Fetoprotein (AFP) Hep Par 1 (hepatocyte) Polyclonal carcinoembryonic antigen
Cholangiocarcinoma	Cytokertain 7/19 pair (+/+ staining) Cytokeratin 7/20 pair (+/+ staining)[†]
Angiomyolipoma	HMB-45
Epithelioid	CD34
Haemangioendothelioma	CD31 Factor VIII
Metastatic carcinoma	
Neuroendocrine	Chromogranin Synaptophysin Neuron-specific enolase
Pancreas	Cytokeratin 7/20 pair (+/+ staining)[†]
Colorectal	Cytokeratin 7/20 pair (−/+ staining)[†]
Breast	Cytokeratin 7/20 pair (+/− staining)[†]
Lung (non-small cell)	Cytokeratin 7/20 pair (+/− staining)[†]

*Staining is canalicular or apical.
[†]See reference 213.
[‡]GPC-3, glypican-3; GS, glutamine synthetase; HSP70, heat shock protein 70. At least two of the three should be positive (see reference 219).

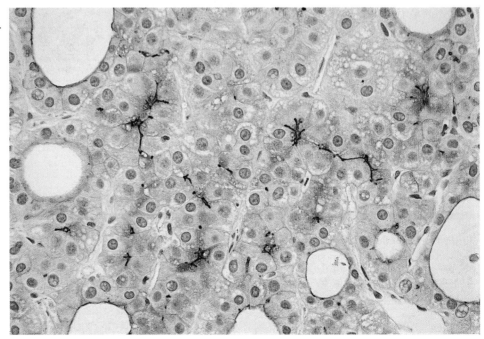

Figure 11.19 Immunohistochemical demonstration of bile canalicular structures in a hepatocellular carcinoma. The branching spaces are here outlined by the use of polyclonal anti-CEA.

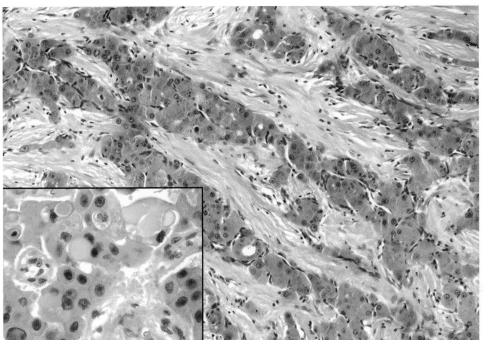

**Figure 11.20
Hepatocellular
carcinoma:
fibrolamellar type.**
Groups of large,
eosinophilic tumour
cells are surrounded
by fibrous septa in
parallel arrays.
(Needle biopsy, H&E.)
Inset: Tumour cells
contain 'pale bodies'
(top centre). Several
hyaline bodies are
also evident in
tumour cells at top,
left of centre.
(Explant liver, H&E.)

as well as cytoplasmic 'pale bodies' which are reactive for fibrinogen.[236] Additional features include bile production (as in other forms of HCC), copper and copper-associated protein within tumour cells,[244,245] and stainable CEA in bile canaliculi.[246] Some fibrolamellar carcinomas have neuroendocrine features,[247,248] mucicarmine-positive pseudoglands[249] or show features of both fibrolamellar and typical HCC.[250] CD68 immunostain shows positive granular stippling of the lysosomes and endosomes within the neoplastic cells.[251] (see Cytopathological diagnosis, below; **Fig. 11.51**). Despite isolated reports such as the association of Fanconi's anaemia with fibrolamellar carcinoma,[252] the pathogenesis of this tumour is uncertain and risk factors are not apparent.

Bile-duct carcinoma (cholangiocarcinoma)

Carcinoma of the bile ducts can arise anywhere between the papilla of Vater and the smaller branches of the biliary tree within the liver. It is not usually associated with cirrhosis. Three types are recognised by anatomical site of involvement, including distal bile duct, perihilar bile ducts (so-called Klatskin tumour[253]) and intrahepatic bile ducts.[254,255] The incidence of intrahepatic cholangiocarcinoma has been rising worldwide in recent decades.[256,257] The most common known predisposing factors to bile-duct cancer are infestation with hepatobiliary flukes (*Opisthorchis viverrini* and *Clonorchis sinensis*), primary sclerosing cholangitis[258] and congenital cystic lesions of the biliary tree.[259,260] Of these, Caroli's disease and choledochal cysts are important precursors, but carcinoma may also arise in von Meyenburg complexes (bile-duct microhamartomas)[261] and in congenital hepatic fibrosis.[262] Development of carcinoma in bile-duct adenoma is also reported.[263] In Japan, hepatitis B and C virus infections have been suggested as a risk factor[264] and intrahepatic cholangiocarcinoma is a known consequence of hepatolithiasis.[265,266] Current genomic and molecular studies of cholangiocarcinoma[267] have demonstrated the importance of mutational events affecting inflammatory,[268,269] oncogene (*KRAS* and *BRAF* especially[270,271]) and metabolic (e.g. *isocitrate dehydrogenase 1* and *2* genes[272]) pathways in the aetiopathogenesis of this tumour.

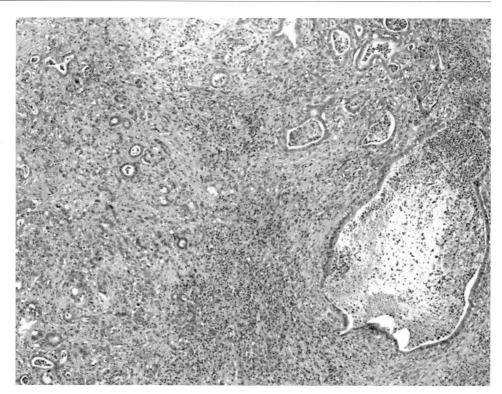

Figure 11.21 Bile-duct carcinoma (cholangiocarcinoma).
There are many medium- and small-sized neoplastic glands invading the desmoplastic fibrous stroma. The neoplastic cells of cholangiocarcinoma are typically cuboidal to low columnar. The adjacent native bile duct is dilated and contains neutrophils due to associated cholangitis. The appearances are different from those of the hepatocellular carcinoma of adenoid pattern shown in **Fig. 11.15**. (Operative specimen, H&E.)

Specification of the genomic derangement by molecular profiling studies is important in targeted tumour therapy.[271] Lesions suspicious for cholangiocarcinoma are often evaluated by endoscopic cholangiography with retrieval of brushings and cytopathological specimens. Fluorescent *in situ* hybridisation (FISH) evaluation for polysomy in tandem with routine morphology and, where indicated, immunohistochemistry, should be considered in the pathological work-up of these frequently difficult diagnostic lesions.

Microscopically, bile-duct carcinomas are mucin-secreting adenocarcinomas with a reactive, desmoplastic fibrous stroma (**Fig. 11.21**). A fairly uniform gland size (medium to small) is often maintained within these tumours, in comparison with the wide size variations seen in glands of metastatic pancreatic carcinoma. The **cholangiolocellular carcinoma** subtype shows interanastomosing antler-like ductular structures composed of small cuboidal cells with scant cytoplasm that appear to evolve from progenitor cells in the region of the canal of Hering (**Fig. 11.22**).[273,274] The tumour cells are cuboidal or columnar and may assume a papillary pattern. Adenosquamous, squamous, mucinous,[275] clear-cell[276] and anaplastic histological types are less common.[277] Intraneural and perineural invasion is common. The presence of free stromal mucin, small groups and isolated tumour cells in fibrous stroma and the concurrence of apparently normal epithelium and abnormal tumour cells within a duct-like structure all help to distinguish cholangiocarcinoma from metastatic tumour.[278] Cholangiocarcinoma must be distinguished from the acinar type of HCC, a distinction usually made with confidence on the basis of mucin or bile secretion,

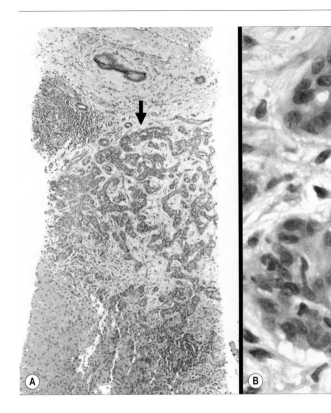

Figure 11.22 Cholangiolocellular carcinoma.
A: These tumours typically grow from periportal regions (arrow), the sites of hepatic progenitor cells. The neoplastic glands grow with an 'antler-like', branching pattern, infiltrating the adjacent liver tissue within a fibrous stroma. **B:** Nuclear atypia and mitotic figures (arrow) are present.

respectively. In difficult cases positive staining for epithelial membrane antigen,[279] tissue polypeptide antigen,[280] biliary cytokeratins[210] (7 and 19), Lewis(x) and Lewis(y) blood group-related antigens[281] and α-amylase[282] helps to exclude HCC. In the uncommon tumour which shows combined hepatocellular–cholangioarcinoma, cytokeratins 7 and 19 and epithelial membrane antigen immunostaining is positive in the cholangiocellular component.[283,284] Other rare mixed tumours show sarcomatoid[285] or fibrolamellar regions.[286] Bile-duct tumours are very occasionally of neuroendocrine type, with characteristic neurosecretory granules in their cytoplasm. The differential diagnosis of bile-duct cancer includes epithelioid haemangioendothelioma and metastatic adenocarcinoma. No specific immunohistochemical stain is currently available for definitive identification of cholangiocarcinoma. Positivity for cytokeratins 7 and 20 (or cytokeratin 7 alone) and CA19.9 is supportive evidence for cholangiocarcinoma, but such positivity does not, for example, exclude metastasis to the liver of a primary pancreatic adenocarcinoma.

Cystadenocarcinomas are rare malignant tumours which sometimes develop from benign cystadenomas.[84,86] Although these have been considered distinct from the more aggressive carcinomas arising from pre-existing congenital cystic lesions,[287] occasional tumours with features of cystadenocarcinoma develop in fibropolycystic disease.[288]

Angiosarcoma

This uncommon, highly malignant tumour forms multiple or, less often, solitary haemorrhagic masses. Predisposing factors include treatment with arsenic,[289] injection of the radioactive contrast medium Thorotrast[290–292] and industrial exposure to vinyl chloride.[293] Other postulated factors include copper-containing vineyard sprays,[294] steroid hormones,[295–297] phenelzine[298] and urethane.[299] Positive staining of tumour cells for factor

**Figure 11.23
Angiosarcoma.**
Elongated tumour cells surround islands of hepatocytes (centre) in this highly vascular tumour. Inset: Pleomorphic endothelial cells line the vascular spaces. (Operative specimen, H&E.)

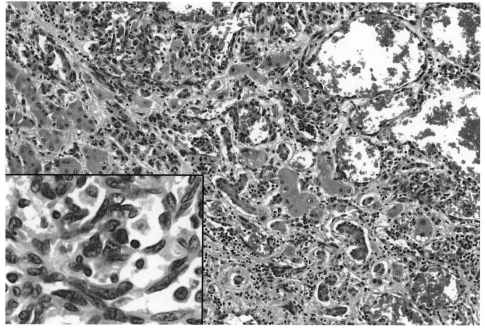

VIII-related antigen and other endothelial markers is evidence of their endothelial origin.[300,301] Their growth is characteristically along sinusoids and around surviving hyperplastic hepatocytes (**Fig. 11.23**). The presence of the latter may lead to confusion with HCC, with which angiosarcoma, however, occasionally coexists. Infiltration of sinusoids beyond the main tumour mass makes the outlines of the tumour indistinct. Both cavernous and solid areas may be present. Other features include islands of haemopoietic cells, and areas of thrombosis and infarction.

The non-neoplastic liver tissue is usually not cirrhotic, but may show fibrosis and other changes attributable to the predisposing factors listed above, including deposits of refractile Thorotrast granules in macrophages. Features seen irrespective of the cause include focal dilatation of sinusoids, hyperplasia of hepatocytes, sinusoid-lining cells and perisinusoidal cells and increased perisinusoidal reticulin.[302] These changes may precede the development of the tumour.[303]

Epithelioid haemangioendothelioma

This endothelial tumour of soft tissues or the lung (intravascular bronchioloalveolar tumour) may uncommonly present as a primary liver tumour. In the liver it is seen in patients from the second to eighth decades of life, with women more commonly affected.[304–306] Its prognosis varies very widely: some patients survive for decades while others die within months of diagnosis.[307] Histologically, it may be confused with adenocarcinoma or with veno-occlusive disease. Its causes are unknown, but a relationship to oral contraceptive use has been postulated.[308]

The lesion consists of proliferated endothelial cells with pleomorphic nuclei, arranged in clusters or singly, some of them with rounded lumens (**Fig. 11.24**). The lumens may be mistaken for lipid or for mucin droplets in a signet-ring cell adenocarcinoma. Two types of tumour cells have been described,[304,306] dendritic and epithelioid, the latter giving rise to the adenocarcinoma-like appearance. The tumour cells should be positive on immunostaining for one or more endothelial markers (CD34, CD31, factor VIII[306]). CD34

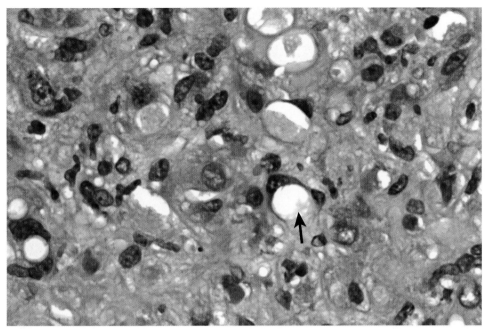

**Figure 11.24
Epithelioid
haemangioen-
dothelioma.**
Individual tumour
cells and small
groups are set in a
dense fibrous
stroma. Some of the
tumour cells have
formed vascular
lumens (arrow).
(Operative specimen,
H&E.)

immunostaining is more sensitive than factor VIII.[309] Further evidence of vascular differentiation is seen ultrastructurally where Weibel–Palade bodies in tumour cells and a tumour tissue component of pericytes have been noted.[310] High cellularity is a predictor of unfavourable prognosis, whereas nuclear pleomorphism and mitotic count are not.[306]

Vascular occlusion by dense fibrous tissue containing tumour cells, a characteristic feature, is seen in both portal and hepatic vein branches. This is best seen with connective tissue stains. The problem of confusion with veno-occlusive disease or even steatohepatitis is compounded by the fact that the tumour sometimes has a zonal distribution, affecting perivenular regions of each lobule in a more or less regular fashion (**Fig. 11.25**).

Extrahepatic malignancy and the liver

Patients with extrahepatic tumour may have biochemical evidence of hepatic dysfunction in the absence of liver metastases, particularly when the tumour is a renal adenocarcinoma. Liver biopsies in such patients have shown Kupffer-cell proliferation, hepatocellular swelling, focal necrosis, fatty change and mild inflammation.[311,312] Granulomas are occasionally found and there may be cholestasis, especially in Hodgkin's disease (see below).

Metastatic tumour

Blind percutaneous needle biopsy may reveal metastatic tumour, but the yield of correct diagnoses is increased if the needle is guided by means of an imaging method. Multiple punctures may be needed to sample the tumour. Guided fine-needle aspiration is a helpful diagnostic procedure,[313,314] and cytological examination of aspiration fluid and touch preparations of biopsy specimens increase the yield of positive results.[315] Step sections of biopsy specimens should be examined if tumour is suspected clinically but initial sections are negative. The primary site of a tumour can sometimes be determined histologically. Some metastases, notably from renal adenocarcinoma, can mimic HCC, and metastatic

Figure 11.25 Epithelioid haemangioen- dothelioma.

In this example the tumour has a zonal distribution, mimicking the fibrosis of venous outflow obstruction. The tumour stroma is predominantly seen in the perivenu- lar and mid-zonal regions, while surviving periportal hepatocytes and ductular reaction are evident at left and at lower right. (Opera- tive specimen, H&E.)

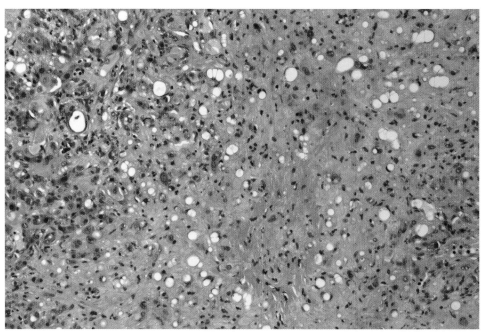

Figure 11.26 Metastatic tumour.

Cells of a carcinoid tumour (arrows) have invaded liver-cell plates (L), giving a false impression of origin from the latter. (Needle biopsy, H&E.)

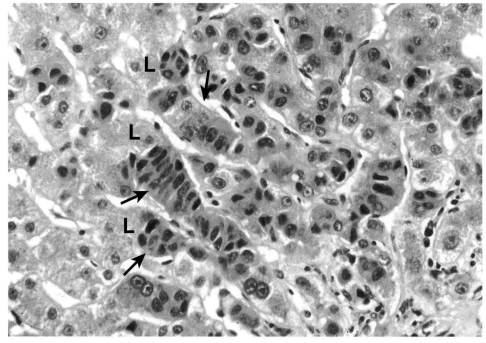

tumour may invade liver-cell plates, giving a false impression of primary carcinoma arising within them (**Fig. 11.26**). Primary extrahepatic carcinomas of the stomach, sex cord-stromal tumours of the ovary and other sites[185] may closely resemble HCC in both their primary sites and in metastatic foci. These 'hepatoid carcinomas' may produce bile or be positive with pCEA or α-fetoprotein immunostains.

Biopsy specimens from the vicinity of a metastasis typically show portal oedema, ductular reaction and infiltration by neutrophils, as well as focal sinusoidal dilatation[316] (**see Fig. 1.5**). The ductular structures sometimes have abnormal epithelium with atypical, hyperchromatic nuclei. The portal changes are reminiscent of those seen in biliary obstruction.

Lymphomas and leukaemias

Hodgkin's disease

Liver biopsy plays an important part in staging; wedge biopsies are more likely than multiple needle biopsies to reveal deposits, and either may be positive in spite of normal macroscopic appearances of the liver at laparotomy.[317] Negative biopsy does not rule out liver involvement. Hepatic involvement by Hodgkin's disease is usually associated with splenic involvement.[318] Step sections of initially negative small biopsies should be examined because the infiltrates of Hodgkin's disease are unevenly distributed and may be sparse. Correct diagnosis of an infiltrate may be difficult because Reed–Sternberg cells are often very scanty, so that the correct diagnosis must be suspected on the basis of other features. These include an abnormal population of cells with deeply stained angular nuclei or vesicular nuclei with prominent nucleoli (**Fig. 11.27**), irregular infiltration beyond portal tracts with destruction of hepatocytes and abundant reticulin fibres. There is a variable component of reactive lymphoid cells, eosinophils and histiocytes. The differential diagnosis of Hodgkin's disease in the liver includes reactive infiltrates and other lymphomas, especially of the T-cell type.

A variety of non-specific changes may be seen in parts of the liver adjacent to the malignant deposits. Even in the absence of malignant deposits there may be lobular lymphoid aggregates with some degree of cellular atypia[319] or epithelioid-cell granulomas.[320] Sinusoidal dilatation with or without Hodgkin's infiltrates in the liver has been reported, most

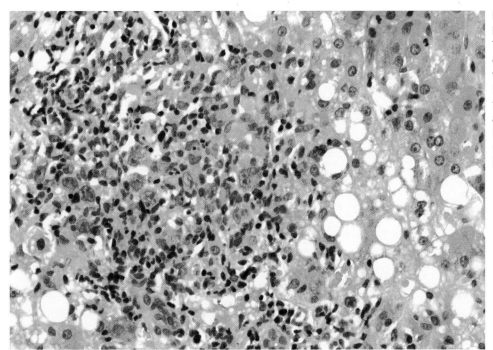

**Figure 11.27
Hodgkin's disease.**
The portal infiltrate is composed of a variety of cells, including large tumour cells with angular, hyperchromatic nuclei. (Needle biopsy, H&E.)

often in patients with general symptoms.[321] The lesion is most severe in acinar zones 2 and 3. **Cholestasis** in Hodgkin's disease is uncommon, seen in the absence of hepatic infiltration in some patients[322] but more often as a feature of advanced disease. In some cases cholestasis is explained by destruction of interlobular bile ducts (ductopenia) related directly to the malignant infiltrates or resembling that seen in ductopenic rejection after liver transplantation.[323,324]

Non-Hodgkin's lymphoma and other haemopoietic malignancies

Non-Hodgkin's lymphomas primarily involve portal tracts, but may spread to periportal parenchyma and sinusoids.[325] Predominantly sinusoidal infiltration is also recognised.[326] Tumour deposits and fibrosis may cause portal hypertension[327] and, rarely, massive infiltration presents clinically as liver failure.[328] Vasculitis is another rare presentation. Malignant infiltrates can usually be distinguished from inflammatory ones by their dense and homogeneous appearance, and by the total or near-total involvement of portal tracts. Substantial apoptosis and necrotic debris may also be seen in lymphoma (**Fig. 11.28**) but are not characteristic of benign infiltrates. Immunohistochemical stains are important in establishing the type of lymphoma.[329] The disease is usually systemic, with involvement of lymphoid tissues as well as liver. **Primary hepatic lymphoma** is quite rare, representing less than 1% of extranodal lymphomas.[330–332] Both B-cell lymphomas, including **mucosa-associated lymphoid tissue (MALT) lymphoma**,[333,334] and T-cell lymphomas are seen, with B-cell tumours predominating.[331,335] Many B-cell lymphomas (splenic marginal B-cell lymphoma, follicular and diffuse large B-cell lymphoma[336]) and proliferative diseases (mixed cryoglobulinaemia, monoclonal gammopathy) and, rarely, T-cell lymphoma[337] are associated with underlying chronic hepatitis C virus infection.[338] Chronic hepatitis C with concomitant B-cell lymphoma and HCC may also occur.[339] **Peripheral γ-δ**[340] and rare **α-β**[341] **T-cell lymphomas** with hepatic sinusoidal infiltration and splenic involvement have also

Figure 11.28 Non-Hodgkin's lymphoma. Tumour cells are seen irregularly infiltrating the adjacent periportal liver parenchyma. Extensive tumour cell necrosis is apparent. (Wedge biopsy, H&E.)

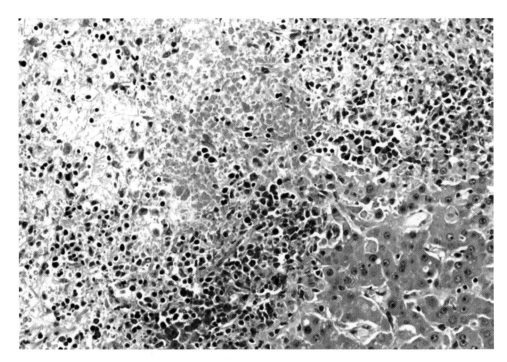

been described. Primary hepatic lymphomas present as solitary or multiple masses, as diffuse hepatic involvement with hepatomegaly, or as liver failure with elevated serum lactate dehydrogenase activity.[331]

The liver may be diffusely or focally infiltrated in **multiple myeloma**.[342] Solitary primary hepatic plasmacytoma has also been reported.[343] In **macroglobulinaemia**,[344] mononuclear cells, some with pyroninophilic cytoplasm, may be found in portal tracts and sinusoids. Both diseases are sometimes complicated by amyloid deposition. **Langerhans' cell histiocytosis** involving only the liver may rarely occur.[345,346] The infiltrating Langerhans' cells, positive on immunostains for S-100 and CD1a, may invade and destroy interlobular bile ducts, leading to ductopenia, chronic cholestasis and features resembling primary sclerosing cholangitis.[347] In **systemic mast-cell disease** with liver involvement, infiltration of portal tracts by mast cells is associated with fibrosis.[348] Parenchymal infiltrates are also seen. The infiltrating cells may be rounded, histiocyte-like or spindle-shaped. Their nature may not be suspected on routine stains of paraffin sections; plastic sections or special mast-cell stains make the diagnosis clear.

The infiltrates of various **leukaemias** are often seen in the liver and are frequently accompanied by steatosis and/or fibrosis.[349] Schwartz and co-workers[350] reported hepatic involvement in nearly all cases of **chronic lymphocytic leukaemia** examined, and noted marked widening of portal tracts with portal–portal linking and a variable degree of fibrosis. In **hairy cell leukaemia** the hepatic sinusoids are infiltrated by the leukaemic cells, often identifiable by the halo-like, clear cytoplasm around rounded or indented nuclei.[351] However, these are not always present.[352] Another histological characteristic is the formation of angiomatous lesions, in which vascular channels in portal tracts or acini are lined by leukaemic cells rather than by endothelium. Endothelial disruption with communication of sinusoids with the perisinusoidal space of Disse is seen by electron microscopy.[353] Staining for tartrate-resistant acid phosphatase in paraffin sections has sometimes been helpful in diagnosis.[354]

Neoplasms and nodules in children

Benign lesions

Rarely, **liver-cell adenoma** may develop spontaneously in children with no underlying disease or exposure to hormones.[355] In this age group it has also been associated with Fanconi's anaemia,[26] type I glycogen storage disease, Hurler's disease, severe combined immunodeficiency,[356] the antiepileptic agent oxcarbazepine[357] and mutations in hepatocyte nuclear factor-1α (see Liver-cell adenoma in adults, below). The vast majority pursue a benign course, but transformation to HCC after many years of observation has been reported.[358] The identification of **FNH** in infancy as well as adulthood has been taken as additional evidence that it is a tumour-like malformation rather than a true neoplasm. **NRH** is unusual in childhood. It occurs as early as 7 months of age and shows the same histological features as in adults.[359] Hepatosplenomegaly and portal hypertension may be present and in some patients there is a history of prior chemotherapy or anticonvulsant medication.

Mesenchymal hamartoma

This is an uncommon lesion of infancy and childhood, rarely seen in older subjects. Loose, oedematous connective tissue rich in blood vessels contains lymphangioma-like cystic spaces, bile ducts and hepatocytes[360,361] (**Fig. 11.29**). Haemopoietic cells are often present. The edge of the lesion is irregular, gradually merging with adjacent normal liver. In adults the bile-duct elements may be difficult to find and the collagenous stroma is densely

Figure 11.29 Mesenchymal hamartoma.
The combination of tissues seen in this benign neoplasm includes loose connective tissue with cystically dilated lymphatics (*), bile ductular structures (arrows) and geographic islands of liver parenchyma (centre). (Operative specimen, H&E.)

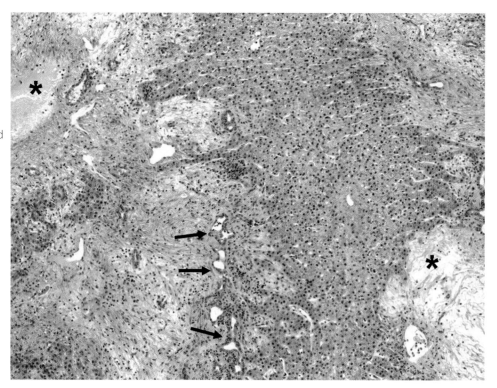

hyalinised.[362] An undifferentiated embryonal sarcoma arising in mesenchymal hamartoma has been reported.[363]

Infantile haemangioendothelioma

This solitary or multicentric tumour is composed of capillary-like vascular channels lined by plump endothelium (**Fig. 11.30**), which with time undergo progressive maturation, scarring and eventual involution.[92,364,365] Central portions of the tumour may show increased fibrous stroma, and thrombosis and dystrophic calcification are sometimes present. The margin of the tumour often merges into adjacent liver parenchyma. Dehner and Ishak[364] described type I tumours with cytologically bland endothelium and type II tumours capable of aggressive behaviour and metastasis, with atypical, hyperchromatic endothelium and intravascular budding. The latter are now considered angiosarcomas.[366] Most cases present in the first 6 months of life with hepatomegaly, abdominal mass or diffuse abdominal enlargement.[92,364,367] There may be high-output cardiac failure due to shunting through the tumour, liver failure or tumour rupture. The possibility that some of these tumours will pursue a malignant course should be kept in mind in evaluating the histopathology of individual cases.

Malignant lesions

Hepatoblastoma

Hepatoblastoma is the most common liver tumour in childhood,[368] usually presenting at less than 2 years of age. The prognosis depends on surgical resectability and histological type. These tumours are usually solitary and histologically classified in two essential

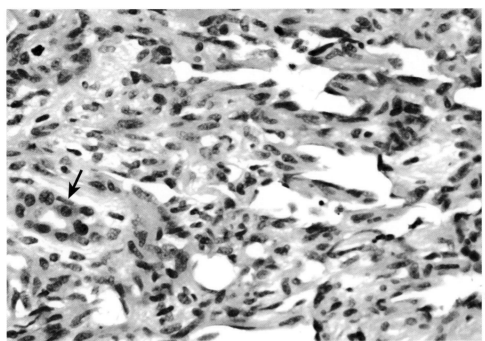

Figure 11.30 Infantile haemangioen-dothelioma. The tumour is composed of vascular channels lined by plump endothelium. Entrapped bile ducts are often present (arrow). (Operative specimen, H&E.)

categories, **epithelial** and **mixed epithelial–mesenchymal**, with a variety of histologic subtypes therein (see **Table 11.4**).[369–373]

The epithelial type consists of fetal or embryonal liver cells, or both. Fetal cells somewhat resemble adult hepatocytes in appearance but are smaller (**Fig. 11.31**). The fat and glycogen content in some fetal cells gives them a pale appearance, thereby rendering a 'light-and-dark' pattern to fetal areas at low magnification. These areas are also characterised by foci of extramedullary haemopoiesis and an absence of mitoses. By histological pattern, the purely fetal type has the best prognosis.[374] Embryonal cells have less cytoplasm, higher nucleus–cytoplasm ratios, higher cell proliferative indices,[375] poorly defined cellular margins and mitotic activity (**Fig. 11.32**). They may form rosettes, acini or tubules. Squamous differentiation may be present in epithelial hepatoblastomas. Gonzalez-Crussi et al.[376] described a **'macrotrabecular'** pattern reminiscent of HCC but containing fetal or embryonal cells. Mixed epithelial–mesenchymal hepatoblastomas, now referred to as 'teratoid hepatoblastoma,'[373] contain mesenchymal elements such as osteoid and cartilage in addition to epithelium. Staining for α-fetoprotein is common in hepatoblastoma. Hep Par 1 is positive in fetal portions of hepatoblastoma (but may be negative in embryonal regions) while GPC-3 immunostain and β-catenin (nuclear positivity) are usually positive (except in the less common histological variants).

Table 11.4 Histological classification of hepatoblastoma*

Epithelial variants
   Pure fetal with low mitotic activity
   Fetal, mitotically active
   Pleomorphic, poorly differentiated
   Embryonal
   Small-cell undifferentiated
      INI-1-negative**
      INI-1-positive
   Epithelial mixed (any/all above)
   Cholangioblastic
   Epithelial macrotrabecular pattern
Mixed epithelial and mesenchymal
   Without teratoid features
   With teratoid features
Hepatocellular carcinoma
   Classic HCC
   Fibrolamellar HCC
   Hepatocellular neoplasm NOS***

*Recommended classification[373] from the COG (Children's Oncology Group)
**INI-1 (integrase interactor 1, involved in chromatin remodeling and cellular transcriptional regulation).
***Indicates provisional entity. Tumors previously designated as transitional liver cell tumors may be included in this category.

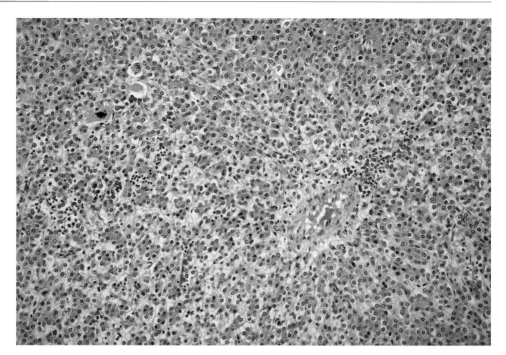

Figure 11.31 Hepatoblastoma, fetal epithelial type.
The tumour grows in cords of small hepatocytes with a 'light-and-dark' herringbone pattern due to the admixed clear (glycogenated) and eosinophilic liver cells. Foci of extramedullary haemopoiesis, including several megakaryocytes and clusters of erythrocyte precursors, are seen at upper left. (Operative specimen, H&E.)

**Figure 11.32
Hepatoblastoma,
embryonal
epithelial type.**
Tumour cells grow in
tubules and show an
increased nucleus–
cytoplasm ratio.
Darkly stained
mitotic figures can
be identified in some
cells. (Operative
specimen, H&E.)

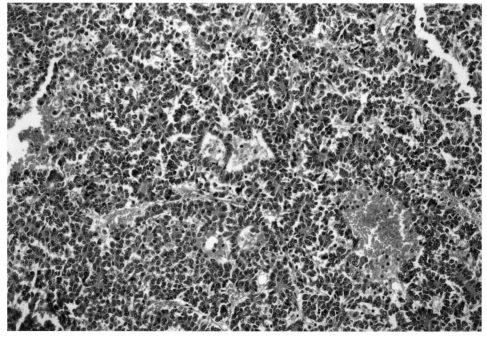

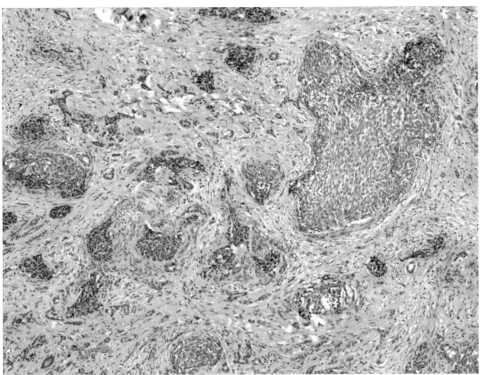

Figure 11.33
Calcifying nested stromal–epithelial tumour.
The desmoplastic stroma contains epithelial nests arranged in a 'zig-zag' pattern. The epithelium varies from larger eosinophilic cells (nest at right) to more basophilic and spindled. Bile-duct structures are in close proximity to the nests. (Partial hepatectomy, H&E.)

Sarcoma and lymphoma

Undifferentiated sarcomas with a poor prognosis occasionally develop in the liver in children.[377] Epithelium trapped within the tumour may give rise to confusion. Light microscopic and ultrastructural features suggest malignant fibrous histiocytoma[378,379] or myoblastic differentiation.[379] Immunohistochemical results are inconsistent, with reports of staining for histiocytic markers, desmin, vimentin and even cytokeratin.[379,380] Another form of sarcoma, arising in the biliary tract, is the **embryonal rhabdomyosarcoma** or **sarcoma botryoides**.[374] The histologically distinctive **calcifying nested stromal–epithelial tumour** is a mixed stromal and epithelial low-grade malignant neoplasm with foci of calcification or ossification.[381–386] This tumour usually grows indolently and shows nests of small, round spindled and large eosinophilic epithelioid cells arranged in irregular zig-zag patterns surrounded by desmoplastic stroma with interspersed bile ducts (**Fig. 11.33**). The tumour shows nuclear and cytoplasmic positivity for β-catenin and mutations in the *β-catenin* gene.[386] Exceptionally rare **primary non-Hodgkin's lymphoma** in the liver has been reported in childhood.[387]

Hepatocellular carcinoma

HCC in children resembles the adult type histologically. Cirrhosis due to tyrosinaemia type 1, bile-salt export pump deficiency (progressive familial intrahepatic cholestasis type 2), biliary atresia and prolonged total parenteral nutrition may be present, as well as other predisposing causes such as type I glycogenosis. EpCAM appears to be an important immunohisochemical marker of this tumour, as well as cytokeratin 19 and GPC-3.[388] The fibrolamellar type of carcinoma has been described in older children, with better prognosis than HCC in general.[235]

Cytopathological diagnosis

FNAB is often used to investigate hepatic masses, particularly for patients with cirrhosis in whom HCC is suspected.[389] This technique may demonstrate lesional tissue as well as components of normal or non-neoplastic liver. In the latter regard, the interpreter must be familiar with the cytological appearances of normal liver, cirrhosis or dysplasia, which are discussed below.

Normal or reactive liver

Aspirates from non-neoplastic liver will contain **normal** or **reactive hepatocytes,** which are present as single cells, clusters or two-dimensional monolayer sheets (**Fig. 11.34**). Normal hepatocytes may be arranged in trabeculae, but these should consist of three or fewer cells, without enveloping endothelium (**Fig. 11.35**). Individual hepatocytes are polygonal cells with well-defined borders and centrally placed, round nuclei which often have conspicuous nucleoli and occasionally show intranuclear cytoplasmic pseudoinclusions (vesicular inclusions). The latter may also be seen in HCC and are therefore not diagnostic. The nuclei of benign hepatocytes may vary considerably in size (not shape) and this is a helpful diagnostic sign which contrasts with the more monomorphic nuclei seen in HCC.[390] The appearance of pigment in the liver varies according to the staining method used.[390,391] The presence of lipofuscin in hepatocytes is indicative of a benign process.

Benign aspirates may also contain **bile-duct epithelium,** which is usually not resent in specimens from liver-cell adenoma and HCC.[392] Bile-duct epithelial cells are smaller than hepatocytes, are arranged in monolayers with a 'honeycomb' glandular pattern (**Fig. 11.36**) and have eccentrically located nuclei in a pale, non-granular cytoplasm.

Figure 11.34 Normal hepatocytes.

A cluster of normal liver cells includes several binucleated hepatocytes and an enlarged, polyploid cell at top. Prominent nucleoli are visible. (Papanicolaou.)

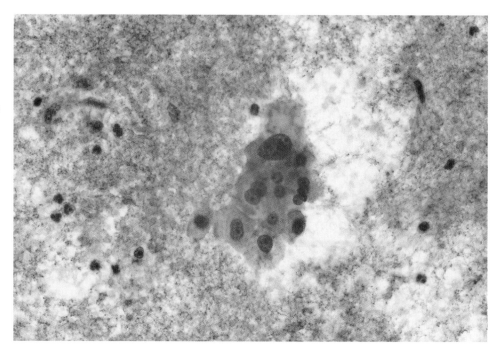

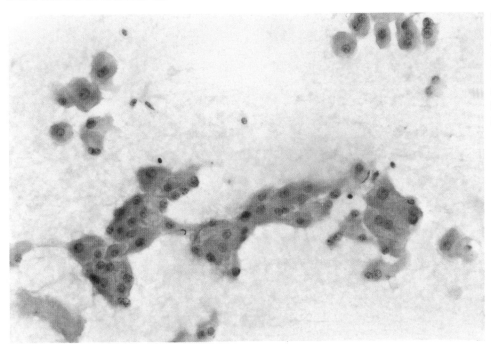

**Figure 11.35
Normal hepatocyte
trabeculae.**
Normal trabeculae of
hepatocytes on
aspirate contain up
to two or three cells.
(Papanicolaou.)

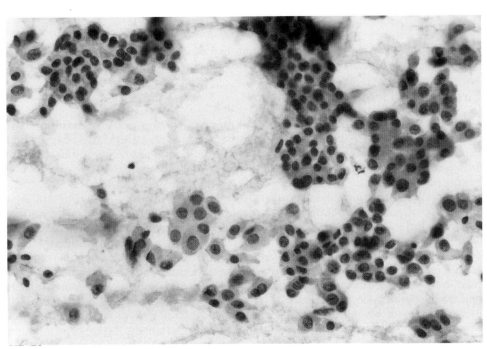

**Figure 11.36
Bile-duct
epithelium.**
Clusters of bile-duct
epithelial cells are
distinguishable from
the group of
hepatocytes near the
centre by their
smaller size and
round, non-descript
nuclei.
Microglandular
structures are also
focally present.
(Papanicolaou.)

Figure 11.37 Mesothelium.
A sheet of mesothelial cells from the peritoneum shows a characteristic clear 'window' at right. (Papanicolaou.)

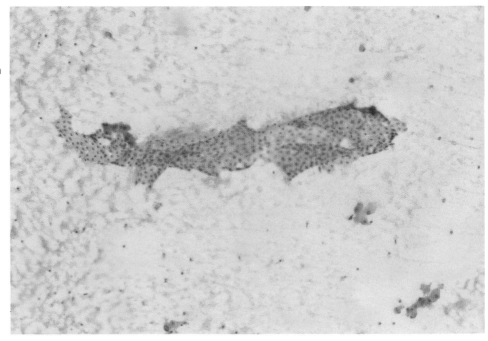

The nuclei have fine chromatin and no prominent nucleoli. Aspirates may also contain sheets of benign **mesothelium** derived from the peritoneum (**Fig. 11.37**).

Cirrhosis and liver-cell dysplasia

Aspirates from cirrhotic liver may contain portions of connective tissue and fibroblasts (**Fig. 11.38**), bile-duct epithelium, reactive hepatocytes arranged in clusters with jagged edges (rather than smooth-edged trabeculae as in HCC) and mixed chronic inflammatory cells (mostly lymphocytes). A definitive diagnosis of cirrhosis based only on FNAB is usually not possible.[393]

Large-cell and small-cell dysplasia (**Ch. 10**) can also be identified on FNAB. The type and degree of nuclear atypia distinguish dysplastic hepatocytes from normal or reactive liver cells. In large-cell dysplasia, nuclei are enlarged, hyperchromatic and pleomorphic, with one or more prominent nucleoli (**Fig. 11.39**). Coarse nuclear chromatin and pseudoinclusions of invaginated cytoplasm are often present. The presence of cellular enlargement with ample cytoplasm maintains a relatively normal nucleus–cytoplasm ratio. In small-cell dysplasia this ratio is increased because the atypical nuclei are found in cells that are smaller than normal hepatocytes (**Fig. 11.40**). The aspirated cell clusters in which dysplastic hepatocytes may be found are accompanied by normal or reactive hepatocytes with heterogeneous nuclear features and cell sizes, an important distinction from aspirates of HCC, which typically show a relatively monomorphous population of hepatocytes.[394]

Hepatocellular adenoma

The cytological diagnosis rendered from the FNAB smear of hepatocellular adenoma is typically 'compatible with' this tumour, since the specimen usually shows single hepatocytes or clusters which resemble benign, normal liver cells.[392] Bile-duct epithelium and connective tissue should be absent, in contrast to FNH.

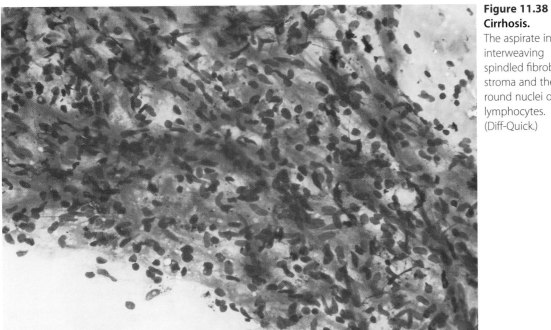

Figure 11.38 Cirrhosis.
The aspirate includes interweaving spindled fibroblasts, stroma and the round nuclei of lymphocytes. (Diff-Quick.)

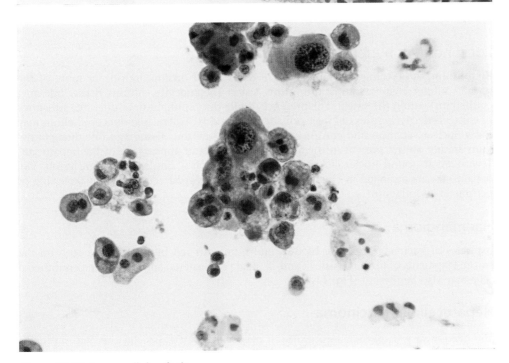

Figure 11.39 Large-cell dysplasia.
Two groups of hepatocytes (top and centre) contain large dysplastic cells intermixed with smaller reactive hepatocytes. The dysplastic cells have hyperchromatic nuclei, coarse chromatin and prominent nucleoli. Normal hepatocytes are seen at left and at bottom. (Papanicolaou.) (Illustration kindly provided by Dr Alastair Deery, London, UK.)

**Figure 11.40
Small-cell
dysplasia.**
The cluster of small
hepatocytes slightly
below centre shows
hyperchromatic
atypical nuclei.
(Papanicolaou.)
(Illustration kindly
provided by Dr
Alastair Deery,
London, UK.)

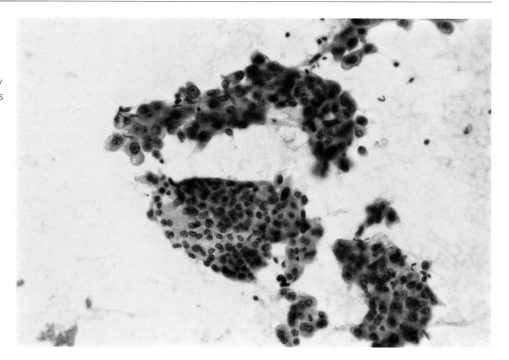

Focal nodular hyperplasia

Establishing the cytological diagnosis of FNH is based on finding one or more of the several cellular elements constituting this lesion (hepatocytes, fibrous tissue, bile-duct epithelium) within the smear. The presence of bile-duct epithelium in duct-like structures or clusters effectively rules out liver-cell adenoma and HCC. The bile-duct epithelium may show nuclear variation and conspicuous nucleoli.[395] Fibrous tissue and bile-duct epithelium are not always present in the aspirate but the bland appearance of the hepatocytes – with small, round nuclei lacking prominent nucleoli – implies a benign lesion. The hepatocytes are arranged in clusters with irregular or jagged edges without traversing or peripheral endothelium.

Haemangioma

Aspirates of haemangiomas are bloody, and numerous red blood cells are seen on the smear. Fragments of fibrous tissue[396] and/or single or clustered spindle-shaped endothelial cells may also be present (**Fig. 11.41**).

Hepatocellular carcinoma

The low-power microscopic appearance of smears from HCC provides several important diagnostic features, especially the rounded edges of tumour cells in clusters or trabeculae (in contrast to the ragged edges of normal or reactive hepatocyte clusters) and endothelial cells which traverse clusters of tumour cells as well as wrap around the periphery of clusters or trabeculae (**Figs 11.42, 11.43**). The paucireticulin pattern of HCC is helpful in FNABs where low-power examination of glass slides shows a finely granular smear (in contrast to the preserved cores or larger tissue fragments seen with benign liver diseases and masses[397]). Tumour cells are polygonal with central nuclei that may have either coarse or fine chromatin and prominent nucleoli or macronucleoli (**Fig. 11.44**). There is usually less

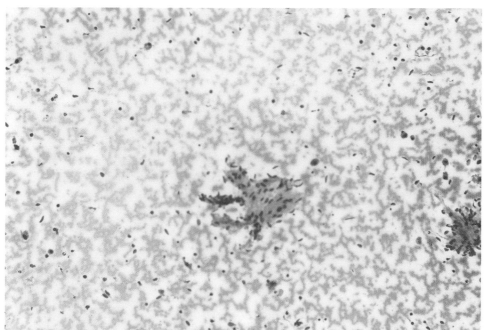

**Figure 11.41
Haemangioma.**
A focus of stromal cells is present with an extensive background of red blood cells. Scattered spindle-shaped endothelial or fibroblast nuclei are seen amid the erythrocytes. (Papanicolaou.)

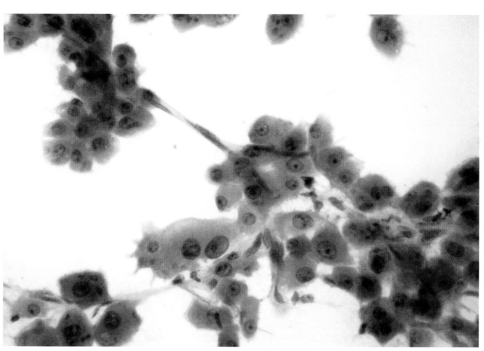

**Figure 11.42
Hepatocellular carcinoma.**
Malignant hepatocytes in clusters are traversed by slender strings of endothelium. (Papanicolaou.)

**Figure 11.43
Hepatocellular
carcinoma.**
Flattened
endothelium is seen
peripherally at the
edge of a trabecula
of hepatocellular
carcinoma.
(Papanicolaou.)

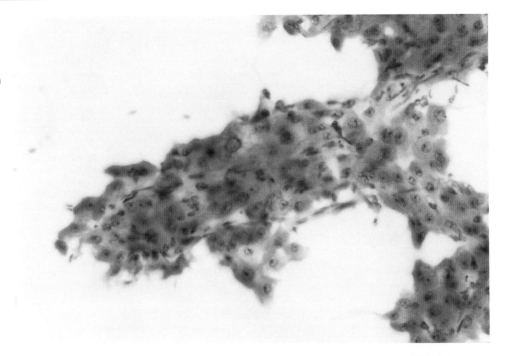

**Figure 11.44
Hepatocellular
carcinoma.**
Malignant
hepatocytes have
fairly uniform nuclei
which are centrally
or peripherally
located. Prominent
nucleoli are seen
throughout and
a mitotic figure
is present at
right centre.
(Papanicolaou.)

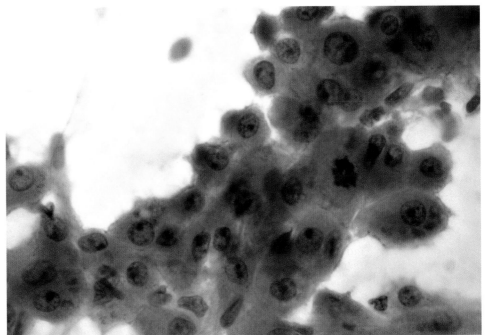

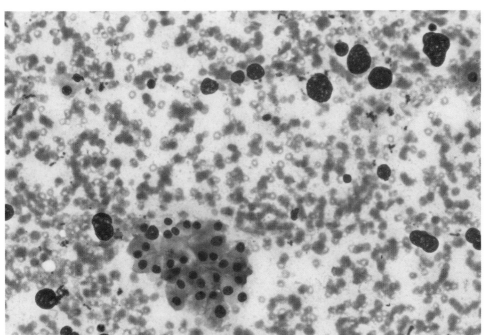

**Figure 11.45
Hepatocellular
carcinoma.**
A cluster of
malignant
hepatocytes is
present along with
'naked nuclei'.
(Diff-Quick.)

variability in the features of HCC cells on smear than in normal or reactive hepatocytes.

Atypical naked nuclei[398] (exceptionally large and irregular nuclei without visible cytoplasm) are also an important diagnostic feature (**Fig. 11.45**). A step-wise logistic regression study showed that the three features which best differentiate HCC from normal or reactive liver are: (1) increased nucleus–cytoplasm ratio; (2) a trabecular pattern of tumour cells enclosed by endothelium; and (3) atypical naked nuclei.[390,399] **Box 11.1** summarises some of the major FNAB cytological features of HCC. The presence of bile within or between tumour cells is indicative of their hepatocellular origin, but bile may be seen in only half the cases[400] and can also be present in smears from non-neoplastic liver.

Box 11.1 Major fine-needle aspiration biopsy features of hepatocellular carcinoma
Polygonal cells with central or paracentral nuclei
Relative homogeneity of tumour cells
High nucleus–cytoplasm ratio
Cell nests and trabeculae with smooth edges
Traversing and/or peripheral endothelium
Atypical naked nuclei

Variants of HCC which may be present include acinar, clear-cell and fibrolamellar carcinoma. As with typical HCC, the presence of peripheral endothelial wrapping or traversal of endothelium across tumour cell clusters favours HCC. When **clear cells** are identified, there are also usually non-clear-cell HCC cells present which help distinguish the tumour from renal, adrenal and ovarian neoplasms.[401] **Fibrolamellar carcinoma** can be diagnosed if the smear includes fibrous tissue or fibroblasts and the distinctive polygonal cells with granular, eosinophilic cytoplasm[402] (**Fig. 11.46**). The tumour cells of fibrolamellar carcinoma are often dispersed or discohesive, in comparison with the cell clusters and trabeculae of typical HCC.[404] Immunohistochemistry for CD68 may be helpful in selected cases.[251]

When metastatic carcinoma must be differentiated from HCC on FNAB, the cytopathologist should bear in mind that nearly all HCCs will have two or three of the following key diagnostic criteria[390]: polygonal cells with centrally placed nuclei; malignant cells traversed by sinusoidal capillaries; and bile.

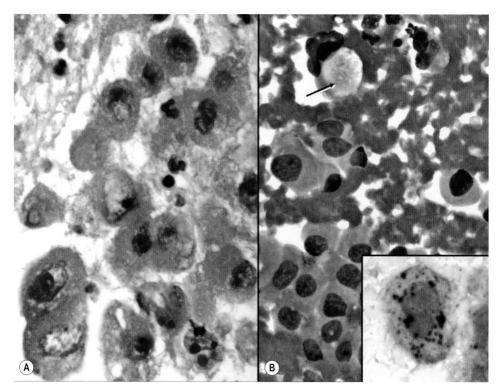

Figure 11.46 Fibrolamellar carcinoma.
A cell block obtained from a fine-needle biopsy aspirate (**A**) shows neoplastic cells with ample eosinophilic and granular ('oncocytic') cytoplasm and pleomorphic nuclei. (H&E stain.) The Diff-Quick stain of the aspirate (**B**) shows plump tumour cells, one of which (at top) contains a 'pale body' (arrow). Inset: CD68 (KP1) immunostain of the cell block shows a tumour cell with positive stippled-granular staining of endosomes and lysosomes, as described in fibrolamellar carcinoma. (Specific immunoperoxidase.)

Hepatoblastoma

The **epithelial type** of hepatoblastoma cytologically resembles HCC and on smear shows cohesive nests, sheets or trabeculae of malignant hepatocytes (**Fig. 11.47**). The tumour cells have hyperchromatic nuclei which may overlap and show prominent nucleoli. Fetal and embryonal subtypes are difficult to distinguish on FNAB alone.[403] There may be extramedullary haemopoiesis, formation of acini and naked tumour-cell nuclei.[403,405] The **mesenchymal type** of hepatoblastoma, or the mixed epithelial–mesenchymal variant, may be represented by spindle cells in the smear.

Cholangiocarcinoma

Aspirate smears from cholangiocarcinoma demonstrate three-dimensional clusters of atypical cells having a small amount of cytoplasm and nuclei with granular chromatin and one or more prominent nucleoli. Tumour cells may also be arranged in acini and cannot be readily distinguished on routine stains from metastatic pancreatic or other adenocarcinomas.[402]

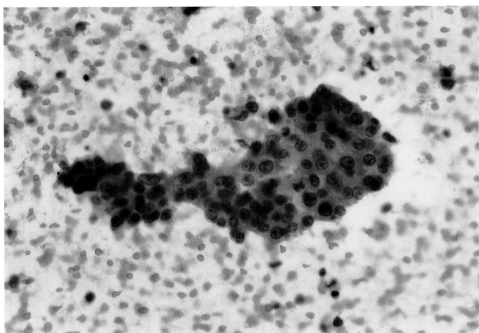

Figure 11.47 Hepatoblastoma. The cell cluster is packed with malignant epithelium. Nuclear features resemble those seen in hepatocellular carcinoma. (Papanicolaou.)

Angiosarcoma

The smear of this tumour is typically bloody, and features a necrotic background with discohesive, pleomorphic spindle cells. Factor VIII and CD34 immunostains are diagnostically helpful.[406]

Lymphoma

Lymphoid proliferations in the liver, including lymphoma and posttransplant lymphoproliferative disease,[407] can be diagnosed on FNAB according to cytological criteria used for aspirates from extrahepatic sites. Smears show dispersed single, monomorphous lymphoid cells with 'blue blobs' of stripped cytoplasm (lymphoglandular bodies[408]) in the background (**Fig. 11.48**). Blue blobs may also be present in smears containing non-neoplastic lymphocytes.

Metastatic tumours

Adenocarcinoma from the colon and pancreas on aspirate smears presents as cell clusters with round or oval vesicular nuclei, prominent nucleoli and delicate cytoplasm. The presence of columnar cells with cigar-shaped, palisaded nuclei and apical cytoplasm or vacuoles (goblet cells) is characteristic of **colon carcinoma** (**Fig. 11.49**). The cytological features of **breast carcinoma** include the tendency to smear as discohesive cell groups or single cells with eccentric nuclei and cone-shaped cytoplasm. Relative uniformity of cell size and shape, prominent small nucleoli and the absence of marked atypia are seen in infiltrating duct carcinoma. Lobular carcinoma may show single-file lines of cells with nuclear moulding. **Neuroendocrine carcinomas** on smear feature organoid nests (carcinoid tumours) or loose groups or sheets (islet-cell carcinoma). The coarse 'salt-and-pepper' chromatin

**Figure 11.48
Lymphoma.**
Dissociated malignant lymphoid cells are present with a background of smaller 'blue blobs' (lymphoglandular bodies). (Diff-Quick.)

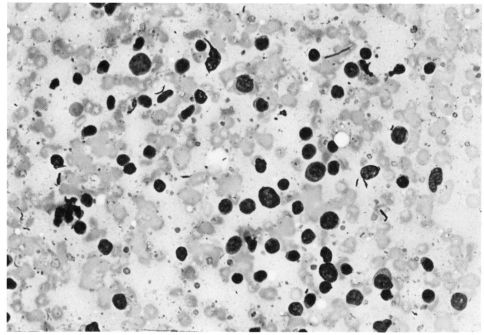

**Figure 11.49
Metastatic colonic adenocarcinoma.**
Several rows of columnar cells are present and the cluster at upper right contains a goblet cell with a large cytoplasmic vacuole. (Papanicolaou.)

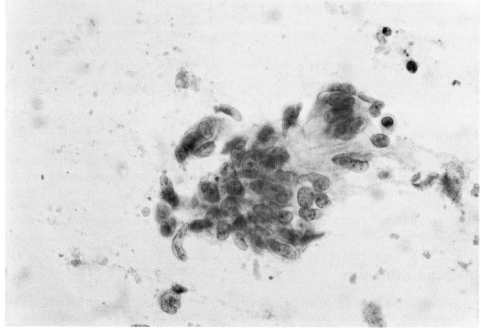

pattern is characteristic of these neoplasms, with islet cell carcinomas often showing more nuclear pleomorphism with prominent nucleoli than carcinoid tumours (**Fig. 11.50**). **Malignant melanoma** often metastasises to the liver and may be confused with HCC on FNAB because of features in common, including eosinophilic macronucleoli, nuclear pseudoinclusions, polygonal cell shape and cohesive cell groups. However, in contrast to

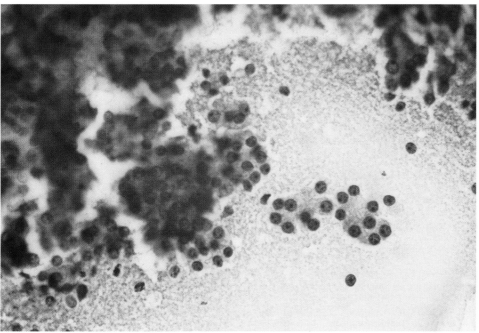

Figure 11.50 Metastatic neuroendocrine carcinoma. Clusters of fairly homogeneous small cells with regular nuclei and substantial cytoplasm are seen. The patient had a pancreatic islet cell carcinoma. Thick trabecular structures are seen at left. (Diff-Quick.)

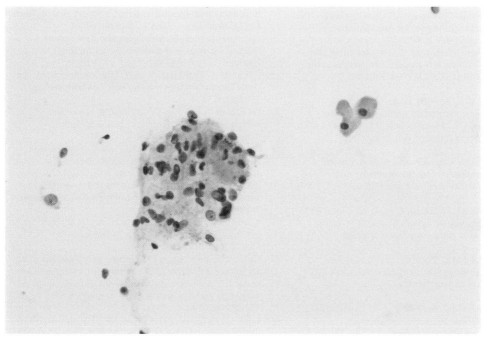

Figure 11.51 Metastatic uveal melanoma. A cluster of melanoma cells with intracellular melanin pigment is present. Several normal hepatocytes are seen at upper right. (Papanicolaou.) (Illustration kindly provided by Dr Alastair Deery, London, UK.)

HCC, aspirates of melanoma are more likely to show single, discohesive cells with eccentric nuclei and intracellular melanin pigment (**Fig. 11.51**). If cell grouping is present, it is unlikely to be accompanied by the traversing or peripheral endothelium seen in HCC. Immunostains for HMB-45 and S-100 should be undertaken if melanoma is a possible diagnosis, particularly if pigment is absent.

References

1 Tao L-C. Oral contraceptive-associated liver cell adenoma and hepatocellular carcinoma. Cytomorphology and mechanism of malignant transformation. Cancer 1991;68:341–7.

2 Greaves WOC, Bhattacharya B. Hepatic adenomatosis. Arch Pathol Lab Med 2008;132:1951–5.

3 Lepreux S, Laurent C, Blanc JF, et al. The identification of small nodules in liver adenomatosis. J Hepatol 2003;39:77–85.

4 Hasan N, Coutts M, Portmann B. Pigmented liver cell adenoma in two male patients. Am J Surg Pathol 2000;24:1429–32.

5 Heffelfinger S, Irani DR, Finegold MJ. 'Alcoholic hepatitis' in a hepatic adenoma. Hum Pathol 1987;18:751–4.

6 Le Bail B, Jouhanole H, Deugnier Y, et al. Liver adenomatosis with granulomas in two patients on long-term oral contraceptives. Am J Surg Pathol 1992;16:982–7.

7 Bieze M, Bioulac-Sage P, Verheij J, et al. Hepatocellular adenomas associated with hepatic granulomas: experience in five cases. Case Rep Gastroenterol 2012;6:677–83.

8 Bioulac-Sage P, Rebouissou S, Thomas C, et al. Hepatocellular adenoma subtype classification using molecular markers and immunohistochemistry. Hepatology 2007;46:740–8.

9 Bioulac-Sage P, Blanc JF, Rebouissou S, et al. Genotype phenotype classification of hepatocellular adenoma. World J Gastroenterol 2007;13:2649–54.

10 Bioulac-Sage P, Cubel G, Balabaud C, et al. Revisiting the pathology of resected benign hepatocellular nodules using new immunohistochemical markers. Semin Liver Dis 2011;31:79–91.

11 Bioulac-Sage P, Cubel G, Taouji S, et al. Immunohistochemical markers on needle biopsies are helpful for the diagnosis of focal nodular hyperplasia and hepatocellular adenoma subtypes. Am J Surg Pathol 2012;36:1691–9.

12 Shafizadeh N, Kakar S. Diagnosis of well-differentiated hepatocellular lesions: role of immunohistochemistry and other ancillary techniques. Adv Anat Pathol 2011;18:438–45.

13 van Aalten SM, Verheij J, Terkivatan T, et al. Validation of a liver adenoma classification system in a tertiary referral centre: implications for clinical practice. J Hepatol 2011;55:120–5.

14 Bioulac-Sage P, Balabaud C, Zucman-Rossi J. Will the pathomolecular classification of hepatocellular adenomas improve their clinical management? J Hepatol 2011;55:8–10.

15 Bioulac-Sage P, Balabaud C, Bedossa P, et al. Pathological diagnosis of liver cell adenoma and focal nodular hyperplasia: Bordeaux update. J Hepatol 2007;46:521–7.

16 Nault J-C, Bioulac-Sage P, Zucman-Rossi J. Hepatocellular benign tumors – from molecular classification to personalized clinical care. Gastroenterology 2013;144:888–902.

17 Evason KJ, Grenert JP, Ferrell LD, et al. Atypical hepatocellular adenoma-like neoplasms with β-catenin activation show cytogenetic alterations similar to well-differentiated hepatocellular carcinomas. Hum Pathol 2013;44:750–8.

18 Farges O, Ferreira N, Dokmak S, et al. Changing trends in malignant transformation of hepatocellular adenoma. Gut 2011;60:85–9.

19 Rebouissou S, Amessou M, Couchy G, et al. Frequent in-frame somatic deletions activate gp130 in inflammatory hepatocellular tumours. Nature 2009;457:200–4.

20 Shafizadeh N, Genrich G, Ferrell L, et al. Hepatocellular adenomas in a large community population, 2000 to 2010: reclassification per current World Helath Organization classification and results of long-term follow up. Hum Pathol 2014;45:976–83.

21 Bellamy COC, Maxwell RS, Prost S, et al. The value of immunophenotyping hepatocellular adenomas: consecutive resections at one UK centre. Histopathology 2013;62:431–45.

22 Micchelli STL, Vivekanandan P, Boitnott JK, et al. Malignant transformation of hepatic adenomas. Mod Pathol 2008;21:491–7.

23 Rooks JB, Ory HW, Ishak KG, et al. Epidemiology of hepatocellular adenoma. The role of oral contraceptive use. JAMA 1979;242:644–8.

24 Sánchez-Osorio M, Duarte-Rojo A, Martinez-Benitez B, et al. Anabolic–androgenic steroids and liver injury. Liver Int 2008;28:278–82.

25 Ozenne V, Paradis V, Vullierme M-P, et al. Liver tumours in patients with Fanconi anaemia: a report of three cases. Eur J Gastrol Hepatol 2008;20:1036–9.

26 Velazquez I, Alter BP. Androgens and liver tumors: Fanconi's anemia and non-Fanconi's conditions. Am J Hematol 2004;77:257–67.

27 Flejou JF, Barge J, Menu Y, et al. Liver adenomatosis. An entity distinct from liver adenoma? Gastroenterology 1985;89:1132–8.

28 Vetaläinen R, Erdogan D, de Graaf W, et al. Liver adenomatosis: re-evaluation of aetiology and management. Liver Int 2008;28:499–508.

29 Bacq Y, Jacquemin E, Balabaud C, et al. Familial liver adenomatosis associated with hepatocyte nuclear factor 1α inactivation. Gastroenterology 2003;125:1470–5.

30 Zucman-Rossi J. Genetic alterations in hepatocellular adenomas: recent findings and new challenges. J Hepatol 2004;40:1036–9.

31 Kahn H, Manzarbeitia C, Theise N, et al. Danazol-induced hepatocellular adenomas. Arch Pathol Lab Med 1991;115:1054–7.

32 Gokhale R, Whitington PR. Hepatic adenomatosis in an adolescent. J Pediatr Gastroenterol Nutr 1996;23:482–6.

33 Foster JH, Donohue TA, Berman MM. Familial liver-cell adenomas and diabetes mellitus. N Engl J Med 1978;299:239–41.

34 Coire CI, Qizilbash AH, Castelli MF. Hepatic adenomata in type Ia glycogen storage disease. Arch Pathol Lab Med 1987;111:166–9.

35 Calderaro J, Labrune P, Morcrette G, et al. Molecular characterization of hepatocellular adenomas developed in patients with glycogen storage disease type I. J Hepatol 2013;58:350–7.

36 Liu T-C, Vachharajani N, Chapman WC, et al. Noncirrhotic hepatocellular carcinoma: derivation from hepatocellular adenoma? Clinicopathologic analysis. Mod Pathol 2014;27:420–32.

37   Paradis V, Laurent A, Flejou J-F, et al. Evidence for the polyclonal nature of focal nodular hyperplasia of the liver by the study of X-chromosome inactivation. Hepatology 1997;26:891–5.

38   Wanless IR, Mawdsley C, Adams R. On the pathogenesis of focal nodular hyperplasia of the liver. Hepatology 1985;5:1194–200.

39   Fukukura Y, Nakashima O, Kusaba A, et al. Angioarchitecture and blood circulation in focal nodular hyperplasia of the liver. J Hepatol 1998;29:470–5.

40   Roskams T, De Vos R, Desmet V. 'Undifferentiated progenitor cells' in focal nodular hyperplasia of the liver. Histopathology 1996;28:291–9.

41   Scoazec J-Y, Flejou J-F, D'Errico A, et al. Focal nodular hyperplasia of the liver: composition of the extracellular matrix and expression of cell–cell and cell–matrix adhesion molecules. Hum Pathol 1995;26:1114–25.

42   Nime F, Pickren JW, Vana J, et al. The histology of liver tumors in oral contraceptive users observed during a national survey by the American College of Surgeons Commission on Cancer. Cancer 1979;44:1481–9.

43   Mathieu D, Kobeiter H, Maison P, et al. Oral contraceptive use and focal nodular hyperplasia of the liver. Gastroenterology 2000;118:560–4.

44   Sadowski DC, Lee SS, Wanless IR, et al. Progressive type of focal nodular hyperplasia characterized by multiple tumors and recurrence. Hepatology 1995;21:970–5.

45   Friedman LS, Gang DL, Hedberg SE, et al. Simultaneous occurrence of hepatic adenoma and focal nodular hyperplasia: report of a case and review of the literature. Hepatology 1984;4:536–40.

46   Wanless IR, Albrecht S, Bilbao J, et al. Multiple focal nodular hyperplasia of the liver associated with vascular malformations of various organs and neoplasia of the brain: a new syndrome. Mod Pathol 1989;2:456–62.

47   Portmann B, Stewart S, Higenbottam TW, et al. Nodular transformation of the liver associated with portal and pulmonary arterial hypertension. Gastroenterology 1993;104:616–21.

48   Haber M, Reuben A, Burrell M, et al. Multiple focal nodular hyperplasia of the liver associated with hemihypertrophy and vascular malformations. Gastroenterology 1995;108:1256–62.

49   Sato Y, Harada K, Ikeda H, et al. Hepatic stellate cells are activated around central scars of focal nodular hyperplasia of the liver – a potential mechanism of central scar formation. Hum Pathol 2009;40:181–8.

50   Butron Vila MM, Haot J, Desmet VJ. Cholestatic features in focal nodular hyperplasia of the liver. Liver 1984;4:387–95.

51   Ahmad I, Iyer A, Marginean CE, et al. Diagnostic use of cytokeratins, CD34, and neuronal cell adhesion molecule staining in focal nodular hyperplasia and hepatic adenoma. Hum Pathol 2009;40:726–34.

52   Ruschenburg I, Droese M. Fine needle aspiration cytology of focal nodular hyperplasia of the liver. Acta Cytol 1989;33:857–60.

53   Makhlouf HR, Abdul-AL HM, Goodman ZD. Diagnosis of focal nodular hyperplasia of the liver by needle biopsy. Hum Pathol 2005;36:1210–16.

54   Schilling MK, Zimmermann A, Redaelli C, et al. Liver nodules resembling focal nodular hyperplasia after hepatic venous thrombosis. J Hepatol 2000;33:673–6.

55   Ibarrola C, Castellano VM, Colina F. Focal hyperplastic hepatocellular nodules in hepatic venous outflow obstruction: a clinicopathological study of four patients and 24 nodules. Histopathology 2004;44:172–9.

56   Wanless IR. Epithelioid hemangioendothelioma, multiple focal nodular hyperplasias, and cavernous hemangiomas of the liver. Arch Pathol Lab Med 2000;124:1105–7.

57   Ra SH, Kaplan JB, Lassman CR. Focal nodular hyperplasia after orthotopic liver transplantation. Liver Transplant 2010;16:98–103.

58   Joseph NM, Ferrell LD, Jain D, et al. Diagnostic utility and limitations of glutamine synthetase and serum amyloid-associated protein immunohistochemistry in the distinction of focal nodular hyperplasia and inflammatory hepatocellular adenoma. Mod Pathol 2014;27:62–72.

59   Reshamwala PA, Kleiner DE, Heller T. Nodular regenerative hyperplasia: not all nodules are created equal. Hepatology 2006;44:7–14.

60   Stromeyer FW, Ishak KG. Nodular transformation (nodular 'regenerative' hyperplasia) of the liver. A clinicopathologic study of 30 cases. Hum Pathol 1981;12:60–71.

61   Thorne C, Urowitz MB, Wanless I, et al. Liver disease in Felty's syndrome. Am J Med 1982;73:35–40.

62   Wanless IR. Micronodular transformation (nodular regenerative hyperplasia) of the liver: a report of 64 cases among 2,500 autopsies and a new classification of benign hepatocellular nodules. Hepatology 1990;11:787–97.

63   Dubinsky MC, Vasiliauskas EA, Singh H, et al. 6-Thioguanine can cause serious liver injury in inflammatory bowel disease patients. Gastroenterology 2003;125:298–303.

64   Paradinas FJ, Bull TB, Westaby D, et al. Hyperplasia and prolapse of hepatocytes into hepatic veins during longterm methyltestosterone therapy: possible relationships of these changes to the development of peliosis hepatis and liver tumours. Histopathology 1977;1:225–46.

65   Baker BL, Axiotis C, Hurwitz ES, et al. Nodular regenerative hyperplasia of the liver in idiopathic hypereosinophilic syndrome. J Clin Gastroenterol 1991;13:452–6.

66   Solis-Herruzo JA, Vidal JV, Colina F, et al. Nodular regenerative hyperplasia of the liver associated with the toxic oil syndrome: report of five cases. Hepatology 1986;6:687–93.

67   Bloxham CA, Henderson DC, Hampson J, et al. Nodular regenerative hyperplasia of the liver in Behçet's disease. Histopathology 1992;20:452–4.

68   Colina F, Pinedo F, Solís A, et al. Nodular regenerative hyperplasia of the liver in early histological stages of primary biliary cirrhosis. Gastroenterology 1992;102:1319–24.

69   Cancado ELR, Medeiros DM, Deguti MM, et al. Celiac disease associated with nodular regenerative hyperplasia, pulmonary abnormalities, and IgA anticardiolipin antibodies. J Clin Gastroenterol 2006;40:135–9.

70   Minato H, Nakanuma Y. Nodular regenerative hyperplasia of the liver associated with metastases of pancreatic endocrine tumour: report of two autopsy cases. Virchows Arch [A] 1992;421:171–4.

71   Kobayashi S, Saito K, Nakanuma Y. Nodular regenerative hyperplasia of the liver in hepatocellular carcinoma. J Clin Gastroenterol 1993;16:155–9.

72   Wanless IR, Godwin TA, Allen F, et al. Nodular regenerative hyperplasia of the liver in hematologic disorders: a possible response to obliterative portal

venopathy. A morphometric study of nine cases with an hypothesis on the pathogenesis. Medicine 1980;59:367–79.

73 Wanless IR, Lentz JS, Roberts EA. Partial nodular transformation of liver in an adult with persistent ductus venosus. Review with hypothesis on pathogenesis. Arch Pathol Lab Med 1985;109:427–32.

74 Terayama N, Terada T, Hoso M, et al. Partial nodular transformation of the liver with portal vein thrombosis. J Clin Gastroenterol 1995;20:71–6.

75 Wanless IR. Vascular disorders. In: MacSween RNM, Anthony PP, Scheuer PJ, et al., editors. Pathology of the Liver. 3rd ed. Edinburgh: Churchill Livingstone; 1994. p. 535–62 [Ch. 14].

76 Allaire GS, Rabin L, Ishak KG, et al. Bile duct adenoma. A study of 152 cases. Am J Surg Pathol 1988;12:708–15.

77 Bhathal PS, Hughes NR, Goodman ZD. The so-called bile duct adenoma is a peribiliary gland hamartoma. Am J Surg Pathol 1996;20:858–64.

78 Hughes NR, Goodman ZD, Bhathal PS. An immunohistochemical profile of the so-called bile duct adenoma. Clues to the pathogenesis. Am J Surg Pathol 2010;34:1312–18.

79 Cho C, Rullis I, Rogers LS. Bile duct adenomas as liver nodules. Arch Surg 1978;113:272–4.

80 Gold JH, Guzman IJ, Rosai J. Benign tumors of the liver. Pathologic examination of 45 cases. Am J Clin Pathol 1978;70:6–17.

81 Govindarajan S, Peters RL. The bile duct adenoma. A lesion distinct from Meyenburg complex. Arch Pathol Lab Med 1984;108:922–4.

82 Scheele PM, Bonar MJ, Zumwalt R, et al. Bile duct adenomas in heterozygous (MZ) deficiency of α1-protease inhibitor. Arch Pathol Lab Med 1988;112:945–7.

83 Varnholt H, Vauthey J-N, Dal Cin P, et al. Biliary adenofibroma. A rare neoplasm of bile duct origin with an indolent behavior. Am J Surg Pathol 2003;27:693–8.

84 Wheeler DA, Edmondson HA. Cystadenoma with mesenchymal stroma (CMS) in the liver and bile ducts. A clinicopathologic study of 17 cases, 4 with malignant change. Cancer 1985;56:1434–45.

85 Gourley WK, Kumar D, Bouton MS, et al. Cystadenoma and cystadenocarcinoma with mesenchymal stroma of the liver. Immunohistochemical analysis. Arch Pathol Lab Med 1992;116:1047–50.

86 Ishak KG, Willis GW, Cummins SD, et al. Biliary cystadenoma and cystadenocarcinoma: report of 14 cases and review of the literature. Cancer 1977;39:322–38.

87 Tung GA, Cronan JJ. Percutaneous needle biopsy of hepatic cavernous hemangioma. J Clin Gastroenterol 1993;16:117–22.

88 Kim GE, Thung SN, Tsui WMS, et al. Hepatic cavernous hemangioma: underrecognized associated histologic features. Liver Int 2006;26:334–8.

89 Berry CL. Solitary 'necrotic nodule' of the liver: a probable pathogenesis. J Clin Pathol 1985;38:1278–80.

90 Van Steenbergen W, Joosten E, Marchal G, et al. Hepatic lymphangiomatosis. Report of a case and review of the literature. Gastroenterology 1985;88:1968–72.

91 Peters WM, Dixon MF, Williams NS. Angiomyelolipoma of the liver. Histopathology 1983;7:99–106.

92 Goodman ZD. Benign tumors of the liver. In: Okuda K, Ishak KG, editors. Neoplasms of the Liver. Tokyo: Springer-Verlag; 1990. p. 105–26.

93 Hytiroglou P, Linton P, Klion F, et al. Benign schwannoma of the liver. Arch Pathol Lab Med 1993;117:216–18.

94 Lederman SM, Martin EC, Laffey KT, et al. Hepatic neurofibromatosis, malignant schwannoma and angiosarcoma in von Recklinghausen's disease. Gastroenterology 1987;92:234–9.

95 Andreu V, Elizalde I, Mallafré C, et al. Plexiform neurofibromatosis and angiosarcoma of the liver in Von Recklinghausen disease. Am J Gastroenterol 1997;92:1229–30.

96 Moran CA, Ishak KG, Goodman ZD. Solitary fibrous tumor of the liver: a clinicpathologic and immunohistochemical study of nine cases. Ann Diagn Pathol 1998;2:19–24.

97 Fried RH, Wardzala A, Willson RA, et al. Benign cartilaginous tumor (chondroma) of the liver. Gastroenterology 1992;103:678–80.

98 Nonomura A, Mizukami Y, Isobe M, et al. Smallest angiomyolipoma of the liver in the oldest patient. Liver 1993;13:51–3.

99 Tsui WMS, Colombari R, Portmann BC, et al. Hepatic angiomyolipoma. A clinicopathologic study of 30 cases and delineation of unusual morphologic variants. Am J Surg Pathol 1999;23:34–48.

100 Nonomura A, Enomoto Y, Takeda M, et al. Angiomyolipoma of the liver: a reappraisal of morphological features and delineation of new characteristic histological features from the clinicopathological findings of 55 tumours in 47 patients. Histopathology 2012;61:863–80.

101 Nonomura A, Mizukami Y, Kadoya M, et al. Multiple angiomyolipoma of the liver. J Clin Gastroenterol 1995;20:248–51.

102 Kyokane T, Akita Y, Katayama M, et al. Multiple angiomyolipomas of the liver (case report). Hepatol Gastroenterol 1995;42:510–15.

103 Pounder DJ. Hepatic angiomyolipoma. Am J Surg Pathol 1982;6:677–81.

104 Goodman ZD, Ishak KG. Angiomyolipomas of the liver. Am J Surg Pathol 1984;8:745–50.

105 Hoffman AL, Emre S, Verham RP, et al. Hepatic angiomyolipoma: two case reports of caudate-based lesions and review of the literature. Liver Transplant Surg 1997;3:46–53.

106 Terris B, Fléjou J-F, Picot R, et al. Hepatic angiomyolipoma. A report of four cases with immunohistochemical and DNA-flow cytometric studies. Arch Pathol Lab Med 1996;120:68–72.

107 Karhunen PJ. Hepatic pseudolipoma. J Clin Pathol 1985;38:877–9.

108 Hastir D, Verset L, Lucidi V, et al. IgG4 positive lymphoplasmacytic inflammatory pseudotumour mimicking hepatocellular carcinoma. Liver Int 2014;34(6):961.

109 Shek TWH, Ng IOL, Chan KW. Inflammatory pseudotumor of the liver. Report of four cases and review of the literature. Am J Surg Pathol 1993;17:231–8.

110 Lawrence B, Perez-Atayde A, Hibbard MK, et al. TPM3-ALK and TPM4-ALK oncogenes in inflammatory myofibroblastic tumors. Am J Pathol 2000;157:377–84.

111 Cessna MH, Zhou H, Sanger WG, et al. Expression of ALK1 and p80 in inflammatory myofibroblastic tumor and its mesenchymal mimics: a study of 135 cases. Mod Pathol 2002;15:931–8.

112 Shek TWH, Ho FCS, Ng GOL, et al. Follicular dendritic cell tumor of the liver. Evidence for an Epstein–Barr virus-related clonal proliferation of follicular dendritic cells. Am J Surg Pathol 1996;20:313–24.

113 Stone JH, Zen Y, Deshpande V. IgG4-related disease. N Engl J Med 2012;366:539–41.

114 Carruthers MN, Stone JH, Khosroshahi A. The latest on IgG4-RD: a rapidly emerging disease. Curr Opin Rheumatol 2012;24:60–9.

115 Balabaud C, Bioulac-Sage P, Goodman ZD, et al. Inlammatory pseudotumor of the liver: a rare but distinct tumor-like lesion. Gastroenterol Hepatol 2012;8:633–4.

116 Park YN. Update on precursor and early lesions of hepatocellular carcinomas. Arch Pathol Lab Med 2011;135:704–15.

117 Ferrell LD, Crawford JM, Dhillon AP, et al. Proposal for standardized criteria for the diagnosis of benign, borderline, and malignant hepatocellular lesions arising in chronic advanced liver disease. Am J Surg Pathol 1993;17:1113–23.

118 International Working Party. Terminology of nodular hepatocellular lesions. Hepatology 1995;22:983–93.

119 International Consensus Group for Hepatocellular Neoplasia. Pathologic diagnosis of early hepatocellular carcinoma: a report of the international consensus group for hepatocellular neoplasia. Hepatology 2009;49:658–64.

120 Park YN, Roncalli M. Large liver cell dysplasia: a controversial entity. J Hepatol 2006;45:734–43.

121 Anthony PP, Vogel CL, Barker LF. Liver cell dysplasia: a premalignant condition. J Clin Pathol 1973;26:217–23.

122 Anthony PP. Hepatocellular carcinoma: an overview. Histopathology 2001;39:109–18.

123 Borzio M, Bruno S, Roncalli M, et al. Liver cell dysplasia is a major risk factor for hepatocellular carcinoma in cirrhosis: a prospective study. Gastroenterology 1995;108:812–17.

124 Ganne-Carrié N, Chastang C, Chapel F, et al. Predictive score for the development of hepatocellular carcinoma and additional value of liver large cell dysplasia in Western patients with cirrhosis. Hepatology 1996;23:1112–18.

125 Thomas RM, Berman JJ, Yetter RA, et al. Liver cell dysplasia: a DNA aneuploid lesion with distinct morphologic features. Hum Pathol 1992;23:496–503.

126 Terris B, Ingster O, Rubbia L, et al. Interphase cytogenetic analysis reveals numerical chromosome aberrations in large liver cell dysplasia. J Hepatol 1997;27:313–19.

127 Natarajan S, Theise ND, Thung SN, et al. Large-cell change of hepatocytes in cirrhosis may represent a reaction to prolonged cholestasis. Am J Surg Pathol 1997;21:312–18.

128 Lee RG, Tsamandas AC, Demetris AJ. Large cell change (liver cell dysplasia) and hepatocellular carcinoma in cirrhosis: matched case–control study, pathological analysis, and pathogenetic hypothesis. Hepatology 1997;26:1415–22.

129 Libbrecht L, Craninx M, Nevens F, et al. Predictive value of liver cell dysplasia for development of hepatocellular carcinoma in patients with non-cirrhotic and cirrhotic chronic viral hepatitis. Histopathology 2001;39:66–71.

130 Koo JS, Kim H, Park BK, et al. Predictive value of liver cell dysplasia for development of hepatocellular carcinoma in patients with chronic hepatitis B. J Clin Gastroenterol 2008;42:738–43.

131 Watanabe S, Okita K, Harada T, et al. Morphologic studies of the liver cell dysplasia. Cancer 1983;51:2197–205.

132 Adachi E, Hashimoto H, Tsuneyoshi M. Proliferating cell nuclear antigen in hepatocellular carcinoma and small cell liver dysplasia. Cancer 1993;72:2902–9.

133 Plentz RR, Park YN, Lechel A, et al. Telomere shortening and inactivation of cell cycle checkpoints characterize human hepatocarcinogenesis. Hepatology 2007;45:968–76.

134 Terada T, Hoso M, Nakanuma Y. Mallory body clustering in adenomatous hyperplasia in human cirrhotic livers. Hum Pathol 1989;20:886–90.

135 Ueno Y, Moriyama M, Uchida T, et al. Irregular regeneration of hepatocytes is an important factor in the hepatocarcinogenesis of liver disease. Hepatology 2001;33:357–62.

136 Terada T, Nakanuma Y. Iron-negative foci in siderotic macroregenerative nodules in human cirrhotic liver. Arch Pathol Lab Med 1989;113:916–20.

137 Deugnier YM, Charalambous P, Le Quilleuc D, et al. Preneoplastic significance of hepatic iron-free foci in genetic hemochromatosis: a study of 185 patients. Hepatology 1993;18:1363–9.

138 Nakanuma Y, Terada T, Ueda K, et al. Adenomatous hyperplasia of the liver as a precancerous lesion. Liver 1993;13:1–9.

139 Furuya K, Nakamura M, Yamamoto Y, et al. Macroregenerative nodule of the liver. A clinicopathologic study of 345 autopsy cases of chronic liver disease. Cancer 1988;61:99–105.

140 Terada T, Ueda K, Nakanuma Y. Histopathological and morphometric analysis of atypical adenomatous hyperplasia of human cirrhotic livers. Virchows Arch [A] 1993;422:381–8.

141 Le Bail B, Bernard P-H, Carles J, et al. Prevalence of liver cell dysplasia and association with HCC in a series of 100 cirrhotic liver explants. J Hepatol 1997;27:835–42.

142 Ferrell LD. Hepatocellular nodules in the cirrhotic liver: diagnostic features and proposed nomenclature. In: Ferrell LD, editor. Diagnostic Problems in Liver Pathology. Philadelphia, PA: Hanley & Belfus; 1994. p. 105–18.

143 Gastaldi M, Massacrier A, Planells R, et al. Detection by in situ hybridization of hepatitis C virus positive and negative RNA strands using digoxigenin-labeled cRNA probes in human liver cells. J Hepatol 1995;23:509–18.

144 Terasaki S, Kaneko S, Kobayashi K, et al. Histological features predicting malignant transformation of nonmalignant hepatocellular nodules: a prospective study. Gastroenterology 1998;115:1216–22.

145 Theise ND, Schwartz M, Miller C, et al. Macroregenerative nodules and hepatocellular carcinoma in forty-four sequential adults liver explants with cirrhosis. Hepatology 1992;16:949–55.

146 Eguchi A, Nakashima O, Okudaira S, et al. Adenomatous hyperplasia in the vicinity of small hepatocellular carcinoma. Hepatology 1992;15:843–8.

147 Aihara T, Noguchi S, Sasaki Y, et al. Clonal analysis of precancerous lesion of hepatocellular carcinoma. Gastroenterology 1996;111:455–61.

148 Donato MF, Arosio E, Del Ninno E, et al. High rates of hepatocellular carcinoma in cirrhotic patients with high liver cell proliferative activity. Hepatology 2001;34:523–8.

149 Di Bisceglie AM, Carithers RL, Gores GJ. Hepatocellular carcinoma. Hepatology 1998;28:1161–5.

150 Schirmacher P, Rogler CE, Dienes HP. Current pathogenetic and molecular concepts in viral liver carcinogenesis. Virchows Arch [B] 1993;63:71–89.

151 Popper H, Thung SN, McMahon BJ, et al. Evolution of hepatocellular carcinoma associated with chronic hepatitis B virus infection in Alaskan eskimos. Arch Pathol Lab Med 1988;112:498–504.

152 Mandishona E, MacPhail AP, Gordeuk VR, et al. Dietary iron overload as a risk factor for hepatocellular carcinoma in black Africans. Hepatology 1998;27:1563–6.

153 Sun Z, Lu P, Gail MH, et al. Increased risk of hepatocellular carcinoma in male hepatitis B surface antigen carriers with chronic hepatitis who have detectable urinary aflatoxin metabolite M1. Hepatology 1999;30:379–83.

154 Nair S, Mason A, Eason J, et al. Is obesity an independent risk factor for hepatocellular carcinoma in cirrhosis? Hepatology 2002;36:150–5.

155 Marrero JA, Fontana RJ, Su GL, et al. NAFLD may be a common underlying liver disease in patients with hepatocellular carcinoma in the United States. Hepatology 2002;36:1349–54.

156 Shimada M, Hashimoto E, Taniai M, et al. Hepatocellular carcinoma in patients with non-alcoholic steatohepatitis. J Hepatol 2002;37:154–60.

157 Paradis V, Bièche I, Dargère D, et al. Molecular profiling of hepatocellular carcinomas (HCC) using a large-scale real-time RT-PCR approach. Determination of a molecular diagnostic index. Am J Pathol 2003;163:733–41.

158 Chen Q, Seol D-W, Carr B, et al. Co-expression and regulation of met and ron proto-oncogenes in human hepatocellular carcinoma tissues and cell lines. Hepatology 1997;26:59–66.

159 Nalesnik MA, Tseng G, Ding Y, et al. Gene deledtions and amplifications in human hepatocellular carcinomas. Correlation with hepatocyte growth regulation. Am J Pathol 2012;180:1495–508.

160 Tannapfel A, Wittekind C. Genes involved in hepatocellular carcinoma: deregulation in cell cycling and apoptosis. Virchows Arch 2002;44:345–52.

161 Park YN, Yang C-P, Fernandez GJ, et al. Neoangiogenesis and sinusoidal 'capillarization' in dysplastic nodules of the liver. Am J Surg Pathol 1998;22:656–62.

162 Kimura H, Nakajima T, Kagawa K, et al. Angiogenesis in hepatocellular carcinoma as evaluated by CD34 immunohistochemistry. Liver 1998;18:14–19.

163 El-Assal ON, Yamanoi A, Soda Y, et al. Clinical significance of microvessel density and vascular endothelial growth factor expression in hepatocellular carcinoma and surrounding liver: possible involvement of vascular endothelial growth factor in the angiogenesis of cirrhotic liver. Hepatology 1998;27:1554–62.

164 Yamaguchi R, Yano H, Iemura A, et al. Expression of vascular endothelial growth factor in human hepatocellular carcinoma. Hepatology 1998;28:68–77.

165 Torimura T, Sata M, Ueno T, et al. Increased expression of vascular endothelial growth factor is associated with tumor progression in hepatocellular carcinoma. Hum Pathol 1998;29:986–91.

166 Nehrbass D, Klimek F, Bannasch P. Overexpression of insulin receptor substrate-1 emerges early in hepatocarcinogenesis and elicits preneoplastic hepatic glycogenosis. Am J Pathol 1998;152:341–5.

167 Hsia CC, Evarts RP, Nakatsukasa H, et al. Occurrence of oval-type cells in hepatitis B virus-associated human hepatocarcinogenesis. Hepatology 1992;16:1327–33.

168 Desmet V, De Vos R. Ultrastructural characteristics of novel epithelial cell types identified in human pathologic liver specimens with chronic ductular reaction. Am J Pathol 1992;140:1441–50.

169 Kim H, Yoo JE, Cho JY, et al. Telomere length, TERT and shelterin complex proteins in hepatocellular carcinomas expressing "stemness"-related markers. J Hepatol 2013;59:746–52.

170 Anthony PP. Tumours and tumour-like lesions of the liver and biliary tract. In: MacSween RNM, Anthony PP, Scheuer PJ, et al., editors. Pathology of the Liver. 3rd ed. Edinburgh: Churchill Livingstone; 1994. p. 635–712 [Ch. 16].

171 Nzeako UC, Goodman ZD, Ishak KG. Hepatocellular carcinoma in cirrhotic and noncirrhotic livers. A clinico-histopathologic study of 804 North American patients. Am J Clin Pathol 1996;105:65–75.

172 Bralet M-P, Régimbeau J-M, Pineau P, et al. Hepatocellular carcinoma occurring in nonfibrotic liver: epidemiologic and histopathologic analysis of 80 French cases. Hepatology 2000;32:200–4.

173 Shikata T, Yamazaki S, Uzawa T. Hepatocellular carcinoma and chronic persistent hepatitis. Acta Pathol Japon 1977;27:297–304.

174 Tabarin A, Bioulac-Sage P, Boussarie L, et al. Hepatocellular carcinoma developed on noncirrhotic livers. Arch Pathol Lab Med 1987;111:174–80.

175 El-Refaie A, Savage K, Bhattacharya S, et al. HCV-associated hepatocellular carcinoma without cirrhosis. J Hepatol 1996;24:277–85.

176 Guzman G, Brunt EM, Petrovic LM, et al. Does nonalcoholic fatty liver disease predispose patients to hepatocellular carcinoma in the absence of cirrhosis? Arch Pathol Lab Med 2008;132:1761–6.

177 Le Bail B, Carles J, Saric J, et al. Ectopic liver and hepatocarcinogenesis. Hepatology 1999;30:585–6.

178 Miyagawa S, Kawasaki S, Makuuchi M. Comparison of the characteristics of hepatocellular carcinoma between hepatitis B and C viral infection: tumor multicentricity in cirrhotic liver with hepatitis C. Hepatology 1996;24:307–10.

179 Kondo Y, Wada K. Intrahepatic metastasis of hepatocellular carcinoma: a histopathologic study. Hum Pathol 1991;22:125–30.

180 van Halteren HK, Salemans JMJI, Peters H, et al. Spontaneous regression of hepatocellular carcinoma. J Hepatol 1997;27:211–15.

181 Kaczynski J, Hansson G, Remotti H, et al. Spontaneous regression of hepatocellular carcinoma. Histopathology 1998;32:147–50.

182 Libbrecht L, Bielen D, Verslype C, et al. Focal lesions in cirrhotic explant livers: pathological evaluation and accuracy of pretransplantation imaging examinations. Liver Transplant 2002;8:749–61.

183 Lauwers GY, Terris B, Balis UJ, et al. Prognostic histologic indicators of curatively resected hepatocellular carcinomas. Am J Surg Pathol 2002;26:25–34.

184 Cillo U, Bassanello M, Vitale A, et al. The critical issue of hepatocellular carcinoma prognostic classification: which is the best tool available? J Hepatol 2004;40:124–31.

185 Lopez-Beltran A, Luque RJ, Quintero A, et al. Hepatoid adenocarcinoma of the urinary bladder. Virchows Arch 2003;442:381–7.

186 Liu X, Cheng Y, Sheng W, et al. Analysis of clinicopathologic features and prognostic factors in hepatoid adenocarcinoma of the stomach. Am J Surg Pathol 2010;34:1465–71.

187 Dhillon AP, Colombari R, Savage K, et al. An immunohistochemical study of the blood vessels within primary hepatocellular tumours. Liver 1992;12:311–18.

188 Krings G, Ramachandran R, Jain D, et al. Immunohistochemical pitfalls and the importance of glypican 3 and arginase in the diagnosis of scirrhous hepatocellular carcinoma. Mod Pathol 2013;26:782–91.

189 Omata M, Peters RL, Tatter D. Sclerosing hepatic carcinoma: relationship to hypercalcemia. Liver 1981;1:33–49.

190 Salomao MA, Yu WM, Brown RS, et al. Steatohepatitic hepatocellular carcinoma (SH-HCC): a distinctive histological variant of HCC in hepatitis C virus-related cirrhosis with associated NAFLD/NASH. Am J Surg Pathol 2010;34:1630–6.

191 Emile J-F, Adam R, Sebagh M, et al. Hepatocellular carcinoma with lymphoid stroma: a tumor with good prognosis after liver transplantation. Histopathology 2000;37:523–9.

192 Nemolato S, Fanni D, Naccarato AG, et al. Lymphoepithelioma-like hepatocellular carcinoma: a case report and a review of the literature. World J Gastroenterol 2008;14:4694–6.

193 Si MW, Thorson JA, Lauwers GY, et al. Hepatocellular lymphoepithelioma-like carcinoma associated with Epstein Barr virus. Diagn Mol Pathol 2004;13:183–9.

194 Park HS, Jang KY, Kim YK, et al. Hepatocellular carcinoma with massive lymphoid infiltration: a regressing phenomenon? Pathol Res Prac 2009;205:648–52.

195 Wood LD, Heaphy CM, Daniel HD-J, et al. Chromophobe hepatocellular carcinoma with abrupt anaplasia: a proposal for a new subtype of hepatocellular carcinoma with unique morphological and molecular features. Mod Pathol 2013;26:1586–93.

196 Yeh MM. Pathology of combined hepatocellular-cholangiocarcinoma. J Gastroenterol Hepatol 2010;25:1485–92.

197 Theise ND, Yao JL, Harada K, et al. Hepatic 'stem cell' malignancies in adults: four cases. Histopathology 2003;43:263–71.

198 Nzeako UC, Goodman ZD, Ishak KG. Comparison of tumor pathology with duration of survival of North American patients with hepatocellular carcinoma. Cancer 1995;76:579–88.

199 Kakizoe S, Kojiro M, Nakashima T. Hepatocellular carcinoma with sarcomatous change. Cancer 1987;59:310–16.

200 Haratake J, Horie A. An immunohistochemical study of sarcomatoid liver carcinomas. Cancer 1991;68:93–7.

201 Buchanan TF Jr, Huvos AG. Clear-cell carcinoma of the liver. A clinicopathologic study of 13 patients. Am J Clin Pathol 1974;61:529–39.

202 Wu PC, Lai CL, Lam KC, et al. Clear cell carcinoma of liver. An ultrastructural study. Cancer 1983;52:504–7.

203 Ajdukiewicz A, Crowden A, Hudson E, et al. Liver aspiration in the diagnosis of hepatocellular carcinoma in the Gambia. J Clin Pathol 1985;38:185–92.

204 Noguchi S, Yamamoto R, Tatsuta M, et al. Cell features and patterns in fine-needle aspirates of hepatocellular carcinoma. Cancer 1986;58:321–8.

205 Pedio G, Landolt U, Zöbeli L, et al. Fine needle aspiration of the liver. Significance of hepatocytic naked nuclei in the diagnosis of hepatocellular carcinoma. Acta Cytol 1988;32:437–42.

206 Bottles K, Cohen MB, Holly EA, et al. A step-wise logistic regression analysis of hepatocellular carcinoma. An aspiration biopsy study. Cancer 1988;62:558–63.

207 Ishak KG, Goodman ZD, Stocker JT. Tumors of the Liver and Intrahepatic Bile Ducts. Washington, DC: Armed Forces Institute of Pathology; 2001. p. 199–230.

208 Nakanuma Y, Ohta G. Expression of Mallory bodies in hepatocellular carcinoma in man and its significance. Cancer 1986;57:81–6.

209 Hurlimann J, Gardiol D. Immunohistochemistry in the differential diagnosis of liver carcinomas. Am J Surg Pathol 1991;15:280–8.

210 Van Eyken P, Sciot R, Paterson A, et al. Cytokeratin expression in hepatocellular carcinoma: an immunohistochemical study. Hum Pathol 1988;19:562–8.

211 Lai Y-S, Thung SN, Gerber MA, et al. Expression of cytokeratins in normal and diseased livers and in primary liver carcinomas. Arch Pathol Lab Med 1989;113:134–8.

212 Thung SN, Gerber MA, Sarno E, et al. Distribution of five antigens in hepatocellular carcinoma. Lab Invest 1979;41:101–5.

213 Ordonez NG, Manning JT Jr. Comparison of alpha-1-antitrypsin and alpha-1-antichymotrypsin in hepatocellular carcinoma: an immunoperoxidase study. Am J Gastroenterol 1984;79:959–63.

214 Chu PG, Weiss LM. Keratin expression in human tissues and neoplasms. Histopathology 2002;40:403–39.

215 Fan Z, van de Rijn M, Montgomery K, et al. Hep Par 1 antibody stain for the differential diagnosis of hepatocellular carcinoma: 676 tumors tested using tissue microarrays and conventional tissue sections. Mod Pathol 2003;16:137–44.

216 Morrison C, Marsh W, Frankel WL. A comparison of CD10 to pCEA, MOC-31, and hepatocyte for the distinction of malignant tumors in the liver. Mod Pathol 2002;15:1279–87.

217 Lau SK, Prakash S, Geller SA, et al. Comparative immunohistochemical profile of hepatocellular carcinoma, cholangiocarcinoma, and metastatic adenocarcinoma. Hum Pathol 2002;33:1175–81.

218 Yan BC, Gong C, Song J, et al. Arginase-1. A new immunohistochemical marker of hepatocytes and hepatocellular neoplasms. Am J Surg Pathol 2010;34:1147–54.

219 Lei J-Y, Bourne PA, diSant'Agnese PA, et al. Cytoplasmic staining of TTF-1 in the differential diagnosis of hepatocellular carcinoma vs. cholangiocarcinoma and metastatic carcinoma of the liver. Am J Clin Pathol 2006;125:519–25.

220 Di Tommaso L, Destro A, Seok JY, et al. The application of markers (HSP70 GPC3 and GS) in liver biopsies is useful for detection of hepatocellular carcinoma. J Hepatol 2009;50:746–54.

221 Ligato S, Mandich D, Cartun RW. Utility of glypican-3 in differentiating hepatocellular carcinoma from other primary and metastatic lesions in FNA of the liver: an immunocytochemical study. Mod Pathol 2008;21:626–31.

222 Shafizadeh N, Ferrell LD, Kakar S. Utility and limitations of glypican-3 expression for the diagnosis of hepatocellular carcinoma at both ends of the differentiation spectrum. Mod Pathol 2008;21:1011–18.

223 Abdul-AL HM, Makhlouf HR, Wang G, et al. Glypican-3 expression in benign liver tissue with active hepatitis C: implications for the diagnosis of hepatocellular carcinoma. Hum Pathol 2008;39:209–12.

224 Zynger DL, Everton MJ, Dimov ND, et al. Expression of glypican 3 in ovarian and extragonadal germ cell tumors. Am J Clin Pathol 2008;130:224–30.

225 Maeda D, Ota S, Takazawa Y, et al. Glypican-3 expression in clear cell adenocarcinoma of the ovary. Mod Pathol 2009;22:824–32.

226 Aviel-Ronen S, Lau SK, Pintilie M, et al. Glypican-3 is overexpressed in lung squamous cell carcinoma, but not in adenocarcinoma. Mod Pathol 2008;21:817–25.

227 Mounajjed T, Zhang L, Wu T-T. Glypican-3 expression in gastrointestinal and pancreatic epithelial neoplasms. Hum Pathol 2013;44:542–50.

228 Roskams T, Katoonizadeh A, Komuta M. Hepatic progenitor cells: an update. Clin Liver Dis 2010;14:705–18.

229 Kim H, Yoo JE, Cho JY, et al. Telomere length, TERT and shelterin complex proteins in hepatocellular carcinomas expressing 'stemness'-related markers. J Hepatol 2013;59:746–52.

230 Gouw ASH, Clouston AD, Theise ND. Ductular reactions in human liver: diversity at the interface. Hepatology 2011;54:1853–63.

231 Govaere O, Komuta M, Berkers J, et al. Keratin 19: a key role player in the invasion of human hepatocellular carcinomas. Gut 2014;63:674–85.

232 Nagorney DM, Adson MA, Weiland LH, et al. Fibrolamellar hepatoma. Am J Surg 1985;149:113–19.

233 Kakar S, Burgart LJ, Batts KP, et al. Clinicopathologic features and survival in fibrolamellar carcinoma: comparison with conventional hepatocellular carcinoma with and without cirrhosis. Mod Pathol 2005;18:1417–23.

234 Berman MM, Libbey NP, Foster JH. Hepatocellular carcinoma. Polygonal cell type with fibrous stroma – an atypical variant with a favorable prognosis. Cancer 1980;46:1448–55.

235 Craig JR, Peters RL, Edmondson HA, et al. Fibrolamellar carcinoma of the liver: a tumor of adolescents and young adults with distinctive clinico-pathologic features. Cancer 1980;46:372–9.

236 Berman MA, Burnham JA, Sheahan DG. Fibrolamellar carcinoma of the liver: an immunohistochemical study of nineteen cases and a review of the literature. Hum Pathol 1988;19:784–94.

237 El-Serag HB, Davila JA. Is fibrolamellar carcinoma different from hepatocellular carcinoma? A US population-based study. Hepatology 2004;39:798–803.

238 Ward SC, Waxman S. Fibrolamellar carcinoma: a review with focus on genetics and comparison to other malignant primary lilver tumors. Semin Liver Dis 2011;31:61–70.

239 Buckley AF, Burgart LJ, Kakar S. Epidermal growth factor receptor expression and gene copy number iin fibrolamellar hepatocellular carcinoma. Hum Pathol 2006;37:410–14.

240 Vecchio FM, Fabiano A, Ghirlanda G, et al. Fibrolamellar carcinoma of the liver: the malignant counterpart of focal nodular hyperplasia with oncocytic change. Am J Clin Pathol 1984;81:521–6.

241 Vecchio FM. Fibrolamellar carcinoma of the liver: a distinct entity within the hepatocellular tumors. A review. Appl Pathol 1988;6:139–48.

242 Orsatti G, Hytiroglou P, Thung SN, et al. Lamellar fibrosis in the fibrolamellar variant of hepatocellular carcinoma: a role for transforming growth factor beta. Liver 1997;17:152–6.

243 Farhi DC, Shikes RH, Silverberg SG. Ultrastructure of fibrolamellar oncocytic hepatoma. Cancer 1982;50:702–9.

244 Lefkowitch JH, Muschel R, Price JB, et al. Copper and copper-binding protein in fibrolamellar liver cell carcinoma. Cancer 1983;51:97–100.

245 Vecchio FM, Federico F, Dina MA. Copper and hepatocellular carcinoma. Digestion 1986;35:109–14.

246 Teitelbaum DH, Tuttle S, Carey LC, et al. Fibrolamellar carcinoma of the liver. Review of three cases and the presentation of a characteristic set of tumor markers defining this tumor. Ann Surg 1985;202:36–41.

247 Payne CM, Nagle RB, Paplanus SH, et al. Fibrolamellar carcinoma of liver: a primary malignant oncocytic carcinoid? Ultrastruct Pathol 1986;10:539–52.

248 Subramony C, Herrera GA, Lockard V. Neuroendocrine differentiation in hepatic neoplasms: report of four cases. Surg Pathol 1993;5:17–33.

249 Torbenson M. Review of the clinicopathologic features of fibrolamellar carcinoma. Adv Anat Pathol 2007;14:217–23.

250 Okano A, Hajiro K, Takakuwa H, et al. Fibrolamellar carcinoma of the liver with a mixture of ordinary hepatocellular carcinoma: a case report. Am J Gastroenterol 1998;93:1144–5.

251 Ross HM, Daniel HDJ, Vivekanandan P, et al. Fibrolamellar carcinomas are positive for CD68. Mod Pathol 2011;24:390–5.

252 LeBrun DP, Silver MM, Freedman MH, et al. Fibrolamellar carcinoma of the liver in a patient with Fanconi anemia. Hum Pathol 1991;22:396–8.

253 Klatskin G. Adenocarcinoma of the hepatic duct at its bifurcation within the porta hepatis. An unusual tumor with distinctive clinical and pathological features. Am J Med 1965;38:241–56.

254 American Joint Committee on Cancer. AJCC Cancer Staging Handbook. 7th ed. New York: Springer; 2010: p. 237–76.

255 Bosman FT, Carneiro F, Hruban RH, et al., editors. WHO Classification of Tumours of the Digestive System. 4th ed. Geneva: WHO Press; 2010.

256 Khan SA, Taylor-Robinson SD, Toledano MB, et al. Changing international trends in mortality rates for liver, biliary and pancreatic tumours. J Hepatol 2002;37:806–13.

257 Bridgewater J, Galle PR, Khan SA, et al. Guidelines for the diagnosis and management of intrahepatic cholangiocarcinoma. J Hepatol 2014;60:1268–89.

258 Case records of the Massachusetts General Hospital. Case 29-1987. N Engl J Med 1987;317:153–60.

259 Bloustein PA. Association of carcinoma with congenital cystic conditions of the liver and bile ducts. Am J Gastroenterol 1977;67:40–6.

260 Tyson GL, El-Serag HB. Risk factors for cholangiocarcinoma. Hepatology 2011;54:173–84.

261 Burns CD, Kuhns JG, Wieman J. Cholangiocarcinoma in association with multiple biliary microhamartomas. Arch Pathol Lab Med 1990;114:1287–9.

262 Yamato T, Sasaki M, Hoso M, et al. Intrahepatic cholangiocarcinoma arising in congenital hepatic fibrosis: report of an autopsy case. J Hepatol 1998;28:717–22.

263 Hasebe T, Sakamoto M, Mukai K, et al. Cholangiocarcinoma arising in bile duct adenoma with focal area of bile duct hamartoma. Virchows Arch 1995;426:209–13.

264 Yu T-H, Yuan R-H, Chen Y-L, et al. Viral hepatitis is associated with intrahepatic cholangiocarcinoma with cholangiolar differentiation and N-cadherin expression. Mod Pathol 2011;24:810–19.

265 Zhu QD, Zhou MT, Zhou QQ, et al. Diagnosis and surgical treatment of intrahepatic hepatolithiasis combined with cholangiocarcinoma. World J Surg 2014;38:2097–104.

266 Guglielmi A, Ruzzenente A, Valdegamberi A, et al. Hepatolithiasis-associated cholangiocarcinoma: results from a multi-institutional national database on a case series of 23 patients. Eur J Surg Oncol 2014;40:567–75.

267 Rizvi S, Gores GJ. Pathogenesis, diagnosis, and management of cholangiocarcinoma. Gastroenterology 2013;145:1215–29.

268 Sia D, Hoshida Y, Villanueva A, et al. Integrative molecular analysis of intrahepatic cholangiocarcinoma reveals 2 classes that have different outcomes. Gastroenterology 2013;144:829–40.

269 Andersen JB, Thorgeirsson SS. Genomic decoding of intrahepatic cholangiocarcinoma reveals therapeutic opportunities. Gastroenterology 2013;144:687–90.

270 Robertson S, Hyder O, Dodson R, et al. The frequency of KRAS and BRAF mutations in intrahepatic cholangiocarcinomas and their correlation with clinical outcome. Hum Pathol 2013;44:2768–73.

271 Voss JS, Holtegaard LM, Kerr SE, et al. Molecular profiling of cholangiocarcinoma shows potential for targeted therapy treatment decisions. Hum Pathol 2013;44:1216–22.

272 Kipp BR, Voss JS, Kerr SE. Isocitrate dehydrogenase 1 and 2 mutations in cholangiocarcinoma. Hum Pathol 2012;43:1552–8.

273 Komuta M, Spee B, Borght SV, et al. Clinicopathological study on cholangiolocellular carcinoma suggesting hepatic progenitor cell origin. Hepatology 2008;47:1544–56.

274 Komuta M, Govaere O, Vandecaveye V, et al. Histological diversity in cholangiocellular carcinoma reflects the different cholangiocyte phenotypes. Hepatology 2012;55:1876–88.

275 Chow LTC, Ahuja AT, Kwong KH, et al. Mucinous cholangiocarcinoma: an unusual complication of hepatolithiasis and recurrent pyogenic cholangitis. Histopathology 1997;30:491–4.

276 Tihan T, Blumgart L, Klimstra DS. Clear cell papillary carcinoma of the liver: an unusual variant of peripheral cholangiocarcinoma. Hum Pathol 1998;29:196–200.

277 Nakajima T, Knodo Y, Miyazaki M, et al. A histopathologic study of 102 cases of intrahepatic cholangiocarcinoma: histologic classification and modes of spreading. Hum Pathol 1988;19:1228–34.

278 Weinbren K, Mutum SS. Pathological aspects of cholangiocarcinoma. J Pathol 1983;139:217–38.

279 Bonetti F, Chilosi M, Pisa R, et al. Epithelial membrane antigen expression in cholangiocarcinoma. A useful immunohistochemical tool for differential diagnosis with hepatocarcinoma. Virchows Arch A Pathol Anat Histopathol 1983;401:307–13.

280 Pastolero GC, Wakabayashi T, Oka T, et al. Tissue polypeptide antigen – a marker antigen differentiating cholangiolar tumors from other hepatic tumors. Am J Clin Pathol 1987;87:168–73.

281 Jovanovic R, Jagirdar J, Thung SN, et al. Blood-group-related antigen Lewis-X and Lewis-Y in the differential diagnosis of cholangiocarcinoma and hepatocellular carcinoma. Arch Pathol Lab Med 1989;113:139–42.

282 Terada T, Nakanuma Y. An immunohistochemical survey of amylase isoenzymes in cholangiocarcinoma and hepatocellular carcinoma. Arch Pathol Lab Med 1993;117:160–2.

283 Maeda T, Adachi E, Kajiyama K, et al. Combined hepatocellular and cholangiocarcinoma: proposed criteria according to cytokeratin expression and analysis of clinicopathologic features. Hum Pathol 1995;26:956–64.

284 Haratake J, Hashimoto H. An immunohistochemical analysis of 13 cases with combined hepatocellular and cholangiocellular carcinoma. Liver 1995;15:9–15.

285 Papotti M, Sambataro D, Marchesa P, et al. A combined hepatocellular/cholangiocellular carcinoma with sarcomatoid features. Liver 1997;17:47–52.

286 Goodman ZD, Ishak KG, Langloss JM, et al. Combined hepatocellular-cholangiocarcinoma. A histologic and immunohistochemical study. Cancer 1985;55:124–35.

287 Azizah N, Paradinas FJ. Cholangiocarcinoma coexisting with developmental liver cysts: a distinct entity different from liver cystadenocarcinoma. Histopathology 1980;4:391–400.

288 Theise ND, Miller F, Worman HJ, et al. Biliary cystadenocarcinoma arising in a liver with fibropolycystic disease. Arch Pathol Lab Med 1993;117:163–5.

289 Lander JJ, Stanley RJ, Sumner HW, et al. Angiosarcoma of the liver associated with Fowler's solution (potassium arsenite). Gastroenterology 1975;68:1582–6.

290 Horta JS. Late effects of thorotrast on the liver and spleen, and their efferent lymph nodes. Ann N Y Acad Sci 1967;145:676–99.

291 Visfeldt J, Poulsen H. On the histopathology of liver and liver tumours in thorium- dioxide patients. Acta Pathol Microbiol Scand [A] 1972;80:97–108.

292 Winberg CD, Ranchod M. Thorotrast induced hepatic cholangiocarcinoma and angiosarcoma. Hum Pathol 1979;10:108–12.

293 Thomas LB, Popper H, Berk PD, et al. Vinyl-chloride-induced liver disease. From idiopathic portal hypertension (Banti's syndrome) to angiosarcomas. N Engl J Med 1975;292:17–22.

294 Pimentel JC, Menezes AP. Liver disease in vineyard sprayers. Gastroenterology 1977;72:275–83.

295 Hoch-Ligeti C. Angiosarcoma of the liver associated with diethylstilbestrol. JAMA 1978;240:1510–11.

296 Falk H, Thomas LB, Popper H, et al. Hepatic angiosarcoma associated with androgenic–anabolic steroids. Lancet 1979;2:1120–3.

297 Monroe PS, Riddell RH, Siegler M, et al. Hepatic angiosarcoma. Possible relationship to long-term oral contraceptive ingestion. JAMA 1981;246:64–5.

298 Daneshmend TK, Scott GL, Bradfield JW. Angiosarcoma of liver associated with phenelzine. BMJ 1979;1:1679.

299 Cadranel JF, Legendre C, Desaint B, et al. Liver disease from surreptitious administration of urethane. J Clin Gastroenterol 1993;17:52–6.

300 Fortwengler HP Jr, Jones D, Espinosa E, et al. Evidence for endothelial cell origin of vinyl chloride-induced hepatic angiosarcoma. Gastroenterology 1981;80:1415–19.

301 Manning JT Jr, Ordonez NG, Barton JH. Endothelial cell origin of thorium oxide-induced angiosarcoma of liver. Arch Pathol Lab Med 1983;107:456–8.

302 Popper H, Thomas LB, Telles NC, et al. Development of hepatic angiosarcoma in man induced by vinyl chloride, thorotrast, and arsenic. Comparison with cases of unknown etiology. Am J Pathol 1978;92:349–69.

303 Tamburro CH, Makk L, Popper H. Early hepatic histologic alterations among chemical (vinyl monomer) workers. Hepatology 1984;4:413–18.

304 Ishak KG, Sesterhenn IA, Goodman ZD, et al. Epithelioid hemangioendothelioma of the liver: a clinicopathologic and follow-up study of 32 cases. Hum Pathol 1984;15:839–52.

305 Ishak KG. Malignant mesenchymal tumors of the liver. In: Okuda K, Ishak KG, editors. Neoplasms of the Liver. Tokyo: Springer-Verlag; 1987. p. 159–76.

306 Makhlouf HR, Ishak KG, Goodman ZD. Epithelioid hemangioendothelioma of the liver. A clinicopathologic study of 137 cases. Cancer 1999;85:562–82.

307 Ekfors TO, Joensuu K, Toivio I, et al. Fatal epithelioid haemangioendothelioma presenting in the lung and liver. Virchows Arch [A] 1986;410:9–16.

308 Dean PJ, Haggitt RC, O'Hara CJ. Malignant epithelioid hemangioendothelioma of the liver in young women. Relationship to oral contraceptive use. Am J Surg Pathol 1985;9:695–704.

309 Demetris AJ, Minervini M, Raikow RB, et al. Hepatic epithelioid hemangioendothelioma. Biological questions based on pattern of recurrence in an allograft and tumor immunophenotype. Am J Surg Pathol 1997;21:263–70.

310 Scoazec J-Y, Degott C, Reynes M, et al. Epithelioid hemangioendothelioma of the liver: an ultrastructural study. Hum Pathol 1989;20:673–81.

311 Utz DC, Warren MM, Gregg JA, et al. Reversible hepatic dysfunction associated with hypernephroma. Mayo Clin Proc 1970;45:161–9.

312 Strickland RC, Schenker S. The nephrogenic hepatic dysfunction syndrome: a review. Am J Dig Dis 1977;22:49–55.

313 Tao LC, Donat EE, Ho CS, et al. Percutaneous fine-needle aspiration biopsy of the liver. Cytodiagnosis of hepatic cancer. Acta Cytol 1979;23:287–91.

314 Axe SR, Erozan YS, Ermatinger SV. Fine-needle aspiration of the liver. A comparison of smear and rinse preparations in the detection of cancer. Am J Clin Pathol 1986;86:281–5.

315 Atterbury CE, Enriquez RE, Desuto-Nagy GI, et al. Comparison of the histologic and cytologic diagnosis of liver biopsies in hepatic cancer. Gastroenterology 1979;76:1352–7.

316 Gerber MA, Thung SN, Bodenheimer HC Jr, et al. Characteristic histologic triad in liver adjacent to metastatic neoplasm. Liver 1986;6:85–8.

317 Glees JP, Thomas M, Redding WH, et al. Liver biopsy at lymphoma laparotomy [letter]. Lancet 1978;1:210–11.

318 Kim H, Dorfman RF, Rosenberg SA. Pathology of malignant lymphomas of the liver: application in staging. In: Popper H, Schaffner F, editors. Progress in Liver Diseases, vol. V. New York: Grune & Stratton; 1976. p. 683–98 [Ch. 40].

319 Leslie KO, Colby TV. Hepatic parenchymal lymphoid aggregates in Hodgkin's disease. Hum Pathol 1984;15:808–9.

320 Abt AB, Kirschner RH, Belliveau RE, et al. Hepatic pathology associated with Hodgkin's disease. Cancer 1974;33:1564–71.

321 Bruguera M, Caballero T, Carreras E, et al. Hepatic sinusoidal dilatation in Hodgkin's disease. Liver 1987;7:76–80.

322 Perera DR, Greene ML, Fenster LF. Cholestasis associated with extrabiliary Hodgkin's disease. Report of three cases and review of four others. Gastroenterology 1974;67:680–5.

323 Hubscher SG, Lumley MA, Elias E. Vanishing bile duct syndrome: a possible mechanism for intrahepatic cholestasis in Hodgkin's lymphoma. Hepatology 1993;17:70–7.

324 Lefkowitch JH, Falkow S, Whitlock RT. Hepatic Hodgkin's disease simulating cholestatic hepatitis with liver failure. Arch Pathol Lab Med 1985;109:424–6.

325 De Wolf-Peeters C. Liver involvement in lymphomas. Ann Diagn Pathol 1998;2:363–9.

326 Trudel M, Aramendi T, Caplan S. Large-cell lymphoma presenting with hepatic sinusoidal infiltration. Arch Pathol Lab Med 1991;115:821–4.

327 Dubois A, Dauzat M, Pignodel C, et al. Portal hypertension in lymphoproliferative and myeloproliferative disorders: hemodynamic and histological correlations. Hepatology 1993;17: 246–50.

328 Saló J, Nomdedeu B, Bruguera M, et al. Acute liver failure due to non-Hodgkin's lymphoma. Am J Gastroenterol 1993;88:774–6.

329 Verdi CJ, Grogan TM, Protell R, et al. Liver biopsy immunotyping to characterize lymphoid malignancies. Hepatology 1986;6:6–13.

330 Freeman C, Berg JW, Cutler SJ. Occurrence and prognosis of extranodal lymphomas. Cancer 1972;29:252–60.

331 Zafrani ES, Gaulard P. Primary lymphoma of the liver. Liver 1993;13:57–61.

332 Stemmer S, Geffen DB, Goldstein J, et al. Primary small noncleaved cell lymphoma of the liver. J Clin Gastroenterol 1993;16:65–9.

333 Maes M, Depardieu C, Dargent J-L, et al. Primary low-grade B-cell lymphoma of MALT-type occurring in the liver: a study of two cases. J Hepatol 1997;27:922–7.

334 Isaacson PG, Banks PM, Best PV, et al. Primary low-grade hepatic B-cell lymphoma of mucosa-associated lymphoid tissue (MALT)-type. Am J Surg Pathol 1995;19:571–5.

335 Scoazec J-Y, Degott C, Brousse N, et al. Non-Hodgkin's lymphoma presenting as a primary tumor of the liver: presentation, diagnosis and outcome in eight patients. Hepatology 1991;13:870–5.

336 Mollejo M, Menárguez J, Guisado-Vasco P, et al. Hepatitis C virus-related lylmphoproliferative disorders encompass a broader clinical and morphological spectrum than previously recognized: a clinicopathological study. Mod Pathol 2014;27:281–93.

337 Kim JH, Kim HY, Kang I, et al. A case of primary hepatic lymphoma with hepatitis C liver cirrhosis. Am J Gastroenterol 2000;95:2377–80.

338 Rasul I, Shepherd FA, Kamel-Reid S, et al. Detection of occult low-grade B-cell non-Hodgkin's lymphoma in patient's with chronic hepatitis C infection and mixed cryoglobulinemia. Hepatology 1999;29:543–7.

339 Lin A, Kadam JS, Bodenheimer HC, et al. Concomitant diffuse large B-cell lymphoma and hepatocellular

carcinoma in chronic hepatitis C virus liver disease: a study of two cases. J Med Virol 2008;80:1350–3.

340 Ohshima K, Haraoka S, Harada N, et al. Hepatosplenic γδ T-cell lymphoma: relation to Epstein–Barr virus and activated cytotoxic molecules. Histopathology 2000;36:127–35.

341 Suarez F, Wlodarski I, Rigal-Huguet F, et al. Hepatosplenic αβ T-cell lymphoma. An unusual case with clinical, histologic, and cytogenetic features of γδ hepatosplenic T-cell lymphoma. Am J Surg Pathol 2000;24:1027–32.

342 Thomas FB, Clausen KP, Greenberger NJ. Liver disease in multiple myeloma. Arch Intern Med 1973;132:195–202.

343 Weichhold W, Labouyrie E, Merlio JPH, et al. Primary extramedullary plasmacytoma of the liver. A case report. Am J Surg Pathol 1995;19:1197–202.

344 Brooks AP. Portal hypertension in Waldenstrom's macroglobulinaemia. BMJ 1976;1:689–90.

345 Lévy S, Capron D, Joly J-P, et al. Hepatic nodules as single organ involvement in an adult with Langerhans cell granulomatosis. J Clin Gastroenterol 1998;26:69–73.

346 Foschini MP, Milandri GL, Dina RE, et al. Benign regressing histiocytosis of the liver. Histopathology 1995;26:363–6.

347 Kaplan KJ, Goodman ZD, Ishak KG. Liver involvement in Langerhans' cell histiocytosis: a study of nine cases. Mod Pathol 1999;12:370–8.

348 Yam LT, Chan CH, Li CY. Hepatic involvement in systemic mast cell disease. Am J Med 1986;80:819–26.

349 Scheimberg IB, Pollock DJ, Collins PW, et al. Pathology of the liver in leukaemia and lymphoma. A study of 110 autopsies. Histopathology 1995;26:311–21.

350 Schwartz JB, Shamsuddin AM. The effects of leukemic infiltrates in various organs in chronic lymphocytic leukemia. Hum Pathol 1981;12:432–40.

351 Roquet ML, Zafrani ES, Farcet JP, et al. Histopathological lesions of the liver in hairy cell leukemia: a report of 14 cases. Hepatology 1985;5:496–500.

352 Yam LT, Janckila AJ, Chan CH, et al. Hepatic involvement in hairy cell leukemia. Cancer 1983;51:1497–504.

353 Zafrani ES, Degos F, Guigui B, et al. The hepatic sinusoid in hairy cell leukemia: an ultrastructural study of 12 cases. Hum Pathol 1987;18:801–7.

354 Grouls V, Stiens R. Hepatic involvement in hairy cell leukemia: diagnosis by tartrate-resistant acid phosphatase enzyme histochemistry on formalin fixed and paraffin-embedded liver biopsy specimens. Pathol Res Pract 1984;178:332–4.

355 Wheeler DA, Edmondson HA, Reynolds TB. Spontaneous liver cell adenoma in children. Am J Clin Pathol 1986;85:6–12.

356 Resnick MB, Kozakewich HPW, Perez-Atayde AR. Hepatic adenoma in the pediatric age group. Clinicopathological observations and assessment of cell proliferative activity. Am J Surg Pathol 1995;19:1181–90.

357 Lautz TB, Finegold MJ, Chin AC, et al. Giant hepatic adenoma with atypical features in a patient on oxcarbazepine therapy. J Pediatr Surg 2008;42:751–4.

358 Janes CH, McGill DB, Ludwig J, et al. Liver cell adenoma at the age of 3 years and transplantation 19 years later after development of carcinoma: a case report. Hepatology 1993;17:583–5.

359 Moran CA, Mullick FG, Ishak KG. Nodular regenerative hyperplasia of the liver in children. Am J Surg Pathol 1991;15:449–54.

360 Srouji MN, Chatten J, Schulman WM, et al. Mesenchymal hamartoma of the liver in infants. Cancer 1978;42:2483–9.

361 Stocker JT, Ishak KG. Mesenchymal hamartoma of the liver: report of 30 cases and review of the literature. Pediatr Pathol 1983;1:245–67.

362 Cook JR, Pfeifer JD, Dehner LP. Mesenchymal hamartoma of the liver in the adult: association with distinct clinical features and histological changes. Hum Pathol 2002;33:893–8.

363 Lauwers GY, Grant LD, Donnelly WH, et al. Hepatic undifferentiated (embryonal) sarcoma arising in a mesenchymal hamartoma. Am J Surg Pathol 1997;21:1248–54.

364 Dehner LP, Ishak KG. Vascular tumors of the liver in infants and children. A study of 30 cases and review of the literature. Arch Pathol 1971;92:101–11.

365 Selby DM, Stocker JT, Waclawiw MA, et al. Infantile hemangioendothelioma of the liver. Hepatology 1994;20:39–45.

366 Dimashkieh HH, Mo JQ, Wyatt-Ashmead J, et al. Pediatric hepatic angiosarcoma: case report and review of the literature. Pediatr Dev Pathol 2004;7:527–32.

367 Dachman AH, Lichtenstein JE, Friedman AC, et al. Infantile hemangioendothelioma of the liver: a radiologic–pathologic–clinical correlation. AJR Am J Roentgenol 1983;140:1091–6.

368 Darbari A, Sabin KM, Shapiro CN, et al. Epidemiology of primary hepatic malignancies in US children. Hepatology 2003;38:560–6.

369 Stocker JT, Ishak KG. Hepatoblastoma. In: Okuda K, Ishak KG, editors. Neoplasms of the Liver. Tokyo: Springer-Verlag; 1987. p. 127–36 [Ch. 9].

370 Ishak KG, Glunz PR. Hepatoblastoma and hepatocarcinoma in infancy and childhood. Report of 47 cases. Cancer 1967;20:396–422.

371 Lack EE, Neave C, Vawter GF. Hepatoblastoma. A clinical and pathologic study of 54 cases. Am J Surg Pathol 1982;6:693–705.

372 Kasai M, Watanabe I. Histologic classification of liver cell carcinoma in infancy and childhood and its clinical evaluation. Cancer 1970;25:551–63.

373 López-Terrada D, Alaggio R, de Dávila MT, et al. Towards an international pediatric liver tumor consensus classification: proceedings of the Los Angeles COG liver tumors symposium. Mod Pathol 2014;27:472–91.

374 Weinberg AG, Finegold MJ. Primary hepatic tumors of childhood. Hum Pathol 1983;14:512–37.

375 Rugge M, Sonego F, Pollice L, et al. Hepatoblastoma: DNA nuclear content, proliferative indices, and pathology. Liver 1998;18:128–33.

376 Gonzalez-Crussi F, Upton MP, Maurer HS. Hepatoblastoma. Attempt at characterization of histologic subtypes. Am J Surg Pathol 1982;6:599–612.

377 Stocker JT, Ishak KG. Undifferentiated (embryonal) sarcoma of the liver: report of 31 cases. Cancer 1978;42:336–48.

378 Keating S, Taylor GP. Undifferentiated (embryonal) sarcoma of the liver: ultrastructural and immunohistochemical similarities with malignant fibrous histiocytoma. Hum Pathol 1985;16:693–9.

379 Aoyama C, Hachitanda Y, Sato JK, et al. Undifferentiated (embryonal) sarcoma of the liver. A tumor of uncertain histogenesis showing divergent differentiation. Am J Surg Pathol 1991;15:615–24.

380 Lack EE, Schloo BL, Azumi N, et al. Undifferentiated (embryonal) sarcoma of the liver. Clinical and pathologic study of 16 cases with emphasis on immunohistochemical features. Am J Surg Pathol 1991;15:1–16.

381 Heerema-McKenney A, Leuschner I, Smith N, et al. Nested stromal epithelial tumor of the liver. Six cases of a distinctive pediatric neoplasm with frequent calcifications and association with Cushing syndrome. Am J Surg Pathol 2005;29:10–20.

382 Hill DA, Swanson PE, Anderson K, et al. Desmoplastic nested spindle cell tumor of liver. Report of four cases of a proposed new entity. Am J Surg Pathol 2005;29:1–9.

383 Makhlouf HR, Abdul-AL HM, Wang G, et al. Calcifying nested stromal–epithelial tumors of the liver. A clinicopathologic, immunohistochemical, and molecular genetic study of 9 cases with a long-term follow-up. Am J Surg Pathol 2009;33:976–83.

384 Wang Y, Zhou J, Huang W-B, et al. Calcifying nested stroma-epithelial tumor of the liver: a case report and review of literature. Int J Surg Pathol 2011;19:268–72.

385 Malowany JI, Merritt NH, Chan NG, et al. Nested stromal epithelial tumor of the liver in Beckwith–Wiedemann syndrome. Ped Dev Pathol 2013;16:312–17.

386 Assmann G, Kappler R, Zeindl-Eberhart E, et al. β-catenin mutations in 2 nested stromal epithelial tumors of the liver – a neoplasia with defective mesenchymal-epithelial transition. Hum Pathol 2012;43:1815–27.

387 Mills AE. Undifferentiated primary hepatic non-Hodgkin's lymphoma in childhood. Am J Surg Pathol 1988;12:721–6.

388 Zen Y, Vara R, Portmann B, et al. Childhood hepatocellular carcinoma: a clinicopathological study of 12 cases with special reference to EpCAM. Histopathology 2014;64:671–82.

389 Caturelli E, Solmi L, Anti M, et al. Ultrasound guided fine needle biopsy of early hepatocellular carcinoma complicating liver: a multicentre study. Gut 2004;53:1356–62.

390 Bottles K, Cohen MB. An approach to fine-needle aspiration biopsy diagnosis of hepatic masses. Diagn Cytopathol 1991;7:204–10.

391 Frias-Hidvegi D. Guides to Clinical Aspiration Biopsy. Liver and Pancreas. New York & Tokyo: Igaku-Shoin; 1988. p. 27–42.

392 Suen KC. Diagnosis of primary hepatic neoplasms by fine needle aspiration cytology. Diagn Cytopathol 1986;2:99–109.

393 Perry MD, Johnson WW. Needle biopsy of the liver for the diagnosis of nonneoplastic liver disease. Acta Cytol 1985;29:385–90.

394 Tao L-C. Are oral contraceptive-associated liver cell adenomas premalignant? Acta Cytol 1992;36:338–44.

395 Ruschenberg I, Droese M. Fine needle aspiration cytology of focal nodular hyperplasia of the liver. Acta Cytol 1989;33:857–60.

396 Taavitsainen M, Airaksinin T, Kreula J, et al. Fine-needle aspiration biopsy of liver hemangioma. Acta Radiol 1990;31:69–71.

397 Yang GCH, Yang G-Y, Tao L-C. Distinguishing well-differentiated hepatocellular carcinoma from benign liver by the physical features of fine-needle aspirates. Mod Pathol 2004;17:798–802.

398 Pedio G, Landolt U, Zobeli L, et al. Fine needle aspiration of the liver. Significance of hepatocytic naked nuclei in the diagnosis of hepatocellular carcinoma. Acta Cytol 1988;32:437–42.

399 Cohen MB, Haber MM, Holly EA, et al. Cytologic criteria to distinguish hepatocellular carcinoma from non-neoplastic liver. Am J Clin Pathol 1991;95:125–30.

400 Wee A, Nilsson B, Chan-Wilde C, et al. Fine needle aspiration biopsy of hepatocellular carcinoma: some unusual features. Acta Cytol 1991;35:661–70.

401 Donat EE, Anderson V, Tao L-C. Cytodiagnosis of clear cell hepatocellular carcinoma. A case report. Acta Cytol 1991;35:671–5.

402 Nguyen G-K. Fine-needle aspiration biopsy cytology of hepatic tumors in adults. Pathol Annu 1986;21:321–49.

403 Davenport RD. Cytologic diagnosis of fibrolamellar carcinoma of the liver by fine-needle aspiration. Diagn Cytopathol 1990;6:275–9.

404 Wakely PEJ, Silverman JF, Geisinger KR, et al. Fine needle aspiration cytology of hepatoblastoma. Mod Pathol 1990;3:688–93.

405 Dekmezian R, Sneigi N, Papok S, et al. Fine needle aspiration cytology of pediatric patients with primary hepatic tumors. Diagn Cytopathol 1988;4:162–8.

406 Saleh HA, Tao LC. Hepatic angiosarcoma: aspiration biopsy cytology and immunocytochemical contribution. Diagn Cytopathol 1998;18:208–11.

407 Siddiqui MT, Reddy VB, Castelli MJ, et al. Role of fine-needle aspiration in clinical management of transplant patients. Diagn Cytopathol 1997;17:429–35.

408 Flanders E, Kornstein M, Wakely P, et al. Lymphoglandular bodies in fine-needle aspiration cytology smears. Am J Clin Pathol 1993;99:566–9.

General reading

Bioulac-Sage P, Cubel G, Balabaud C, et al. Revisiting the pathology of resected benign hepatocellular nodules using new immunohistochemical markers. Semin Liver Dis 2011;31:91–103.

Bosman FT, Carneiro F, Hruban RH, et al., editors. WHO Classification of Tumours of the Digestive System. 4th ed. Geneva: WHO Press; 2010.

DeMay RM. Practical Principles of Cytopathology. Chicago, IL: ASCP Press; 1999. p. 307–20.

El-Serag HB. Hepatocellular carcinoma. N Engl J Med 2011;365:1118–27.

Goodman ZD, Terracciano L, Wee A. Tumours and tumour-like lesions of the liver. In: Burt AD, Portmann BC, Ferrell LD, editors. Pathology of the Liver. 6th ed. Edinburgh: Churchill Livingstone/Elsevier; 2001. p. 761–852.

Kakar S, Gown AM, Goodman ZD, et al. Best practices in diagnostic immunohistochemistry. Hepatocellular carcinoma versus metastatic neoplasms. Arch Pathol Lab Med 2007;131:1648–54.

Knudsen ES, Gopal P, Singal AG. The changing landscape of hepatocellular carcinoma. *Etiology, genetics, and therapy.* Am J Pathol 2014;184:574–83.

López-Terrada D, Alaggio R, de Dávila MT, et al. Towards an international pediatric liver tumor consensus classification: proceedings of the Los Angeles COG liver tumors symposium. Mod Pathol 2014;27:472–91.

Okuda K, Ishak KG, editors. Neoplasms of the Liver. Tokyo: Springer-Verlag; 1987.

Pitman MB, Szyfelbein WM, editors. Fine Needle Aspiration Biopsy of the Liver. A Color Atlas. Boston: Butterworth-Heinemann; 1994.

Rizvi S, Gores GJ. Pathogenesis, diagnosis, and management of cholangiocarcinoma. Gastroenterology 2013;145L:1215–22.

Tao L-C. Liver and pancreas. In: Bibbo M, editor. Comprehensive Cytopathology. 2nd ed. Philadelphia, PA: WB Saunders; 1997. p. 827–64.

Vascular Disorders

The hepatic arteries

The effects of occlusion of hepatic artery branches are unpredictable because of the liver's double blood supply and variable collateral flow. Potential effects of thrombotic or other occlusion include infarction, and ischaemic damage to the biliary tree leading to stricture formation, cholangitis or duct rupture.[1-3] The branches of the hepatic artery are sometimes involved in **polyarteritis nodosa,**[2,4,4a] the arteritis of **systemic lupus erythematosus,**[5] **Schönlein–Henoch purpura**[3] and **giant-cell arteritis.**[6] In the last the liver may contain granulomas of classical[7] or fibrin-ring type.[8] The arterial lesions of these systemic diseases are not often seen in needle biopsies of the liver. Vasculitis affecting small intrahepatic vessels is sometimes a manifestation of infection or neoplasia.

In some older patients, especially those with systemic hypertension, small arteries and arterioles in portal tracts appear thickened and hyaline.[9] **Amyloidosis** can give rise to thickening of arterial walls in the absence of sinusoidal deposits.

The arteriovenous malformations and telangiectases of **hereditary haemorrhagic telangiectasia** are sometimes found in the liver, with or without surrounding fibrosis.[10] The presentation is as portal hypertension (accompanied by hepatic encephalopathy and nodular regeneration[11,12]), biliary disease (sometimes resembling primary sclerosing cholangitis or Caroli's disease) or cardiac failure due to arteriovenous shunting.[13] Patients with liver involvement may have raised serum alkaline phosphatase levels without jaundice ('anicteric cholestasis'), attributed to abnormal blood supply to the biliary tree.[14] Severely damaged medium-sized bile ducts are occasionally seen histologically.

Infarcts of the liver result from arteritis, aneurysms, thrombosis, embolism or surgical ligation. They may complicate pregnancy or liver transplantation. Infarction can also follow occlusion of portal-vein branches,[15] and may even be found in the absence of demonstrable vascular obstruction. The pathological features are as in other organs: there are well-defined zones of coagulative necrosis with congested and inflamed borders (**Fig. 12.1**). Portal tracts may survive within the infarcted areas. Coagulative necrosis of the centres of cirrhotic nodules following hypoperfusion is sometimes called nodular infarction.

Shock, heart failure and heatstroke

Severe hypoperfusion of the hepatic parenchyma leads to necrosis, usually in perivenular regions (acinar zone 3) but also, additionally or alternatively, in mid-zonal regions

Figure 12.1 Infarct. The dead parenchyma to the right is intensely congested. Surviving liver tissue (left) is fatty. (Postmortem liver, H&E.)

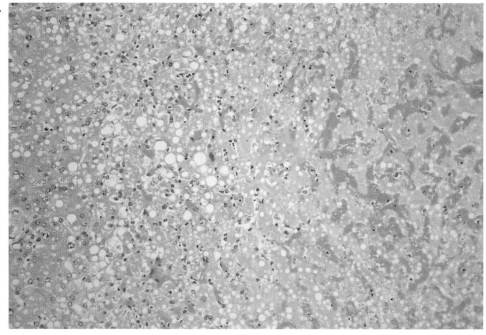

(zone 2).[16] Portal tracts and the periportal parenchyma typically remain normal. However, there are uncommon instances where interlobular bile ducts are injured due to hepatic hypoperfusion, especially in severely ill individuals with prolonged intensive care hospitalisations, and changes similar to sclerosing cholangitis may develop.[17,18] In contrast to the necrosis of acute hepatitis there is usually little or no inflammation, but in some patients neutrophils accumulate in limited numbers, particularly if the individual has received pressor support for 1 day or more.[19] Affected areas may be congested, and contain large, ceroid-laden macrophages. There may be cholestasis and evidence of regenerative hyperplasia in the surviving parenchyma. The reticulin network shows regular condensation in the necrotic areas. Similar changes are seen in patients with heatstroke (**Fig. 12.2**). There may be steatosis in the surviving parenchyma. Inflammation ranges from absent in mild cases[20] to severe when the damage is extensive.[21] Systemic candidiasis is a complication.

One of the most important causes of this type of necrosis is heart failure with consequent hypoperfusion of the liver. The term ischaemic hepatitis is commonly used for the viral hepatitis-like clinical picture which may ensue.[22] Congestive heart failure leads to sinusoidal dilatation (see Venous congestion and outflow obstruction, below).

The portal veins

Thrombosis of the main portal veins may result from infection (local or in the portal venous drainage area), cirrhosis,[23] liver transplantation, disorders of coagulation and venous outflow obstruction.[24] Invasion by hepatocellular carcinoma is a common cause. In some patients no reason for the thrombosis can be discovered, but an underlying thrombophilic condition should always be excluded.[23] In the acute phase of pylephlebitis, septic thrombi may be seen in portal-vein branches in portal tracts (**Fig. 12.3**).

Possible results of portal-vein thrombosis include diffuse or focal parenchymal atrophy, increase in the number of apoptotic hepatocytes,[25] parenchymal nodularity (see Nodular

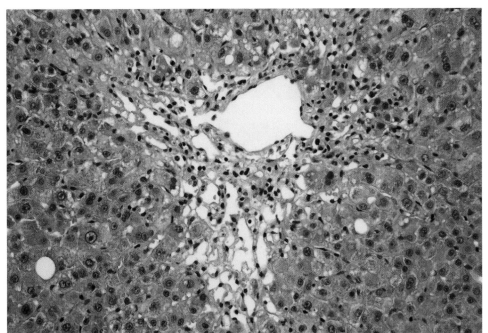

Figure 12.2
Heatstroke.
There has been confluent necrosis in acinar zone 3. (Needle biopsy, H&E.) (Section kindly provided by Professor Helmut Denk, Graz, Austria.)

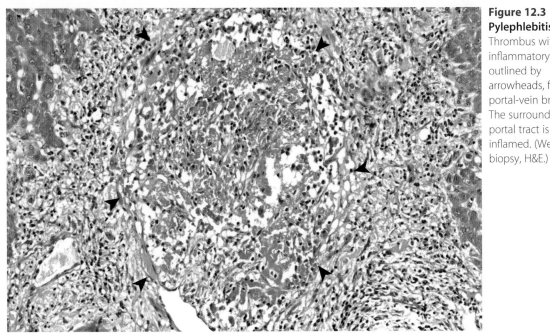

Figure 12.3
Pylephlebitis.
Thrombus with inflammatory cells, outlined by arrowheads, fills a portal-vein branch. The surrounding portal tract is also inflamed. (Wedge biopsy, H&E.)

regenerative hyperplasia, **Ch. 11**), and a mild degree of portal fibrosis. Focal atrophy, also known as Zahn's infarction, is often found at the margins of tumour nodules. Occasionally portal venous obstruction leads to true infarction of the hepatic parenchyma.[15] In many patients with thrombosis of the main portal veins the liver remains histologically normal.

Portal vein branches are absent from portal tracts in the rare **Abernethy malformation** (congenital extrahepatic portosystemic shunts). In this condition the extrahepatic portal

Figure 12.4
Portal-vein absence in Abernethy malformation.
The portal tract shows an interlobular bile duct and two cross-sectional cuts of the hepatic arteriole, but no typical large-calibre portal vein is present. The prominent spaces adjacent to the portal tract are dilated lymphatics (L), which showed endothelial positivity with D2-40 immunostain. (Explant liver, H&E.)

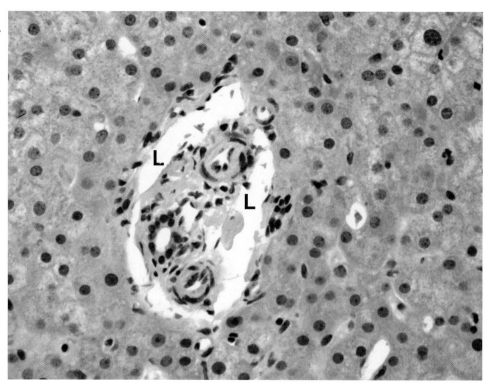

vein is either absent or severely atrophic, and portal blood is diverted to the inferior vena cava, rather than returning to the heart via the liver. Intrahepatic small portal tracts show absent veins, fibrous vein remnants, dilated lymphatics and arteriolar changes (**Fig. 12.4**).[26]

Portal hypertension

Portal hypertension is most often the result of cirrhosis. Other causes include schisto-somiasis, alcohol-related liver disease, non-alcoholic steatohepatitis, congenital hepatic fibrosis, the tropical splenomegaly syndrome, hepatic venous outflow obstruction and portal venous thrombosis. The last probably contributes to portal hypertension in poly-cythaemia and other haematological diseases.[27] In lymphoproliferative and myelopro-liferative disorders, the portal infiltration may be a further pathogenetic factor.[28] The anatomical subdivision of portal hypertension into prehepatic, intrahepatic and posthe-patic forms should be considered in conjunction with specific structural alterations in classifying the individual case.[29]

There remains a somewhat ill-defined group of patients with portal hypertension not attributable to cirrhosis or to the other causes mentioned above (**non-cirrhotic portal hypertension**[30]). These cases represent an intrahepatic type of portal hypertension[31] which is a category separate from prehepatic causes such as thrombosis of the major portal vein and from posthepatic causes such as congenital webs of the inferior vena cava. Several different labels have been used to describe aspects of this group (**hepatoportal sclerosis, non-cirrhotic portal fibrosis, idiopathic portal hypertension**). The term **obliterative portal venopathy** has also been used[32] and indicates that there may be demonstrable thrombosis or narrowing of portal-vein branches, but this is not always the case, and it is

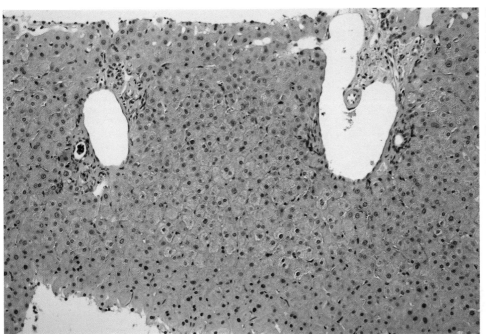

**Figure 12.5
Non-cirrhotic portal
hypertension.**
The portal-vein
branches in the two
portal tracts are
widely dilated and
appear to have
herniated into the
parenchyma. (Needle
biopsy, H&E.)
(Section kindly
provided by
Professor Helmut
Denk, Graz, Austria.)

not clear whether the portal venous narrowing or occlusion is primary or secondary. Non-cirrhotic portal hypertension is most prevalent in India and Japan, but is also described in Western countries.[31] Certain cases have been attributed to a toxin or toxins such as arsenic,[31,33] vinyl chloride,[34,35] azathioprine,[31] cytotoxic drugs[36] and didanosine therapy in HIV disease.[32] Thrombophilic/pro-coagulant states need to be excluded as possible causes. In many patients no cause is found. Variceal bleeding and portal vein thrombosis are important longterm complications.[36a]

Needle liver biopsies from patients with non-cirrhotic portal hypertension are often normal or show only non-specific changes. Abnormalities are more likely to be seen in operative wedge biopsies. Portal-vein branches are sometimes thickened and narrowed, unusually inconspicuous or replaced by multiple small, thin-walled channels. Their overall area is reduced, while portal tract lymphatics increase in number.[37] Dilated venules appear to herniate into the adjacent parenchyma[38,39] (**Fig. 12.5**). There may be portal fibrosis and enlargement, with or without inflammatory-cell infiltration (**Fig. 12.6**). Slender fibrous septa extending from the portal tracts give an appearance indistinguishable from incomplete septal cirrhosis.[40] These septa sometimes connect with bridge-like zones of necrosis.[38] There may be randomly distributed thin-walled vessels in the lobules ('megasinusoids'), and sclerosis or dilatation of efferent veins.[38]

Diffuse or localised nodular hyperplasia of the parenchyma is commonly seen in these patients. There is thus overlap between hepatoportal sclerosis, nodular regenerative hyperplasia, incomplete septal cirrhosis[40,41] and, rarely, partial nodular transformation.[42] Nodular regenerative hyperplasia, however, is also found in the absence of clinically evident portal hypertension.

In patients exposed to vinyl chloride monomer and other carcinogens there may be, in addition to the above features, perisinusoidal fibrosis and an increase in the number and size of sinusoidal cells.[34,35] Perisinusoidal fibrosis may also contribute to the portal hypertension which develops in some patients after renal transplantation.[43] Prolonged drug therapy has been suggested as a possible mechanism.

**Figure 12.6
Non-cirrhotic portal
hypertension.**
An enlarged,
sclerotic portal tract
contains arteries (a)
and bile ducts (b),
but portal-vein
branches are
inconspicuous.
(Wedge biopsy, H&E.)

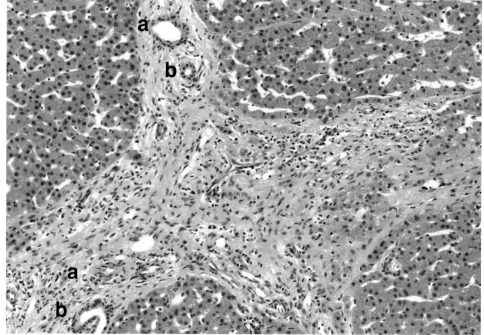

The hepatic sinusoids

The sinusoids may show a spectrum of pathological changes, from dilatation and congestion to lesions affecting the subendothelial spaces of Disse.[44] The width of the sinusoids
in liver biopsy specimens is very variable. It is influenced not only by the state of the
patient's circulation at the time of biopsy, but also by fixation and tissue processing. Slight
variations in width are therefore of doubtful significance.

The amount of connective tissue in sinusoidal walls should also be assessed critically,
since its appearance varies with section thickness. A definite increase in fibres is characteristic of chronic venous outflow obstruction and of steatohepatitis. In the former the pattern
of fibrosis is usually linear (peri- or parasinusoidal fibrosis), while in steatohepatitis the
fibrosis surrounds hepatocytes (pericellular fibrosis). Increased sinusoidal type IV collagen
in diabetic hepatosclerosis[45] is also in the differential diagnosis (**see Ch. 7**). Other
causes and associations, some of them already mentioned above, include congenital
syphilis, vinyl chloride toxicity, heroin addiction,[46] hypervitaminosis A,[47] diabetes,[48]
renal transplantation, myeloid metaplasia[49] and thrombocytopenic purpura.[50] Endothelial
cells lining the hepatic sinusoids sometimes contain iron-rich granules of uncertain significance, especially in viral hepatitis[51] and alcoholic liver disease. Immunoglobulin-
containing eosinophilic granules have been reported, particularly in chronic hepatitis[52,53]
(**see Fig. 9.12**).

Definite and regular **dilatation** of the sinusoidal network is associated with several conditions, the most important being venous outflow obstruction (see below). It has been
reported in patients with tumours or granulomas, even when these did not involve the
liver,[54] in Crohn's disease,[55] in patients with anticardiolipin antibodies and features of the
antiphospholipid syndrome,[56] haemophagocytic syndrome[57] and in heroin addicts.[58] Sinusoidal dilatation and congestion in the absence of venous outflow obstruction may also
be seen with portal-vein thrombosis and congenital absence, rheumatoid arthritis, Still's
disease, and in wedge biopsies taken during abdominal surgery.[59] Dilatation of periportal

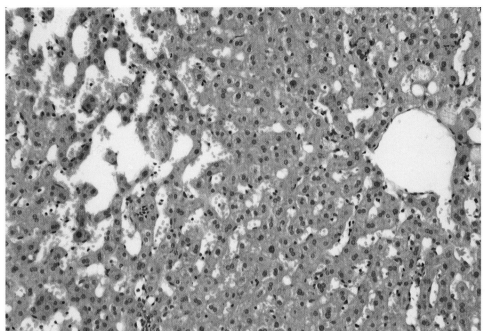

Figure 12.7
Sinusoidal
dilatation.
Dilated periportal and mid-zonal sinusoids are seen to the left, and a terminal hepatic venule to the right. The dilatation was attributed to an oral contraceptive steroid. (Needle biopsy, H&E.) (Section kindly provided by Professor Hemming Poulsen, Copenhagen, Denmark.)

and mid-zonal sinusoids has been described in a small number of patients taking oral contraceptives[60,61] (**Fig. 12.7**). In some patients with renal cell carcinoma there is focal dilatation of mid-zonal sinusoids.[62]

Peliosis hepatis

The borderline between regular diffuse dilatation and the focal dilatation known as peliosis hepatis is not always sharp.[62,63] In peliosis, blood-filled cysts are found in the parenchyma (**Fig. 12.8**), ranging in size from less than 1 mm to several millimetres in diameter. The endothelial lining is usually incomplete.[64] Peliosis is found in association with many different conditions and circumstances, including wasting diseases, asphyxia,[65] neoplasia,[66] liver and renal transplantation,[67,68] drug therapy[69,70] and bacterial infection.[71] The lesion is often discovered incidentally, but rupture leading to haemoperitoneum has been reported.[71,72] Bacillary peliosis hepatis (**see Ch. 15**) is a different lesion, and is attributed to the bacteria which cause cutaneous bacillary angiomatosis in patients with AIDS. Their presence in silver preparations distinguishes the condition from simple peliosis.

Disseminated intravascular coagulation

This commonly involves the liver.[73] Sinusoids and small portal vessels contain fibrin thrombi (**Fig. 12.9**), but the fibrin is often difficult to identify with certainty in conventional sections. Similar changes are seen in eclampsia, in association with periportal necrosis and acute inflammation. In congestive cardiac failure thrombi may form in the sinusoids.[74]

Sickle-cell disease

In most patients with sickle-cell disease clumps of sickled erythrocytes are found in dilated sinusoids[75] (**Fig. 12.10**). Lesions of peliosis may develop, and there is often some degree

**Figure 12.8
Peliosis.**
There are blood-filled spaces within the parenchyma. (Needle biopsy, H&E.)

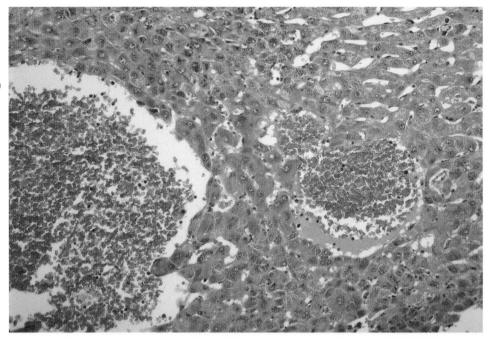

**Figure 12.9
Disseminated intravascular coagulation.**
Periportal sinusoids are filled with fibrin and neutrophils. (Needle biopsy, H&E.)

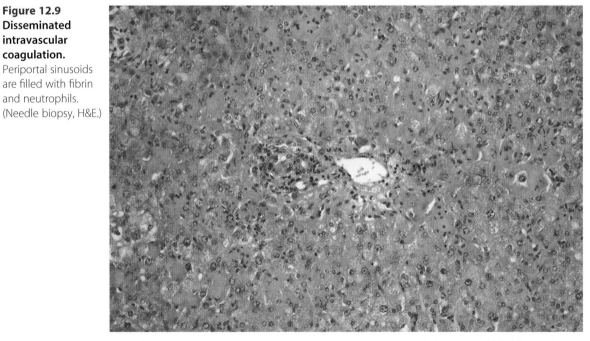

of perisinusoidal fibrosis. There is erythrophagocytosis, and hypertrophied Kupffer cells and hepatocytes contain iron. Hepatocytes may show atrophy and ischaemic necrosis[76] as well as evidence of regeneration. The degree of sickling seen does not correlate with biochemical or clinical evidence of liver damage, and some hepatic manifestations in patients with sickle-cell disease are thought to be the result of complications such as transfusion-related hepatitis,[77] siderosis, cholelithiasis and venous outflow obstruction. Cirrhosis occasionally develops, possibly as a consequence of viral hepatitis.

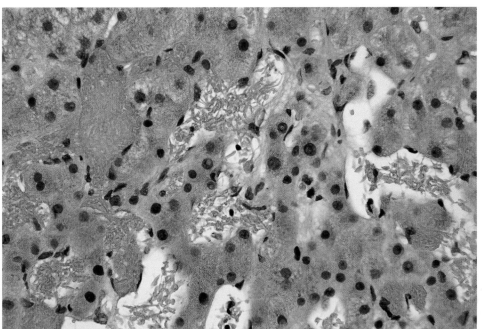

**Figure 12.10
Sickle-cell disease.**
Clumped and sickled
erythrocytes are seen
in distended
sinusoids. (Needle
biopsy, H&E.)

Venous congestion and outflow obstruction

Interference with the venous outflow of the liver results from a multitude of causes, ranging from congestive cardiac failure to occlusion of the smallest tributaries of the hepatic veins within the liver. Space-occupying lesions such as tumours may cause localised obstruction affecting only parts of the liver. The term **Budd–Chiari syndrome** is often used to describe the clinical findings when the inferior vena cava or main hepatic veins are obstructed, and is sometimes extended to obstruction at the level of the heart.[78] Further classification should be based on the nature and location of the obstruction.[79] The pathologist faced with a severely congested liver biopsy is often unsure about the level and nature of the block. Use of the term **venous outflow obstruction** is then appropriate. Chronic venous outflow leads to fibrosis surrounding efferent veins and within nearby perisinusoidal spaces, eventually with variable degrees of bridging fibrosis (central-to-central or central-to-portal) and hepatocellular regenerative hyperplasia. The degree of fibrosis in chronic congestive hepatopathy should be stated in the biopsy report since it is an important parameter to correlate with cardiopulmonary and hepatic vascular pressures and with the possible need for double organ (i.e., heart-liver) transplantation.[79a,79b] Centrilobular regions may also demonstrate unusual changes, including ingrowth of microvessels,[80] aberrant immunohistochemical positivity of perivenular hepatocytes for biliary-type keratins[80,81] (cytokeratin 7) and altered glutamine synthetase immunostain results (either loss of usual expression in centrilobular hepatocytes or relocalisation of positivity to periportal/periseptal regions).[82] Hepatocellular carcinoma is an uncommon late outcome of chronic venous outflow obstruction in Budd-Chiari syndrome[82a] and in young adults with single ventricle-type congenital heart diseases who have undergone Fontan procedures.[82b]

Congestive cardiac failure

The terminal hepatic venules and adjacent sinusoids show variable combinations of dilatation and congestion in patients with congestive failure.[83] The degree of dilatation or congestion can vary from lobule to lobule in a given tissue section. As already noted, the

Figure 12.11
Venous congestion.
Perivenular sinusoids
are dilated. The pale
zone of necrosis
indicates an element
of hypoperfusion.
Kupffer cells in and
around this area are
loaded with brown
ceroid pigment.
(Needle biopsy, H&E.)

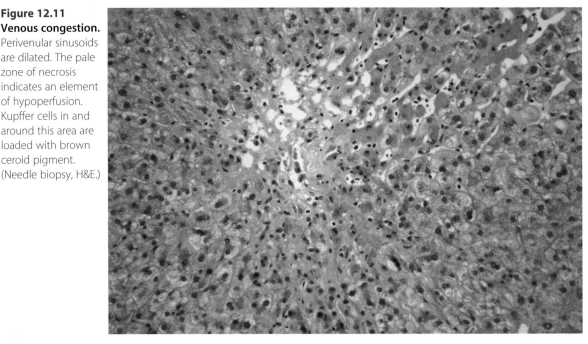

congestion may be accompanied by hepatocellular necrosis if there is also a significant element of hypoperfusion (**Fig. 12.11**), as in the combination of right- and left-sided heart failure. Sinusoidal and venous thrombosis may also contribute to hepatocellular damage.[74] Blood may infiltrate the liver-cell plates.[84] Canalicular cholestasis is sometimes seen, and must be distinguished from the commonly found ceroid pigment in Kupffer cells. Inflammation is typically mild or absent, and portal tracts usually remain normal. Periportal necrosis occurs rarely.[83] There may be regenerative hyperplasia of hepatocytes; chronic venous congestion is one cause of nodular regenerative hyperplasia and, very rarely, cirrhosis.[83] Perivenular and perisinusoidal fibrosis ('cardiac sclerosis') reflects prior episodes of failure.[19,83] In some patients hepatocytes contain periodic acid–Schiff (PAS)-positive globules which probably represent phagosomes containing imbibed plasma proteins.[85] The globules are usually located in or near the congested areas. They can be distinguished from the globules of α_1-antitrypsin deficiency by their location and, if necessary, by immunochemical staining.

Obstruction to large veins

Obstruction of the inferior vena cava or the main hepatic veins typically causes severe congestion. The many causes include thrombosis related to myeloproliferative disorders,[10,86] predisposing coagulopathies[87] and other haematological diseases. Disorders characterised by vasculitis, such as Behçet's disease, may be complicated by either venous outflow obstruction[88,89] or portal-vein obstruction.[90] An association of outflow obstruction with the use of oral contraceptives lacks conclusive proof.[91] Fibrous webs may represent a late consequence of thrombosis,[92,93] but there is some evidence to support an alternative, non-thrombotic pathogenesis.[94] Occasionally the obstruction results from administration of chemotherapeutic agents[10] or infection.[95] In some patients no cause can be discovered. While in Western countries primary hepatic vein thrombosis is more common than obliterative disease of the inferior vena cava ('obliterative cavopathy'), the reverse is true in the developing world.[96] Caval obstruction is often complicated by hepatocellular carcinoma.

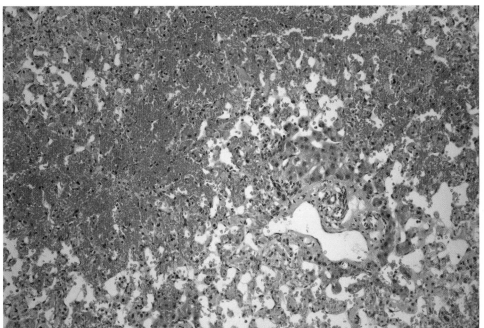

Figure 12.12 Acute venous outflow obstruction.
In this example, owing to obstruction of major veins (Budd–Chiari syndrome), much of the parenchyma has been replaced by blood. A few hepatocytes have survived around the portal tract (below right). (Wedge biopsy, H&E.)

In the acute stages much of the parenchyma may be replaced by blood. Sinusoids at the border between the haemorrhagic zones and the surviving parenchyma are dilated and empty (**Fig. 12.12**). Small efferent veins may be narrowed or blocked, depending on the cause of the obstruction (see discussion of veno-occlusive disease, below). Portal-vein branches may also be thrombosed.[97] In acute or chronic venous outflow obstruction it is common to find normal-appearing portal tracts, but there may also be portal features that mimic biliary tract disease, including a ductular reaction, inflammation and portal and/or periportal fibrosis, typically unassociated with cholestasis.[98] Eventually the haemorrhage and congestion lead to fibrosis or even cirrhosis (**Fig. 12.13**). The pattern of cirrhosis following venous outflow obstruction is influenced by the presence or absence of concomitant portal venous thrombosis; this is associated with extensive portal–central–portal bridging, with presence of portal tracts within the fibrous septa.[24] In some cases parenchymal nodularity is due to nodular regenerative hyperplasia rather than true cirrhosis, and isolated nodules resembling focal nodular hyperplasia (**see Ch. 11**) can develop as a result of locally increased arterial blood flow.[97]

Fibrosis is often difficult to distinguish from simple acute condensation of pre-existing reticulin and collagen. Stains for elastic fibres are then sometimes helpful, as in the distinction between bridging necrosis and fibrosis (**see Ch. 4**). Two further diagnostic problems should be noted. First, blocked veins may be missed in haematoxylin and eosin-stained sections so that a collagen stain should be examined if venous outflow obstruction is suspected. Thin-walled bypass channels should not be mistaken for patent veins. Second, the obstruction may not affect all the hepatic veins, so that parts of the liver escape serious congestion. As a result, biopsy samples may show considerable regional variability, which can lead to diagnostic confusion. It follows that a near-normal liver biopsy does not exclude a diagnosis of venous outflow obstruction.

Sinusoidal obstruction syndrome/veno-occlusive disease

The recent term **sinusoidal obstruction syndrome** (SOS) has been used to describe the spectrum of sinusoidal congestion, dilatation, thrombosis and fibrous occlusion of

Figure 12.13 Chronic venous outflow obstruction.
Late in the disease fibrous tissue has been laid down in the congested areas, top left. Surviving parenchyma shows 'reversed lobulation' around a portal tract. (Needle biopsy, H&E.)

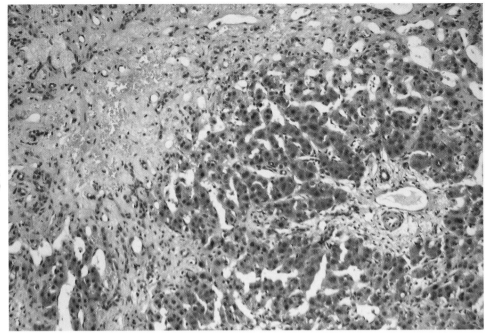

efferent venules which developed due to injury to sinusoidal endothelial injury of varying aetiology, often chemical.[10,99] **Veno-occlusive disease** (VOD) – in which the smallest tributaries of the hepatic veins, the terminal hepatic venules and sublobular veins are occluded by fibrous tissue (**Fig. 12.14**) – is a manifestation of SOS. The venous lesions can thus be detected in needle biopsies. There is often associated fibrosis of sinusoidal walls (perisinusoidal fibrosis), probably mediated by hepatic stellate cells.[100] Apart from these lesions the changes are as for obstruction of large veins. As already noted, the borderline between obstruction to large and small veins is not sharp, since both may be affected by thrombosis, for example in patients with coagulation disorders. Furthermore, thrombosis of large or medium-sized hepatic veins may lead to fibrous intimal thickening of smaller vessels. Rarely, an exuberant form of fibrous obliteration involves veins of all calibres and has been shown to recur after liver transplantation.[101] Careful inspection of the congested sinusoids in SOS in liver biopsy specimens may disclose loss or discontinuity of endothelium from the vascular lining, endothelial and/or hepatocyte extrusion into the sinusoidal lumen and intravasation of red blood cells into the space of Disse (**see Fig. 16.23**).

As in the case of obstruction to larger veins, there are many causes of SOS and VOD. The classical cause, ingestion of pyrrolizidine alkaloids, remains a hazard.[102] Sinusoidal endothelium in general is also susceptible to similar toxic injury, particularly in individuals receiving chemotherapy or myeloablative conditioning therapy prior to haematopoietic cell transplantation.[10,103] Among these agents are 6-thioguanine, busulfan, gemtuzimab–ozogamicin and oxaliplatin.[10] Venous occlusion is also seen following renal or liver transplantation.[100,104–106] Other associations and causes are irradiation of the liver,[107] AIDS,[108] heroin addiction,[46] primary vascular disease,[109] Hodgkin's disease,[110,111] drug therapy[70,112] and arsenic poisoning.[113] Epithelioid haemangioendothelioma of the liver can mimic VOD because of the characteristic vascular occlusions produced by tumour invasion, and can also give rise to clinical and histological features of the Budd–Chiari syndrome.[114] Finally, careful examination of connective tissue stains may reveal occluded veins in the livers of patients with alcoholic and non-alcoholic fatty liver disease[115,116] and indeed in cirrhosis from any cause.[117]

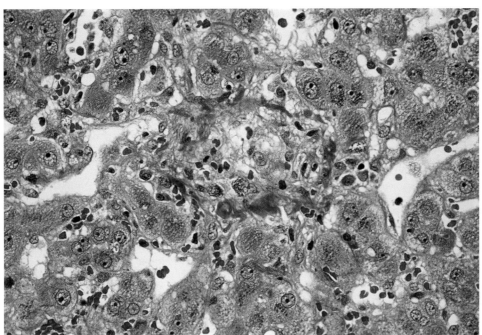

**Figure 12.14
Veno-occlusive disease.**
A terminal hepatic venule has been occluded by recently formed collagen and cells, following liver transplantation. (Needle biopsy, chromotrope–aniline blue.) (Section kindly provided by Professor AP Dhillon, London, UK.)

References

1 Valente JF, Alonso MH, Weber FL, et al. Late hepatic artery thrombosis in liver allograft recipients is associated with intrahepatic biliary necrosis. Transplantation 1996;61:61–5.

2 Goritsas CP, Repanti M, Papadaki E, et al. Intrahepatic bile duct injury and nodular regenerative hyperplasia of the liver in a patient with polyarteritis nodosa. J Hepatol 1997;26:727–30.

3 Viola S, Meyer M, Fabre M, et al. Ischemic necrosis of bile ducts complicating Schönlein–Henoch purpura. Gastroenterology 1999;117:211–14.

4 Parangi S, Oz MC, Blume RS, et al. Hepatobiliary complications of polyarteritis nodosa. Arch Surg 1991;126:909–12.

4a Choi HL, Sung RH, Kang MH, et al. Polyarteritis nodosa presented as a dilatation of the intrahepatic bile duct. Ann Surg Treat Res 2014;87:273–5.

5 Matsumoto T, Yoshimine T, Shimouchi K, et al. The liver in systemic lupus erythematosus: pathologic analysis of 52 cases and review of Japanese autopsy registry data. Hum Pathol 1992;23:1151–8.

6 Rousselet M-C, Kettani S, Rohmer V, et al. A case of temporal arteritis with intrahepatic arterial involvement. Pathol Res Pract 1989;185:329–31.

7 Heneghan MA, Feeley KM, DeFaoite N, et al. Granulomatous liver disease and giant-cell arteritis. Dig Dis Sci 1998;43:2164–7.

8 De Bayser L, Roblot P, Ramassamy A, et al. Hepatic fibrin-ring granulomas in giant cell arteritis. Gastroenterology 1993;105:272–3.

9 Fiel MI, Deniz K, Elmali F, et al. Increasing hepatic arteriole wall thickness and decreased luminal diameter occur with increasing age in normal livers. J Hepatol 2011;55:582–6.

10 DeLeve LD, Valla D-C, Garcia-Tsao G. Vascular disorders of the liver. Hepatology 2009;49:1729–64.

11 Martini GA. The liver in hereditary haemorrhagic telangiectasia: an inborn error of vascular structure with multiple manifestations: a reappraisal. Gut 1978;19:531–7.

12 Wanless IR, Gryfe A. Nodular transformation of the liver in hereditary hemorrhagic telangiectasia. Arch Pathol Lab Med 1986;110:331–5.

13 Larson AM. Liver disease in hereditary hemorrhagic telangiectasia. J Clin Gastroenterol 2003;36:149–58.

14 Bernard G, Mion F, Henry L, et al. Hepatic involvement in hereditary hemorrhagic telangiectasia: clinical, radiological, and hemodynamic studies of 11 cases. Gastroenterology 1993;105:482–7.

15 Saegusa M, Takano Y, Okudaira M. Human hepatic infarction: histopathological and postmortem angiological studies. Liver 1993;13:239–45.

16 de la Monte SM, Arcidi JM, Moore GW, et al. Midzonal necrosis as a pattern of hepatocellular injury after shock. Gastroenterology 1984;86:627–31.

17 Gelbmann CM, Rümmele P, Wimmer M, et al. Ischemic-like cholangiopathy with secondary sclerosing cholangitis in critically ill patients. Am J Gastroenterol 2007;102:1221–9.

18 Voigtländer T, Negm AA, Schneider AS, et al. Secondary sclerosing cholangitis in critically ill patients: model of end-stage liver disease score and renal function predict outcome. Endoscopy 2012;44:1055–8.

19 Lefkowitch JH, Mendez L. Morphologic features of hepatic injury in cardiac disease and shock. J Hepatol 1986;2:313–27.

20 Sort P, Mas A, Salmeron JM, et al. Recurrent liver involvement in heatstroke. Liver 1996;16:334–7.

21 Hassanein T, Perper JA, Tepperman L, et al. Liver failure occurring as a component of exertional heatstroke. Gastroenterology 1991;100:1442–7.

22 Gitlin N, Serio KM. Ischemic hepatitis: widening horizons. Am J Gastroenterol 1992;87:831–6.

23 Amitrano L, Guardascione MA, Brancaccio V, et al. Risk factors and clinical presentation of portal vein thrombosis in patients with liver cirrhosis. J Hepatol 2004;40:736–41.

24 Tanaka M, Wanless IR. Pathology of the liver in Budd–Chiari syndrome: portal vein thrombosis and the histogenesis of veno-centric cirrhosis, veno-portal cirrhosis, and large regenerative nodules. Hepatology 1998;27:488–96.

25 Shimamatsu K, Wanless IR. Role of ischemia in causing apoptosis, atrophy, and nodular hyperplasia in human liver. Hepatology 1997;26:343–50.

26 Lisovsky M, Konstas AA, Misdraji J. Congenital extrahepatic portosystemic shunts (Abernethy malformation): a histopathologic evaluation. Am J Surg Pathol 2011;35:1381–90.

27 Wanless IR, Peterson P, Das A, et al. Hepatic vascular disease and portal hypertension in polycythemia vera and agnogenic myeloid metaplasia: a clinicopathological study of 145 patients examined at autopsy. Hepatology 1990;12:1166–74.

28 Dubois A, Dauzat M, Pignodel C, et al. Portal hypertension in lymphoproliferative and myeloproliferative disorders: hemodynamic and histological correlations. Hepatology 1993;17:246–50.

29 Roskams T, Baptista A, Bianchi L, et al. Histopathology of portal hypertension: a practical guideline. Histopathology 2003;42:2–13.

30 Khanna R, Sarin SK. Non-cirrhotic portal hypertension – diagnosis and management. J Hepatol 2014;60:421–41.

31 Verheij J, Schouten JNL, Komuta M, et al. Histological features in western patients with idiopathic non-cirrhotic portal hypertension. Histopathology 2013;62:1083–91.

32 Aggarwal S, Fiel MI, Schiano TD. Obliterative portal venopathy: a clinical and histopathological review. Dig Dis Sci 2013;58:2767–76.

33 Nevens F, Fevery J, Van Steenbergen W, et al. Arsenic and non-cirrhotic portal hypertension. A report of eight cases. J Hepatol 1990;11:80–5.

34 Thomas LB, Popper H, Berk PD, et al. Vinyl-chloride-induced liver disease. From idiopathic portal hypertension (Banti's syndrome) to angiosarcomas. N Engl J Med 1975;292:17–22.

35 Popper H, Thomas LB, Telles NC, et al. Development of hepatic angiosarcoma in man induced by vinyl chloride, thorotrast, and arsenic. Comparison with cases of unknown etiology. Am J Pathol 1978;92:349–69.

36 Shepherd P, Harrison DJ. Idiopathic portal hypertension associated with cytotoxic drugs. J Clin Pathol 2004;43:206–10.

36a Siramolpiwat S, Seijo S, MiquelR, et al. Idiopathic portal hypertension: natural history and long-term outcome. Hepatology 2014;59:2276–85.

37 Oikawa H, Masuda T, Sato S-I, et al. Changes in lymph vessels and portal veins in the portal tract of patients with idiopathic portal hypertension: a morphometric study. Hepatology 1998;27:1607–10.

38 Ludwig J, Hashimoto E, Obata H, et al. Idiopathic portal hypertension: a histopathological study of 26 Japanese cases. Histopathology 1993;22:227–34.

39 Ohbu M, Okudaira M, Watanabe K, et al. Histopathological study of intrahepatic aberrant vessels in cases of noncirrhotic portal hypertension. Hepatology 1994;20:302–8.

40 Nakanuma Y, Hoso M, Sasaki M, et al. Histopathology of the liver in non-cirrhotic portal hypertension of unknown etiology. Histopathology 1996;28:195–204.

41 Bernard P-H, Le Bail B, Cransac M, et al. Progression from idiopathic portal hypertension to incomplete septal cirrhosis with liver failure requiring liver transplantation. J Hepatol 2004;22:495–9.

42 Ibarrola C, Colina F. Clinicopathological features of nine cases of non-cirrhotic portal hypertension: current definitions and criteria are inadequate. Histopathology 2003;42:251–64.

43 Nataf C, Feldmann G, Lebrec D, et al. Idiopathic portal hypertension (perisinusoidal fibrosis) after renal transplantation. Gut 1979;20:531–7.

44 Brunt EM, Gouw ASH, Hubscher SG, et al. Pathology of the liver sinusoids. Histopathology 2014;64:907–20.

45 Harrison SA, Brunt EM, Goodman ZD, et al. Diabetic hepatosclerosis: a novel entity or a rare form of nonalcoholic fatty liver disease? Arch Pathol Lab Med 2006;130:27–32.

46 Trigueiro de Araújo MS, Gerard F, Chossegros P, et al. Vascular hepatotoxicity related to heroin addiction. Virchows Arch [A] 1990;417:497–503.

47 Bioulac-Sage P, Quinton A, Saric J, et al. Chance discovery of hepatic fibrosis in patient with asymptomatic hypervitaminosis A. Arch Pathol Lab Med 1988;112:505–9.

48 Latry P, Bioulac-Sage P, Echinard E, et al. Perisinusoidal fibrosis and basement membrane-like material in the livers of diabetic patients. Hum Pathol 1987;18:775–80.

49 Degott C, Capron J, Bettan L, et al. Myeloid metaplasia, perisinusoidal fibrosis, and nodular regenerative hyperplasia of the liver. Liver 1985;5:276–81.

50 Lafon ME, Bioulac-Sage P, Grimaud JA, et al. Perisinusoidal fibrosis of the liver in patients with thrombocytopenic purpura. Virchows Arch [A] 1987;411:553–9.

51 Bardadin KA, Scheuer PJ. Endothelial cell changes in acute hepatitis. A light and electron microscopic study. J Pathol 1984;144:213–20.

52 Iwamura S, Enzan H, Saibara T, et al. Appearance of sinusoidal inclusion-containing endothelial cells in liver disease. Hepatology 1994;20:604–10.

53 Iwamura S, Enzan H, Saibara T, et al. Hepatic sinusoidal endothelial cells can store and metabolize serum immunoglobulin. Hepatology 1995;22:1456–61.

54 Bruguera M, Aranguibel F, Ros E, et al. Incidence and clinical significance of sinusoidal dilatation in liver biopsies. Gastroenterology 1978;75:474–8.

55 Capron JP, Lemay JL, Gontier MF, et al. Hepatic sinusoidal dilatation in Crohn's disease. Scand J Gastroenterol 1979;14:987–92.

56 Saadoun D, Cazals-Hatem D, Denninger M-H, et al. Association of idiopathic hepatic sinusoidal dilatation with the immunological features of the antiphospholipid syndrome. Gut 2004;53:1516–19.

57 de Kerguenec C, Hillaire S, Molinié V, et al. Hepatic manifestations of hemophagocytic syndrome: a study of 30 cases. Am J Gastroenterol 2001;96:852–7.

58 Trigueiro de Araújo MS, Gerard F, Chossegros P, et al. Lack of hepatocyte involvement in the genesis of the sinusoidal dilatation related to heroin addiction: a morphometric study. Virchows Arch [A] 1992;420:149–53.

59 Kakar S, Kamath PS, Burgart LJ. Sinusoidal dilatation and congestion in liver biopsy. Is it always due to venous outflow impairment? Arch Pathol Lab Med 2004;128:901–4.

60 Winkler K, Poulsen H. Liver disease with periportal sinusoidal dilatation. A possible complication to contraceptive steroids. Scand J Gastroenterol 1975;10:699–704.

61 Winkler K, Christoffersen P. A reappraisal of Poulsen's disease (hepatic zone 1 sinusoidal dilatation). APMIS 1991;(Suppl. 23):86–90.

62 Aoyagi T, Mori I, Ueyama Y, et al. Sinusoidal dilatation of the liver as a paraneoplasticmanifestation of renal cell carcinoma. Hum Pathol 1989;20:1193–7.

63 Oligny LL, Lough J. Hepatic sinusoidal ectasia. Hum Pathol 1992;23:953–6.

64 Wold LE, Ludwig J. Peliosis hepatis: two morphologic variants? Hum Pathol 1981;12:388–9.

65 Selby DM, Stocker JT. Focal peliosis hepatis, a sequela of asphyxial death? Pediatr Pathol Lab Med 1995;15:589–96.

66 Fine KD, Solano M, Polter DE, et al. Malignant histiocytosis in a patient presenting with hepatic dysfunction and peliosis hepatis. Am J Gastroenterol 1995;90:485–8.

67 Degott C, Rueff B, Kreis H, et al. Peliosis hepatis in recipients of renal transplants. Gut 1978;19:748–53.

68 Scheuer PJ, Schachter LA, Mathur S, et al. Peliosis hepatis after liver transplantation. J Clin Pathol 1990;43:1036–7.

69 Soe KL, Soe M, Gluud C. Liver pathology associated with the use of anabolic-androgenic steroids. Liver 1992;12:73–9.

70 Modzelewski JRJ, Daeschner C, Joshi VV, et al. Veno-occlusive disease of the liver induced by low-dose cyclophosphamide. Mod Pathol 1994;7:967–72.

71 Jacquemin E, Pariente D, Fabre M, et al. Peliosis hepatis with initial presentation as acute hepatic failure and intraperitoneal hemorrhage in children. J Hepatol 1999;30:1146–50.

72 Takiff H, Brems JJ, Pockros PJ, et al. Focal hemorrhagic necrosis of the liver. A rare cause of hemoperitoneum. Dig Dis Sci 1992;37:1910–14.

73 Shimamura K, Oka K, Nakazawa M, et al. Distribution patterns of microthrombi in disseminated intravascular coagulation. Arch Pathol Lab Med 1983;107:543–7.

74 Wanless IR, Liu JJ, Butany J. Role of thrombosis in the pathogenesis of congestive hepatic fibrosis (cardiac cirrhosis). Hepatology 1995;21:1232–7.

75 Banerjee S, Owen C, Chopra S. Sickle cell hepatopathy. Hepatology 2001;33:1021–8.

76 Charlotte F, Bachir D, Nénert M, et al. Vascular lesions of the liver in sickle cell disease. A clinicopathological study in 26 living patients. Arch Pathol Lab Med 1995;119:46–52.

77 Comer GM, Ozick LA, Sachdev RK, et al. Transfusion-related chronic liver disease in sickle cell anemia. Am J Gastroenterol 1991;86:1232–4.

78 Valla D-C. Budd Chiari syndrome and veno-occlusive disease/sinusoidal obstruction syndrome. Gut 2008;57:1469–78.

79 Ludwig J, Hashimoto E, McGill DB, et al. Classification of hepatic venous outflow obstruction: ambiguous terminology of the Budd–Chiari syndrome. Mayo Clin Proc 1990;65:51–5.

79a Dai D-F, Swanson PE, Krieger EV, et al. Congestive hepatic fibrosis score: a novel histologic assessment of clinical severity. Mod Pathol 2014;27:1552–8.

79b Farr M, Mithcell J, Lippel M, et al. The combination of liver biopsy with MELD-XI scores for post-transplant outcome prediction in patients with advanced heart failure and suspected liver dysfunction. J Heart Lung Transplant 2015; (In press).

80 Krings G, Can B, Ferrell L. Aberrant centrizonal features in chronic hepatis venous outflow obstruction. Am J Surg Pathol 2014;38:205–14.

81 Pai RK, Hart JA. Aberrant expression of cytokeratin 7 in perivenular hepatocytes correlates with a cholestatic chemistry profile in patients with heart failure. Mod Pathol 2010;23:1650–6.

82 Fleming KE, Wanless IR. Glutamine synthetase expression in activated hepatocyte progenitor cells and loss of hepatocellular expression in congestion and cirrhosis. Liver Int 2013;33:525–34.

82a Moucari R, Rautou P-E, Cazals-Hatem D, et al. Hepatocellular carcinoma in Budd-Chiari syndrome: characteristics and risk factors. Gut 2008;57:828–35.

82b Asrani SK, Warnes CA, Kamath PS. Hepatocellular carcinoma after the Fontan procedure. N Engl J Med 2013;368:1756–7.

83 Myers RP, Cerini R, Sayegh R, et al. Cardiac hepatopathy: clinical, hemodynamic, and histologic characteristics and correlations. Hepatology 2003;37:393–400.

84 Kanel GC, Ucci AA, Kaplan MM, et al. A distinctive perivenular hepatic lesion associated with heart failure. Am J Clin Pathol 1980;73:235–9.

85 Klatt EC, Koss MN, Young TS, et al. Hepatic hyaline globules associated with passiv*congestion. Arch Pathol Lab Med 1988;112:510–13.

86 Boughton BJ. Hepatic and portal vein thrombosis. Closely associated with chronic myeloproliferative disorders. BMJ 1991;302:192–3.

87 Valla D-C. The diagnosis and management of the Budd–Chiari syndrome: consensus and controversies. Hepatology 2003;38:793–803.

88 Bismuth E, Hadengue A, Hammel P, et al. Hepatic vein thrombosis in Behçet's disease. Hepatology 1990;11:969–74.

89 Bayraktar Y, Balkanci F, Bayraktar M, et al. Budd–Chiari syndrome: a common complication of Behcet's disease. Am J Gastroenterol 1997;92:858–62.

90 Bayraktar Y, Balkanci F, Kansu E, et al. Cavernous transformation of the portal vein: a common manifestation of Behcet's syndrome. Am J Gastroenterol 1995;90:1476–9.

91 Maddrey WC. Hepatic vein thrombosis (Budd–Chiari syndrome): possible association with the use of oral contraceptives. Semin Liver Dis 1987;7:32–9.

92 Blanshard C, Dodge G, Pasi J, et al. Membranous obstruction of the inferior vena cava in a patient with factor V Leiden: evidence for a post-thrombotic aetiology. J Hepatol 1997;26:731–5.

93 Valla D, Hadengue A, el Younsi M, et al. Hepatic venous outflow block caused by short-length hepatic vein stenoses. Hepatology 1997;25:814–19.

94 Riemens SC, Haagsma EB, Kok T, et al. Familial occurrence of membranous obstruction of the inferior vena cava: arguments in favor of a congenital etiology. J Hepatol 1995;22:404–9.

95 Vallaeys JH, Praet MM, Roels HJ, et al. The Budd–Chiari syndrome caused by a zygomycete. A new pathogenesis of hepatic vein thrombosis. Arch Pathol Lab Med 1989;113:1171–4.

96 Okuda K, Kage M, Shrestha SM. Proposal of a new nomenclature for Budd–Chiari syndrome: hepatic vein thrombosis versus thrombosis of the inferior vena cava at its hepatic portion. Hepatology 1998;28:1191–8.

97 Cazals-Hatem D, Vilgrain V, Genin P, et al. Arterial and portal circulation and parenchymal changes in Budd–Chiari syndrome: a study in 17 explanted livers. Hepatology 2003;37:510–19.

98 Kakar S, Batts KP, Poterucha JJ, et al. Histologic changes mimicking biliary disease in liver biopsies with venous outflow impairment. Mod Pathol 2004;17:874–8.

99 DeLeve LD, Shulman HM, McDonald GB. Toxic injury to hepatic sinusoids: sinusoidal obstruction syndrome (veno-occlusive disease). Semin Liver Dis 2002;22:27–42.

100 Sato Y, Asada Y, Hara S, et al. Hepatic stellate cells (Ito cells) in veno-occlusive disease of the liver after allogeneic bone marrow transplantation. Histopathology 1999;34:66–70.

101 Fiel MI, Schiano TD, Klion FM, et al. Recurring fibro-obliterative venopathy in liver allografts. Am J Surg Pathol 1999;23:734–7.

102 Chojkier M. Hepatic sinusoidal-obstruction syndrome: toxicity of pyrrolizidine alkaloids. J Hepatol 2003;39:437–46.

103 Sakai M, Strasser SI, Shulman HM, et al. Severe hepatocellular injury after hematopoietic cell transplant: incidence, etiology and outcome. Bone Marrow Transplant 2009;56:1–7.

104 Katzka DA, Saul SH, Jorkasky D, et al. Azathioprine and hepatic venocclusive disease in renal transplant patients. Gastroenterology 1986;90:446–54.

105 Shulman HM, FIsher LB, Schoch HG, et al. Venoocclusive disease of the liver after marrow transplantation: histological correlates of clinical signs and symptoms. Hepatology 1994;19:1171–80.

106 Dhillon AP, Burroughs AK, Hudson M, et al. Hepatic venular stenosis after orthotopic liver transplantation. Hepatology 1994;19:106–11.

107 Lawrence TS, Robertson JM, Anscher MS, et al. Hepatic toxicity resulting from cancer treatment. Int J Radiat Oncol Biol Phys 1995;31:1237–48.

108 Buckley JA, Hutchins GM. Association of hepatic veno-occlusive disease with the acquired immunodeficiency syndrome. Mod Pathol 1995;8:398–401.

109 Ito N, Kimura A, Nishikawa M, et al. Veno-occlusive disease of the liver in a patient with allergic granulomatous angiitis. Am J Gastroenterol 1988;83:316–19.

110 Lohse AW, Dienes HP, Wolfel T, et al. Veno-occlusive disease of the liver in Hodgkin's disease prior to and resolution following chemotherapy (letter). J Hepatol 1995;22:378.

111 Palladino M, Miele L, Pompili M, et al. Severe veno-occlusive disease after autologous peripheral blood stem cell transplantation for high-grade non-Hodgkin lymphoma: report of a successfully managed case and a literature review of veno-occlusive disease. Clin Transplant 2008;22:837–41.

112 Nakhleh RE, Wesen C, Snover DC, et al. Venoocclusive lesions of the central veins and portal vein radicles secondary to intraarterial 5-fluoro-2'-deoxyuridine infusion. Hum Pathol 1989;20:1218–20.

113 Labadie H, Stoessel P, Callard P, et al. Hepatic venoocclusive disease and perisinusoidal fibrosis secondary to arsenic poisoning. Gastroenterology 1990;99:1140–3.

114 Walsh MM, Hytiroglou P, Thung SN, et al. Epithelioid hemangioendothelioma of the liver mimicking Budd–Chiari syndrome. Arch Pathol Lab Med 1998;122:846–8.

115 Burt AD, MacSween RN. Hepatic vein lesions in alcoholic liver disease: retrospective biopsy and necropsy study. J Clin Pathol 1986;39:63–7.

116 Wanless IR, Shiota K. The pathogenesis of nonalcoholic steatohepatitis and other fatty liver diseases: a four-step model including the role of lipid release and hepatic venular obstruction in the progression to cirrhosis. Semin Liver Dis 2004;24:99–106.

117 Nakanuma Y, Ohta G, Doishita K. Quantitation and serial section observations of focal venocclusive lesions of hepatic veins in liver cirrhosis. Virchows Arch [A] 1985;405:429–38.

General reading

Brunt EM, Gouw ASH, Hubscher SG, et al. Pathology of the liver sinusoids. Histopathology 2014;64:907–20.

Cazals-Hatem D, Vilgrain V, Genin P, et al. Arterial and portal circulation and parenchymal changes in Budd–Chiari syndrome: a study in 17 explanted livers. Hepatology 2003;37:510–19.

DeLeve LD, Shulman HM, McDonald GB. Toxic injury to hepatic sinusoids: sinusoidal obstruction syndrome (veno-occlusive disease). Semin Liver Dis 2002;22:27–42.

DeLeve LD, Valla D-C, Garcia-Tsao G. Vascular disorders of the liver. Hepatology 2009;49:1729–64.

Okudaira M, Ohbu M, Okuda K. Idiopathic portal hypertension and its pathology. Semin Liver Dis 2002;22:59–72.

Roskams T, Baptista A, Bianchi L, et al. Histopathology of portal hypertension: a practical guideline. Histopathology 2003;42:2–13.

Wanless IR, Huang W-Y. Vascular disorders. In: Burt AD, Portmann BC, Ferrell LD, editors. MacSween's Pathology of the Liver. 6th ed. Edinburgh: Churchill Livingstone/ Elsevier; 2012. p. 601–44.

Childhood Liver Disease and Metabolic Disorders

Introduction

Paediatric liver biopsies present a unique set of diagnostic problems for the pathologist,[1] many of which become clinically apparent in the first few months of life as **neonatal cholestasis**.[2] Among the important disorders one must consider in evaluating neonatal liver biopsies are **extrahepatic biliary atresia**, **paucity of intrahepatic bile ducts** (syndromatic and non-syndromatic types), **metabolic diseases**, **viral hepatitis** and the hepatic effects of **parenteral nutrition (Table 13.1)**. Common to many of these conditions are the histological features of **cholestasis** and **giant-cell hepatitis** (formation of multinucleated hepatocytes). Because these features are not specifically diagnostic of any one neonatal liver disease, the pathologist must be acquainted with other biopsy changes by which to establish or suggest the diagnosis. In many instances, assays of metabolic enzymes and products in serum and liver tissue take diagnostic precedence over routine histopathological interpretation. Electron microscopy may be required to assess the structure of organelles or storage material in hepatocytes or Kupffer cells, particularly when lysosomal storage disorders are being considered. Consultation with investigators dealing with mitochondriopathies,[3,4] mutations of bile-salt transport proteins[5] and expression of proteins involved in blood vessel and bile-duct morphogenesis (e.g. Jagged proteins and Notch receptors) should be considered if special studies are needed to determine the cause of neonatal cholestasis. Childhood liver tumours are discussed in **Chapter 11**.

Diagnostic approach to neonatal liver biopsy

Histopathological examination of neonatal liver biopsies may benefit from a systematic checklist of questions by which the major diagnostic concerns in neonatal liver disease can be evaluated. A simplified, stepwise set of seven questions can be asked:

1 *Is the acinar structure normal for age?* As described in **Chapter 3**, the hepatic plates are two cells thick until 5 or 6 years of age and should not be misconstrued as a pathological change. As with adult biopsies, the presence of fibrosis, nodularity or cirrhosis should be noted early in the biopsy evaluation and correlated with other histological features which may define the aetiology.

2 *Are cholestasis and giant cells present?* As indicated above, neither of these is diagnostically specific. If present, the next interpretive steps should be examination of portal tracts for evidence of biliary tract obstruction (e.g. atresia) and of portal tracts and parenchyma for evidence of hepatitis.

Table 13.1 Liver biopsy interpretation in neonatal cholestasis*

Aetiology	Histological features
Extrahepatic biliary atresia	Ductular reaction; ductular cholestasis; portal and periportal fibrosis
Paucity of intrahepatic bile ducts	Loss of interlobular bile ducts (bile duct–hepatic artery ratio <1)
Neonatal hepatitis	Portal and lobular mononuclear cell inflammation; apoptotic bodies
Metabolic disorders	Steatosis; fibrosis or cirrhosis; storage product in liver cells or Kupffer cells (see specific disorder)
Parenteral nutrition	Ductular reaction; portal fibrosis or cirrhosis

*Many of the conditions shown in **Table 13.1** are associated with histological cholestasis and formation of giant multinucleated hepatocytes, in addition to the diagnostic features listed.

3 *Are histological changes of hepatitis present?* Mononuclear cell infiltrates within acini and portal tracts associated with liver-cell degeneration should be sought when considering cytomegalovirus, Epstein–Barr virus, rubella or hepatitis virus infections.

4 *Are the interlobular bile ducts normal?* This question has three major ramifications. **Abundance of bile ducts** usually signifies some form of biliary obstruction, such as extrahepatic atresia or choledochal cyst. **Paucity of bile ducts** (**ductopenia, vanishing bile-duct syndrome**) may be due to developmental, metabolic or infectious causes. Last, **malformations of bile ducts** comprise a spectrum of problems related to abnormal remodelling of the embryonic bile-duct plate (fibropolycystic diseases).

5 *Does the biopsy specimen contain iron or copper?* Although rare, neonatal haemochromatosis[6] and Indian childhood cirrhosis (copper toxicosis in young children) are serious liver diseases with high mortality rates that must be excluded. In the older child and adolescent, Wilson's disease (**Ch. 14**) must not be overlooked. It should be noted, however, that fetal and neonatal liver contains much higher copper levels than adults, with an irregular tissue distribution.[7] Mild siderosis is also within the spectrum of normal findings in the fetal and neonatal liver.[8]

6 *Has the biopsy specimen been studied by diastase–periodic acid–Schiff (PAS) or immunoperoxidase staining to exclude α_1-antitrypsin deficiency?* The expression of α_1-antitrypsin deficiency is variable, and biopsies may not show diagnostic staining of retained enzyme within liver cells prior to 13–15 weeks of age. This condition should be histologically excluded whenever possible.

7 *Are storage cells present?* Abnormal storage products in liver cells or Kupffer cells may be seen in various metabolic diseases which cause hepatomegaly and failure to thrive. These should be sought on routine haematoxylin and eosin (H&E) as well as special stains.

Neonatal hepatitis

Inflammation and hepatocellular damage in the neonatal period may result from infections and from inborn errors of metabolism. Infections include type B hepatitis,

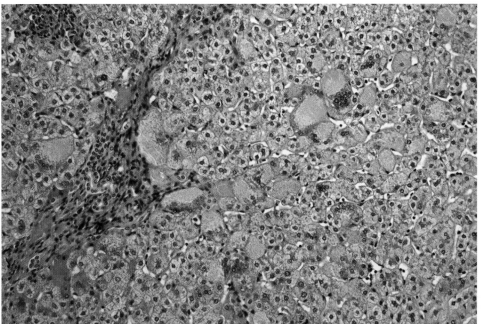

Figure 13.1 Neonatal (giant-cell) hepatitis. The parenchyma consists of multinucleated giant liver cells and the portal tract shown is infiltrated by lymphocytes. (Wedge biopsy, H&E.)

cytomegalovirus infection and rubella among others; inborn errors of metabolism include α_1-antitrypsin deficiency, galactosaemia and bile-acid synthetic defects.[9] Disorders at the ultrastructural or molecular level may also need to be considered, such as neonatal hepatitis due to depletion of mitochondrial DNA.[10-16] A diagnosis of neonatal hepatitis is therefore a signal for further investigation. The histological picture is broadly similar whatever the cause. There is a variable degree of hepatocellular swelling and multinucleation, cholestasis and portal inflammation (**Fig. 13.1**). Lobular inflammation may be mild. Liver-cell necrosis and swelling result in collapse and distortion of the reticulin framework. Fibrosis is sometimes already well developed, as in neonatal haemochromatosis (**see Ch. 14**) or the severe perinatal liver disease which may rarely be seen in Down's syndrome.[17] Giant multinucleated hepatocytes are commonly seen, whatever the cause of the hepatitis (**Fig. 13.2**). The outcome of neonatal giant-cell hepatitis is resolution, liver failure, cirrhosis or a chronic cholestatic course. The variety of different outcomes is well illustrated in α_1-antitrypsin deficiency.[18]

From a histological point of view, the main differential diagnosis of neonatal hepatitis is extrahepatic biliary obstruction, which may require surgical treatment. Giant multinucleated hepatocytes, an altered reticulin structure and little or no ductular reaction are more prominent in hepatitis than in biliary obstruction, while cholestasis is usually more severe in atresia and there is typically a ductular reaction.

Extrahepatic biliary atresia

Extracellular biliary atresia results from inflammation and destruction of all or part of the extrahepatic bile-duct system *in utero* or in the perinatal period.[19] Pathological studies of atretic bile-duct segments[20-22] show chronic inflammation and obliterative fibrosis, sometimes with a few remaining bile-duct cells[23] seen on routine stains or cytokeratin immunostaining. Satisfactory bile drainage and an improved outcome after the Kasai

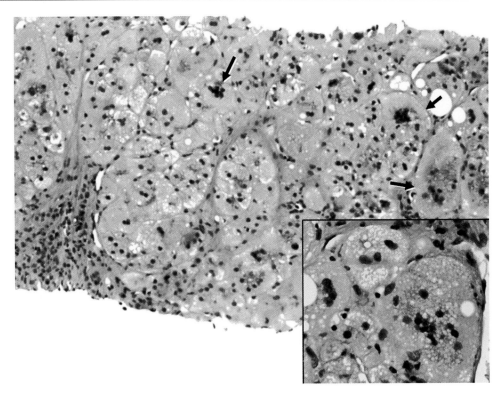

Figure 13.2 Neonatal (giant-cell) hepatitis.
Multinucleated giant hepatocytes are present (arrows) and there is mild parenchymal disarray and inflammation. The portal tract at left shows mild periportal fibrosis and inflammation. Hepatocytes contain finely divided lipid vacuoles (microvesicular steatosis), as seen in the inset. This neonate also had neurological deficits and genetic analysis demonstrated a mitochondriopathy associated with mitochondrial DNA depletion. (Needle biopsy, H&E.)

portoenterostomy[24] have sometimes been associated with identification of bile ducts with lumens of 150 μm or greater at the proximal resection margin.[21] Optimal surgical results are obtained if the Kasai procedure (hepatic portoenterostomy) is performed within the first 8 weeks of life,[25] with approximately 30% surviving into adulthood with their native liver.[26] Many patients, nevertheless, later require liver transplantation.[27]

The trigger for the destructive process in extrahepatic atresia is unknown, but considerations have included viral infections (reovirus type 3, rotavirus), exposure to toxins, abnormalities in regulatory T cells,[28] abnormal remodelling of the embryonic bile-duct plate and disorders of Jagged protein/Notch receptor and Hedgehog signalling.[19,29] DNA microarray studies suggest a gene profile of abnormal cell signalling and transcription regulation.[30] There may be associated congenital abnormalities, including polysplenia,[31] intrahepatic biliary cysts,[32] laterality defects and cardiovascular, musculoskeletal and genitourinary defects[33,34] in approximately 20% of cases with more severe and earlier disease (the 'embryonic' form of biliary atresia). In contrast, the majority of patients have the 'perinatal' form without such anomalies. Expression of various regulatory genes appears to differentiate the two types.[35] The process of biliary atresia is a dynamic one which may also involve the intrahepatic bile ducts,[36,37] and result in progressive fibrosis[38] even after Kasai surgery.[39]

Liver biopsy shows cholestasis and portal tract changes resembling those of large bile-duct obstruction in the adult (**see Ch. 5**). Portal tracts are enlarged by oedema and fibrosis

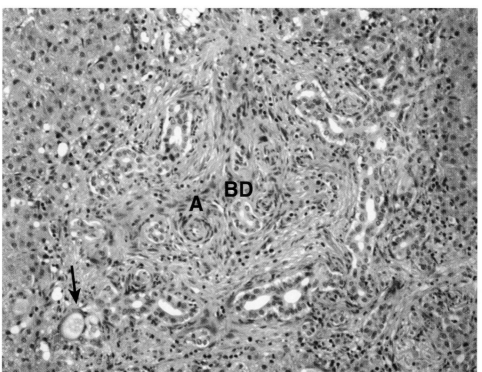

Figure 13.3
Extrahepatic biliary atresia.
The portal tract shows the characteristic diagnostic changes of fibrosis and prominent ductular reaction, with numerous proliferated bile ductular structures circumferentially surrounding the tract. Focal bile ductular cholestasis is evident (arrow). Note the intact hepatic arteriole (A) and similar-calibre bile duct (BD) at the centre of the tract. (Needle biopsy, H&E.)

(which varies depending on the age at biopsy), a striking ductular reaction and infiltrating neutrophils with fewer chronic inflammatory cells (**Fig. 13.3**). Native interlobular bile ducts are usually intact and can be identified near hepatic arterioles. Bile-containing portal macrophages are often also present. Ductular structures may contain inspissated bile ('ductular cholestasis') (**Fig. 13.3**) and occasionally resemble the embryonic bile-duct plate described by Jörgensen[40] (**Figs 13.4, 13.5**). A prominent ductular reaction is the major histological point of distinction from neonatal hepatitis.[41] There is panlobular cholestasis with accentuation in zone 3. Giant cells are common, but not as numerous or as striking as in neonatal hepatitis. The lobular architecture remains intact, except in patients diagnosed late in the disease who may then show secondary biliary cirrhosis (**see Fig. 5.11**). Overall, the most reliable diagnostic features that predict the presence of biliary atresia are the combination of ductular reaction, portal fibrosis and absence of sinusoidal fibrosis.[42] α_1-Antitrypsin deficiency and total parenteral nutrition cause identical changes[42] and therefore require appropriate exclusion before rendering a pathological diagnosis of biliary atresia.

Paucity of intrahepatic bile ducts in childhood

Two varieties of intrahepatic bile duct paucity (formerly called intrahepatic biliary atresia) are recognised in childhood: **syndromatic** and **non-syndromatic**.[43] In syndromatic paucity[44,45] (Alagille syndrome or ALGS, arteriohepatic dysplasia), loss of small intrahepatic bile ducts is associated with abnormal facies, vertebral anomalies and various other malformations. The pathogenesis is linked to mutations in the *Jagged 1* gene that produce a structurally abnormal ligand for binding to the Notch 1 receptor which is involved in cell–cell interactions in differentiation and the development of intrahepatic bile ducts.[46,47,47a]

**Figure 13.4
Extrahepatic biliary
atresia with
bile-duct plate-like
structures.**
The proliferating
bile-duct structures
in this case resemble
the embryonic
bile-duct plate.
(Wedge biopsy, H&E.)

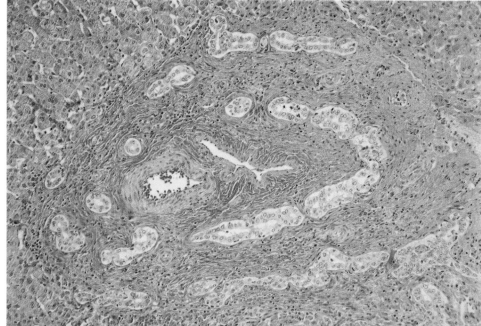

**Figure 13.5
Extrahepatic biliary
atresia with
bile-duct plate-like
structures.**
The field shown in
Fig. 13.4 stained
with antibodies to
cytokeratin
highlights the
circumferential portal
bile-duct structures
resembling the
embryonic bile-duct
plate. (Wedge
biopsy, specific
immunoperoxidase.)

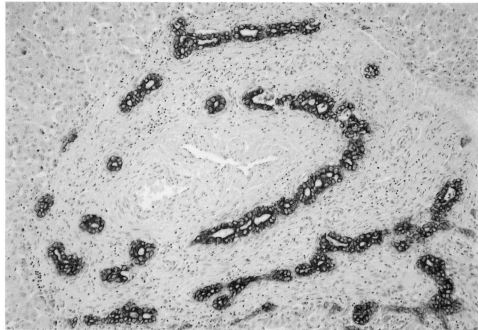

There is associated impairment of branching and elongation of hilar ducts distally into the liver periphery.[48] Increased mortality in these patients is linked to the presence of intracardiac congenital heart disease.[49] In non-syndromatic paucity, duct loss is not associated with facial or other anomalies. In some patients it may be related to a definable cause such as α_1-antitrypsin deficiency or cytomegalovirus infection,[50] while in others there is

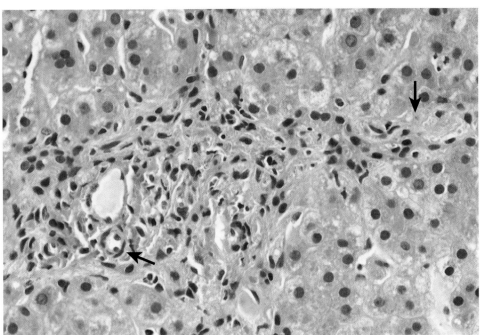

**Figure 13.6
Paucity of bile
ducts in childhood.**
The portal tract
shows an artery (left
arrow) but no
corresponding bile
duct of similar
calibre. There is
periportal cholestasis
(right arrow). (Needle
biopsy, H&E.)

no detectable aetiological factor. The exact time of onset of bile-duct injury is difficult to establish accurately and probably varies from case to case. Some patients have active destruction of ducts in the first few weeks of life[45] and later stabilise, potentially with few symptoms or only mild chronic cholestasis, into young adulthood. In others, cirrhosis and liver failure may develop within months or many years later.[51] It has been speculated that there may be a small subgroup of patients with non-syndromatic paucity in which chole-static disease first presents in adulthood[51] ('**idiopathic adulthood ductopenia**').[52]

Histologically, in both forms of intrahepatic duct paucity there is canalicular cholestasis and chronic periportal cholestasis. Portal tracts show a variable degree of fibrosis and small bile ducts are scanty or absent[53] (**Fig. 13.6**). Step sections and cytokeratin 7 or 19 immu-nostaining may be needed for thorough assessment of duct numbers which, as in primary biliary cirrhosis, should approximately correspond to the number of arteries of similar size. A ductular reaction is usually not a prominent feature, in contrast to extrahepatic biliary atresia.[54] Immunohistochemical staining for clusters of differentiation marker CD10 (neutral endopeptidase) is normally identified on bile canaliculi, but is absent before the age of 24 months and also in Alagille's syndrome,[55] which can be helpful when used in the appropriate clinical setting. Inflammation is often slight or even absent, but lymphoid aggregates may be seen in the place of bile ducts (**Fig. 13.7**). Secondary biliary cirrhosis develops in some patients.[51,56] α_1-Antitrypsin deficiency should be looked for in all patients with paucity of ducts. Duct paucity has also been described in association with Langerhans' cell histiocytosis.[57,58] As primary sclerosing cholangitis can also present in childhood,[59] it should be considered in the differential diagnosis.

Fibropolycystic diseases

The term fibropolycystic diseases covers a number of congenital abnormalities involving bile ducts, many of them related to an abnormal remodelling of the embryonic 'bile-duct plate'.[60–70] They include congenital hepatic fibrosis, Caroli's disease (congenital dilatation

**Figure 13.7
Paucity of bile
ducts in childhood.**
A lymphoid
aggregate is present
at the former site of
the bile duct.
(Needle biopsy, H&E.)

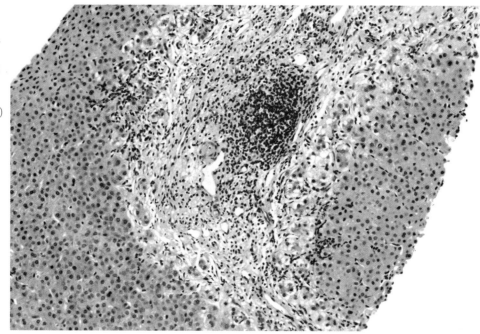

of the intrahepatic bile ducts), microhamartoma (von Meyenburg complex), choledochal cyst,[70a] and both infantile and adult forms of polycystic disease. The first four of these carry an increased risk of carcinoma of the biliary tree.[71-74] The bile-duct plate, first seen at approximately 8 weeks of gestation, is a layer of primitive small cells encircling the portal tract mesenchyme (**Figs 13.4, 13.5**). Progressive involution of most of these cells, with acquisition of strong cytokeratin 7 and 19 positivity in those remaining, is the process by which mature interlobular bile ducts of the portal tracts are formed.[61-64] Persistence of portions of the ductal plate and abnormal remodelling (the 'ductal plate malformation' described by Jörgensen[40]) lead to ectatic and irregularly shaped bile ducts set in dense fibrous stroma, the basic histopathological feature common to all fibropolycystic diseases. Mutations in genes encoding proteins found on primary cilia of bile duct epithelium and resultant ciliary defects in mechanical, chemical and osmotic sensing underlie the characterisation of many of these diseases as **'ciliopathies'**.[65-68]

Congenital hepatic fibrosis

Congenital hepatic fibrosis is a recessively inherited condition, which presents as hepatomegaly or the effects of portal hypertension, usually in childhood but occasionally in adults.[75] Some cases have been associated with phosphomannose isomerase deficiency in which the resultant hypoglycosylation may affect remodelling of the bile-duct plate.[76] The liver is enlarged and very hard. Islands of normal liver parenchyma with unaltered vascular relationships are separated by broad and narrow septa of dense, mature fibrous tissue containing elongated or cystic spaces lined by regular biliary epithelium (**Fig. 13.8**). These represent cross-sections of the hollow structures constituting the ductal plate malformation. Two separate sets of duct-like structures can often be identified, one lying centrally in the septa, the other near the parenchyma. The lumens may contain inspissated bile. Portal-vein branches are small and inconspicuous in some cases. There is usually no cholestasis, necrosis, inflammation or hepatocellular regeneration. In older patients with

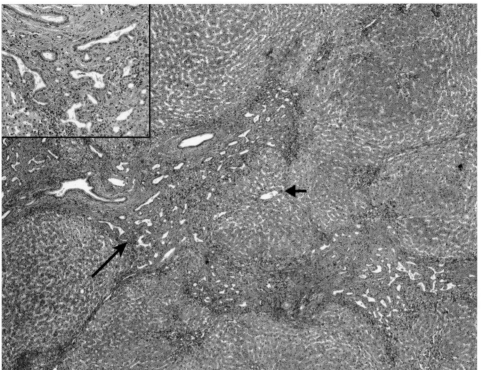

**Figure 13.8
Congenital
hepatic fibrosis.**
Several portal tracts
are interconnected
by bridging fibrous
septa containing
ductal-plate
malformations. The
fibrosis surrounds
normal parenchyma
with a terminal
venule (short arrow)
preserved in a
central position.
Inset: Higher
magnification of the
abnormal duct
structures seen at
lower left (long
arrow). (Explant liver,
H&E.)

congenital hepatic fibrosis, the abnormal duct-like structures may be less apparent because of atrophy.

Congenital hepatic fibrosis must be differentiated from cirrhosis, in which there is nodular regeneration and often inflammation and necrosis, and in which the abnormal biliary channels are not seen. The shape of the parenchymal islands in congenital hepatic fibrosis is very similar to that seen in secondary biliary cirrhosis (**see Fig. 5.11**). In this condition the septa contain irregular, newly proliferated bile ducts rather than congenitally abnormal plates; the connective tissue of the septa is loose and inflamed and there may be cholestatic features. Histological cholangitis, other types of inflammation or cholestasis in a liver with the characteristic features of congenital hepatic fibrosis should raise the possibility of coexisting Caroli's disease. The combination constitutes Caroli's syndrome.

Caroli's disease (congenital dilatation of the intrahepatic bile ducts)

This cystic malformation can affect different parts of the intrahepatic biliary tree and is seen alone or in combination with other congenital abnormalities, notably congenital hepatic fibrosis.[77] Because the cysts communicate with the rest of the biliary tree, there is a risk of ascending bacterial infection. Liver biopsy then shows the changes of cholangitis, with or without associated congenital hepatic fibrosis. The lesion of Caroli's disease must be distinguished from the acquired cholangiectases sometimes found in primary sclerosing cholangitis.[78]

Microhamartoma

Microhamartomas (von Meyenburg complexes, bile-duct malformations) are rounded nodules closely related to portal tracts, containing multiple biliary channels lined by

Figure 13.9 Microhamartoma. A cluster of duct-like structures with irregular contours and focal dilatations is seen in a portal tract. Note resemblance to congenital hepatic fibrosis, shown in **Fig. 13.8**. (Wedge biopsy, H&E.)

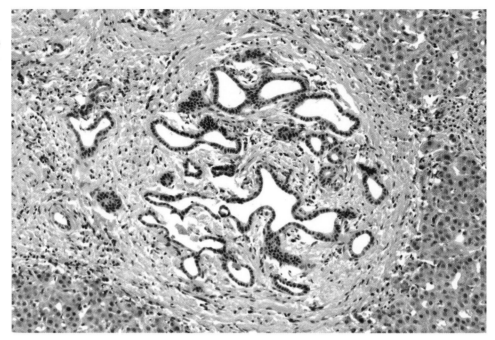

regular epithelium and set in a stroma of dense fibrous tissue (**Fig. 13.9**). They may be grossly visible on the liver surface as white nodules 1–2 mm across. The lumens of the biliary structures sometimes contain inspissated bile. Serial sectioning shows that they are interconnected.[79] Microhamartomas are usually found incidentally and do not normally give rise to symptoms or abnormalities of liver function. They are often multiple, in which case they may very occasionally be associated with portal hypertension; distinction from congenital hepatic fibrosis is then difficult. Multiple lesions may be mistaken for metastatic tumour.[80] If a small nodule on the liver surface is seen during surgery, frozen section may occasionally be requested in order to exclude metastatic carcinoma. The irregularly dilated duct structures, inspissated bile and circumscription seen in microhamartomas are helpful in making this distinction.

Polycystic disease

The infantile type of polycystic disease is regularly associated with renal involvement.[61,81] Portal tracts contain multiple cystic channels set in a fibrous stroma. In the adult type the cysts are lined by epithelium of biliary type (**Fig. 13.10**) but are not connected with the rest of the biliary tree. Solitary congenital cysts are histologically similar. The cuboidal or flattened epithelial lining helps distinguish these cysts from **ciliated hepatic foregut cysts** which are lined by ciliated cells and mucin-secreting goblet cells.[82] The presence of micro-hamartomas and features of Caroli's disease in individuals with polycystic disease favours a continuum in the expression of fibropolycystic disease.[83–85]

Inherited metabolic disorders

Cystic fibrosis

Cystic fibrosis is an inherited disease in which abnormally viscous exocrine secretions are present in the pancreas, salivary glands, alimentary tract and lungs. Liver disease is present

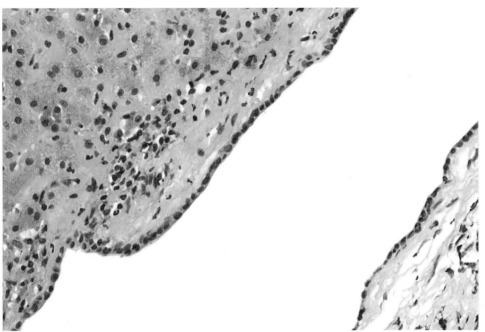

Figure 13.10
Cystic liver.
A cyst (top left) is lined by a single layer of low cuboidal epithelium. (Wedge biopsy, H&E.)

in up to 10% of children but is very uncommon in adults with cystic fibrosis.[86-88] Jaundice in the neonatal period has been attributed to bile-duct obstruction by abnormally viscous bile and to gastrointestinal obstruction by meconium. Intercurrent hepatitis may also be responsible. Steatosis is common, although not always related to malnutrition.[89] Paucity of intrahepatic bile ducts in cystic fibrosis has also been reported.[90] In a proportion of older children a characteristic lesion of intrahepatic bile ducts is found.[91] Dense plugs of PAS-positive material are seen within dilated, proliferated ducts (**Fig. 13.11**). Bile-duct cells may undergo degeneration and necrosis.[89] There is surrounding fibrosis[92] and a variable degree of inflammatory infiltration which may be associated with abnormal intrahepatic ducts on cholangiography.[93] Eventually the fibrous areas may join, separating parenchymal islands. The term **focal biliary fibrosis** expresses the uneven involvement of the intrahepatic bile ducts in this process, with parts of the liver remaining unaffected. In some patients the disease evolves to secondary biliary cirrhosis.[91]

Storage disorders: general remarks

Inherited metabolic defects leading to the abnormal accumulation of lipids, proteins and carbohydrates in the liver are many and varied; for a full description of the morphological changes, reviews should be consulted.[94-96] Ishak[94] helpfully discusses the differential diagnosis of individual histological features. Liver biopsy is sometimes useful in diagnosis, though by no means always decisive. The following points are offered as practical suggestions for occasions when biopsy is contemplated in children suspected of having storage disorders.

1   Storage disorders can involve hepatocytes (e.g. glycogenoses, α_1-antitrypsin deficiency), macrophages (e.g. Gaucher's disease), or both (e.g. Niemann–Pick disease, mucopolysaccharidoses,[97] cholesterol ester storage disease). When Kupffer cells are involved, they may swell to the size of hepatocytes and their involvement may not at first be apparent; the use of stains other than H&E, especially PAS and trichrome stains, then usually makes the Kupffer-cell involvement obvious.

Figure 13.11 Cystic fibrosis. Proliferated bile ducts in an enlarged, fibrosed portal tract contain dense inspissated material (arrows). (Postmortem liver, H&E.)

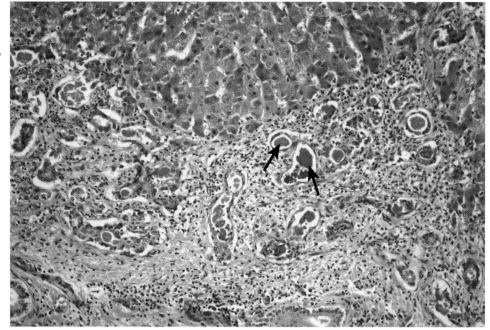

2 Suspicion of a possible storage disorder is one of the few indications for electron microscopy of part of the biopsy specimen as a diagnostic procedure, because characteristic ultrastructural appearances sometimes enable a correct diagnosis to be established quickly.[98] Even when the changes are not diagnostic they can direct attention to a particular group of diseases, and suggest the next line of investigation. Arrangements for electron microscopy should be made beforehand, so that part of the specimen can be put into the correct fixative without delay. In centres without facilities for electron microscopy, part of the specimen should still be correctly fixed and/or embedded, and sent to a referral centre later if light microscopic findings warrant this.

3 Arrangements should also be made to freeze part of the specimen and to store it in liquid nitrogen for possible biochemical analysis and histochemical staining of frozen sections. Speed is essential to avoid loss of enzyme activity. Again, a specialist centre may need to be consulted, because few centres or pathologists have the necessary expertise to investigate the rarer metabolic diseases.

Many inherited metabolic diseases affect the liver and several may lead to **cirrhosis**[94] (glycogenosis types III, IV and VI, galactosaemia, tyrosinaemia type I, α_1-antitrypsin deficiency, Wilson's disease, hereditary haemochromatosis). Liver transplantation may be indicated in some patients.[27,99,100] The discussion in this chapter will be limited primarily to the disorders mentioned under point 1 above. Haemochromatosis and Wilson's disease are described in **Chapter 14**.

Glycogen storage diseases (glycogenoses)

Most forms of glycogen storage disease involve the liver.[101,102] In type I glycogenosis (von Gierke's disease), fat and glycogen accumulate in the cytoplasm of hepatocytes. These appear swollen, pale-staining and sometimes vacuolated with H&E and have centrally placed nuclei (**Fig. 13.12**). Mallory–Denk bodies may be found in the cytoplasm.[103] The abundant glycogen displaces the organelles of affected cells to the periphery, giving them

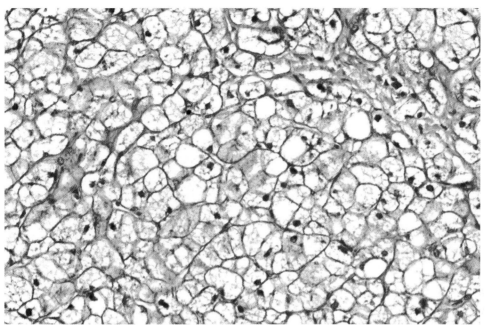

Figure 13.12 Glycogenosis. In this example of type I glycogen storage disease, hepatocytes are swollen and resemble plant cells. (Wedge biopsy, H&E.)

a plant-cell-like appearance. Some liver-cell nuclei also contain glycogen. Sinusoids are compressed. The overall appearance has been described as a uniform mosaic pattern.[101] Slender periportal fibrous scars often develop. Hepatocellular adenomas[104,105] or even, rarely, carcinomas[106] may develop. Rapid fixation in buffered formal saline usually enables abundant glycogen to be demonstrated in hepatocytes in paraffin sections, but it should be noted that the diagnosis does not rest only on the demonstration of glycogen, which is plentiful in normal liver. Features closely resembling type I glycogenosis can be seen in poorly controlled diabetics with **Mauriac syndrome** and **glycogenic hepatopathy (see Ch. 7)**.

In type II glycogenosis (Pompe's disease), the highly soluble storage material is contained in enlarged lysosomes, visible as vacuoles in hepatocytes and Kupffer cells by light microscopy. Many other tissues are involved. Type III glycogenosis has been subdivided into several biochemical subtypes. Histological appearances are like those of type I, but fat is less abundant and there may be fibrosis or cirrhosis.[107] Type IV (amylopectinosis) is characterised by abnormal glycogen in the form of well-defined cytoplasmic inclusions in hepatocytes[108] **(see Ch. 4)**. The glycogen is only incompletely removed by diastase digestion. The inclusions have a ground-glass appearance and must be distinguished from hepatitis B virus surface antigen and other similar cytoplasmic inclusions[109] **(see Fig. 4.4 and Box 4.1)**. In other types of glycogenosis there is often much variation in the degree of hepatocellular swelling in different areas, in contrast to the regular distribution of the changes in type I.[101]

α_1-Antitrypsin deficiency

Individuals with decreased levels of the serum protease inhibitor α_1-antitrypsin (α_1-antitrypsin deficiency) may present with liver disease as neonates (neonatal cholestasis), in adolescence or in adulthood, even beyond 60 years of age.[110–112] There are over 100 different alleles of the α_1-antitrypsin (AAT) gene,[113] two of which determine an individual's phenotype. The most common phenotype, PiMM, is associated with normal serum levels of AAT. Individuals with heterozygous (PiMZ) and homozygous (PiZZ) deficiency have

Figure 13.13
α₁-Antitrypsin
deficiency.

Hepatocytes near a
portal tract (PT)
contain many
magenta globules of
different sizes.
(Explant liver,
diastase–PAS.)

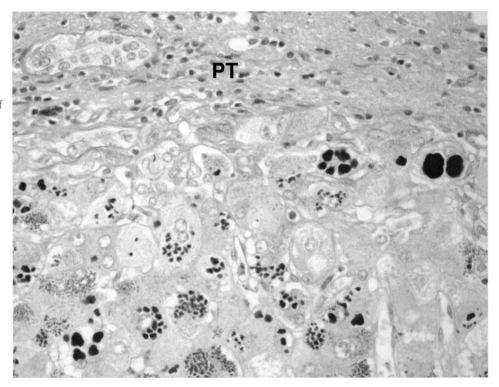

moderately and profoundly reduced serum levels of AAT, respectively. The accumulation of characteristic PAS-positive, diastase-resistant globules in the hepatocytes of AAT-deficient individuals (**Fig. 13.13**) is based on a structural change in the glycoprotein which is encoded by the mutant Z gene.[114] An amino acid substitution (lysine for glutamic acid at position 342) results in abnormal folding and polymerisation[115] of the protein and failure of both its secretion from the endoplasmic reticulum[114] and its subsequent degradation. In this regard AAT deficiency is conceptually similar to Alzheimer's and Parkinson's diseases, where inclusions result from conformational disorders of serine proteases ('serpinopathies').[116]

The globules of AAT which accumulate range from less than 1 μm to 10 μm or more in diameter. They are mainly found in periportal hepatocytes, a similar distribution to the much smaller granules of copper-associated protein and haemosiderin, from which they need to be distinguished. In doubtful cases, immunohistochemical staining enables AAT to be identified with certainty (**Fig. 13.14**). Moreover, immunohistochemical staining is more sensitive than diastase–PAS positivity, and is helpful when diastase–PAS-positive globules are scanty or unevenly distributed. Conversely, immunohistochemically positive material is found in some patients without the genetic deficiency, usually with a panlobular or perivenular rather than a periportal distribution,[117,118] and particularly in livers with sinusoidal congestion and hypoxia.[119] From a practical point of view, it is wise to regard the presence of diastase-resistant PAS-positive globules in periportal liver cells as evidence for α₁-antitrypsin deficiency until proved otherwise.[120] Intracellular AAT globules have been vividly demonstrated in a transgenic mouse model of the disease.[121]

Some children with homozygous AAT deficiency develop neonatal cholestasis. Histological changes include a ductular reaction and fibrosis, but the typical globules may not be seen until the age of 3 or 4 months.[122] The subsequent course varies: many children improve, while others develop a chronic cholestatic syndrome with paucity of bile ducts

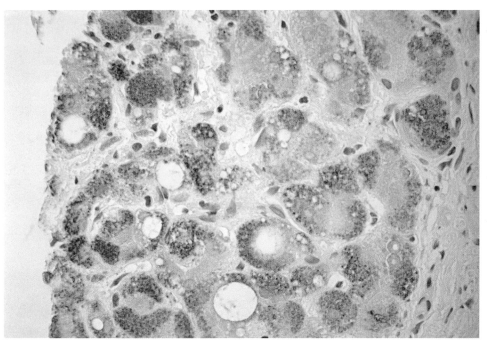

Figure 13.14 α₁-Antitrypsin deficiency. Periportal hepatocytes contain numerous globules of α₁-antitrypsin, stained brown by the immunoperoxidase method. Typically, each globule is stained around the perimeter, with a central unstained region. (Needle biopsy, specific immunoperoxidase.)

or cirrhosis.[18,112,123] Cirrhosis in children with AAT deficiency often has 'biliary' features, such as a ductular reaction and partial preservation of lobular architecture.

Adults carrying two Z alleles present with pulmonary emphysema or liver disease, but may also be symptom-free and healthy. Liver biopsy may show little apart from the PAS-positive globules, or varying degrees of fibrosis. Cirrhosis develops in approximately one-third of homozygotes[113] and is either inactive or shows features of chronic hepatitis. An increased prevalence of hepatitis B and C viral infections in AAT deficiency may contribute to this picture.[124] The characteristic globules are found predominantly in periportal or periseptal hepatocytes. They are seen most easily in sections stained with diastase–PAS, phosphotungstic acid–haematoxylin or specific immunoperoxidase, but are also seen in trichrome preparations and, when large and abundant, are faintly visible with H&E. Similar globules are seen in some hepatocellular carcinomas in patients with or without the Z allele.[125,126] Furthermore, an increased risk of hepatocellular carcinoma has been reported in male patients with AAT deficiency.[127] Chronic hepatitis, cirrhosis, large-cell liver-cell dysplasia and hepatocellular carcinoma may also be seen in heterozygous (PiMZ) AAT deficiency[128] and in individuals with other allelic variants such as Mmalton.[129–131]

Brief mention should be made of several other endoplasmic reticulum inclusions found in hepatocytes in patients who may have chronic hepatitis or cirrhosis. Diastase–PAS-negative periportal granules of α₁-antichymotrypsin can be identified by specific immuno-histochemical staining in **partial α₁-antichymotrypsin deficiency.**[132,133] In **fibrinogen storage disease** there are diastase–PAS-negative intracellular pale inclusions resembling ground-glass hepatocytes.[132,134]

Gaucher's disease (glycosyl ceramide lipidosis)

Cerebrosides accumulate in Kupffer cells and portal macrophages, which are enlarged, moderately diastase–PAS-positive and have a finely striated appearance (**Fig. 13.15**). The affected cells compress hepatocytes and sinusoids and may give rise to portal hypertension. Pericellular fibrosis is a common finding.[135]

Figure 13.15
Gaucher's disease.
Pale-staining, striated Kupffer cells containing stored lipid are present within sinusoids. (Wedge biopsy, H&E.)

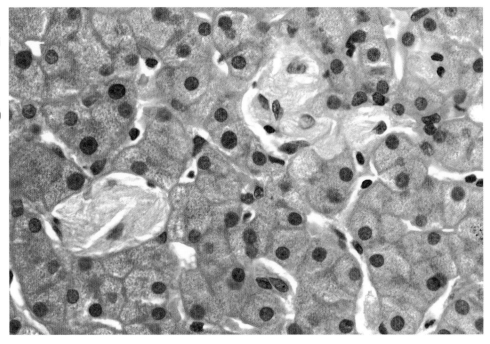

Niemann–Pick disease (sphingomyelin lipidosis)

There are several variants of Niemann–Pick disease, and the clinical features range from severe and fatal neurological disease in infancy to symptomless hepatosplenomegaly in adults. The typical morphological feature of this disorder is the accumulation of sphingo-myelin in both hepatocytes and macrophages. The latter are greatly swollen, foamy and diastase–PAS-positive to a variable extent. They can readily be distinguished from glycogen-rich liver cells in sections stained by the PAS method (**Fig. 13.16**). In addition to sphingomyelin, portal phagocytes, especially in the adult form, may also contain a brown lipofuscin-like pigment; these, as well as similar cells in bone marrow, stain a sea-blue colour by the Giemsa method. Niemann–Pick disease is thus one cause of the so-called sea-blue histiocyte syndrome.[136] Type B Niemann–Pick disease may progress to cirrhosis.[100,137]

Wolman's disease and cholesterol ester storage disease

In these apparently related conditions – the first a severe and usually fatal disease of infants, the second a milder disease of older children – cholesterol esters accumulate in hepatocytes and macrophages.[138,139] Hepatocytes also contain much triglyceride. The diag-nosis may be suspected from the bright-orange colour of the liver biopsy core. By light microscopy, hepatocytes show microvesicular steatosis, and macrophages are enlarged and foamy.[140] Crystalline deposits may be seen within affected cells, particularly in frozen sec-tions. The excess lipid is birefringent. Other features which may be found include ductular proliferation, pericellular fibrosis and even cirrhosis.[139]

Galactosaemia

Severe fatty change appears early in children with an inherited deficiency of galactose-1-phosphate uridyl transferase. Ductular reaction and cholestasis may also be present. Within

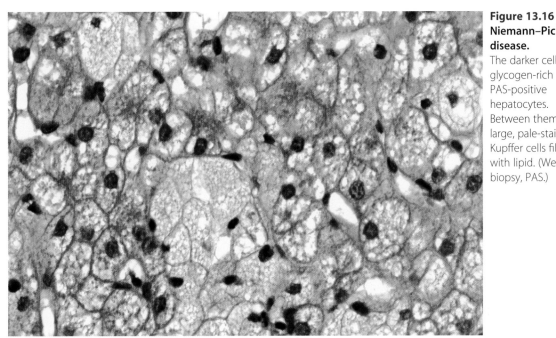

**Figure 13.16
Niemann–Pick
disease.**
The darker cells are
glycogen-rich
PAS-positive
hepatocytes.
Between them are
large, pale-staining
Kupffer cells filled
with lipid. (Wedge
biopsy, PAS.)

a few weeks, liver-cell plates become transformed into tubular, duct-like structures (cholestatic rosettes) which dominate the histological picture, and there is siderosis and extramedullary haemopoiesis. Fibrosis and cirrhosis then develop. Institution of a galactose-free diet may result in substantial histological improvement.[141]

Histologically, the differential diagnosis includes **hereditary fructose intolerance**, in which the changes are somewhat similar but less severe. Also similar but more severe are the histological changes of **tyrosinaemia**. In this condition adenoma-like nodules are often seen, containing much fat.[94,95] Siderosis is also prominent. Hepatocellular carcinoma can develop, particularly in children over the age of 2 years, and liver transplantation is an important therapeutic option to forestall this event.[142]

Disorders of ureagenesis

Deficiencies in enzymes of the urea cycle, including ornithine transcarbamylase and carbamyl-phosphate synthase, may produce fatal hyperammonaemia in children and, rarely, in adults.[143] In these disorders the liver shows microvesicular steatosis which may be accompanied by aggregates of clear hepatocytes (**focal glycogenosis**[144]) (**Fig. 13.17**). These glycogen-enriched regions stain brightly with PAS and are diagnostically helpful in excluding other causes of paediatric microvesicular fatty liver such as Reye's syndrome (see below).

Reye's syndrome

This is a serious and often fatal condition of encephalopathy and fatty change in the viscera of children under the age of 18 years. Viral infections (influenza B or A, varicella), salicylate ingestion and endotoxaemia have been implicated in the pathogenesis.[145–147] The incidence of Reye's syndrome declined throughout the 1980s, parallel with a decrease in the use of salicylates for childhood viral illnesses. Rarely, it is still seen in some parts of the world.[148,149]

Figure 13.17
Focal glycogenosis.
Two foci of glycogen-containing hepatocytes with clear cytoplasm are seen near the portal tract. The patient had undergone partial hepatectomy for metastatic adenocarcinoma. In individuals with deficiencies of urea cycle enzymes, this lesion is accompanied by microvesicular steatosis. (Partial hepatectomy, H&E.)

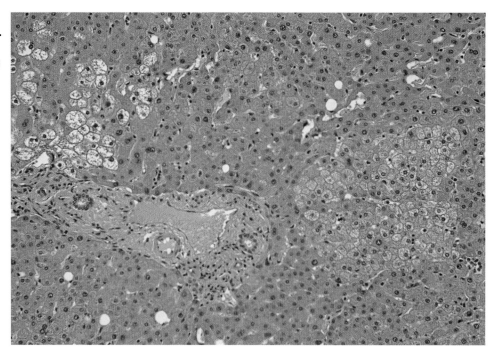

Liver biopsy is an important part of the investigation. The specimen is abnormally pale or yellow on naked-eye examination, and on light microscopy there is fine-droplet fatty change. This is panlobular in distribution and may be difficult to see without specific staining for fat, because of the small size of the vacuoles. Droplets are smaller in perivenular regions than elsewhere. Necrosis and inflammation are usually slight or absent, but in a few patients there is periportal ballooning or necrosis of hepatocytes.[150,151] Electron microscopy shows characteristic degenerative changes in liver-cell mitochondria; these are swollen and irregular in shape, with flocculent, electron-lucent matrix and reduced numbers of granules.[152] Succinic dehydrogenase activity is reduced. The differential diagnosis includes other conditions with microvesicular fat such as drug hepatotoxicity, urea cycle defects and mitochondrial hepatopathies associated with respiratory chain[153] and fatty acid oxidation defects.[4]

Parenteral nutrition

The effects of parenteral nutrition have been briefly mentioned in **Chapters 7 and 8**. It is pertinent to note here that in infants **cholestasis** is the major lesion associated with parenteral nutrition[154,155]; this may occasion diagnostic difficulties when other causes of cholestasis such as sepsis or biliary obstruction are also under clinical consideration. These difficulties are compounded by the fact that with prolonged administration of parenteral nutrition the portal tracts show progressive changes which are very similar to those of bile-duct obstruction and biliary atresia (**Fig. 13.18**). A ductular reaction may be present after 3 weeks of parenteral nutrition,[156] followed by portal fibrosis at 8–12 weeks and cirrhosis after 12 weeks.[157] Correlation of biopsy features with detailed clinical information regarding the duration of parenteral nutrition is clearly paramount in establishing the cause of jaundice in this population. Steatosis is less common in infants than in older children and adults who receive parenteral nutrition.[158] Even after parenteral nutrition is discontinued, steatosis as well as portal fibrosis may persist.[159]

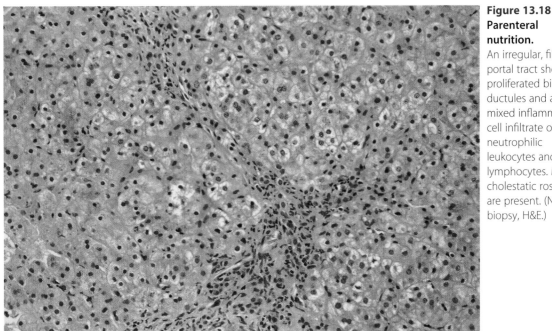

Figure 13.18 Parenteral nutrition.
An irregular, fibrotic portal tract shows proliferated bile ductules and a mixed inflammatory cell infiltrate of neutrophilic leukocytes and lymphocytes. Many cholestatic rosettes are present. (Needle biopsy, H&E.)

Hyperbilirubinaemias

In **Gilbert's syndrome**, a common form of familial unconjugated hyperbilirubinaemia (the most common hereditary hyperbilirubinaemia affecting approximately 5–10% of Caucasians),[160-162] the liver is histologically normal by light microscopy except for increased hepatocellular lipofuscin. In the **Dubin–Johnson syndrome**, in which the serum bilirubin is mainly conjugated, canalicular excretion of bilirubin and some other organic substances is defective[163] because of a mutation in the gene for canalicular multispecific-organic-anion transporter.[161,164] Other constituents of bile are excreted normally and there is no cholestasis. A complex dark brown pigment accumulates in hepatocytes, especially in perivenular areas, giving the liver a dark, speckled appearance to the naked eye. The pigment granules somewhat resemble normal lipofuscin pigment and occupy a similar pericanalicular site in hepatocytes, but are darker, more abundant, larger and more variable in size (**Fig. 13.19**). When the pigment is very abundant, its pericanalicular location is no longer evident. Simple histochemical characteristics such as PAS-positivity and acid-fastness do not reliably distinguish between Dubin–Johnson pigment and lipofuscin because both stain variably (**see Table 3.1**), but the distinction is usually clear on the basis of the above morphological features. When there is doubt, this may be resolved by electron microscopy, which shows the Dubin–Johnson pigment granules to be composed of characteristic strands of electron-dense material in an electron-lucent background, together with scanty lipid droplets (**see Fig. 17.2**).

Inherited cholestatic syndromes

Consideration of this group of disorders should be prompted when bland canalicular or canalicular and hepatocellular cholestasis with or without giant-cell transformation are the predominant histological features. This picture may develop owing to a variety of

Figure 13.19 Dubin–Johnson syndrome.
Hepatocytes contain abundant coarse, dark-brown pigment granules. (Needle biopsy, H&E.)

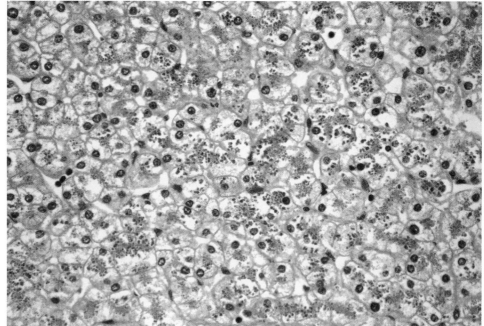

mutations of bile transport proteins or inborn errors of bile acid synthesis. The morphological assessment should take into account not only the presence or absence of giant cells, but also whether native bile ducts are injured or absent and whether a mild ductular reaction and/or portal/periportal fibrosis or cirrhosis are present, since such features may help to distinguish among aetiologies.[1] Electron microscopy to assess the appearance of the bile and immunohistochemical staining to evaluate preservation or absence of specific bile transport proteins (e.g. bile-salt export pump (BSEP),[165] multidrug resistance protein 3 (MDR3)[166]) provide additional diagnostic information.

The cholestatic group of diseases termed **progressive familial intrahepatic cholestasis (PFIC)** – currently subdivided into three types: PFIC-1, -2, and -3 – are autosomal recessive disorders in which gene mutations result in defective bile-salt transporter proteins on the canalicular membrane[164,166–173] (**Table 13.2**). Affected infants have jaundice, pruritus and intrahepatic cholestasis which may progress to cirrhosis early, or in later childhood. An unusually low or normal serum gamma glutamyl transferase (GGT) level should raise the possibility of PFIC type 1 or 2 (**Table 13.2**). The best known of these is **PFIC-1 (Byler disease)**, which was originally described in kindred of the Amish settler Jacob Byler.[169] PFIC-1 is caused by mutations in *ATP8B1* (chromosome 18q21–q22) that encode FIC-1 protein, which is expressed on bile canaliculi and intestinal epithelium. In **PFIC-2 (Byler syndrome)**, there are mutations in *ABCB11* (chromosome 2q24.3-2q31.1) which encode BSEP, which is selectively expressed on bile canaliculi. The presence of normal to low levels of serum γ-glutamyl transferase relative to the degree of cholestasis is an important diagnostic feature of both PFIC types 1 and 2. The bland bile canalicular cholestasis of PFIC-1 (**Fig. 13.20**) contrasts with the features of 'neonatal hepatitis' (giant cells, inflammation, lobular disturbance) and progressive periportal fibrosis seen in PFIC-2 (**Fig. 13.21**). Electron microscopy shows distinctive coarsely granular bile in PFIC-1 (Byler disease) and filamentous or amorphous bile in PFIC-2 (BSEP deficiency; Byler syndrome)[169] (**see Fig. 17.11**). Portal fibrosis, ductular reaction and cirrhosis eventually develop in PFIC-2, sometimes in very young infants less than a year of age.[168] Hepatocellular carcinoma[165,165a] and

Table 13.2 Histological features of progressive familial intrahepatic cholestasis (PFIC)

Disorder	Liver histopathology
(Synonyms)	(Serum GGT level)
Gene/protein	
PFIC-1 (Byler disease) (FIC-1 deficiency) ATB8B1/FIC-1	Bland canalicular cholestasis Giant cell-transformation uncommon Little or no ductular reaction Occasional paucity of intrahepatic bile ducts (late) Slower progression than PFIC-2 Coarse bile ('Byler bile') on electron microscopy (**Low or normal GGT**)

PFIC-2
(Byler syndrome)
(BSEP deficiency)
ABCB11/BSEP
	Bile canalicular and hepatocellular cholestasis (zone 3>zone1)
	Giant-cell transformation common
	Greater lobular disturbance than PFIC-1
	Perivenular, pericellular and periportal fibrosis with progression to cirrhosis
	    (sometimes <1 year of age)
	Mild ductular reaction (later)
	Occasional interlobular bile-duct paucity (later)
	Hepatocellular carcinoma and cholangiocarcinoma have been reported
	Recurrent cholestasis after liver transplant in some who develop IgG
	    anti-BSEP antibodies
	Negative immunostain for BSEP
	Hepatocellular carcinomas and cholangiocarcinomas may develop as sequelae
	(**Low or normal GGT**)

PFIC-3 (MDR3 deficiency) ABCB4/MDR3	Hepatocellular cholestasis with occasional canalicular and ductular cholestasis Ductular reaction prominent (resembles biliary obstruction) Portal/periportal fibrosis with cirrhosis Negative immunostain for MDR3 (**High GGT**)

BSEP, bile-salt export pump; GGT, gamma glutamyl transferase; MDR3, multidrug resistance protein 3.

cholangiocarcinoma[174] are other reported sequelae. Many PFIC-1 patients develop graft steatosis after liver transplantation, possibly because of the continued expression of dysfunctional FIC-1 protein on intestinal epithelium.[175,176] Steatohepatitis with cirrhosis are additional complications.[177] **PFIC-3** is associated with mutations in the *ABCB4* gene (chromosome 7q21.1) which encodes MDR3. Biopsy shows bile canalicular cholestasis (occasionally with hepatocellular and/or ductular cholestasis), portal fibrosis and prominent ductular reaction and progression to a biliary-type cirrhosis.[168]

Episodic cholestasis is seen in two subtypes of **benign recurrent intrahepatic cholestasis (BRIC)**.[178] Subtype 1 shows a gene mutation mapped to *ATP8B1* on chromosome 18 (as in PFIC-1) and subtype 2 has a mutation in the *ABCB11* gene (also the target in PFIC-2).[179] Affected patients have multiple attacks of jaundice and itching, often starting in childhood or early adult life[164,166,180] and often triggered by a minor viral infection. Histologically, canalicular cholestasis is seen in attacks, usually unaccompanied by any substantial degree of inflammation (**Fig. 13.22**). Between attacks the liver returns to normal and there is no fibrosis or progression to cirrhosis. A clinical continuum between BRIC and PFIC is suggested in some cases.[181]

Figure 13.20 Progressive familial intrahepatic cholestasis type 1 (PFIC-1) (Byler disease). Bland canalicular bile (arrows) is present, with relatively unperturbed parenchyma. (Needle biopsy, H&E.)

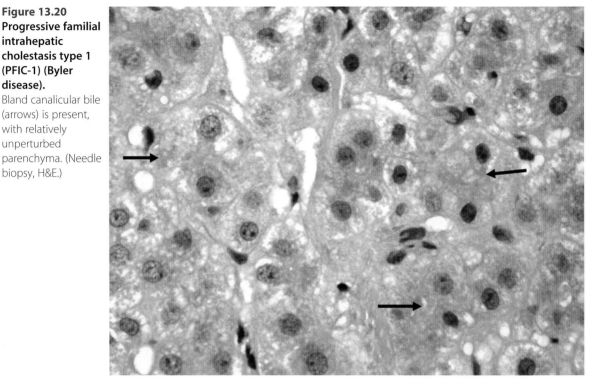

Additional congenital or familial cholestatic syndromes are described,[182] including Norwegian cholestasis, North American Indian cholestasis,[43,170] Navajo neurohepatopathy[3] and recurrent cholestasis in the Faeroe Islands.[183] Some children with microvillous inclusion disease (MVID) of the intestine also develop jaundice, pruritus and bile canalicular cholestasis with abnormally accentuated canalicular and cytoplasmic BSEP expression on immunostain as a result of inherent deficits in endosomal trafficking to epithelial cell membranes.[183a]

Cirrhosis in childhood

Children are susceptible to many of the causal cirrhotic agents affecting adults, including hepatitis virus infections. As already noted, several inherited metabolic disorders lead to cirrhosis, and the possibility of Wilson's disease should always be considered in a child with chronic liver disease. Cirrhosis in young women should raise the question of autoimmune hepatitis, either type I (with anti-actin antibodies) or type II (anti-liver–kidney microsomal antibodies)[184] (**see Ch. 9**). Rare familial forms of cirrhosis have been described.[185] Not infrequently, the aetiology of some forms of childhood cirrhosis is obscure, as for example in the cerebral degenerative disorder Alper's disease,[186] in which microvesicular fat is also present. Cryptogenic cirrhosis due to keratin mutations[187] is another consideration (**see Ch. 10**).

Indian childhood cirrhosis, a disease of high mortality affecting young Indian children (and occasionally reported from outside the Indian subcontinent[188–194]), greatly declined in incidence after the mid-1990s, when brass- and copper-containing vessels used for milk feeding were identified as sources of copper contamination.[195] The major features include

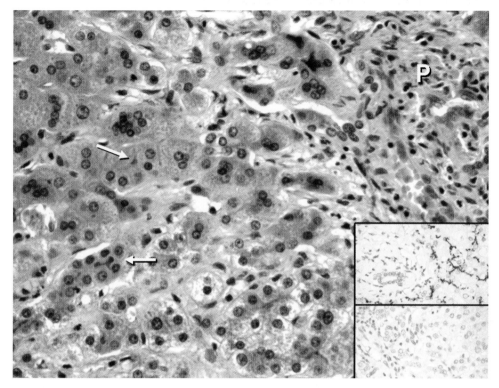

Figure 13.21 Progressive familial intrahepatic cholestasis type 2 (PFIC-2) (bile-salt export pump (BSEP) deficiency).
Cholestasis is present within bile canaliculi (arrows) and hepatocytes, accompanied by numerous multinucleated giant hepatocytes. The portal tract (P) shown is inflamed and fibrotic. Elsewhere in the specimen ductular reaction and developing cirrhosis were seen. (Explant liver, H&E.) Inset: Immunostain for BSEP shows strong bile canalicular positivity in the control (top), but absent staining in this specimen (below). (Explant liver, specific immunohistochemistry.)

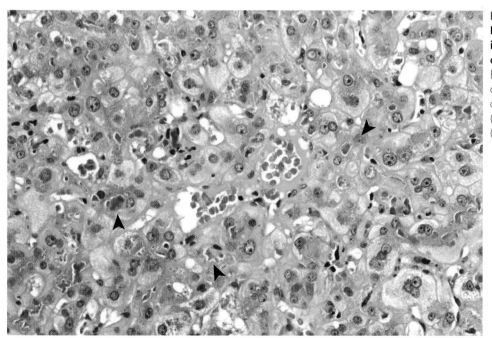

Figure 13.22 Benign recurrent intrahepatic cholestasis.
Bile canalicular cholestasis is diffusely prominent (arrowheads). (Needle biopsy, H&E.)

Figure 13.23
Indian childhood
cirrhosis.
Many liver cells are swollen (centre), and surrounded by fibrosis and mononuclear cells. Mallory–Denk bodies are present within some hepatocytes (arrow). Regenerating hepatocytes are organised into small clusters. (Postmortem liver, H&E.)

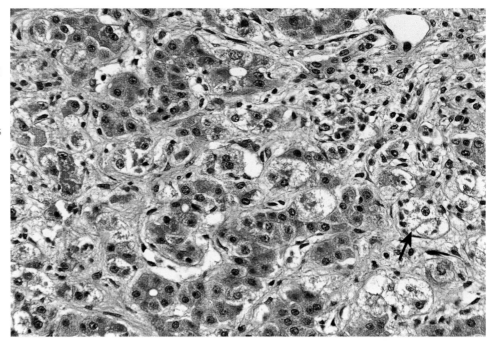

hepatocellular swelling at an early stage followed by ballooning, Mallory–Denk body formation and necrosis. Focal accumulations of neutrophils and pericellular fibrosis resemble steatohepatitis, but there is little or no fatty change (**Fig. 13.23**). Large amounts of copper and copper-associated protein accumulate in affected hepatocytes[196,197] and chelation therapy with D-penicillamine therapy is effective in some patients.[198] The small clusters of damaged hepatocytes surrounded by fibrosis eventually evolve to a cirrhosis characterised by very small nodules ('micro-micronodular cirrhosis').

References

1 Ovchinsky N, Moreira RK, Lefkowitch JH, et al. Liver biopsy in modern clinical practice: a pediatric point-of-view. Adv Anat Pathol 2012;19:250–62.

2 Balistreri WF, Bezerra JA, Jansen P, et al. Intrahepatic cholestasis: summary of an American Association for the Study of Liver Diseases Single-Topic Conference. Hepatology 2005;42:222–35.

3 Vu TH, Tanji K, Holve SA, et al. Navajo neurohepatopathy: a mitochondrial DNA depletion syndrome? Hepatology 2001;34:116–20.

4 Lee WS, Sokol RJ. Mitochondrial hepatopathies: advances in genetics and pathogenesis. Hepatology 2007;45:1555–65.

5 Jansen PLM, Sturm E. Genetic cholestasis, causes and consequences for hepatobiliary transport. Liver Int 2003;23:315–22.

6 Knisely AS, Mieli-Vergani G, Whitington PF. Neonatal hemochromatosis. Gastroenterol Clin North Am 2003;32:877–89.

7 Faa G, Liguori C, Columbano A, et al. Uneven copper distribution in the human newborn liver. Hepatology 1987;7:838–42.

8 Faa G, Sciot R, Farci AMG, et al. Iron concentration and distribution in the newborn liver. Liver 1994;14:193–9.

9 Bove KE, Daugherty CC, Tyson W, et al. Bile acid synthetic defects and liver disease. Pediatr Devel Pathol 2000;3:1–16.

10 Müller-Höcker J, Muntau A, Schäfer S, et al. Depletion of mitochondrial DNA in the liver of an infant with neonatal giant cell hepatitis. Hum Pathol 2002;33:247–53.

11 Karadimas CL, Vu TH, Holve SA, et al. Navajo neurohepatopathy is caused by a mutation in the *MPV17* gene. Am J Hum Gen 2006;79:544–8.

12 Spinazzola A, Santer R, Akman OH, et al. Hepatocerebral form of mitochondrial depletion syndrome. Novel MPV17 mutations. Arch Neurol 2008;65:1108–13.

13 El-Hattab AW, Li F-Y, Schmitt E, et al. *MPV17*-associated hepatocerebral mitochondrial DNA depletion syndrome: new patients and novel mutations. Mol Gen Metab 2010;99:300–8.

14 Labarthe F, Dobbelaere D, Devisme L, et al. Clinical, biochemical and morphological features of hepatocerebral syndrome with mitochondrial DNA depletion due to deoxyguanosine kinase deficiency. J Hepatol 2005;43:333–41.

15 Lee WS, Sokol RJ. Mitochondrial hepatopathies: advances in genetics, therapeutic approaches, and outcomes. J Peds 2013;163:942–8.

16 Fellman V, Kotarsky H. Mitochondrial hepatopathies in the newborn period. Semin Fetal Neonatal Med 2011;16:222–8.

17 Ruchelli ED, Uri A, Dimmick JE, et al. Severe perinatal liver disease and Down syndrome: an apparent relationship. Hum Pathol 1991;22:1274–80.

18 Hadchouel M, Gautier M. Histopathologic study of the liver in the early cholestatic phase of alpha-1-antitrypsin deficiency. J Pediatr 1976;89:211–15.

19 Perlmutter DH, Shepherd RW. Extrahepatic biliary atresia: a disease or a phenotype. Hepatology 2002;35: 1297–304.

20 Gautier M, Eliot N. Extrahepatic biliary atresia. Morphological study of 98 biliary remnants. Arch Pathol Lab Med 1981;105:397–402.

21 Chandra RS, Altman RP. Ductal remnants in extrahepatic biliary atresia: a histopathologic study with clinical correlation. J Pediatr 1978;93:196–200.

22 Gautier M, Jehan P, Odièvre M. Histologic study of biliary fibrous remnants in 48 cases of extrahepatic biliary atresia: correlation with postoperative bile flow restoration. J Pediatr 1976;89:704–9.

23 Haas JE. Bile duct and liver pathology in biliary atresia. World J Surg 1978;2:561–9.

24 Kasai M, Suzuki S. A new operation for 'non-correctable' biliary atresia. Shujitsu 1959;13:173–9.

25 Logan S, Stanton A. Screening for biliary atresia. Lancet 1993;342:256.

26 Chardot C, Buet C, Serinet M-O, et al. Iimproving outcomes of biliary atresia: French national series 1986–2009. J Hepatol 2013;58:1209–17.

27 Whitington PF, Balistreri WF. Liver transplantation in pediatrics: indications, contraindications, and pretransplant management. J Pediatr 1991;118:169–77.

28 Alvarez F. Is biliary atresia an immune mediated disease? J Hepatol 2013;59:648–50.

29 Cui S, Layva-Vega M, Tsai EA, et al. Evidence from human and zebrafish that *GPC1* is a biliary atresia susceptibility gene. Gastroenterology 2013;144:1107–15.

30 Chen L, Goryachev A, Sun J, et al. Altered expression of genes involved in hepatic morphogenesis and fibrogenesis are identified by cDNA microarray analysis in biliary atresia. Hepatology 2003;38:567–76.

31 Silveira TR, Salzano FM, Howard ER, et al. Congenital structural abnormalities in biliary atresia: evidence for etiopathogenic heterogeneity and therapeutic implications. Acta Paediatr Scand 1991;80:1192–9.

32 Fain JS, Lewin KJ. Intrahepatic biliary cysts in congenital biliary atresia. Arch Pathol Lab Med 1989;113:1383–6.

33 Schwarz KB, Haber BH, Rosenthal P, et al. Extrahepatic anomalies in infants with biliary atresia: results of a large prospective North American multicentre study. Hepatology 2013;58:1724–31.

34 Desai MS, Zainuer S, Kennedy C, et al. Cardiac structural and functional alterations in infants and children with biliary atresia, listed for liver transplantation. Gastroenterology 2011;141: 1264–72.

35 Zhang D-Y, Sabla G, Shivakumar P, et al. Coordinate expression of regulatory genes differentiates embryonic and perinatal forms of biliary atresia. Hepatology 2004;39:954–62.

36 Raweily EA, Gibson AAM, Burt AD. Abnormalities of intrahepatic bile ducts in extrahepatic biliary atresia. Histopathology 1990;17:521–7.

37 Nietgen GW, Vacanti JP, Perez-Atayde AR. Intrahepatic bile duct loss in biliary atresia despite portoenterostomy: a consequence of ongoing obstruction? Gastroenterology 1992;102:2126–33.

38 Lampela H, Kosola S, Heikkilä P. Native liver histology after successful portoenterostomy in biliary atresia. J Clin Gastroenterol 2014;48:721–8.

39 Alagille D. Extrahepatic biliary atresia. Hepatology 1984;4:7S–10S.

40 Jörgensen MJ. The ductal plate malformation: a study of the intrahepatic bile-duct lesion in infantile polycystic disease and congenital hepatic fibrosis. Acta Pathol Microbiol Scand 1977;257(Suppl.):1–88.

41 Brough AJ, Bernstein J. Conjugated hyperbilirubinemia in early infancy. A reassessment of liver biopsy. Hum Pathol 1974;5:507–16.

42 Russo P, Magee JC, Boitnott J, et al. Design and validation of the biliary atresia research consortium histologic assessment system for cholestasis in infancy. Cliln Gastroenterol Hepatol 2011;9:357–62.

43 Riely CA. Familial intrahepatic cholestatic syndromes. Semin Liver Dis 1987;7:119–33.

44 Dahms BB, Petrelli M, Wyllie R, et al. Arteriohepatic dysplasia in infancy and childhood: a longitudinal study of six patients. Hepatology 1982;2:350–8.

45 Kahn EI, Daum F, Markowitz J, et al. Arteriohepatic dysplasia. II. Hepatobiliary morphology. Hepatology 1983;3:77–84.

46 Nijjar SS, Crosby HA, Wallace L, et al. Notch receptor expression in adult human liver: a possible role in bile duct formation and hepatic neovascularisation. Hepatology 2001;34:1184–92.

47 Turnpenny PD, Ellard S. Alagille syndrome: pathogenesis, diagnosis and management. Eur J Hum Gen 2012;20:251–7.

47a Geisler F, Strazzabosco M. Emerging roles of Notch signaling in liver disease. Hepatology 2015;61: 382–92.

48 Libbrecht L, Spinner NB, Moore EC, et al. Peripheral bile duct paucity and cholestasis in the liver of a patient with Alagille syndrome. Further evidence supporting a lack of postnatal bile duct branching and elongation. Am J Surg Pathol 2005;29:820–6.

49 Emerick KM, Rand EB, Goldmuntz E, et al. Features of Alagille syndrome in 92 patients: frequency and relation to prognosis. Hepatology 1999;29:822–9.

50 Finegold MJ, Carpenter RJ. Obliterative cholangitis due to cytomegalovirus: a possible precursor of paucity of intrahepatic bile ducts. Hum Pathol 1982;13:662–5.

51 Bruguera M, Llach J, Rodés J. Nonsyndromic paucity of intrahepatic bile ducts in infancy and idiopathic ductopenia in adulthood: the same syndrome? Hepatology 1992;15:830–4.

52 Ludwig J, Wiesner RH, La Russo NF. Idiopathic adulthood ductopenia: a cause of chronic cholestatic liver disease and biliary cirrhosis. J Hepatol 1988;7:193–9.

53 Kahn E, Daum F, Markowitz J, et al. Nonsyndromatic paucity of interlobular bile ducts: light and electron microscopic evaluation of sequential liver biopsies in early childhood. Hepatology 1986;6:890–901.

54 Fabris L, Cadamuro M, Guido M, et al. Analysis of liver repair mechanisms in Alagille syndrome and biliary atresia reveals a role for Notch signaling. Am J Pathol 2007;171:641–53.

55 Byrne JA, Meara NJ, Rayner AC, et al. Lack of hepatocellular CD10 along bile canaliculi is physiologic in early childhood and persistent in Alagille syndrome. Lab Invest 2007;87:1138–48.

56 Heathcote J, Deodhar KP, Scheuer PJ, et al. Intrahepatic cholestasis in childhood. N Engl J Med 1976;295:801–5.

57 Leblanc A, Hadchouel M, Jehan P, et al. Obstructive jaundice in children with histiocytosis X. Gastroenterology 1981;80:134–9.

58 Kaplan KJ, Goodman ZD, Ishak KG. Liver involvement in Langerhans' cell histiocytosis: a study of nine cases. Mod Pathol 1999;12:370–8.

59 Gregorio GV, Portmann B, Karani J, et al. Autoimmune hepatitis/sclerosing cholangitis overlap syndrome in childhood: a 16-year prospective study. Hepatology 2001;33:544–53.

60 Summerfield JA, Nagafuchi Y, Sherlock S, et al. Hepatobiliary fibropolycystic diseases. A clinical and histological review of 51 patients. J Hepatol 1986;2: 141–56.

61 Desmet VJ. Congenital diseases of intrahepatic bile ducts: variations on the theme 'ductal plate malformation'. Hepatology 1992;16:1069–83.

62 Strazzabosco M, Fabris L. Development of the bile ducts: essentials for the clinical hepatologist. J Hepatol 2012;56:1159–70.

63 Raynaud P, Tate J, Callens C, et al. A classification of ductal plate malformations based on distinct pathogenic mechanisms of biliary dysmorphogenesis. Hepatology 2011;53:1959–66.

64 Huppert SS. A new set of classifications for ductal plate malformations. Hepatology 2011;53:1795–7.

65 Gunay-Aygun M. Liver and kidney disease in ciliopathies. Am J Med Genet Part C Semin Med Genet 2009;151C:296–306.

66 Gunay-Aygun M, Font-Montgomery E, Lukose L, et al. Characteristics of congenital hepatic fibrosis in a large cohort of patients with autosomal recessive polycystic kidney disease. Gastroenterology 2013;144:112–21.

67 Masyuk AI, Masyuk TV, LaRusso NF. Chlangiocyte primary cilia in liver health and disease. Dev Dyn 2006;237:2007–12.

68 O'Hara SP, Tabibian JH, Splinter PL, et al. The dynamic biliary epithelia: molecules, pathways, and disease. J Hepatol 2013;58:575–82.

69 Desmet VJ. What is congenital hepatic fibrosis? Histopathology 1992;20:465–77.

70 Desmet VJ. Pathogenesis of ductal plate abnormalities. Mayo Clin Proc 1998;73:80–9.

70a Katabi N, Pillarisetty VG, DeMatteo R, et al. Choledochal cysts: a clinicopathologic study of 36 cases with emphasis on the morphologic and the immunohistochemical features of premalignant and malignant alterations. Hum Pathol 2014;45:2107–14.

71 Scott J, Shousha S, Thomas HC, et al. Bile duct carcinoma: a late complication of congenital hepatic fibrosis. Case report and review of literature. Am J Gastroenterol 1980;73:113–19.

72 Chaudhuri PK, Chaudhuri B, Schuler JJ, et al. Carcinoma associated with congenital cystic dilation of bile ducts. Arch Surg 1982;117:1349–51.

73 Honda N, Cobb C, Lechago J. Bile duct carcinoma associated with multiple von Meyenburg complexes in the liver. Hum Pathol 1986;17:1287–90.

74 Case records of the Massachusetts General Hospital. Case 48-1988. N Engl J Med 1988;319:1465–74.

75 Hodgson HJF, Davies DR, Thompson RPH. Congenital hepatic fibrosis. J Clin Pathol 1976;29:11–16.

76 de Koning TJ, Nikkels PGJ, Dorland L, et al. Congenital hepatic fibrosis in 3 siblings with phosphomannose isomerase deficiency. Virchows Arch 2000;437:101–5.

77 Nakanuma Y, Terada T, Ohta G, et al. Caroli's disease in congenital hepatic fibrosis and infantile polycystic disease. Liver 1982;2:346–54.

78 Ludwig J, MacCarty RL, LaRusso NF, et al. Intrahepatic cholangiectases and large-duct obliteration in primary sclerosing cholangitis. Hepatology 1986;6:560–8.

79 Thommesen N. Biliary hamartomas (von Meyenburg complexes) in liver needle biopsies. Acta Pathol Microbiol Scand [A] 1978;86:93–9.

80 Quentin M, Scherer A. The 'von Meyenburg complex'. Hepatology 2010;52:1167–8.

81 Landing BH, Wells TR, Claireaux AE. Morphometric analysis of liver lesions in cystic diseases of childhood. Hum Pathol 1980;11:549–60.

82 Chatelain D, Chailley-Heu B, Terris B, et al. The ciliated hepatic foregut cyst, an unusual bronchiolar foregut malformation: a histological, histochemical, and immunohistochemical study of 7 cases. Hum Pathol 2000;31:241–6.

83 Forbes A, Murray-Lyon IM. Cystic disease of the liver and biliary tract. Gut 1991;32(Suppl.):S116–22.

84 Terada T, Nakanuma Y. Congenital biliary dilatation in autosomal dominant adult polycystic disease of the liver and kidneys. Arch Pathol Lab Med 1988;112:1113–16.

85 Ramos A, Torres VE, Holley KE, et al. The liver in autosomal dominant polycystic kidney disease. Implications for pathogenesis. Arch Pathol Lab Med 1990;114:180–4.

86 Lewindon PJ, Shepherd RW, Walsh MJ, et al. Importance of hepatic fibrosis in cystic fibrosis and the predictive value of liver biopsy. Hepatology 2011;53:193–201.

87 Bhardwaj S, Canlas K, Kahi C, et al. Hepatobiliary abnormalities and disease in cystic fibrosis. Epidemiology and outcomes through adulthood. J Clin Gastroenterol 2009;43:858–64.

88 Rudnick DA. Cystic fibrosis-associated liver disease: when will the future be now? J Ped Gastroenterol Nutr 2012;54:312.

89 Lindblad A, Hultcrantz R, Strandvik B. Bile-duct destruction and collagen deposition: a prominent ultrastructural feature of the liver in cystic fibrosis. Hepatology 1992;16:372–81.

90 Furuya KN, Roberts EA, Canny GJ, et al. Neonatal hepatitis syndrome with paucity of interlobular bile ducts in cystic fibrosis. J Pediatr Gastroenterol Nutr 1991;12:127–30.

91 Isenberg JI. Cystic fibrosis: its influence on the liver, biliary tree, and bile salt metabolism. Semin Liver Dis 1982;4:302–13.

92 Lewindon PJ, Pereira TN, Hoskins AC, et al. The role of hepatic stellate cells and transforming growth factor-beta-1 in cystic fibrosis liver disease. Am J Pathol 2002;160:1705–15.

93 Nagel RA, Westaby D, Javaid A, et al. Liver disease and bile duct abnormalities in adults with cystic fibrosis. Lancet 1989;2:1422–5.

94 Ishak KG. Hepatic morphology in the inherited metabolic diseases. Semin Liver Dis 1986;6:246–58.

95 Ishak KG, Sharp HL. Metabolic errors and liver disease. In: MacSween RNM, Anthony PP, Scheuer PJ, et al., editors. Pathology of the Liver. 3rd ed. Edinburgh: Churchill Livingstone; 1994. p. 123–218 [Ch. 4].

96 Portmann BC. Liver biopsy in the diagnosis of inherited metabolic disorders. In: Anthony PP, MacSween RNM, editors. Recent Advances in Histopathology, vol. 14. Edinburgh: Churchill Livingstone; 1989. p. 139–59.

97 Resnick JM, Whitley CB, Leonard AS, et al. Light and electron microscopic features of the liver in mucopolysaccharidosis. Hum Pathol 1994;25:276–86.

98 Phillips MJ, Poucell S, Patterson J, et al., editors. The Liver. An Atlas and Text of Ultrastructural Pathology. New York: Raven Press; 1987.

99 Resnick JM, Krivit W, Snover DC, et al. Pathology of the liver in mucopolysaccharidosis: light and electron microscopic assessment before and after bone marrow transplantation. Bone Marrow Transplant 1992;10:273–80.

100 Smanik EJ, Tavill AS, Jacobs GH, et al. Orthotopic liver transplantation in two adults with Niemann–Pick and Gaucher's diseases: implications for the treatment of inherited metabolic disease. Hepatology 1993;17:42–9.

101 McAdams AJ, Hug G, Bove KE. Glycogen storage disease, types I to X: criteria for morphologic diagnosis. Hum Pathol 1974;5:463–87.

102 Hicks J, Wartchow E, Mierau G. Glycogen storage diseases: a brief review and update on clinical features, genetic abnormalities, pathologic features, and treatment. Ultrastructural Pathol 2011;35:183–96.

103 Itoh S, Ishida Y, Matsuo S. Mallory bodies in a patient with type Ia glycogen storage disease. Gastroenterology 1987;92:520–3.

104 Howell RR, Stevenson RE, Ben-Menachem Y, et al. Hepatic adenomata with type 1 glycogen storage disease. JAMA 1976;236:1481–4.

105 Coire CI, Qizilbash AH, Castelli MF. Hepatic adenomata in type Ia glycogen storage disease. Arch Pathol Lab Med 1987;111:166–9.

106 Limmer J, Fleig WE, Leupold D, et al. Hepatocellular carcinoma in type I glycogen storage disease. Hepatology 1988;8:531–7.

107 Markowitz AJ, Chen Y-T, Muenzer J, et al. A man with type III glycogenosis associated with cirrhosis and portal hypertension. Gastroenterology 1993;105:1882–5.

108 Bannayan GA, Dean WJ, Howell RR. Type IV glycogen-storage disease. Light-microscopic, electron-microscopic, and enzymatic study. Am J Clin Pathol 1976;66:702–9.

109 Vázquez JJ. Ground glass hepatocytes: light and electron microscopy. Characterization of the different types. Histol Histopathol 1990;5:379–86.

110 Jack CIA, Evans CC. Three cases of alpha-1-antitrypsin deficiency in the elderly. Postgrad Med J 1991;67:840–2.

111 Rakela J, Goldschmiedt M, Ludwig J. Late manifestation of chronic liver disease in adults with alpha-1-antitrypsin deficiency. Dig Dis Sci 1987;32:1358–62.

112 Deutsch J, Becker H, Auböck L. Histopathological features of liver disease in alpha-1-antitrypsin deficiency. Acta Paediatr 1994;393(Suppl.):8–12.

113 Fairbanks KD, Tavill AS. Liver disease in alpha-1-antitrypsin deficiency: a review. Am J Gastroenterol 2008;103:2136–41.

114 Perlmutter DH. The cellular basis for liver injury in α_1-antitrypsin deficiency. Hepatology 1991;13:172–85.

115 Aldonyte R, Jamsson L, Ljungberg O, et al. Polymerized α_1-antitrypsin is present on lung vascular endothelium. New insights into the biological significance of α_1-antitrypsin polymerization. Histopathology 2004;45:587–92.

116 Carrell RW, Lomas DA. Alpha-1-antitrypsin deficiency – a model for conformational diseases. N Engl J Med 2002;346:45–53.

117 Callea F, Fevery J, De Groote J, et al. Detection of Pi Z phenotype individuals by alpha-1-antitrypsin (AAT) immunohistochemistry in paraffin-embedded liver tissue specimens. J Hepatol 1986;2:389–401.

118 Theaker JM, Fleming KA. Alpha-1-antitrypsin and the liver: a routine immunohistological screen. J Clin Pathol 1986;39:58–62.

119 Qizilbash A, Young-Pong O. Alpha 1 antitrypsin liver disease differential diagnosis of PAS-positive, diastase-resistant globules in liver cells. Am J Clin Pathol 1983;79:697–702.

120 Hay CR, Preston FE, Triger DR, et al. Progressive liver disease in haemophilia: an understated problem? Lancet 1985;1:1495–8.

121 Geller SA, Nichols WS, Dycaico MJ, et al. Histopathology of α_1-antitrypsin liver disease in a transgenic mouse model. Hepatology 1990;12:40–7.

122 Talbot IC, Mowat AP. Liver disease in infancy: histological features and relationship to alpha-antitrypsin phenotype. J Clin Pathol 1975;28:559–63.

123 Odièvre M, Martin JP, Hadchouel M, et al. Alpha1-antitrypsin deficiency and liver disease in children: phenotypes, manifestations, and prognosis. Pediatrics 1976;57:226–31.

124 Propst T, Propst A, Dietze O, et al. High prevalence of viral infection in adults with homozygous and heterozygous alpha-1-antitrypsin deficiency and chronic liver disease. Ann Intern Med 1992;117:641–5.

125 Palmer PE, Wolfe HJ. Alpha-antitrypsin deposition in primary hepatic carcinomas. Arch Pathol Lab Med 1976;100:232–6.

126 Reintoft I, Hagerstrand I. Demonstration of alpha 1-antitrypsin in hepatomas. Arch Pathol Lab Med 1979;103:495–8.

127 Eriksson S, Carlson J, Velez R. Risk of cirrhosis and primary liver cancer in alpha 1-antitrypsin deficiency. N Engl J Med 1986;314:736–9.

128 Graziadei IW, Joseph JJ, Wiesner RH, et al. Increased risk of chronic liver failure in adults with heterozygous α_1-antitrypsin deficiency. Hepatology 1998;28:1058–63.

129 Pittschieler K. Liver disease and heterozygous alpha-1-antitrypsin deficiency. Acta Paediatr Scand 1991;80: 323–7.

130 Marwick TH, Cooney PT, Kerlin P. Cirrhosis and hepatocellular carcinoma in a patient with heterozygous (MZ) alpha-1-antitrypsin deficiency. Pathology 1985;17:649–52.

131 Reid CL, Wiener GJ, Cox DW, et al. Diffuse hepatocellular dysplasia and carcinoma associated with the Mmalton variant of α_1-antitrypsin. Gastroenterology 1987;93: 181–7.

132 Callea F, Brisigotti M, Fabbretti G, et al. Hepatic endoplasmic reticulum storage diseases. Liver 1992;12:357–62.

133 Lindmark B, Eriksson S. Partial deficiency of α_1-antichymotrypsin is associated with chronic cryptogenic liver disease. Scand J Gastroenterol 1991;26:508–12.

134 Rubbia-Brandt L, Neerman-Arbez M, Rougemont A-L, et al. Fibrinogen gamma 375 Arg–γtrp mutation (fibrinogen Aguadilla) causes hereditary hypofibrinogenemia, hepatic endoplasmic reticulum storage disease and cirrhosis. Am J Surg Pathol 2006;30:906–11.

135 James SP, Stromeyer FW, Chang C, et al. Liver abnormalities in patients with Gaucher's disease. Gastroenterology 1981;80:126–33.

136 Long RG, Lake BD, Pettit JE, et al. Adult Niemann–Pick disease: its relationship to the syndrome of the sea-blue histiocyte. Am J Med 1977;62:627–35.

137 Tassoni JP, Fawaz KA, Johnston DE. Cirrhosis and portal hypertension in a patient with adult Niemann–Pick disease. Gastroenterology 1991;100:567–9.

138 Lake BD, Patrick AD. Wolman's disease: deficiency of E600-resistant acid esterase activity with storage of lipids in lysosomes. J Pediatr 1970;76:262–6.

139 Beaudet AL, Ferry GD, Nichols BL Jr, et al. Cholesterol ester storage disease: clinical, biochemical, and pathological studies. J Pediatr 1977;90:910–14.

140 Bernstein DL, Hűlkova H, Bialer MG, et al. Cholesteryl ester storage disease: review of the findings in 135 reported patients with an underdiagnosed disease. J Hepatol 2013;58:1230–43.

141 Applebaum MN, Thaler MM. Reversibility of extensive liver damage in galactosemia. Gastroenterology 1975;69:496–502.

142 Mieles LA, Esquivel COO, Van Thiel DH, et al. Liver transplantation for tyrosinemia: a review of 10 cases from the University of Pittsburgh. Dig Dis Sci 1990;35:153–7.

143 Lichtenstein GR, Kaiser LR, Tuchman M, et al. Fatal hyperammonemia following orthotopic lung transplantation. Gastroenterology 1997;112:236–40.

144 Badizadegan K, Perez-Atayde AR. Focal glycogenosis of the liver in disorders of ureagenesis: its occurrence and diagnostic significance. Hepatology 1997;26:365–73.

145 Kilpatrick-Smith L, Hale DE, Douglas SD. Progress in Reye syndrome: epidemiology, biochemical mechanisms and animal models. Dig Dis Sci 1989;7:135–46.

146 Lichtenstein PK, Heubi JE, Daugherty CC, et al. Grade I Reye's syndrome. A frequent cause of vomiting and liver dysfunction after varicella and upper-respiratory-tract infection. N Engl J Med 1983;309:133–9.

147 Mowat AP. Reye's syndrome: 20 years on. BMJ Clin Res 1983;286:1999–2001.

148 Gosalakkal JA, Kamoji V. Reye syndrome and Reye-like syndrome. Ped Neurol 2008;39:198–200.

149 Pugliese A, Beltramo T, Torre D. Reye's and Reye's-like syndromes. Cell Biochem Funct 2008;26:741–6.

150 Brown RE, Ishak KG. Hepatic zonal degeneration and necrosis in Reye's syndrome. Arch Pathol Lab Med 1976;100:123–6.

151 Kimura S, Kobayashi T, Tanaka Y, et al. Liver histopathology in clinical Reye syndrome. Brain Dev 1991;13:95–100.

152 Tonsgard JH. Effect of Reye's syndrome serum on the ultrastructure of isolated liver mitochondria. Lab Invest 1989;60:568–73.

153 Mandel H, Hartman C, Berkowitz D, et al. The hepatic mitochondrial DNA depletion syndrome: ultrastructural changes in liver biopsies. Hepatology 2001;34:776–84.

154 Balistreri WF, Bove KE. Hepatobiliary consequences of parenteral alimentation. In: Popper H, Schaffner F, editors. Progress in Liver Diseases, vol. IX. Philadelphia, PA: WB Saunders; 1990. p. 567–602.

155 Quigley EMM, Marsh MN, Shaffer JL, et al. Hepatobiliary complications of total parenteral nutrition. Gastroenterology 1993;104:286–301.

156 Cohen C, Olsen MM. Pediatric total parenteral nutrition. Liver histopathology. Arch Pathol Lab Med 1981;105:152–6.

157 Mullick FG, Moran CA, Ishak KG. Total parenteral nutrition: a histopathologic analysis of the liver changes in 20 children. Mod Pathol 1994;7:190–4.

158 Naini BV, Lassman CR. Total parenteral nutrition therapy and liver injury: a histopathologic study with clinical correlation. Hum Pathol 2012;43:826–33.

159 Mutanen A, Lohi J, Heikkilä P, et al. Persistnet abnormal liver fibrosis after weaning off parenteral nutrition in pediatric intestinal failure. Hepatology 2013;58:729–38.

160 Bosma PJ. Inherited disorders of bilirubin metabolism. J Hepatol 2003;38:107–17.

161 Sticova E, Jirsa M. New insights in bilirubin metabolism and their clinical implications. World J Gastroenterol 2013;19:6398–407.

162 Cebecauerova D, Jirasek T, Budisova L, et al. Dual hereditary jaundice: simultaneous occurrence of mutations causing Gilbert's and Dubin–Johnson syndrome. Gastroenterology 2005;129:315–20.

163 Berthelot P, Dhumeaux D. New insights into the classification and mechanisms of hereditary, chronic, non-haemolytic hyperbilirubinaemias. Gut 1978;19:474–80.

164 Traunder M, Meier PJ, Boyer JL. Molecular pathogenesis of cholestasis. N Engl J Med 1998;339:1217–27.

165 Knisely AS, Strautnieks SS, Meier Y, et al. Hepatocellular carcinoma in ten children under five years of age with bile salt export pump deficiency. Hepatology 2006;44:478–86.

165a Vilarinho S, Erson-Omay EZ, Harmanci AS, et al. Paediatric hepatocellular carcinoma due to somatic CTNNB1 and NFE212 mutations in the settings of inherited bi-allelic ABCB11 mutations. J Hepatol 2014;61:1178–83.

166 Jacquemin E. Progressive familial intrahepatic cholestasis. Clin Res Hepatol Gastroenterol 2012;36:526–35.

167 Balistreri WF, Bezerra JA, Jansen P, et al. Intrahepatic cholestasis: summary of an American Association for the Study of Liver Diseases Single-Topic Conference. Hepatology 2005;42:222–35.

168 Morotti RA, Suchy FJ, Magid MS. Progressive familial intrahepatic cholestasis (PFIC) type 1, 2 and 3: a review of the liver pathology findings. Semin Liver Dis 2011;31:3–10.

169 Bull LN, Carolton VEH, Stricker NL, et al. Genetic and morphological findings in progressive familial intrahepatic cholestasis (Byler disease [PFIC-1] and Byler syndrome): evidence for heterogeneity. Hepatology 1997;26:155–64.

170 Nicolaou M, Andress EJ, Zolnerciks JK, et al. Canalicular ABC transporters and liver disease. J Pathol 2012;226:300–15.

171 van der Woerd WL, van Mil SWC, Stapelbroek JM, et al. Familial cholestasis: progressive familial intrahepatic cholestasis, benign recurrent intrahepatic cholestasis and intrahepatic cholestasis of pregnancy. Best Pract Res Clin Gastroenterol 2010;24:541–53.

172 van Mil SW, Klomp LW, Bull LN, et al. FIC1 disease: a spectrum of intrahepatic cholestatic disorders. Semin Liver Dis 2001;21:535–44.

173 Lam P, Soroka CJ, Boyer JL. The bile salt export pump: clinical and experimental aspects of genetic and acquired cholestatic liver disease. Semin Liver Dis 2010;30:125–33.

174 Scheimann AO, Strautnieks SS, Knisely AS, et al. Mutations in bile salt export pump (*ABCB11*) in two children with progressive familial intrahepatic cholestasis and cholangiocarcinoma. J Pediatr 2007;150:556–9.

175 Lykavieris P, van Mil S, Cresteil D, et al. Progressive familial intrahepatic cholestasis type 1 and extrahepatic features: no catch-up of stature growth, exacerbation of diarrhea, and appearance of liver steatosis after liver transplantation. J Hepatol 2003;39:447–52.

176 Shneider BL. Liver transplantation for progressive familial intrahepatic cholestasis: the evolving role of genotyping. Liver Transplant 2009;15:565–6.

177 Miyagawa-Hayashino A, Egaqa H, Yorifuji T, et al. Allograft steatohepatitis in progressive familial intrahepatic cholestasis type 1 after living donor liver transplantation. Liver Transplant 2009;15:610–18.

178 Folvik G, Hilde O, Helge GO. Benign recurrent intrahepatic cholestasis: review and long-term follow-up of five cases. Scand J Gastroenterol 2012;47:482–8.

179 van Mil SWC, Van Der Woerd WL, Van Der Brugge G, et al. Benign recurrent intrahepatic cholestasis type 2 is caused by mutations in ABCB11. Gastroenterology 2004;127:379–84.

180 Beaudoin M, Feldmann G, Erlinger S, et al. Benign recurrent cholestasis. Digestion 1973;9:49–65.

181 van Ooteghem NAM, Klomp LWJ, van Berge-Henegouwen GP, et al. Benign recurrent intrahepatic cholestasis progressing to progressive familial intrahepatic cholestasis: low GGT cholestasis is a clinical continuum. J Hepatol 2002;36:439–43.

182 Jansen PLM, Müller M, Sturm E. Genes and cholestasis. Hepatology 2001;34:1067–74.

183 Tygstrup N, Steig BA, Juijn JA, et al. Recurrent familial intrahepatic cholestasis in the Faeroe Islands. Phenotypic heterogeneity but genetic homogeneity. Hepatology 1999;29:506–8.

183a Girard M, Lacaille F, Verkarre V, et al. MYO5B and bile salt export pump contribute to cholestatic liver disorder in microvillous inclusion disease. Hepatology 2014;60:301–10.

184 Johnson PJ, McFarlane IG, Eddleston ALWF. The natural course and heterogeneity of autoimmune-type chronic active hepatitis. Semin Liver Dis 1991;11:187–96.

185 Barnett JL, Appelman HD, Moseley RH. A familial form of incomplete septal cirrhosis. Gastroenterology 1992;102:674–8.

186 Narkewicz MR, Sokol RJ, Beckwith B, et al. Liver involvement in Alpers disease. J Pediatr 1991;119:260–7.

187 Ku N-O, Gish R, Wright TL, et al. Keratin 8 mutations in patients with cryptogenic liver disease. N Engl J Med 2001;344:1580–7.

188 Klass HJ, Kelly JK, Warnes TW. Indian childhood cirrhosis in the United Kingdom. Gut 1980;21:344–50.

189 Lefkowitch JH, Honig CL, King ME, et al. Hepatic copper overload and features of Indian childhood cirrhosis in an American sibship. N Engl J Med 1982;307:271–7.

190 Müller-Höcker J, Meyer U, Wiebecke B, et al. Copper storage disease of the liver and chronic dietary copper intoxication in two further German infants mimicking Indian childhood cirrhosis. Pathol Res Pract 1988;183:39–45.

191 Adamson M, Reiner B, Olson JL, et al. Indian childhood cirrhosis in an American child. Gastroenterology 1992;102:1771–7.

192 Aljajeh IA, Mughal S, Al-Tahou B, et al. Indian childhood cirrhosis-like liver disease in an Arab child. A brief report. Virchows Arch 1994;424:225–7.

193 Baker A, Gormally S, Saxena R, et al. Copper-associated liver disease in childhood. J Hepatol 1995;23:538–43.

194 Müller T, Feichtinger H, Berger H, et al. Endemic Tyrolean infantile cirrhosis: an ecogenetic disorder. Lancet 1996;347:877–80.

195 Tanner MS, Kantarjian AH, Bhave SA, et al. Early introduction of copper-contaminated animal mild feeds as a possible cause of Indian childhood cirrhosis. Lancet 1983;2:992–5.

196 Popper H, Goldfischer S, Sternlieb I, et al. Cytoplasmic copper and its toxic effects. Studies in Indian childhood cirrhosis. Lancet 1979;1:1205–8.

197 Tanner MS, Portmann B, Mowat AP, et al. Increased hepatic copper concentration in Indian childhood cirrhosis. Lancet 1979;1:1203–5.

198 Bhusnurmath SR, Walia BNS, Singh S, et al. Sequential histopathologic alterations in Indian childhood cirrhosis treated with D-penicillamine. Hum Pathol 1991;22:653–8.

General reading

Chandra RS, Stocker JT. The liver, gallbladder, and biliary tract. In: Stocker JT, Dehner LP, editors. Pediatric Pathology. Philadelphia, PA: JB Lippincott; 1992. p. 703–90.

Elferink RPJO, Paulusma CC, Groen AK. Hepatocanalicular transport defects: pathophysiologic mechanisms of rare diseases. Gastroenterology 2006;130:908–25.

Feingold MJ. Common diagnostic problems in pediatric liver pathology. Clin Liver Dis 2002;6:421–54.

Geisler F, Sstraazbosco M. Emerging roles of Notch signaling in liver disease. Hepatology 2015;61:382–92.

Hansen K, Horslen S. Metabolic liver disease in children. Liver Transpl 2008;14:391–411.

Ishak KG. Inherited metabolic diseases of the liver. Clin Liver Dis 2002;6:455–80.

Kelly DA, editor. Diseases of the Liver and Biliary System in Children. 3rd ed. Chichester, West Sussex, UK: Wiley-Blackwell; 2008.

Morotti RA, Suchy FJ, Magid MS. Progressive familial intrahepatic cholestasis (PFIC) type 1, 2 and 3: a review of the liver pathology findings. Semin Liver Dis 2011;31:3–10.

Ovchinsky N, Moreira RK, Lefkowitch JH, et al. Liver biopsy in modern clinical practice: a pediatric point-of-view. Adv Anat Pathol 2012;19:250–62.

Portmann BC, Roberts EA. Developmental abnormalities and liver disease in childhood. In: Burt AD, Portmann BC, Ferrell LD, editors. MacSween's Pathology of the Liver. 6th ed. Edinburgh: Churchill Livingstone/Elsevier; 2012. p. 101–56.

Thompson RJ, Portmann BC, Roberts EA. Genetic and metabolic liver disease. In: Burt AD, Portmann BC, Ferrell LD, editors. MacSween's Pathology of the Liver. 6th ed. Edinburgh: Churchill Livingstone/Elsevier; 2012. p. 157–260.

Disturbances of Copper and Iron Metabolism

Wilson's disease (hepatolenticular degeneration)

Wilson's disease is an autosomal recessive disorder due to mutations in the gene *ATP7B* for copper-transporting ATPase located in the *trans*-Golgi network of the liver.[1] It is uncommon but important and treatable. Normal hepatic copper transport[2] is disrupted owing to various ATP7B mutations,[3] leading to the accumulation of copper in hepatocytes and liver disease. The large number and diverse mutations identified currently preclude simple genetic testing,[4] in contrast to hereditary haemochromatosis (discussed later). Liver biopsy is important for histological diagnosis and monitoring.[5]

Chemical quantitation of copper concentration in the biopsy sample helps to establish the diagnosis and is sometimes used for determination of the genetic status of a patient's siblings.[6,7] Copper determination can be made from specimens obtained by routine liver biopsy or retrieved from paraffin blocks, without special copper-free solutions or instruments.[8] Homozygous individuals have increased liver copper levels from an early age but do not develop symptoms of liver disease in the first few years of life. Increased liver copper levels precede the development of histological abnormalities. Hepatic copper levels are typically greater than 4 µmol/g dry weight (>250 µg/g dry weight).[8]

Histological lesions develop before the disease is clinically apparent. In the early, precirrhotic phase there is fatty change,[7] sometimes with the formation of fat granulomas.[6] Slender fibrous septa extend from portal tracts (**Fig. 14.1**). There may be unusually abundant lipofuscin pigment in hepatocytes and glycogen vacuolation of hepatocyte nuclei, but neither feature is easy to evaluate; both are found in normal individuals, and nuclear vacuolation is particularly common in the young. Lipofuscin granules may be larger and less regular in outline than normal.[9] Inflammation is absent or mild in the early stages. Kupffer cells are sometimes enlarged and may stain for iron as a result of haemolysis. Electron microscopy helps in the diagnosis of both early and late disease because of characteristic changes in mitochondria and lysosomes (**see Ch. 17**).

In some patients a phase of chronic hepatitis develops next that is difficult to distinguish histologically from chronic viral hepatitis. Stains for copper and copper-associated protein may be helpful, as discussed below. Cirrhosis develops in untreated patients, with or without a recognisable preceding phase of chronic hepatitis. A common though not invariable pattern is of active cirrhosis with fatty change, ballooned hepatocytes, focally dense eosinophilic cytoplasm and glycogen vacuolation of nuclei (**Fig. 14.2**). Cholestasis may be present. Hepatocytes often contain Mallory–Denk bodies and these are sometimes very

**Figure 14.1
Wilson's disease.**
At this early stage slender septa extend from portal tracts (P) but acinar architecture is intact. There is steatosis, just visible in this reticulin preparation. (Wedge biopsy, reticulin.)

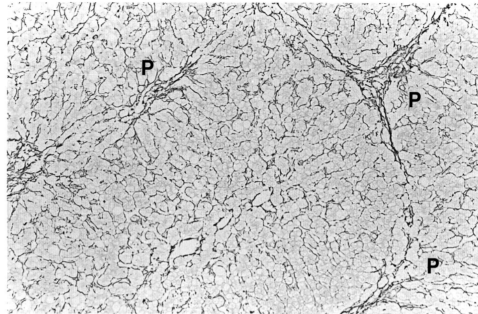

**Figure 14.2
Wilson's disease.**
Active cirrhosis with liver-cell swelling, steatosis (arrowheads) and nuclear vacuolation (arrow). (Wedge biopsy, H&E.)

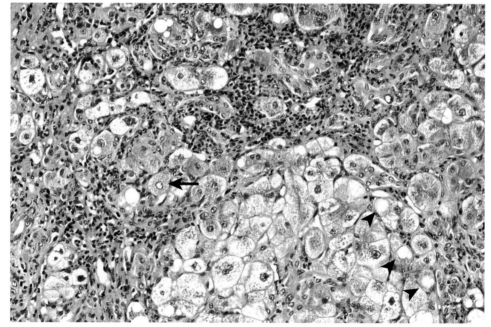

abundant. They are associated with an infiltrate rich in neutrophils, as in steatohepatitis (**Fig. 14.3**). Partial fibrous occlusion of efferent veins has been reported.[9] Hepatocellular carcinoma is a rare sequel of cirrhosis in Wilson's disease.[10,11]

Fulminant hepatic failure may be the first manifestation of Wilson's disease and is a major indication for liver transplantation.[12] The presence of haemolysis in a young individual with acute liver failure should therefore prompt consideration of Wilson's disease.[13] Cirrhosis is usually already present in such cases,[14,15] in contradistinction to acute liver

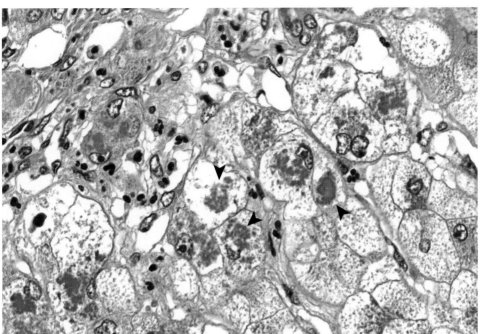

Figure 14.3
Wilson's disease.
Numerous Mallory–Denk bodies (arrowheads) are seen within hepatocytes. (Postmortem liver, H&E.)

failure, owing to viral or drug hepatitis where recent massive necrosis is evident. The cirrhotic nodules are frequently small and separated by septa containing abundant ductular structures and variable chronic inflammatory cells (**Fig. 14.4**). The death of hepatocytes in the fulminant disease occurs by both apoptosis and necrosis,[16] resulting in new zones of confluent necrosis superimposed on the underlying cirrhotic architecture. Cholestasis is often striking and hepatocytes may contain large- or small-droplet fat. The presence of much stainable copper and/or copper-associated protein in hepatocytes and Kupffer cells distinguishes Wilson's disease from other causes of fulminant hepatic failure.

Staining for copper and copper-associated protein plays a part in the diagnosis of Wilson's disease, though staining results (as well as the copper concentration) can vary considerably throughout the liver.[17] Failure to stain in either case is common at some stages of the disease and does not therefore exclude the diagnosis. Conversely, both copper and copper-associated protein are found in other liver diseases, usually as a result of failure to secrete copper into the bile. Thus, in a child with liver disease strong staining for copper might reflect loss of bile ducts rather than Wilson's disease. Other copper storage disorders have been described, including Indian childhood cirrhosis (**see Ch. 13**, **Fig. 13.23**), which is also occasionally seen elsewhere in the world.[18–20] Furthermore, neonatal liver is normally rich in copper.[21]

In the early phases of Wilson's disease, liver copper levels are high, but the copper is difficult to demonstrate histochemically. This is because it is diffusely distributed in hepatocytes and not concentrated in lysosomes. Sensitive histochemical methods (e.g. Timm's silver method or rhodanine) may show faint cytoplasmic staining. Later in the course of the disease copper begins to accumulate in liver-cell lysosomes and is then more easily stained. Once cirrhosis has developed, the distribution of copper is typically uneven, some nodules staining strongly while others are negative (**Fig. 14.5**). Staining for copper and copper–protein may be dissociated, although in most cases both are positive.[22,23] Timm's silver stain appears to be the most sensitive staining method for demonstrating copper in this disease.[24]

Figure 14.4 Fulminant liver failure in Wilson's disease. Fulminant hepatitis in Wilson's disease usually develops on a background of already developed cirrhosis, as seen in this case. **A:** Cirrhotic nodules (N) are surrounded by inflamed fibrous septa with numerous bile ductular structures. The acute illness is related to progressive hepatocyte necrosis, inflammation and ductular reaction at the septal–parenchymal interface, as seen in the upper right field. **B:** Severe bile canalicular and hepatocellular cholestasis with both small- and large-droplet steatosis are present. (Explant liver, H&E.)

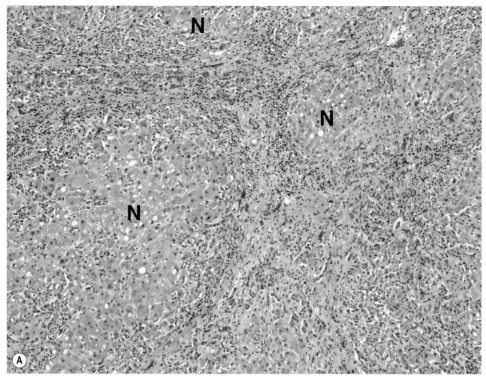

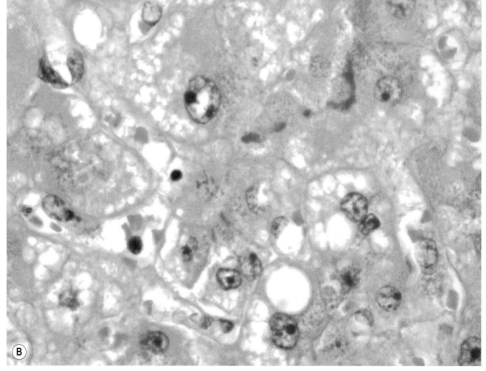

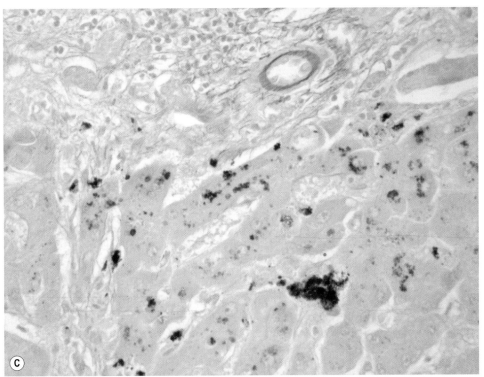

Figure 14.4, cont'd
C: Copper-binding protein is present in both periportal hepatocytes and sinusoidal Kupffer cells. (Explant liver, Victoria blue.)

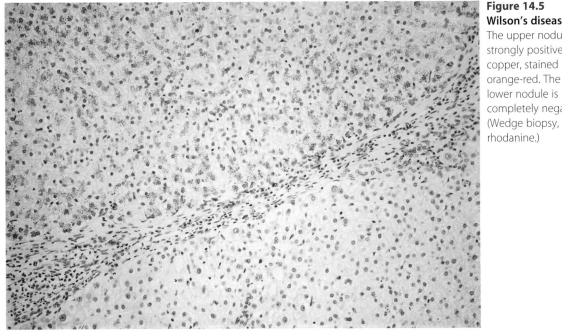

Figure 14.5
Wilson's disease.
The upper nodule is strongly positive for copper, stained orange-red. The lower nodule is completely negative. (Wedge biopsy, rhodanine.)

Because of the great variety of histological lesions in the liver, Wilson's disease can easily be mistaken for other liver disorders. Clinicians and pathologists should consider Wilson's disease in the differential diagnosis of hepatocellular disease, especially in the young, but also at all ages, including (uncommonly) older-aged individuals.[25] The disease can be arrested by treatment and its development prevented in siblings. The penalties for missing the diagnosis are therefore very great.

Iron overload

Siderosis

Siderosis (or haemosiderosis) means the presence of demonstrable iron in tissues, irrespective of cause. The main forms of iron in hepatocytes are ferritin, haemosiderin and haem.[26] Stainable iron is mainly haemosiderin, which is principally located in lysosomes and is seen as granules concentrated towards the biliary poles of the cells. Ferritin gives rise to more diffuse staining, imparting a bluish hue to the liver-cell cytoplasm on iron staining. Hepatocellular siderosis almost always shows a diminishing gradient of intensity from the periphery of lobules towards the central (efferent) veins. It is most severe in periportal regions (acinar zones 1) near small portal tracts, and least severe in centrilobular regions (acinar zones 3). The normal adult liver is usually negative on iron staining or at best shows minimal siderosis.[27] This is also true of the neonatal liver, although some cases may show mild periportal liver-cell siderosis (residual iron storage from the active period of hepatic haemopoiesis of the third trimester).[28]

Since iron stains of liver tissue are expected to be negative in most instances, a positive stain requires explanation. In this regard, two major categories of hepatic iron storage disease need to be considered, designated as **primary and secondary iron overload disorders**[29] (**Box 14.1**). The *primary disorders* are predominantly forms of hereditary haemochromatosis in which genetic mutations alter iron homeostasis in the gastrointestinal tract and liver. The *secondary disorders* are acquired conditions in which increased iron in the liver is due to exogenous sources of iron, abnormal erythrocyte destruction or changes in iron absorption and distribution related to underlying liver disease. The pathologist may be able to suggest the reason for the siderosis, based on the distribution of the stainable iron. For example, in most of the primary iron overload disorders, such as classic *HFE*-related haemochromatosis, the excess iron is mainly hepatocellular. In thalassaemia both hepatocytes and macrophages are positive, while exogenous iron overload leads to Kupffer-cell storage in the first instance. Various types of underlying liver disease are also associated with siderosis. Cirrhotic livers of varied aetiology may contain much iron,[30-32] even within macroregenerative nodules.[33] In viral hepatitis and alcoholic liver disease small amounts of stainable iron are often found. Siderosis in the setting of non-alcoholic fatty liver disease (**dysmetabolic iron**

Box 14.1 Primary and secondary iron overload disorders

Primary

Classic *HFE*-related hereditary haemochromatosis (type 1*)

Non-*HFE* hereditary haemochromatosis

Juvenile hereditary haemochromatosis

Hemojuvelin or *HJV* (*HFE2*)-related (type 2A*)

Hepcidin or *HAMP*-related (type 2B*)

Transferrin receptor 2-related haemochromatosis (type 3*)

Ferroportin-related iron overload (type 4*)

Aceruloplasminaemia

Others

Secondary

Transfusion

Haemolysis

Haemodialysis

Dietary

Underlying liver disease (e.g. chronic hepatitis, fatty liver)

*Types 1–4 are classified as forms of hereditary haemochromatosis in the OMIM (Online Mendelian Inheritance in Man) database.[44]

overload syndrome) is increasingly recognised.[34] Dense, iron-positive granules are common in endothelial cells in a variety of conditions, including acute hepatitis,[35] chronic hepatitis B and C[36] and alcoholic liver disease, but their significance is not known.

The siderotic liver should be evaluated for the **distribution of stainable iron** among the various cell types, the **grade of siderosis**, the **presence of any related tissue damage** (fibrosis, cirrhosis, necrosis or even hepatocellular carcinoma) and **coexisting liver disease of other aetiology**. Various numerical methods of assessing the degree of siderosis (discussed below) are also helpful in evaluating causation and the effectiveness of therapeutic iron removal.

Numerical assessment of tissue iron

Many different systems have been devised for the quantification of iron in tissue sections.[37] **Histological grading of hepatocellular iron** can be simply scored on a scale from 1 to 4, with grade 1 representing minimal deposition (recognisable only with a high-power objective), grade 4 massive deposits with obliteration of the usual lobular gradient, and grades 2 and 3 intermediate amounts. Examples are shown in various illustrations to this chapter. The alternative comprehensive grading system of Deugnier and colleagues[38] measures iron not only in hepatocytes, but also in mesenchymal cells, bile-duct epithelium, blood vessels and connective tissue. Kupffer cell haemosiderin, on the other hand, is not graded numerically, but its presence should be noted in the diagnosis (using modifiers such as 'diffuse', 'minimal' or 'mild' when necessary). The presence of Kupffer cell siderosis is usually *a priori* evidence against classical (*HFE*-related) haemochromatosis, except for certain rare types (discussed later).

Hepatic iron concentration (HIC) can now be determined by magnetic resonance imaging or by measuring the iron concentration directly from a specimen of liver tissue. A separate biopsy core or larger tissue section can be embedded in paraffin and processed for iron quantification, or the concentration can be determined from a biopsy specimen obtained for histology or by fine-needle aspiration biopsy.[39] An actual paraffin block (biopsy, explant, postmortem) can be analysed[3] after histological examination is complete.[40] This has the advantage that the nature of the sample is known.[41] HIC has also been used in conjunction with the subject's age in order to calculate a hepatic iron index,[42] but its diagnostic value has been superseded by current diagnostic algorithms which include genetic testing, global assessment of serum iron indices and other parameters.[43]

Primary iron overload disorders

Molecular genetic studies have now defined a variety of heritable disorders affecting iron handling by the gastrointestinal tract and liver.[44] Several of these are listed in **Box 14.1** and the reader is encouraged to consult the section on General reading at the end of this chapter for further details. The best understood of the primary iron overload disorders was first described in 1889 by von Recklinghausen[45] and is the disease referred to as 'hereditary haemochromatosis'. The majority of these cases are examples of what is currently known to be classic *HFE*-related hereditary haemochromatosis, which is discussed below. However, the identical picture of predominantly periportal hepatocellular iron overload can be found in patients with various combinations of the gene defects listed in **Box 14.1**. There is thus a pathological pattern of **classic haemochromatosis** with more than one possible cause.[44]

Classic *HFE*-related hereditary haemochromatosis

This autosomal recessive disorder is associated with progressive accumulation of iron in the liver, heart, pancreas and other organs. The frequency of homozygous disease is approximately 1 person in 300,[46] while heterozygotes are found in about 1 person in 8–10.[47] Overt disease may be found in as few as 1 in 5000,[26] and even within families homozygous persons may show different rates of iron accumulation.[48] The **HFE gene**, the gene for this type of haemochromatosis, is located on the short arm of chromosome 6 at some distance from the HLA-A locus.[47,49–52] A missense mutation in HFE known as Cys282Tyr (C282Y) has been identified which results in tyrosine substitution for cysteine at position 282 of the gene protein product.[52] The majority (80–100%) of individuals with the typical phenotype of hereditary haemochromatosis are homozygous for this mutation (designated C282Y/C282Y).[46,52] Genetic tests for C282Y can be performed on peripheral blood or on paraffin-embedded tissue.[53] Expression of the mutated HFE protein on duodenal crypt epithelium is one of several factors that have been considered important in the pathogenesis of iron overload in haemochromatosis.[54] A second mutation, His63Asp (H63D), has been identified in fewer patients with haemochromatosis, either in homozygous form or as compound heterozygotes in conjunction with C282Y or the wild-type (normal) protein.[52] In such cases, if stainable iron is present, it is usually only minimal or mild in periportal hepatocytes or in Kupffer cells, and may be due to concurrent liver diseases such as non-alcoholic fatty liver disease or chronic hepatitis.[55,56] Other HFE mutations such as S65C (serine to cysteine) or rarer types are also reported.[57,58] Non-HFE hereditary haemochromatosis[29] and other genetic disorders associated with iron overload are discussed later.

Until recently, a comprehensive panel of **diagnostic tests** combined with liver biopsy findings could be expected to provide a firm diagnosis of hereditary haemochromatosis (**Table 14.1**). However, the availability of genetic testing for HFE-related and other forms of haemochromatosis now sometimes obviates the need for liver biopsy, particularly if certain criteria indicate that the likelihood of hepatic fibrosis is low[59] (i.e. the patient is less than 40 years old, ferritin is less than 1000 ng/ml (<1000 µg/L), serum liver tests are normal and hepatomegaly is absent). However, when there are coexisting liver diseases such as chronic hepatitis C or alcoholism that may accelerate hepatic fibrosis in the presence of a genetic iron overload disorder[60] or there are other reasons for direct morphological assessment of liver tissue, liver biopsy continues to offer considerable information. Moreover, understanding the pathological progression of classic HFE-related hereditary haemochromatosis (discussed below) provides a useful comparative model of iron-related liver damage.

The first histological abnormality in homozygous HFE-related haemochromatosis is the appearance of stainable iron in periportal hepatocytes. This may be found incidentally in the course of investigation for other diseases. The unexplained presence of more than very

Table 14.1 Characteristic diagnostic profile in HFE homozygous hereditary haemochromatosis

Diagnostic modality	Typical result(s)
Serum transferrin saturation	>62% (screening threshold is >45%[46])
Serum ferritin	≥300 µg/l (men); ≥200 µg/l (women)
Hepatic iron concentration	>2200 µg/g dry weight (men) >1600 µg/g dry weight (women)
Hepatic iron index	≥1.9
Genetic testing	C282Y/C282Y *H 36 D*
Liver biopsy	Hepatocellular iron ≥grade 2 Minimal or no Kupffer cell iron

small amounts of iron in hepatocytes should always raise the possibility of early hereditary haemochromatosis. The diagnosis can then be confirmed or refuted by means of genetic testing and/or calculating the hepatic iron index, as discussed previously. Early diagnosis is most important, because cirrhosis can be prevented by appropriate treatment both in patients and in their homozygous relatives, and life expectancy returned to normal.[61] In heterozygotes, stainable liver iron is either absent or very scanty.[45]

As iron stores increase, fibrosis begins to expand the portal tracts and slender septa extend from these to give a pattern of fibrosis resembling holly leaves (**Fig. 14.6**). The enlarged tracts contain iron-rich macrophages and a ductular reaction (which contributes to progressive fibrosis[62]), but usually show only mild or no inflammatory infiltration. Iron may be seen in the ductular structures and in the epithelium of interlobular ducts in small amounts; larger quantities are not found until a later stage, when parenchymal siderosis is severe. It is a challenging paradox that in early haemochromatosis most of the iron is in hepatocytes but there is little or no evidence of liver-cell damage, liver-cell function remains virtually unimpaired and the progressive lesion is portal in location. However, with increasing iron overload foci of sideronecrosis[38] are found, comprising eosinophilic or lytic necrosis of iron-laden hepatocytes, often in close association with clusters of macrophages. The ratio of non-hepatocytic to hepatocytic iron, as assessed histologically, rises progressively. The ultrastructural progression of iron overload has also been examined.[63]

In fully developed hereditary haemochromatosis the lobular gradient of iron staining is obliterated; iron in hepatocytes is now seen throughout the lobules, whereas earlier it is more abundant in periportal and mid-zonal regions.[38] Within individual hepatocytes the iron is seen to be deposited in pericanalicular granules, outlining the bile canalicular system (**Fig. 14.7**). Cirrhosis slowly develops as fibrosis and hepatocellular hyperplasia alter the normal architectural relationships. True nodule formation is, however, a late event and for a long period there is fibrosis rather than cirrhosis, with irregular islands of parenchyma demarcated by fibrous septa (**Fig. 14.8**). The pattern is somewhat like that of chronic biliary tract disease. At this stage some regression of fibrosis as a result of treatment remains possible.[64] Once cirrhosis has developed, biopsy assessment of the effect of treatment on structural changes becomes more difficult because of a tendency for increasing nodule size and compression or remodelling of septa. The onset of cirrhosis marks a fall in life expectancy and an increased risk of hepatocellular carcinoma.[61] The presence of iron-free foci may represent an early stage of malignant transformation.[65,66] Carcinoma has been recorded in non-cirrhotic patients with hereditary haemochromatosis, but is very rare.[65,67]

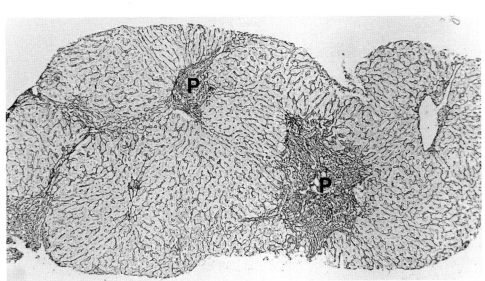

Figure 14.6 Hereditary haemochromatosis. At this early stage of fibrosis lobular architecture is still intact and vascular relationships are maintained. The portal tracts (P) are expanded by fibrous tissue. (Needle biopsy, reticulin.)

Figure 14.7
Hereditary
haemochromatosis.
Grade 4 (maximal)
liver-cell siderosis.
Iron-rich granules in
a pericanalicular
location outline bile
canaliculi (arrow).
(Needle biopsy, Perls'
stain.)

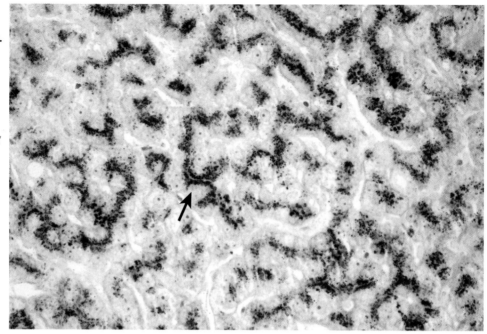

Figure 14.8
Hereditary
haemochromatosis.
Fibrous septa
surround irregular
islands of liver
parenchyma. (Wedge
biopsy, H&E.)

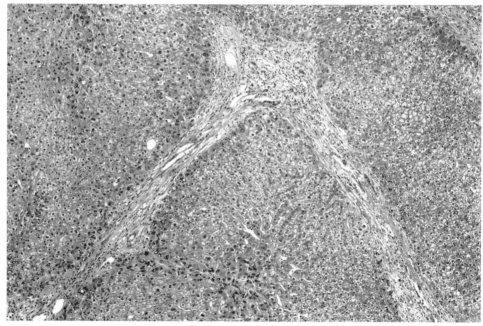

Effective treatment leads to a steady reduction in stainable iron. Iron encrusted on to portal collagen is usually the most resistant to removal and may be the only stainable iron remaining in the liver. Removal of iron unmasks a brown lipofuscin-like pigment in hepatocytes and connective tissue. Following liver transplantation for haemochromatosis, iron may reaccumulate in hepatocytes of the donor liver, but the rate is uncertain.[68]

Other primary iron overload disorders

Several types of **non-*HFE* haemochromatosis**[29] (**Box 14.1**) and other genetic diseases such as **aceruloplasminaemia**[69] result in hepatic iron overload, with marked hepatocellular siderosis present in the majority. However, some of these diseases show an atypical iron distribution. Both early and later stages of **ferroportin-related iron overload** feature abundant Kupffer-cell siderosis[70] (in contrast to *HFE*-related haemochromatosis). Liver-cell haemosiderin is absent or minimal in the early stage and as it progresses it is seen throughout the lobule, without the usual gradient from periportal to centrilobular regions.[29] The importance of ceruloplasmin in mediating egress of iron from cells is demonstrated in **aceruloplasminaemia**, where both hepatocytes and Kupffer cells accumulate haemosiderin.[69,71,72] Excessive Kupffer-cell siderosis that cannot be accounted for by one of the causes of secondary iron overload (see below) should therefore also raise the suspicion of a genetic iron overload disorder.

Secondary iron overload disorders

In routine practice most siderosis is secondary and located in sinusoidal Kupffer cells (**Fig. 14.9**). Haemolysis, transfusions and haemodialysis are common causes. Identification of significant iron overload with this distribution is evidence against most genetic forms of haemochromatosis, with the exception of ferroportin disease.[70] It is only when the threshold for macrophage iron storage is reached in such acquired disorders that liver-cell haemosiderin becomes evident in periportal regions (e.g. thalassaemia, sickle-cell disease).

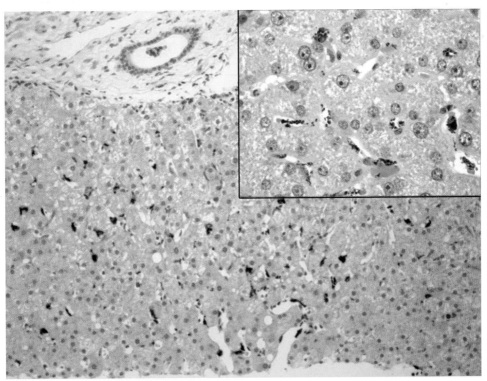

Figure 14.9 Secondary (acquired) iron overload. Diffuse siderosis of sinusoidal Kupffer cells is present. Common causes are haemolysis, transfusions and haemodialysis. (Needle biopsy, Prussian blue iron stain.) Inset: Refractile brown haemosiderin granules are present within sinusoidal Kupffer cells. (Needle biopsy, H&E.)

Neonatal haemochromatosis

This severe liver disease of stillborns or newborns is characterised by marked liver injury and loss of functional parenchyma, a resultant acquired hepcidin deficiency and extensive siderosis of liver and extrahepatic organs (thyroid, pancreas, myocardium, minor salivary glands). It is not related to hereditary haemochromatosis in adults. Many cases are due to gestational alloimmune liver disease (GALD), in which maternal antifetal liver IgG antibodies cross the placenta, activate fetal complement and cause severe hepatocyte necrosis.[73-75] Postmortem and explant livers usually show cirrhosis (or exceptionally severe fibrosis with sparse, small regenerative foci), abundant ductular reaction, variable giant-cell transformation, cholestasis and very few remaining hepatocytes (**Fig. 14.10**). Many of the features resemble those seen in adults with acute liver failure and massive hepatic necrosis. Active Sonic hedgehog signaling by the ductular reaction in GALD mediates the development of extensive fibrosis.[75a] Haemosiderin, when present, is limited to hepatocytes and the ductular reaction and is largely absent from Kupffer cells. The diagnosis may be confirmed by labial minor salivary gland biopsy[76] (**Fig. 14.10C**). The differential diagnosis of neonatal haemochromatosis includes other causes of severe perinatal liver disease and liver failure such as mitochondriopathies and Down syndrome with megakaryocytic

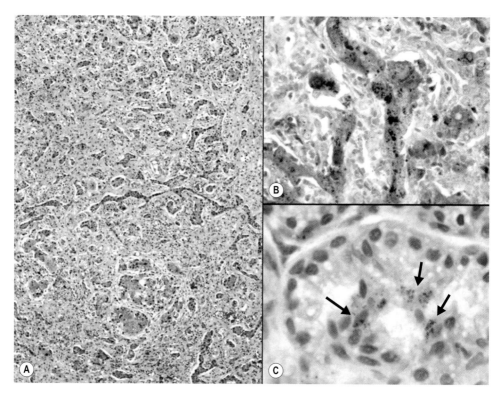

Figure 14.10 Neonatal haemochromatosis.
A: There is massive loss of liver parenchyma, with replacement by fibrosis and numerous bile ductular structures (ductular reaction). A few small clusters of remaining hepatocytes are seen in the lower half of the field. The pigment visible at this magnification includes both bile and haemosiderin. (Explant liver, H&E.) **B:** There is much haemosiderin within the bile ductular epithelium and in the few surviving hepatocytes, without significant Kupffer cell siderosis. (Explant liver, Prussian blue iron stain.) **C:** Biopsy of the patient's labial salivary gland shows intraepithelial haemosiderin granules (arrows). (Needle biopsy, Prussian blue iron stain.)

transient myeloproliferative disorder.[75] A recent French multicentre retrospective study of many cases of neonatal haemochromatosis provides a wealth of clinical and pathologic data.[77]

Iron overload in haematological disorders

Siderosis is found in patients with thalassaemia and, less commonly, other haematological disorders. The iron overload is partly the result of blood transfusion. In addition to the hepatocytic siderosis, portal fibrosis and septum formation seen in hereditary haemochromatosis, there is iron in macrophages from an early stage (**Fig. 14.11**) and haemopoietic cells may be present. There is often more infiltration of portal tracts, septa and sinusoids by lymphocytes than in hereditary haemochromatosis (**Fig. 14.12**). This, together with focal hepatocellular damage in some cases, is attributable to transfusion-related hepatitis, usually hepatitis C.[78,79] The pattern of fibrosis and degree of inflammation in a liver biopsy often help to determine the relative roles of iron overload and hepatitis C in the progression of the disease. Kupffer-cell siderosis is a common finding in haemolysis, haemophagocytic syndrome,[80] haemodialysis and sickle-cell disease.[81]

Liver disease of varied aetiology

Chronic viral hepatitis, alcoholic and non-alcoholic fatty liver disease and cirrhosis of diverse aetiologies unrelated to hereditary haemochromatosis[30,31] are often associated with variable degrees of siderosis (**Fig. 14.13**). In **chronic hepatitis**, levels of serum iron and ferritin are sometimes increased as a result of release of iron from damaged hepatocytes, and iron may be seen on liver biopsy. The iron may be located in periportal hepatocytes, in Kupffer cells or in the endothelium of portal vessels.[36,82] Patchy iron-rich foci of hepatocytes in an otherwise non-siderotic biopsy may occasionally be seen.[83] In chronic hepatitis C, iron overload adversely affects therapy with interferon.[84] The severe siderosis which

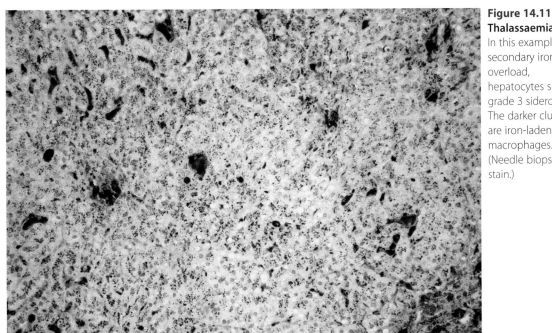

Figure 14.11
Thalassaemia.

In this example of secondary iron overload, hepatocytes show grade 3 siderosis. The darker clumps are iron-laden macrophages. (Needle biopsy, Perls' stain.)

Figure 14.12 Thalassaemia.
There are iron-laden macrophages in the portal tract and in sinusoids. Haemosiderin granules are also evident in hepatocytes. The portal inflammation is probably due to transfusion-transmitted hepatitis C. (Needle biopsy, H&E.)

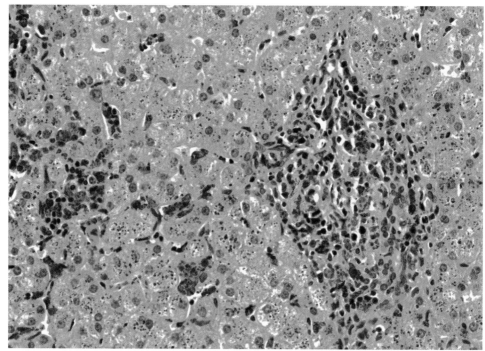

Figure 14.13 Cirrhosis with siderosis.
This case of relatively inactive cirrhosis due to chronic hepatitis C demonstrates considerable variability in the degree of hepatocellular siderosis among the nodules. (Explant liver, Perls' stain.)

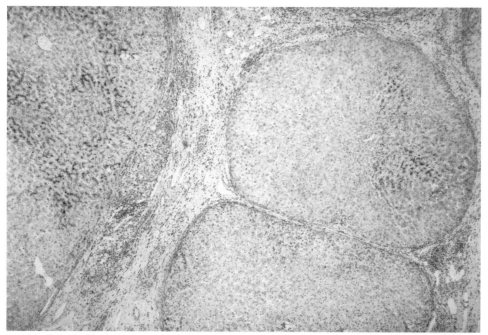

can complicate cirrhosis due to viral hepatitis and alcohol use may sometimes mimic hereditary haemochromatosis,[30,31] with marked elevations in HIC and hepatic iron index. In such cases there may even be siderosis of extrahepatic organs (heart, pancreas, stomach, thyroid, others).[85] Such cases require a comprehensive correlation of the histopathological features, biochemical test results, genetic analysis and other clinical data in order to clarify

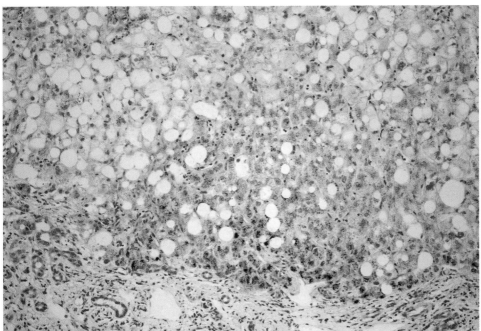

Figure 14.14
Cirrhosis with siderosis.
In this fatty cirrhosis in an alcohol abuser there is grade 2 hepatocellular siderosis, the cause of which needs investigation. (Needle biopsy, Perls' stain.)

the aetiology of the iron overload. Biopsies from patients with **steatosis** sometimes show siderosis in periportal hepatocytes and in Kupffer cells, in which instance the possibility of **dysmetabolic iron overload** syndrome (DIOS) (**see Fig. 7.12**) – associated with metabolic syndrome (central obesity, hypertension, hyperlipidaemia, hyperglycaemia and insulin resistance) – should be considered.[34,86]

The presence of underlying liver disease is not in itself necessarily sufficient to explain the presence of hepatocellular haemosiderosis, nor does it preclude the diagnosis of a coexisting genetic iron overload disorder. An example of this is **porphyria cutanea tarda** in which siderosis is present and increased frequencies of both hepatitis C virus infection[87,88] and *HFE* gene mutations have been identified.[88] Histological siderosis in **alcoholic liver disease** (**Fig. 14.14**) may reflect underlying homozygous or heterozygous haemochromatosis or concomitant spur-cell haemolytic anaemia.[89] Alcohol and chronic hepatitis C are known to accelerate the progression of liver disease in patients with *HFE*-related homozygous hereditary haemochromatosis.[60,90]

References

1   Riordan SM, Williams R. The Wilson's disease gene and phenotypic diversity. J Hepatol 2001;34:165–71.

2   Tao TY, Gitlin JD. Hepatic copper metabolism: insights from genetic disease. Hepatology 2003;37:1241–7.

3   Huster D, Hoppert M, Lutsenko S, et al. Defective cellular localization of mutant ATP7B in Wilson's disease patients and hepatoma cell lines. Gastroenterology 2003;124:335–45.

4   Schmidt HHJ. Role of genotyping in Wilson's disease. J Hepatol 2009;50:449–52.

5   Cope-Yokoyama S, Finegold MJ, Sturniolo GC, et al. Wilson disease: histopathological correlations with treatment on follow-up liver biopsies. World J Gastroenterol 2010;16:1487–94.

6   Scheinberg IH, Sternlieb I. Wilson's Disease. Major Problems in Internal Medicine XXIII. Philadelphia, PA: WB Saunders; 1984.

7   Walshe JM. Diagnosis and treatment of presymptomatic Wilson's disease. Lancet 1988;ii:435–7.

8 Ludwig J, Moyer TP, Rakela J. The liver biopsy diagnosis of Wilson's disease. Methods in pathology. Am J Clin Pathol 1994;102:443–6.

9 Stromeyer FW, Ishak KG. Histology of the liver in Wilson's disease: a study of 34 cases. Am J Clin Pathol 1980;73:12–24.

10 Polio J, Enriquez RE, Chow A, et al. Hepatocellular carcinoma in Wilson's disease. Case report and review of the literature. J Clin Gastroenterol 1989;11:220–4.

11 Cheng WSC, Govindarajan S, Redeker AG. Hepatocellular carcinoma in a case of Wilson's disease. Liver 1992;12:42–5.

12 Schilsky ML, Scheinberg IH, Sternlieb I. Liver transplantation for Wilson's disease: indications and outcome. Hepatology 1994;19:583–7.

13 Eleazar JA, Memeo L, Jhang JS, et al. Progenitor cell expansion: an important source of hepatocyte regeneration in chronic hepatitis. J Hepatol 2004;41:983–91.

14 Roberts EA, Schilsky ML. Diagnosis and treatment of Wilson disease: an update. Hepatology 2008;47: 2089–111.

15 Davies SE, Williams R, Portmann B. Hepatic morphology and histochemistry of Wilson's disease presenting as fulminant hepatic failure: a study of 11 cases. Histopathology 1989;15:385–94.

16 Strand S, Hofmann WJ, Grambihler A, et al. Hepatic failure and liver cell damage in acute Wilson's disease involve CD95 (APO-1/Fas) mediated apoptosis. Nat Med 1998;4:588–93.

17 Faa G, Nurchi V, Demelia L, et al. Uneven hepatic copper distribution in Wilson's disease. J Hepatol 1995;22:303–8.

18 Müller-Höcker J, Meyer U, Wiebecke B, et al. Copper storage disease of the liver and chronic dietary copper intoxication in two further German infants mimicking Indian childhood cirrhosis. Pathol Res Pract 1988;183:39–45.

19 Baker A, Gormally S, Saxena R, et al. Copper-associated liver disease in childhood. J Hepatol 1995;23:538–43.

20 Müller T, Feichtinger H, Berger H, et al. Endemic Tyrolean infantile cirrhosis: an ecogenetic disorder. Lancet 1996;347:877–80.

21 Faa G, Liguori C, Columbano A, et al. Uneven copper distribution in the human newborn liver. Hepatology 1987;7:838–42.

22 Elmes ME, Clarkson JP, Mahy NJ, et al. Metallothionein and copper in liver disease with copper retention – a histopathological study. J Pathol 1989;158:131–7.

23 Mulder TPJ, Janssens AR, Verspaget HW, et al. Metallothionein concentration in the liver of patients with Wilson's disease, primary biliary cirrhosis, and liver metastasis of colorectal cancer. J Hepatol 1992;16:346–50.

24 Pilloni L, Lecca S, Van Eyken P, et al. Value of histochemical stains for copper in the diagnosis of Wilson's disease. Histopathology 1998;33:28–33.

25 Ala A, Borjigin J, Rochwarger A, et al. Wilson disease in septuagenarian siblings: raising the bar for diagnosis. Hepatology 2005;41:668–70.

26 Tavill AS, Sharma BK, Bacon BR. Iron and the liver: genetic hemochromatosis and other hepatic iron overload disorders. In: Popper H, Schaffner F, editors. Progress in Liver Diseases, vol. IX. Philadelphia, PA: WB Saunders; 1990. p. 281–306.

27 Searle J, Leggett BA, Crawford DHG, et al. Iron storage diseases. In: MacSween RNM, Burt AD, Portmann BC, et al., editors. Pathology of the Liver. 4th ed. Edinburgh: Churchill Livingstone; 2002. p. 257–72 [Ch. 5].

28 Faa G, Sciot R, Farci AMG, et al. Iron concentration and distribution in the newborn liver. Liver 1994;14:193–9.

29 Pietrangelo A. Non-*HFE* hemochromatosis. Hepatology 2004;39:21–9.

30 Deugnier Y, Turlin B, Le Quilleuc D, et al. A reappraisal of hepatic siderosis in patients with end-stage cirrhosis: practical implications for the diagnosis of hemochromatosis. Am J Surg Pathol 1997;21:669–75.

31 Ludwig J, Hashimoto E, Porayko MK, et al. Hemosiderosis in cirrhosis: a study of 447 native livers. Gastroenterology 1997;112:882–8.

32 Bergmann OM, Mathahs MM, Broadhurst KA, et al. Altered expression of iron regulatory genes in cirrhotic human livers: clues to the cause of hemosiderosis? Lab Invest 2008;88:1349–57.

33 Terada T, Nakanuma Y. Survey of iron-accumulative macroregenerative nodules in cirrhotic livers. Hepatology 1989;10:851–4.

34 Turlin B, Mendler MH, Moirand R, et al. Histologic features of the liver in insulin resistance-associated iron overload. A study of 139 patients. Am J Clin Pathol 2001;116:263–70.

35 Bardadin KA, Scheuer PJ. Endothelial cell changes in acute hepatitis. A light and electron microscopic study. J Pathol 1984;144:213–20.

36 Kaji K, Nakanuma Y, Sasaki M, et al. Hemosiderin deposition in portal endothelial cells: a novel hepatic hemosiderosis frequent in chronic viral hepatitis B and C. Hum Pathol 1995;26:1080–5.

37 Olynyk J, Hall P, Sallie R, et al. Computerized measurement of iron in liver biopsies: a comparison with biochemical iron measurement. Hepatology 1990;12:26–30.

38 Deugnier YM, Loréal O, Turlin B, et al. Liver pathology in genetic hemochromatosis: a review of 135 homozygous cases and their bioclinical correlations. Gastroenterology 1992;102:2050–9.

39 Olynyk J, Williams P, Fudge A, et al. Fine-needle aspiration biopsy for the measurement of hepatic iron concentration. Hepatology 1992;15:502–6.

40 Olynyk JK, O'Neill R, Britton RS, et al. Determination of hepatic iron concentration in fresh and paraffin-embedded tissue: diagnostic implications. Gastroenterology 1994;106:674–7.

41 Ludwig J, Batts KP, Moyer TP, et al. Liver biopsy diagnosis of homozygous hemochromatosis: a diagnostic algorithm. Mayo Clin Proc 1993;68:263–7.

42 Bassett ML, Halliday JW, Powell LW. Value of hepatic iron measurements in early hemochromatosis and determination of the critical iron level associated with fibrosis. Hepatology 1986;6:24–9.

43 Kanwar P, Kowdley KV. Metal storage disorders. Wilson disease and hemochromatosis. Med Clin N Am 2014;98:87–102.

44 Pietrangelo A. Hereditary hemochromatosis – a new look at an old disease. N Engl J Med 2004;350:2383–97.

45 von Recklinghausen FD. Hemochromatosis. Taggeblatt Versammlung Dtsch Naturforsch Arzte Heidelberg 1889;62:324–5.

46 Powell LW, George K, McDonnell SM, et al. Diagnosis of hemochromatosis. Ann Intern Med 1998;129:925–31.

47 Pietrangelo A. Hemochromatosis 1998: is one gene enough? J Hepatol 1998;29:502–9.

48 Adams PC. Intrafamilial variation in hereditary hemochromatosis. Dig Dis Sci 1992;37:361–3.

49 Riedel H-D, Stremmel W. The haemochromatosis gene. J Hepatol 1997;26:941–4.

50 Ramrakhiani S, Bacon BR. Hemochromatosis. Advances in molecular genetics and clinical diagnosis. J Clin Gastroenterol 1998;27:41–6.

51 Brissot P, Moirand R, Guyader D, et al. Hemochromatosis after the gene discovery: revisiting the diagnostic strategy. J Hepatol 1998;28:14–18.

52 Bacon BR. Diagnosis and management of hemochromatosis. Gastroenterology 1997;113:995–9.

53 Bartolo C, McAndrew PE, Sosolik RC, et al. Differential diagnosis of hereditary hemochromatosis from other liver disorders by genetic analysis. Gene mutation analysis of patients previously diagnosed with hemochromatosis by liver biopsy. Arch Pathol Lab Med 1998;122:633–7.

54 Parkkila S, Niemelä O, Britton RS, et al. Molecular aspects of iron absorption and HFE expression. Gastroenterology 2001;121:1489–96.

55 Cheng R, Barton JC, Morrison ED, et al. Differences in hepatic phenotype between hemochromatosis patients with HFE C282Y homozygosity and other HFE genotypes. J Clin Gastroenterol 2009;43:569–73.

56 Bassett ML, Hickman PE, Dahlstrom JE. The changing role of liver biopsy in diagnosis and management of haemochromatosis. Pathology 2011;43:433–9.

57 Wallace DF, Walker AP, Pietrangelo A, et al. Frequency of the S65C mutation of HFE and iron overload in 309 subjects heterozygous for C282Y. J Hepatol 2002;36:474–9.

58 European Association for the Study of the Liver. EASL clinical practice guidelines for HFE hemochromatosis. J Hepatol 2010;53:3–22.

59 Harrison SA, Bacon BR. Hereditary hemochromatosis: update for 2003. J Hepatol 2003;38:S14–23.

60 Diwarkaran HH, Befeler AS, Britton RS, et al. Accelerated hepatic fibrosis in patients with combined hereditary hemochromatosis and chronic hepatitis C infection. J Hepatol 2002;36:687–91.

61 Niederau C, Fischer R, Sonnenberg A, et al. Survival and causes of death in cirrhotic and in noncirrhotic patients with primary hemochromatosis. N Engl J Med 1985;313:1256–62.

62 Wood MJ, Gadd VL, Powell LW, et al. Ductular reaction in hereditary hemochromatosis: the link between hepatocyte senescence and fibrosis progression. Hepatology 2014;59:848–57.

63 Iancu TC, Deugnier Y, Halliday JW, et al. Ultrastructural sequences during liver iron overload in genetic hemochromatosis. J Hepatol 1997;27:628–38.

64 Falize L, Guillygomarc'h A, Perrin M, et al. Reversibility of hepatic fibrosis in treated genetic hemochromatosis: a study of 36 cases. Hepatology 2006;44:472–7.

65 Deugnier YM, Guyuder D, Crantock I, et al. Primary liver cancer in genetic hemochromatosis: a clinical, pathological, and pathogenetic study of 54 cases. Gastroenterology 1993;104:228–34.

66 Deugnier YM, Charalambous P, Le Quilleuc D, et al. Preneoplastic significance of hepatic iron-free foci in genetic hemochromatosis: a study of 185 patients. Hepatology 1993;18:1363–9.

67 Fellows IW, Stewart M, Jeffcoate WJ, et al. Hepatocellular carcinoma in primary haemochromatosis in the absence of cirrhosis. Gut 1988;29:1603–6.

68 Farrell FJ, Nguyen M, Woodley S, et al. Outcome of liver transplantation in patients with hemochromatosis. Hepatology 1994;20:404–10.

69 Loréal O, Turlin B, Pigeon C, et al. Aceruloplasminemia: new clinical, pathophysiological and therapeutic insights. J Hepatol 2002;36:851–6.

70 Pietrangelo A. Hemochromatosis: an endocrine liver disease. Hepatology 2007;46:1291–301.

71 Kono S, Suzuki H, Takahashi K, et al. Hepatic iron overload associated with a decreased serum ceruloplasmin level in a novel clinical type of aceruloplasminemia. Gastroenterology 2006;131:240–5.

72 Kerkhof M, Honkoop P. Never forget aceruloplasminemia in case of highly suggestive Wilson's disease score. Hepatology 2014;59:1645–7.

73 Whitington PF. Gestational alloimmune liver disease and neonatal hemochromatosis. Semin Liver Dis 2012;32:325–32.

74 Bonilla S, Prozialeck JD, Malladi P, et al. Neonatal iron overload and tissue siderosis due to gestational alloimmune liver disease. J Hepatol 2012;56:1351–5.

75 Zoller H, Knisely AS. Control of iron metabolism – lessons from neonatal hemochromatosis. J Hepatol 2012;56:1226–9.

75a Asai A, Malladi S, Misch J, et al. Elaboration of tubules with active hedgehog drives parenchymal fibrogenesis in gestational alloimmune liver disease. Hum Pathol 2015;46:84–93.

76 Smith SR, Shneider BL, Magid M, et al. Minor salivary gland biopsy in neonatal hemochromatosis. Arch Otolaryngol Head Neck Surg 2004;130:760–3.

77 Collardeau-Frachon S, Heissat S, Bouvier R, et al. French retrospective multicentric study of neonatal hemochromatosis: iimportance of autopsy and autoimmune maternal manifestations. Pediatr Dev Pathol 2012;15:450–70.

78 Wonke B, Hoffbrand AV, Brown D, et al. Antibody to hepatitis C virus in multiply transfused patients with thalassaemia major. J Clin Pathol 1990;43:638–40.

79 Donohue SM, Wonke B, Hoffbrand AV, et al. Alpha interferon in the treatment of chronic hepatitis C infection in thalassaemia major. Br J Haematol 1993;83:491–7.

80 de Kerguenec C, Hillaire S, Molinié V, et al. Hepatic manifestations of hemophagocytic syndrome: a study of 30 cases. Am J Gastroenterol 2001;96:852–7.

81 Banerjee S, Owen C, Chopra S. Sickle cell hepatopathy. Hepatology 2001;33:1021–8.

82 Haque S, Chandra B, Gerber MA, et al. Iron overload in patients with chronic hepatitis C: a clinicopathologic study. Hum Pathol 1996;27:1277–81.

83 Lefkowitch JH, Yee HT, Sweeting J, et al. Iron-rich foci in chronic hepatitis. Hum Pathol 1998;29:116–18.

84 Bonkovsky HL, Banner BF, Rothman AL. Iron and chronic viral hepatitis. Hepatology 1997;25:759–68.

85 Eng SC, Taylor SL, Reyes V, et al. Hepatic iron overload in alcoholic end-stage liver disease is associated with iron deposition in other organs in the absence of HFE-1 hemochromatosis. Liver Int 2005;25:513–17.

86 Deugnier Y, Brissot P, Loréal O. Iron and the liver: update 2008. J Hepatol 2008;48:S113–23.

87 Nagy Z, Kószo F, Pár A, et al. Hemochromatosis (*HFE*) gene mutations and hepatitis C virus infection as risk factors for porphyria cutanea tarda in Hungarian patients. Liver Int 2004;24:16–20.

88 Bonkovsky HL, Poh-Fitzpatrick M, Pimstone N, et al. Polrphyria cutanea tarda, hepatitis C and *HFE* gene mutations in North America. Hepatology 1998;27:1661–9.

89 Pascoe A, Kerlin P, Steadman C, et al. Spur cell anaemia and hepatic iron stores in patients with alcoholic liver disease undergoing orthotopic liver transplantation. Gut 1999;45:301–5.

90 Fletcher LM, Dixon JL, Purdie DM, et al. Excess alcohol greatly increases the prevalence of cirrhosis in hereditary hemochromatosis. Gastroenterology 2002;122:281–9.

General reading

Bacon BR, Adams PC, Kowdley KV, et al. Diagnosis and management of hemochromatosis: 2011 practice guideline by the American Association for the Study of Liver Diseases. Hepatology 2011;54:328–43.

Datz C, Felder TK, Niederseer D, et al. Iron homeostasis in the metabolic syndrome. Eur J Clin Invest 2013;43:215–24.

European Association for the Study of the Liver. EASL clinical practice guidelines for HFE hemochromatosis. J Hepatol 2010;53:3–22.

European Association for the Study of the Liver. EASL clinical practice guidelines: Wilson's disease. J Hepatol 2012;56:671–85.

Ferenci P, Caca K, Loudianos G, et al. Diagnosis and phenotypic classification of Wilson disease. Liver Int 2003;23:139–42.

Kanwar P, Kowdley KV. Metal storage disorders: Wilson disease and hemochromatosis. Med Cliin North Am 2014;98:87–102.

Merle U, Schaefer M, Ferenci P, et al. Clinical presentation, diagnosis and long-term outcome of Wilson's disease: a cohort study. Gut 2007;56:115–20.

Paterson AC, Pietrangelo A. Disorders of iron overload. In: Burt AD, Portmann BC, Ferrell LD, editors. MacSween's Pathology of the Liver. 6th ed. Edinburgh: Churchill Livingstone/Elsevier; 2012. p. 261–92.

Pietrangelo A. Hereditary hemochromatosis – a new look at an old disease. N Engl J Med 2004;350:2383–97.

Pietrangelo A. Non-*HFE* hemochromatosis. Hepatology 2004;39:21–9.

Pietrangelo A. Hemochromatosis: an endocrine liver disease. Hepatology 2007;46:1291–301.

Roberts EA, Schilsky ML. Diagnosis and treatment of Wilson disease: an update. Hepatology 2008;47:2089–111.

Thompson RJ, Portmann BC, Roberts EA. Genetic and metabolic liver disease. In: Burt AD, Portmann BC, Ferrell LD, editors. MacSween's Pathology of the Liver. 6th ed. Edinburgh: Churchill Livingstone/Elsevier; 2012. p. 157–260.

The Liver in Systemic Disease and Pregnancy

Introduction

Liver biopsies are often obtained to evaluate abnormalities of liver function tests in patients with known or suspected systemic disease and in the investigation of pyrexia of unknown origin.[1,2] In the latter, liver biopsy provides diagnostic information in approximately 15–30% of cases.[3] The hepatic changes associated with systemic diseases vary from obvious granulomas or steatosis (discussed in **Ch. 7**) to more subtle findings such as an increase in liver-cell mitoses. The pathologist will want to know, whenever possible, whether or not the biopsy changes are specific for a systemic disease. For example, when granulomas are present, their aetiology usually has important therapeutic implications. Liver biopsy in patients with AIDS may demonstrate suspected hepatotoxicity due to antiretroviral drugs or hepatic involvement by a micro-organism already identified elsewhere in the patient, or may disclose a new diagnosis such as lymphoma. Liver biopsy also provides tissue for culture and special stains. This chapter examines the pathology of hepatic granulomas, hepatic changes in a variety of infectious diseases and liver involvement in gastrointestinal and haemopoietic diseases and the porphyrias.

In the unusual situation where liver dysfunction is found in pregnancy, the histopathologist may be called upon to differentiate intercurrent conditions such as viral hepatitis from several varieties of liver disease unique to pregnancy. This differential diagnosis is discussed later on in this chapter.

Granulomas

There are many causes of hepatic granulomas, including local irritants, infections, infestations and hypersensitivity to drugs. The constituents of these lesions, depending on the aetiology and inflammatory cytokines produced,[4] include large epithelioid cells, multinucleated giant cells, varied numbers of mononuclear cells and eosinophils. Hepatic granulomas can be further morphologically classified as **caseating (necrotising)**, **non-caseating**, **lipogranulomas (Ch. 7)** and **fibrin-ring granulomas**.[5-7] The causes vary in frequency from one country to another. Although the aetiology may be determined from the histological features, from special stains for micro-organisms, from culture of part of the biopsy specimen or polymerase chain reaction of the paraffin-embedded specimen,[8] or from clinical and serological data, the cause of hepatic granulomas may remain unknown in some 10–36% of cases.[9,10]

From a practical point of view biopsies containing granulomas fall into one of four groups:

1 The cause of the granuloma is seen under the microscope. Examples are the granulomas around schistosome ova, and the mineral-oil lipogranulomas found in portal tracts or near terminal hepatic venules.

2 The cause is not seen, but other histological features and clinical circumstances make the diagnosis clear. For example, granulomas near damaged bile ducts in a patient with clinically and immunologically typical primary biliary cirrhosis are almost certainly due to this disease.

3 The cause is uncertain, but appearances favour one particular line of further investigation rather than another. For instance, sarcoidosis should be suspected when clusters of large granulomas with prominent epithelioid cells, large multinucleated giant cells and dense fibrosis are found in portal tracts.

4 The cause of the granulomas cannot be determined from the histological appearances. This is unfortunately common, and the help that the pathologist can then give to the clinician is limited.

These four circumstances can be summarised as **see the cause**, **know the cause**, **suspect the cause** and **don't know the cause**. Some of the histological guidelines for evaluating granulomas are shown in **Table 15.1**.

Granulomas are found in up to 10% of liver biopsies.[11,12] They may be sparse, and suspicion of granulomatous disease is an indication for examining step sections from different levels of a paraffin block, if no lesions are seen initially. Because identifiable granulomas are generally more than 50 μm in diameter, serial sections 5 μm thick are unnecessary unless a single granuloma is to be further investigated.

Table 15.1 Histological features of hepatic granulomas

Aetiology	Favoured site(s)	Special features
Sarcoidosis	Portal/periportal	Clustering Hyalinisation Inclusions in giant cells May destroy bile ducts
Tuberculosis	None	Necrosis
PBC	Portal	Near damaged bile duct Lobular granulomas uncommon
Drug	None	Eosinophils Other lesions often present (hepatitis, fat, cholestasis)
Mineral oil	Portal, perivenous	Oil vacuoles
Q fever, CMV, allopurinol, etc.	None	Fibrin-ring granuloma
CGDC	None	Brown pigment in macrophages May be necrotising
Cat-scratch disease, tularaemia, *Yersinia*	None	Purulent centre

PBC, primary biliary cirrhosis; CMV, cytomegalovirus; CGDC, chronic granulomatous disease of childhood.

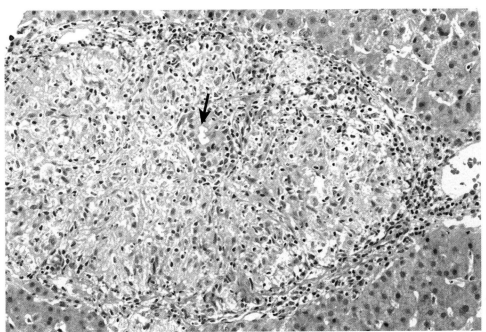

Figure 15.1 Sarcoidosis. A cluster of epithelioid-cell granulomas with giant cells has expanded a portal tract and surrounded a bile duct (arrow). (Needle biopsy, H&E.)

Granulomas are commonly found in the liver in **sarcoidosis** and may even recur following liver transplantation.[13] The liver is usually one of several organs involved, but occasionally extrahepatic lesions are difficult to demonstrate and chest X-ray may be normal.[14] Liver biopsy is helpful for diagnosis, especially in patients with fever and arthralgia.[15] The lesions may be found both in portal tracts and in lobules, and consist of well-defined, rounded granulomas with variable infiltration by inflammatory cells, including plasma cells and eosinophils (**Fig. 15.1**). The granulomas contain reticulin fibres (**Fig. 15.2**). Multinucleated giant cells may contain inclusions of different types.[16] Central necrosis may infrequently be present, but is never as extensive as in tuberculosis. The granulomas often cluster in portal and periportal regions[17] (**Fig. 15.2**) and older lesions show dense hyalinised collagen. The fibrosis may extend to interfere with normal acinar structure, and in more severe cases may progress to cirrhosis.[16,18] A surprising degree of reactive portal and lobular inflammation may occasionally be seen in association with sarcoid granulomas, raising the question of concomitant hepatitis.[18] The lobular component consists predominantly of hyperplastic Kupffer cells; acidophil bodies are rare. The portal tracts show considerable variability in the amount of lymphocytic inflammation and the most active portal inflammation is usually near granulomas. Serological tests for viral hepatitis should be obtained if there is serious diagnostic concern. In those few patients with sarcoidosis who develop portal hypertension,[19,20] it may be related to portal and periportal fibrosis or to broad areas of replacement fibrosis,[16] nodular regenerative hyperplasia[21] or cirrhosis.[16,18] Another rare complication of sarcoidosis is a primary biliary cirrhosis-like lesion, with destruction of bile ducts and a clinical picture of chronic cholestasis.[22] Portal features suggesting biliary obstruction may also be present.[16,18] It should be noted that a diagnosis of sarcoidosis cannot be proved by histological examination of the liver alone, because very similar lesions are found in other granulomatous diseases.

In **chronic granulomatous disease of childhood**, defective neutrophil leukocyte function leads to the development of infective granulomas of different sizes, containing homogeneous eosinophilic material, necrotic debris or pus. Portal tracts are inflamed and there may be fibrosis. A brown pigment of ceroid type accumulates in portal macrophages and to a lesser extent in Kupffer cells.[23-25] Abscesses and bile-duct fibroinflammatory lesions

**Figure 15.2
Sarcoidosis.**
The granulomas are clustered in the portal tract (P) and periportal region, a characteristic feature of sarcoidosis. They are associated with increased reticulin fibres. (Needle biopsy, reticulin.)

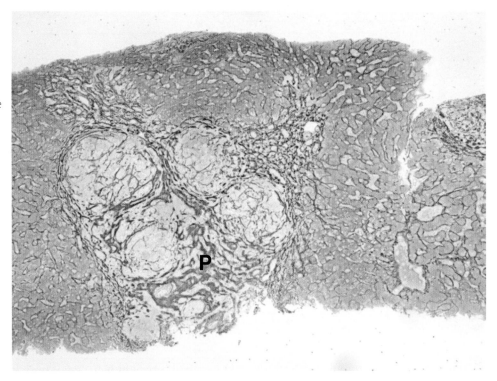

resembling primary sclerosing cholangitis are also seen.[26] The development of non-cirrhotic portal hypertension related to nodular regenerative hyperplasia and obliterative fibrosis of terminal venules and/or portal veins contributes to mortality.[27] **Common variable immunodeficiency** may be associated with portal and/or lobular epithelioid granulomas[28] as well as with nodular regenerative hyperplasia,[29] mild portal lymphocytic infiltrates with mild fibrosis[30] and, rarely, primary biliary cirrhosis or autoimmune hepatitis.[31]

A small number of patients with **chronic hepatitis C** may show non-caseating granulomas in the liver, either portal or lobular in location,[32,33] sometimes recurring after liver transplantation.[34] In one series, nearly 10% of granulomas were ascribed to this infection.[10] Their pathogenesis is unknown. In some instances, other causes such as schistosomiasis may become apparent during a thorough evaluation.[35] Necrotising granulomas at the edges of abscesses due to the Gram-negative bacillus *Achromobacter xylosoxidans* have been reported after cholecystectomy, with multilobulated 'coral-like' masses on computed tomography scan.[36]

Drugs and toxins should be considered in the evaluation of hepatic granulomas (**see Ch. 8**), particularly if eosinophils are prominent.[37] A diverse array of particulate materials may cause granulomas, including aluminium,[38] feldspar[39] and silicone.[40] Biopsies with granulomas should therefore be examined under polarised light for evidence of particulate material. Dense reactive fibrosis may develop in the form of **sclerohyaline nodules** in individuals exposed to silica, chromium, cobalt or magnesium, either in the workplace or by intravenous drug abuse.[41]

The **fibrin-ring granuloma** is a distinctive though non-specific[42] form described in Q fever,[42-47] Hodgkin's disease,[48] allopurinol hypersensitivity,[49] cytomegalovirus (CMV)[50] and Epstein–Barr virus infections,[51] leishmaniasis,[52] toxoplasmosis,[48] hepatitis A,[53,54] giant-cell arteritis[55] and systemic lupus erythematosus.[56] This granuloma is composed of a fat vacuole surrounded by a ring of fibrin, epithelioid cells, giant cells and neutrophils (**Fig. 15.3**). Serial sections may be needed to demonstrate the typical fibrin-ring or 'doughnut' lesion.[44]

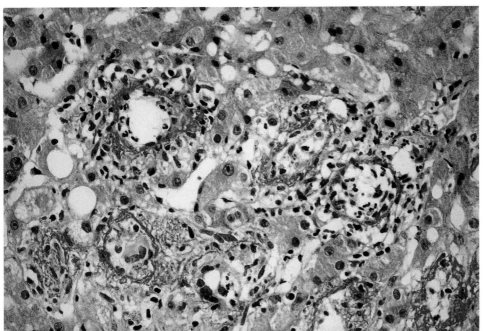

Simon and Wolff[57] described a syndrome characterised by fever, constitutional symptoms and hepatic granulomas, which does not respond to antituberculous drugs but improves on corticosteroid therapy or sometimes with methotrexate.[58] In some patients the syndrome resolves spontaneously without treatment.[59] The cause has not been established.

Viral diseases

The pathological changes in the liver resulting from virus infections other than hepatitis viruses have been reviewed by Lucas.[60] The viral haemorrhagic fevers, such as mosquito-borne **flavivirus** infection (**dengue fever**[61]) and rodent-borne **hantavirus** infections,[62] are characterised by mid-zonal or more extensive hepatic necrosis. In **yellow fever**, acidophil bodies are typically abundant; they were first described in this disease by Councilman over 100 years ago.[63,64]

Several viruses not normally associated with liver disease can occasionally cause liver damage. Examples include **herpes simplex virus** infection leading to irregular and randomly distributed areas of coagulative necrosis[65,66] (**Fig. 15.4**) and **adenovirus** infection.[67,68] In both infections, virus particles or antigens can be identified in hepatocytes. Paramyxovirus-like particles were described in adults with associated syncytial giant-cell hepatitis.[69] Multinucleated giant hepatocytes in liver biopsies from adults (**postinfantile giant-cell hepatitis**) may also be seen in hepatitis C virus mono-infection or co-infection with human immunodeficiency virus (HIV),[70] human herpesvirus-6A infection,[71] in autoimmune hepatitis and in other liver diseases.[72,73]

Cytomegalovirus infection

CMV has been implicated in some children with neonatal hepatitis (**see Ch. 13**). Histological features include giant-cell formation as in other forms of neonatal liver damage,

Figure 15.4 Herpes simplex hepatitis. Pale, ground-glass-like intranuclear inclusions are present in a multinucleated hepatocyte (near centre) and elsewhere (arrows). An adjacent focus of necrosis with neutrophils is seen at the right of the field. (Needle biopsy, H&E.)

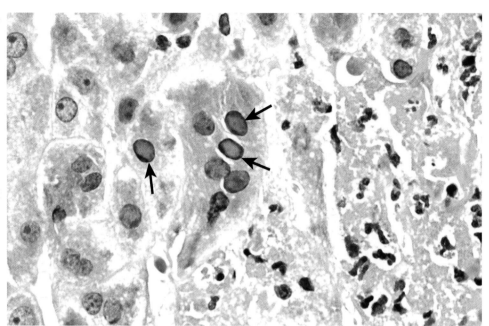

inflammation and cholestasis. Bile ducts are damaged and may be destroyed.[74] The CMV genome can be identified by the polymerase chain reaction in many cases.[75]

In later life, CMV infection can present as a mononucleosis-like illness, but also as hepatitis. Asymptomatic infection is common in immunocompromised patients. In these, the histological changes are often mild, but typical CMV inclusions are found in hepatocytes, bile-duct epithelium and endothelial cells (**Fig. 15.5**). Specific immunocytochemical staining reveals CMV antigens, even in cells without inclusions,[76] but sometimes with an abnormal granular basophilic cytoplasm.[77] Patients with CMV infection may also show aggregation of neutrophils in sinusoids, with or without evidence of CMV in neighbouring cells,[77] an important diagnostic consideration in immunocompromised patients or individuals who have received organ transplants. Larger accumulations of macrophages and lymphocytes can be seen and epithelioid-cell granulomas have been reported.[78] In immunocompetent patients, there are varying degress of focal liver-cell and bile-duct damage, portal inflammation, infiltration of sinusoids with lymphoid cells and increased mitoses in hepatocytes.[79] In such patients, it may not be possible to demonstrate CMV inclusions or antigen, a situation possibly analogous to hepatitis B virus infection, where inclusions and antigen may be scanty or absent during the acute attack while characteristic of the carrier state.[79]

Infectious mononucleosis

The liver is histologically abnormal in infectious mononucleosis even when there is no clinical jaundice.[80] Dense accumulations of atypical lymphocytes are found in portal tracts and sinusoids (**Fig. 15.6**). Sinusoidal aggregates must be distinguished from the more heterogeneous collections of cells found in extramedullary haemopoiesis. The infiltration also mimics that of leukaemia. Kupffer cells are enlarged. Epithelioid-cell granulomas are occasionally present.[12] Small foci of hepatocellular necrosis and acidophil bodies may be seen, but the diffuse hepatocellular damage characteristic of viral hepatitis is usually absent and extensive necrosis[81] is rare. Cholestasis is absent or mild.

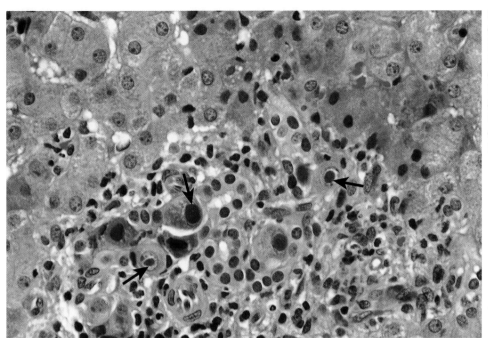

Figure 15.5 Cytomegalovirus hepatitis in AIDS. Numerous cytomegalovirus inclusions (arrows) are seen within bile-duct epithelial cells. (Needle biopsy, H&E.)

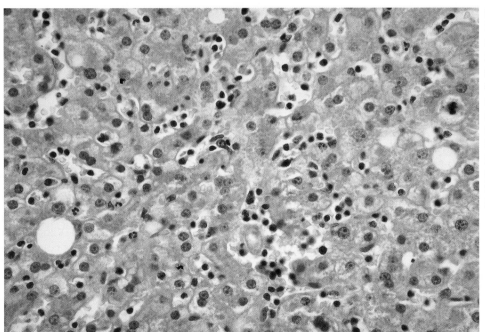

Figure 15.6 Infectious mononucleosis. At left, a prominent sinusoidal 'beads-on-a-string' pattern is seen, consisting of atypical lymphocytes and hyperplastic Kupffer cells. Atypical lymphocytes are also present in the portal tract at right. (Needle biopsy, H&E.)

Acquired immune deficiency syndrome (AIDS)

A spectrum of hepatobiliary lesions has been associated with AIDS and HIV-1 infection since the onset of the epidemic[82–91] (**Table 15.2**). Liver biopsy continues to play an important diagnostic role in the evaluation of abnormal liver function tests in these patients,[84,85,92] particularly in managing the potential hepatotoxicity of highly active antiretroviral therapy

Table 15.2 Hepatobiliary lesions in HIV-1 infection and AIDS

Lesion	Cause(s) or type(s)
Granulomas	Mycobacteria, fungi, drugs
Abscesses	Staphylococci, streptococci, listeria
Bacillary peliosis	*Bartonella henselae*
Biliary tract disease (AIDS cholangiopathy)	CMV, cryptosporidia, microsporidia
Neoplasms	Kaposi's sarcoma, lymphoma, smooth-muscle tumours
Chronic viral hepatitis	HBV, HCV, HDV
Autoimmune hepatitis	Coexistent or following immune reconstitution
Other viral infections	CMV, herpes simplex virus, Epstein–Barr virus, adenovirus
Vascular lesions	Peliosis hepatis, sinusoidal dilatation
Drug toxicity	Sulfa agents, antiretrovirals
Miscellaneous	Steatosis, haemosiderosis, stellate cell hypertrophy, amyloidosis

HIV-1, human immunodeficiency virus; AIDS, acquired immunodeficiency syndrome; CMV, cytomegalovirus; HBV, HCV, HDV, hepatitis B, C, D virus.

(HAART)[93–96] and concurrent chronic hepatitis B and/or C which may be present. Although Kupffer cells and endothelial cells[97–101] are potential target cells for HIV-1 infection, there are no specific hepatic lesions due to HIV-1, a few cases of alleged 'HIV-1 hepatitis'[102,103] notwithstanding.

Despite the reduction in morbidity and mortality due to antiretroviral therapy and prophylactic antibiotics,[104] opportunistic infections and neoplasms such as Kaposi's sarcoma and lymphoma must still be excluded on liver biopsy. Specimens should routinely be studied with acid-fast and silver stains for detection of high-incidence pathogens such as mycobacteria and fungi. Other methods such as Gram or Warthin–Starry stains can be applied, depending on the clinical and histological indications. A portion of the biopsy should be sent for culture.

Drug-related hepatotoxicity

Antiretroviral drugs may need to be excluded as the cause of liver dysfunction in HIV-positive individuals, particularly in those with negative hepatitis virus serology. Combination therapy frequently presents the problem of distinguishing among various medications. Some of the newer antiretroviral agents have been associated with elevated serum liver enzymes, but few morphologic data are available.[105] It is helpful to consider the type of hepatic damage reported with the several classes of **HAART agents**.[94] The nucleoside reverse transcriptase inhibitors cause mitochondrial damage and microvesicular steatosis, while the non-nucleoside reverse transcriptase inhibitors may produce hepatitis and confluent necrosis. The lesions attributed to protease inhibitors are various, including bile-duct damage, hepatocyte necrosis and ballooning, Mallory–Denk body formation, steatohepatitis and perivenular fibrosis.[94,95] Liver biopsy in some individuals receiving combined

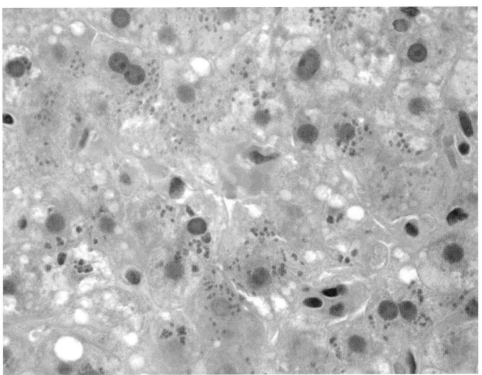

Figure 15.7
Hepatocellular pigment associated with antiretroviral therapy for HIV.
Hepatocytes show coarse brown pigment granules resembling Dubin–Johnson pigment. The pigment is often panlobular in distribution. The specific causative medication is not known. (Needle biopsy, H&E.)

antiretroviral therapy shows coarse brown hepatocellular pigment granules resembling the pigment of Dubin–Johnson syndrome, often panlobular in distribution[106] (**Fig. 15.7**). The specific causative drug has not been identified. Since antiretroviral liver injury is often idiosyncratic, the internet and other sources should be consulted for emerging descriptions of new cases.

Opportunistic infections and infestations

Opportunistic infections and infestations involving the liver and bile ducts in AIDS include *Mycobacterium avium–intracellulare* and *Mycobacterium tuberculosis* infections, CMV infection, cryptococcosis, candidiasis, histoplasmosis, leishmaniasis,[107] malaria, cryptosporidiosis[108] and microsporidiosis.[109–111] Mycobacterial and fungal infections frequently produce **granulomas**. *M. avium–intracellulare* results in numerous granulomas and the organisms are readily demonstrated by staining with diastase–periodic acid–Schiff (PAS) or the Ziehl–Neelsen method[112–115] (**Fig. 15.8**). Each granuloma consists of foamy histiocytes with few lymphocytes. The histiocytes often show a striated appearance on haematoxylin and eosin (H&E) staining due to the abundant packing of organisms in each cell. *M. avium–intracellulare* organisms are also well stained with Gomori methenamine silver. For screening of liver biopsies, particularly for *M. tuberculosis*, which may be present in fewer numbers than *M. avium–intracellulare*, the auramine–rhodamine fluorescent method[116,117] gives excellent results. Careful examination of special stains is of particular importance, as some AIDS patients have mycobacterial infection without typical granuloma formation; scant, single mycobacteria may be present within sinusoids or portal tracts. *Pneumocystis carinii* may disseminate to the liver, producing acellular exudative masses which closely resemble the pulmonary alveolar exudates.[118]

Figure 15.8
Mycobacterium avium–intracellulare **in AIDS.**
Abundant macrophages with densely packed mycobacteria are present within a granuloma. Individual organisms are best seen in the centre of the field. (Postmortem liver, Ziehl–Neelsen.)

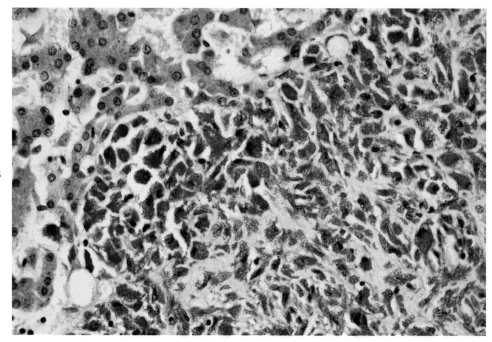

AIDS cholangiopathy

AIDS cholangiopathy resembles sclerosing cholangitis clinically and radiographically and is due to infections of the large bile ducts by several possible pathogens, including CMV, cryptosporidia and microsporidia.[109-111],[119-121] Liver biopsy changes are those of large-duct obstruction. Cryptosporidia and microsporidia are best identified in aspirates obtained at endoscopy, duodenal biopsies or postmortem tissue samples of the major bile ducts.[109-111]

Peliosis hepatis

Peliosis hepatis[114,122,123] in AIDS has been postulated to be due to endothelial damage by HIV-1 infection.[101] Alternatively, **bacillary peliosis hepatis** may develop as a consequence of hepatic infection by the Gram-negative bacillus *Bartonella henselae.*[124-127] Smudge-like or granular pink-to-purple material associated with a myxoid stroma is seen within dilated vascular spaces (**Fig. 15.9**) and the Warthin–Starry stain shows clumped bacilli in these areas.

Lymphomas

Lymphomas involve the liver as nodular masses or portal tract infiltrates (**see Fig. 7.3**) and are high-grade large-cell, immunoblastic and Burkitt types.[128,129]

Chronic hepatitis

AIDS patients have many of the same risk factors for infection by hepatitis viruses, and serum markers of prior infection or active viral hepatitis are often present. While the liver biopsy lesions of **chronic hepatitis B, C and delta** can vary considerably in persons infected with HIV,[130-132] it is now recognised that HIV infection may exert an adverse effect.[133-135] Fulminant hepatitis may occur[136] and in drug addicts a propensity for more

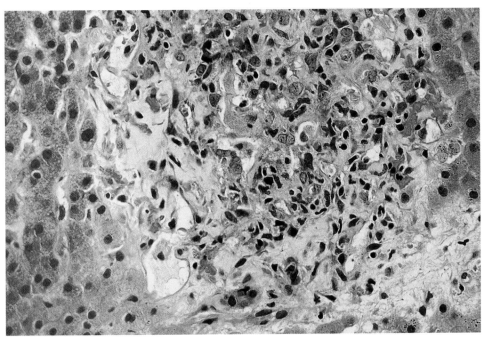

Figure 15.9
Bacillary peliosis in AIDS.
The portal tract is expanded by dilated blood vessels (left and right), chronic inflammatory cells and pink-grey smudge-like material (at centre) which contains bacilli. (Needle biopsy, H&E.)

severe chronic hepatitis with progression to cirrhosis has been noted.[137] Coexistent autoimmune hepatitis may need exclusion when abnormal serum liver tests are found in the HIV-infected individual[138] and rarely *de novo* autoimmune hepatitis may develop because of **immune reconstitution** after antiretroviral therapy has begun.[139]

Steatosis and other changes

Steatosis is common[140] and occasionally is periportal (**see Fig. 7.3**). Severe macrovesicular or microvesicular fat is cause for concern because this may reflect toxicity of antiviral medications[93,94,141,142] and can be associated with liver failure.[143] Non-alcoholic steatohepatitis (NASH) and abnormal liver enzymes may be present because of concomitant insulin resistance and features of metabolic syndrome.[144,145] **Siderosis** of Kupffer cells is related to transfusion or viraemia-associated erythrophagocytosis. In some cases, **non-specific changes** consisting of sparse portal or acinar lymphocytic inflammation with scattered apoptotic bodies are seen, with no apparent aetiology.

Other lesions reported include **nodular regenerative hyperplasia**,[146,147] **amyloidosis**[148] and **hypertrophied perisinusoidal stellate (Ito) cells** containing numerous lipid droplets.[149] In children, **giant-cell hepatitis**,[102,150] **chronic hepatitis** of uncertain cause[151] and **primary leiomyosarcoma**[152] are described.

Rickettsial, bacterial and fungal infections

Q fever

In Q fever, due to infection with *Coxiella burnetii*, liver involvement is common, although only a few patients present clinically with liver disease. Histological changes include focal necrosis, non-specific inflammation and fatty change. The most characteristic lesion is the **fibrin-ring granuloma**[42–48] (**see Fig. 15.3**), a granulomatous lesion also seen in several other infections and in some patients taking allopurinol.[49] Atypical lesions without annular arrangement or a central clear area (but containing irregular fibrin strands) are also found, as are non-specific granulomas without fibrin. In chronic Q fever progressive fibrosis and cirrhosis have been reported.[153]

Brucellosis

In most patients with brucellosis, liver biopsy shows non-specific reactive changes comprising sinusoidal-cell hypertrophy, portal inflammation and focal necrosis.[153a] Non-necrotising granulomas, often small and located within the acini, are more commonly found in the acute phase of the infection.[154]

Typhoid fever

Liver involvement is uncommon, but most patients with 'typhoid hepatitis' are jaundiced.[155] Liver biopsy shows a mild hepatitis with marked hyperplasia of mononuclear phagocytes, and lymphocytoid cells in sinusoids.[156] Characteristic granuloma-like collections of mononuclear cells, the typhoid nodules, are described.[157] Other features include fatty change and portal inflammation.[155,158]

Cat-scratch disease

Infection by a short Gram-negative rod, *Bartonella henselae*, typically produces pyrexia and regional lymphadenopathy in children. Rarely, dissemination to the liver results in hepatic **granulomas with central stellate microabscesses** surrounded by palisaded macrophages, lymphocytes and an outer layer of fibroblasts.[159,160] The Warthin–Starry stain is used to identify the organisms.

Tuberculosis

Tuberculous lesions are present in the liver either as part of a generalised infection[161] or, less often, in the hepatobiliary form of the disease.[162] A normal chest X-ray does not exclude the diagnosis.[163] Granulomas are found randomly scattered in the parenchyma and also in the portal tracts. They range from small accumulations of macrophage-like cells to well-developed, large epithelioid-cell nodules with Langhans giant cells (**Fig. 15.10**). Central necrosis may or may not be present, and its absence does not exclude the diagnosis. Extensive necrosis (**Fig. 15.11**) is more likely to be seen when there are widely disseminated granulomas in the liver. Mycobacteria are seen in a minority of biopsies. Acute lesions contain little reticulin, while chronic ones undergo scarring. Remaining liver tissue shows non-specific reactive features and fatty change. Patients with AIDS sometimes have mycobacterial infection without typical granulomas, or may form tuberculous abscesses.[164] In all patients in whom tuberculosis is suspected, part of the liver biopsy specimen should be cultured. Polymerase chain reaction studies may also be performed on biopsy samples.[165] Lesions similar to those of tuberculosis have been reported in patients given BCG immunotherapy.[166–169]

Leprosy

In lepromatous leprosy specific granuloma-like lesions composed of foam cells are found in the liver and often contain acid-fast bacilli.[170] Organisms are also seen in Kupffer cells. Epithelioid-cell granulomas of tuberculoid type, rare in lepromatous leprosy, are found in the livers of some patients with the tuberculoid form of the disease. Either type of granuloma is seen in borderline leprosy.[171]

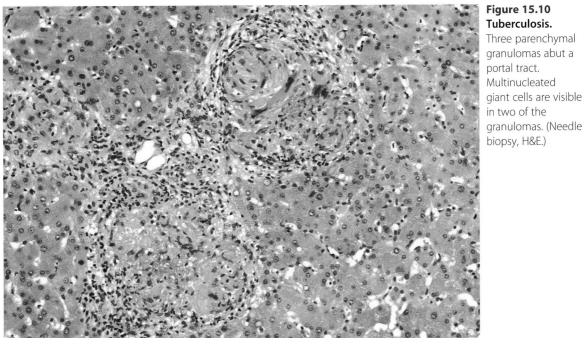

**Figure 15.10
Tuberculosis.**
Three parenchymal
granulomas abut a
portal tract.
Multinucleated
giant cells are visible
in two of the
granulomas. (Needle
biopsy, H&E.)

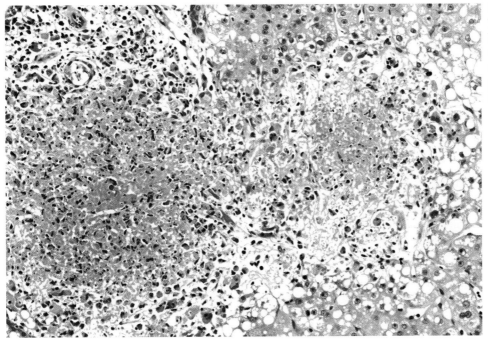

**Figure 15.11
Tuberculosis.**
There is extensive
necrosis with little
residual evidence of
granulomas. (Needle
biopsy, H&E.)

Spirochaetal infection

Syphilis

In congenital syphilis there is widespread fibrosis separating small groups of hepatocytes and spirochaetes are numerous. In early infections in adults, liver biopsies are normal or show non-specific changes.[172] Spirochaetes may be demonstrable histologically. In patients with secondary syphilis and jaundice or abnormal liver function tests, there is a variable degree of focal parenchymal inflammation, granuloma formation,[173] hepatocellular necrosis and portal inflammation. The portal reaction may mimic that of biliary obstruction,[174] and there may be inflammation of bile-duct epithelium as well as of the walls of small arteries and veins.[175,176] Because patients with syphilis often have other infections as well, lesions cannot always be confidently attributed to the syphilis itself.[177] The typical lesion of tertiary syphilis is the gumma, an area of necrosis surrounded by granulomatous tissue in which there is endarteritis. Healing is by fibrosis.

Leptospirosis

Most studies of the pathology of leptospirosis have dealt with autopsy material, in which disorganisation of liver-cell plates is a prominent feature. This is usually absent from liver biopsies.[178] Hepatocytes are swollen, especially in perivenular areas, and there is an increase in mitotic figures. A few acidophil bodies and fat vacuoles may be seen. Kupffer cells are prominent and there is a mild mononuclear-cell infiltrate in portal tracts. Cholestasis is common, and may persist after resolution of the other changes.[179] The diagnosis can be confirmed by demonstrating leptospiral antigen in paraffin sections by immunocytochemistry.[180]

Lyme disease

Hepatomegaly, elevated serum aminotransferase activity and biopsy features resembling viral hepatitis may be seen in patients infected with the tick-borne spirochaete *Borrelia burgdorferi*.[181] Liver-cell ballooning and numerous mitoses are accompanied by sinusoidal inflammation (hyperplastic Kupffer cells, lymphocytes, plasma cells and neutrophilic leukocytes). Rarely, necrotising granulomas with multinucleated giant cells and many eosinophils develop.[182] The organism can be identified in liver tissue by Dieterle silver stain.

Candidiasis

The most common hepatic manifestations of candidiasis in immunocompromised hosts are **microabscesses** and **granulomas**.[183,184] The more acute lesions show microabscess formation with central necrosis, visible on gross examination as 1–2-mm yellow-white nodules. Yeasts and pseudohyphae can be seen in some, but not all, cases with diastase–PAS and Gomori methenamine silver stains. The predominantly neutrophilic infiltrates are replaced by epithelioid histiocytes and granulomas as the lesions evolve, sometimes surrounded by reactive fibrosis. Candidiasis is most often diagnosed postmortem, but should be suspected in the presence of fever, abdominal symptoms and elevated serum alkaline phosphatase activity. Systemic candidiasis has been noted as an important cause of mortality in patients with zone 3 or multilobular hepatic necrosis due to **exertional heatstroke**.[185]

Histoplasmosis

Hepatomegaly is common in disseminated histoplasmosis due to *Histoplasma capsulatum*. The disease is very occasionally seen in countries where it is not endemic.[186] The liver may rarely be the only organ clinically involved.[187] Liver biopsy shows non-specific inflammation as well as granulomas which may be mistaken for the lesions of tuberculosis.[188,189] The organisms may be scanty or abundant, and are found in Kupffer cells and granulomas. They are round or oval, 1–5 μm across, and have a capsule and central chromatin mass. Diastase–PAS and other stains for fungi can be used for their demonstration and differentiation from Leishman–Donovan bodies; the latter are PAS-negative in tissues.[190] Disseminated infection with *Histoplasma duboisii*, seen in Africa, also involves the liver. Nodular lesions contain the much larger and easily demonstrable organisms.[191]

Fibrous, calcified and even bony nodules are sometimes found in and deep to the liver capsule in long-standing histoplasmosis. The nodules, 1–3 mm in diameter, may have a necrotic core surrounded by granulomatous tissue, and the organism is demonstrable in some instances.[192]

The liver in sepsis

Hepatic changes in sepsis are the result of infection of the liver itself, of circulating toxins, of ischaemia, or of a combination of these factors. In many patients the exact cause cannot be established.

Infective lesions include **liver abscess** and **bacterial cholangitis**. Less commonly, infection produces a diffuse bacterial hepatitis in which bacterial colonisation of the liver is associated with portal inflammation.[193] Infection in areas drained by the portal venous system can give rise to **pylephlebitis (see Fig. 12.3)**. Rarely, cholangiographic and histological features resembling primary sclerosing cholangitis develop in sepsis, possibly related to ischaemic damage to large ducts.[194] Postmortem liver sections from septic patients may show neutrophils aggregated within sinusoids and in sparse numbers dispersed throughout the connective tissue of portal tracts.

Patients with extrahepatic sepsis are often jaundiced, especially when the infection is due to Gram-negative organisms.[195] Three histological patterns have been described in such patients. The commonest is **canalicular cholestasis**, most severe in perivenular areas. This is associated with various degrees of Kupffer-cell activation, fatty change and portal inflammation, but usually little or no hepatocellular necrosis.[196]

The second pattern is one of **ductular cholestasis and inflammation**.[195,197] Bile ductular structures and canals of Hering at the margins of portal tracts are dilated and filled with bile, often in the form of dense, highly pigmented deposits, and neutrophils are seen within and around the affected ductules (**Fig. 15.12**). Perivenular cholestasis is usually present. Periportal canalicular bile is also sometimes present. These changes are not seen in uncomplicated bile-duct obstruction. They are common in the terminal stages of fatal acute or chronic liver disease complicated by sepsis. Damage to bile-duct epithelium has been reported[198] but in most instances the interlobular bile ducts are not affected. Patients with the ductular cholestasis pattern have disproportionately elevated serum bilirubin levels compared with alkaline phosphatase and aminotransferases.[199] Because of its dire implications, this biopsy finding should be communicated rapidly to the clinician and sepsis should be investigated.

The third pattern is **non-bacterial cholangitis**, seen in the **toxic-shock syndrome**.[200] The histological features are similar to those of bacterial cholangitis, but the biliary tree is anatomically normal and the lesion is attributed to a circulating staphylococcal toxin rather than to bacteraemia. In many patients, but not all, the underlying lesion is a staphylococcal vaginitis associated with the use of tampons.

Parasitic diseases

Toxoplasmosis

Toxoplasma gondii is occasionally responsible for neonatal liver injury. In adults, hepatic changes include extensive lymphocytic infiltration of sinusoids, evidence of mild liver-cell

Figure 15.12 Bile ductular cholestasis in sepsis. Proliferated bile ductules at the edge of the portal tract contain inspissated bile. The patient died of septicaemia. (Postmortem liver, H&E.)

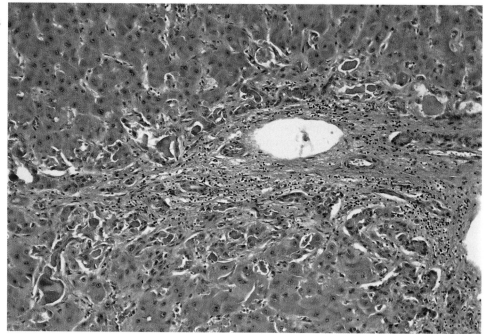

damage and granuloma formation.[12,201] Trophozoites may be seen within necrotic hepatocytes and can be identified by specific immunocytochemical methods.[202,203]

Malaria

In non-immune patients with malaria there is hypertrophy of Kupffer cells and these contain malarial pigment (haemozoin) in the form of fine, dark brown or black pigment granules (**Fig. 15.13**). In acute malaria due to *Plasmodium falciparum* they also contain erythrocytes, parasites and iron. Malarial pigment closely resembles schistosomal pigment. It often gives pinpoint birefringence and, like formalin pigment, is soluble in alcoholic picric acid. This distinguishes it from carbon, with which it may be confused.[204] Other black pigment in Kupffer cells, portal tract macrophages or granulomas can be seen after gold salt therapy or following knee or hip replacement with titanium-containing prostheses.[205] Following an attack of malaria the pigment clears from the acini but can be found in portal macrophages.

The **tropical splenomegaly syndrome (hyperreactive malarial splenomegaly)** probably represents an abnormal immune response of the patient to the malarial parasite.[206] Large numbers of small T lymphocytes are seen in dilated hepatic sinusoids (**Fig. 15.14**). Kupffer cells are enlarged but hepatocytes remain normal. Malarial pigment is scanty or absent. The differential histological diagnosis is from leukaemia, hepatitis C virus infection, infectious mononucleosis, CMV infection and toxoplasmosis.

Visceral leishmaniasis (kala-azar)

Infection by *Leishmania donovani* produces striking hypertrophy of Kupffer cells and portal macrophages. These cells contain variable, sometimes very large numbers of Leishman–Donovan bodies, easily visible in H&E-stained sections (**Fig. 15.15**). The PAS stain after diastase digestion is negative, in contrast to the positive staining obtained with

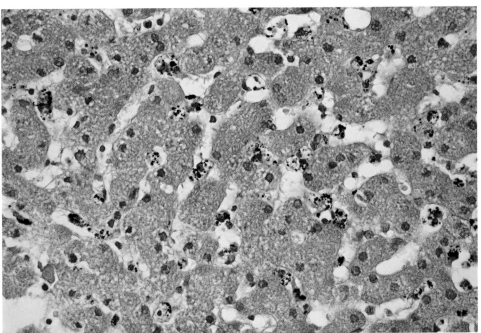

Figure 15.13 Malaria. Kupffer cells contain abundant dark granules of malarial pigment. (Needle biopsy, H&E.)

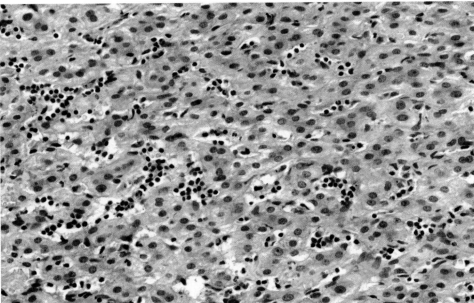

Figure 15.14 Tropical splenomegaly syndrome (hyperreactive malarial splenomegaly). There are groups of lymphocytes in the sinusoids. Kupffer cells are enlarged. Hepatocytes appear normal. (Needle biopsy, H&E.)

Histoplasma. In some patients the liver contains epithelioid-cell granulomas, which heal by fibrosis.[12,207]

Amoebiasis

In patients with liver abscesses due to *Entamoeba histolytica*,[208] the amoebae may be found at the margins of the lesion or, less often, within the necrotic debris. They may also be

Figure 15.15
Kala-azar.
There are many Leishman–Donovan bodies within several hepatocytes, just large enough to give the cells a stippled appearance at this magnification. (Postmortem liver, H&E.)

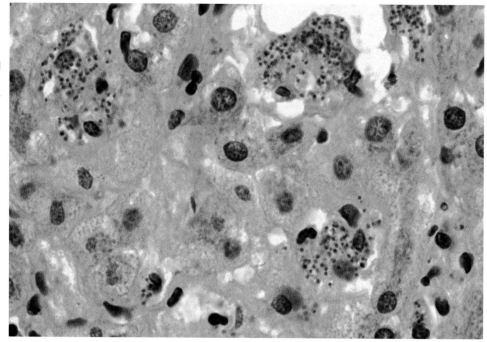

seen in the adjacent liver tissue. They are most easily demonstrated by the PAS or Giemsa methods. Organisms may be identified in fine-needle aspiration biopsy specimens[209] (**Fig. 15.16**).

Schistosomiasis

Liver lesions are usually caused by *Schistosoma mansoni* or *S. japonicum*, and less commonly by other species.[210] In acute schistosomiasis due to *S. mansoni* the portal tracts are infiltrated by eosinophils, lymphocytes and macrophages. Kupffer cells are enlarged and there is focal hepatocellular necrosis. Granulomas around ova are rare.[211]

More commonly schistosomiasis is chronic. Ova, initially containing live miracidia, are trapped in portal tracts where they excite a granulomatous reaction. This is composed of epithelioid cells, multinucleated giant cells, eosinophils and lymphocytes (**Fig. 15.17**). Healing is by fibrosis. When ova are scanty and granulomas are no longer seen, step sections may need to be searched. Ziehl–Neelsen staining is then helpful, because the ova of species other than *S. haematobium* are acid-fast.[212] Schistosomal pigment, found in portal tracts in some patients with chronic or past schistosomiasis, is a fine, dark granular material closely resembling malarial pigment.

There are lesions in portal-vein branches of all sizes.[211] The smallest contain ova and granulomas. Angiomatoids, wide, irregular thin-walled vascular channels, are characteristically found in fibrotic and enlarged portal tracts. Medium-sized veins show intimal thickening which may be eccentric and polypoid, and in large veins there are thrombi and adult worms. In the course of portal scarring, isolated smooth-muscle cells may become separated from the portal-vein wall and entrapped in fibrous tissue, a helpful diagnostic feature.[213] Diffuse hyaline thickening and tortuosity of veins with surrounding fibrosis constitute 'clay pipestem fibrosis', in which hepatic artery branches and bile ducts are preserved[213] (**Fig. 15.18**).

Lobular changes are usually slight, but sinusoidal lining cells are prominent and there is an increase in fibre within the space of Disse.[214,215] Portal tract lymphocytic infiltrates

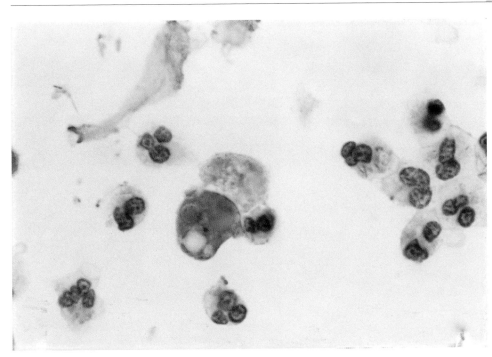

**Figure 15.16
Amoebic abscess.**
A trophozoite of
Entamoeba histolytica
is present in this
fine-needle
aspiration biopsy
sample, with a round
nucleus above
several cytoplasmic
glycogen vacuoles.
Adjacent cells are
neutrophilic
leukocytes.
(Papanicolaou.)
(Illustration kindly
provided by Dr
Alastair Deery,
London, UK.)

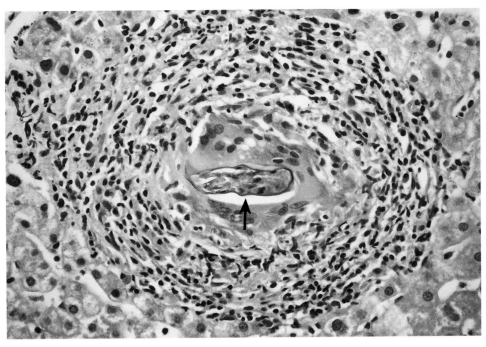

**Figure 15.17
Schistosomiasis.**
An ovum (arrow)
surrounded by giant
cells is seen at the
centre of a
granuloma. The
infiltrate is rich in
eosinophil
leukocytes. (Needle
biopsy, H&E.)

Figure 15.18 Schistosomiasis. Serpiginous septa contain many small blood vessels in this example of 'pipestem' fibrosis. (Wedge biopsy, H&E.)

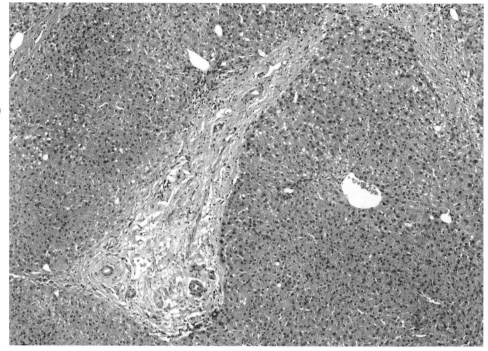

and piecemeal necrosis are likely to reflect the presence of chronic hepatitis, as hepatitis B virus infection is increased in patients with hepatosplenic schistosomiasis,[216,217] as is hepatitis C.

Liver flukes

Invasion of the biliary tree by the trematodes *Clonorchis sinensis* (the Chinese liver fluke), *Opisthorchis viverrini* and *O. felineus* is followed by proliferation of duct-like structures around the large bile ducts. The ductal epithelium may undergo goblet-cell metaplasia.[218] Smaller ducts are surrounded by an eosinophil-rich infiltrate. Complications include bile-duct obstruction, infection, portal fibrosis and hypertension, and bile-duct carcinoma.[219] Infestation may present several years after the patient has left an endemic area.[220]

The liver fluke *Fasciola hepatica* enters the liver from the peritoneal cavity and reaches the biliary tree some weeks later. White nodules are seen on the liver surface at the points of entry and may be mistaken for tumour. Migration tracks extend into the liver. Histologically, capsular and subcapsular lesions are composed of serpiginous areas of necrosis containing eosinophils and Charcot–Leyden crystals and bordered by palisaded histiocytes[221] (**Fig. 15.19**). Elsewhere in the liver, portal tracts are infiltrated with eosinophils. The biliary phase of the infestation is marked by cholangitis with rather less bile-duct hyperplasia than in *Clonorchis* or *Opisthorchis* infections, and both arterial and venous thrombosis. Features of bile-duct obstruction, periductal fibrosis and an ovum within a granuloma have also been reported.[222]

Ascariasis

Focal areas of necrosis with infiltration by eosinophils and neutrophils are seen in the migratory phase, when larvae travel to the lungs via the liver. Adult worms may enter the biliary tree from the duodenum, giving rise to bile-duct obstruction, cholangitis and abscess formation.[212]

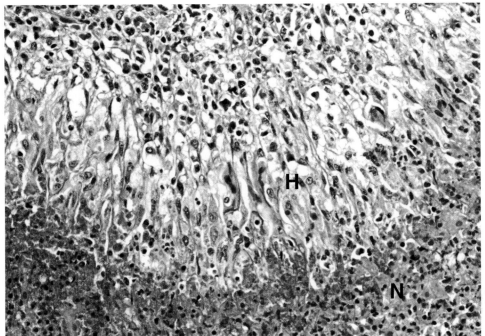

**Figure 15.19
Fascioliasis.**
Part of a nodule near the surface of the liver. A central area of necrosis (N) filled with leukocytes is bordered by palisaded histiocytes (H). (Wedge biopsy, H&E.)

Larval diseases

In several parasitic diseases with larval stages, including infestation by *Toxocara*, the larvae may reach the liver and give rise to eosinophil-rich abscesses or granulomas. Larvae are sometimes seen within these lesions.[12] White capsular and subcapsular liver nodules composed of mature fibrous tissue with calcification and few infiltrating cells surround larval remnants in long-standing disease due to *Toxocara* or to arthropod larvae.[223]

Gastrointestinal disorders and the liver

Patients with **coeliac disease** sometimes have elevated serum aminotransferases with non-specific acinar or portal mononuclear inflammation, fatty liver or infrequently chronic hepatitis, cirrhosis and hepatocellular carcinoma.[224] Occasionally, coeliac disease is associated with primary biliary cirrhosis or, rarely, with autoimmune hepatitis, primary sclerosing cholangitis or autoimmune cholangitis.[224,225] In **Whipple's disease** the characteristic foamy PAS-positive macrophages may be found in the liver[226] and epithelioid-cell granulomas have been reported.[227] Granulomas, associated with a heavy infiltration by eosinophils, have also been described in **eosinophilic gastroenteritis**.[228] Gastrointestinal cancers (colorectal, pancreas, bile duct, small intestine) are sometimes associated with pyogenic liver abscesses.[229]

Chronic inflammatory bowel disease

The spectrum of liver lesions is generally similar in ulcerative colitis and Crohn's disease. In Crohn's disease, serious hepatic complications such as sclerosing cholangitis are much less common and there may be granulomas in the liver[230] or amyloid deposition.[231] Gallstones are more common in patients with Crohn's disease than in the general population.

In both Crohn's disease and ulcerative colitis, malnutrition, anaemia and toxaemia can lead to steatosis.[232]

A minority of patients with ulcerative colitis has persistent abnormalities of liver function tests.[233] Careful examination including cholangiography shows that most of these patients have primary sclerosing cholangitis (**see Ch. 5**). Bile-duct carcinoma, sometimes accompanied by diffuse dysplasia of biliary epithelium[234,235] (**see Fig. 5.18**), is increased in patients with ulcerative colitis, probably reflecting underlying sclerosing cholangitis.[236,237] Portal inflammatory lesions with or without periductal fibrosis in ulcerative colitis have occasioned use of the term 'pericholangitis'. However, patients with such portal inflammation have largely been shown to have typical primary sclerosing cholangitis[238] or its small-duct variant.[239] Furthermore, some examples of so-called pericholangitis probably represent a non-specific inflammatory response to the colitis. The term pericholangitis should therefore be discarded.[239] While liver biopsies from patients with ulcerative colitis may show features of chronic hepatitis, this may be due to intercurrent viral hepatitis (e.g. following blood transfusion). However, it should be noted that interface hepatitis is also common in primary sclerosing cholangitis. From a practical point of view it therefore seems wise to consider the possibility of sclerosing cholangitis in all patients with ulcerative colitis and chronic liver disease.

Haematological disorders and the liver

One of the most common findings in liver biopsies from patients with haematological disorders is diffuse **Kupffer-cell siderosis**, usually reflecting prior transfusion (**Ch. 14**). In **reactive haemophagocytic syndrome**[240,241] diffuse Kupffer-cell hyperplasia with siderosis and phagocytosis of erythrocytes may be seen in patients with systemic infections, disseminated carcinoma, leukaemia and lymphoma. Kupffer-cell erythrophagocytosis in **macrophage activation syndrome** triggered by infection, malignancy or collagen vascular disease[242] is accompanied by portal and parenchymal CD8-positive T lymphocytes which may cause a clinical and histopathological hepatitis, the latter featuring prominent apoptotic bodies and, rarely, bile-duct damage or destruction.[243,244] Phagocytosed red blood cells are well demonstrated on chromotrope–aniline blue stain and the histiocytes stain much less intensely on diastase–PAS than those engaged in necrotising processes such as viral hepatitis. Hepatic involvement by leukaemias and lymphomas is discussed in **Chapter 11**, the effects of thrombosis and sickle-cell disease in **Chapter 12** and graft-versus-host disease following bone marrow transplantation in **Chapter 16**.

Haemophilia

Hepatitis viruses are readily transmitted in blood products, and hepatitis is therefore common in patients with haemophilia.[245-248] Hepatitis C virus and possibly other putative non-A, non-E hepatitis viruses are the most important agents involved, but markers of infection with hepatitis B virus are also present in some patients. Liver histopathology is most often that of a mild chronic hepatitis[248]; cirrhosis is infrequent. The complications of infection by HIV-1 and AIDS have been seen in some haemophiliacs who received blood products contaminated with HIV-1 prior to mandated screening for the virus which was initiated in the 1980s.

Extramedullary haemopoiesis

Haemopoiesis in the liver sinusoids is normal in fetal and neonatal life. In adults it is seen mainly in the myeloproliferative disorders and when tumours invade bone marrow. Foci of haemopoiesis may also be seen in the congested liver of patients with cardiac failure,[249]

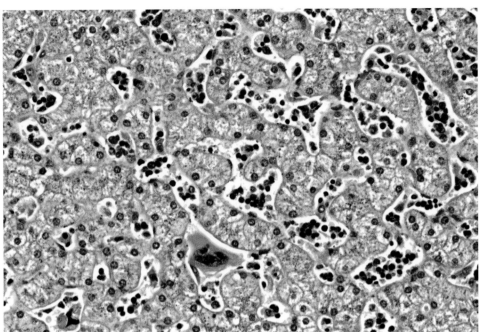

Figure 15.20
Extramedullary haemopoiesis. Clumps of haemopoietic cells are seen in the sinusoids, including a megakaryocyte at the bottom of the field. (Needle biopsy, H&E.)

in massive hepatic necrosis,[250] in transplant livers with zone 3 necrosis[251] or in the rare situation of graft-versus-host disease in liver transplant recipients.[252] The sinusoids and spaces of Disse of the enlarged liver contain discrete clumps of haemopoietic cells (**Fig. 15.20**), and there are similar cells in portal tracts. Features which distinguish haemopoiesis from the infiltrates of leukaemias, infectious mononucleosis, other infections and the tropical splenomegaly syndrome are the variety of cells in the aggregates and the presence of recognisable marrow cells such as normoblasts and eosinophil myelocytes. Megakaryocytes are commonly seen (**Fig. 15.20**) and are sometimes the only marrow elements found. Owing to the restraints of space, these cells are more elongated than in a section or smear of bone marrow. In the liver of neonates or stillborn infants with **Down's syndrome**, megakaryocytes may be the predominant form of extramedullary haemopoiesis[253,254] and perisinusoidal fibrosis may also be present.[255]

The liver in rheumatoid, immune-complex and collagen diseases

Liver pathology is uncommon in this group of diseases, but when present is most often **steatosis**.[256] **Nodular regenerative hyperplasia** is also seen in many connective tissue diseases.[257,258] The presence of multisystem disordered immunity in these conditions may be reflected in some cases by associated immune damage to bile ducts (**primary biliary cirrhosis**) or in the form of hepatic vasculitis.[258,259]

Polyarteritis nodosa in small hepatic arteries can lead to infarction. Immune complexes containing hepatitis B surface antigen are sometimes demonstrable in vessel walls in this disease.[260] Both hepatitis B and C virus antigen–antibody complexes have been implicated in the pathogenesis of **essential (type II) mixed cryoglobulinaemia**.[261–264] In the **polymyalgia rheumatica-giant-cell arteritis syndrome** the liver may contain granulomas.[265,266] Other findings reported include fatty change, venous congestion, non-specific hepatitis and prominent stellate cells.[267,268]

Patients with **rheumatoid arthritis** often have abnormal liver function tests, but liver biopsy more often shows non-specific changes or normal liver than definitive liver disease.[269-271] Amyloidosis or necrotising arteritis may be found, and rheumatoid nodules in the liver such as those typically found in subcutaneous tissue have been reported.[272] In **Felty's syndrome**[273] (rheumatoid arthritis, leucopenia and splenomegaly), the nodular lesions may be attributable to arteritis involving small intrahepatic vessels.[274]

Scleroderma and the **CRST syndrome** (calcinosis, Raynaud's phenomenon, sclerodactyly and telangiectasia) may be associated with primary biliary cirrhosis.[275,276] Giant, dense mitochondria on electron microscopy, with normal liver or non-specific changes on light microscopy, have been described in patients with **systemic sclerosis**.[277]

Most patients with **systemic lupus erythematosus** (SLE) do not have significant liver pathology but chronic hepatitis, cirrhosis and hepatic granulomas have been reported.[278,279] Abnormal liver function tests may be present without serious lesions.[280,281] Other changes described in SLE include steatosis,[282] cholestasis, nodular regenerative hyperplasia and necrotising arteritis involving arteries of 100–400 μm diameter.[279] An unusual case of **malacoplakia** involving the liver in a steroid-treated patient with SLE and Gram-negative bacterial infection showed aggregates of histiocytes with typical Michaelis–Gutmann bodies.[283] Although there appears to be no close relationship between systemic lupus and autoimmune ('lupoid') hepatitis, SLE with autoimmune hepatitis or with primary biliary cirrhosis may coexist.[282] The case of a patient with chronic hepatitis and **mixed connective tissue disease** has been reported.[284]

Amyloidosis and light-chain deposition

The liver is commonly involved in systemic amyloidosis. 'Primary' (AL) and reactive (AA) amyloidosis cannot definitively be distinguished by the pattern of liver involvement,[285,286] although sinusoidal deposition in AL and vascular involvement in AA are consistent patterns reported in several studies.[285,287] Histological distinction is made by the resistance of AL amyloid to potassium permanganate before Congo red staining[288] and by immunohistochemistry for immunoglobulin light chains, AA protein, transthyretin and other proteins.[286,289,290] In most patients the amyloid is deposited in portal arteries (**Figs 15.21 and 15.22**) or diffusely in the perisinusoidal space of Disse (**Fig. 15.23**). The two patterns are often combined. The perisinusoidal deposits compress both the sinusoids and the liver-cell plates, occasionally leading to portal hypertension or to cholestasis.[291-293] Rarely, AL or AA amyloid may be in the form of globular deposits[294] in the space of Disse (**Fig. 15.24**), within or surrounding portal arteries and veins or terminal venules, or within hepatocytes. Globular amyloid may be histologically contiguous with sinusoidal (linear) amyloid and thus be the precursor of the latter type.[295]

Amorphous perisinusoidal and portal deposits that are somewhat like amyloid are seen when the liver is involved in light-chain deposit disease.[296] Immunoglobulin light chains, usually kappa, can be identified immunochemically. The characteristic green birefringence of amyloid after Congo red staining is absent. Occasionally, amyloid and light-chain deposits are found in the same patient.[297,298]

The liver in the porphyrias

Liver lesions are found in **porphyria cutanea tarda** (PCT) and **protoporphyria**.[299] Red porphyrin fluorescence can be demonstrated in both diseases using unfixed liver tissue.

In **PCT**, hepatocytes contain needle-shaped birefringent porphyrin crystals, sufficiently water-soluble to make their demonstration difficult or impossible in routinely prepared

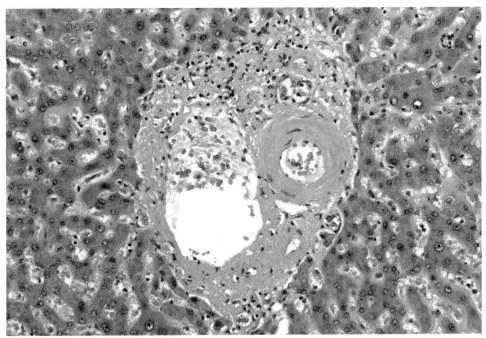

**Figure 15.21
Amyloidosis.**
The artery at right within this portal tract is thickened by amyloid deposit. (Needle biopsy, H&E.)

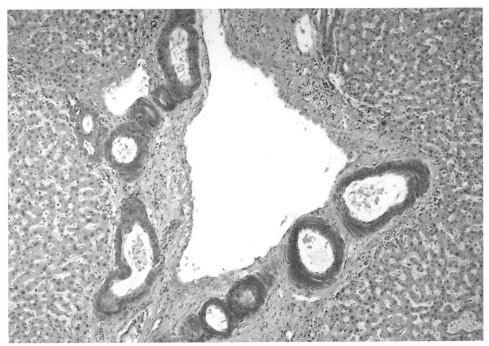

**Figure 15.22
Amyloidosis.**
Arterial amyloid deposits in this large-calibre portal tract are highlighted by Congo red staining. (Wedge biopsy, Congo red.)

paraffin sections. They can be seen in unstained paraffin sections, with a ferric ferricyanide reduction stain[300] and in H&E-stained sections prepared with minimal exposure to water.[301] Fatty change and hepatocellular siderosis are common[302] and intra-acinar clumps of iron- and ceroid-containing macrophages, fat droplets and inflammatory cells may also be present.[303] The role of *HFE* mutations in PCT varies geographically.[304-306] Alcohol

Figure 15.23 Amyloidosis. Amyloid has been laid down in the space of Disse. Liver-cell plates have undergone atrophy and sinusoids are narrowed. Cholestasis, an unusual complication of hepatic amyloidosis, is seen at upper right. (Explant liver, H&E.)

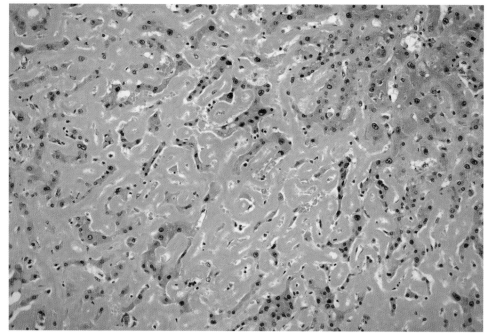

Figure 15.24 Globular amyloid. There are rounded deposits of amyloid (A) in the space of Disse. (Needle biopsy, Congo red.)

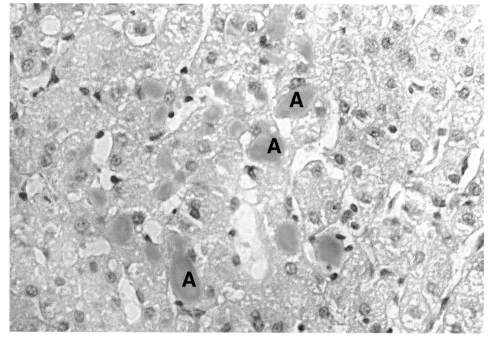

contributes to the pathogenesis of PCT and biopsies should be critically examined for alcohol-related injury. More importantly, **chronic hepatitis** and **cirrhosis** are common in patients with PCT and the majority have hepatitis C virus infection.[307–310] The prevalence of chronic hepatitis C in this population is approximately 50%,[311,312] which may also explain the development of **hepatocellular carcinoma**.[299]

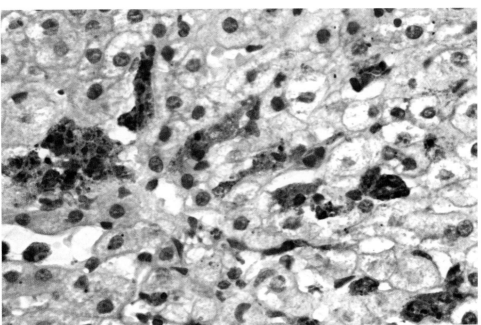

Figure 15.25 Erythropoietic protoporphyria. Dense brown protoporphyrin deposits are seen within sinusoids. (Needle biopsy, H&E.)

In **protoporphyria** (erythropoietic or erythrohepatic protoporphyria) dense, dark brown deposits of poorly soluble protoporphyrin accumulate in the liver (**Fig. 15.25**). These give a diagnostic red birefringence under polarised light, with a characteristic dark Maltese cross centrally.[313] There may be serious liver damage, with cholestasis, perisinusoidal and perivenular fibrosis and cirrhosis developing in some patients.[314,315]

Non-specific reactive changes

A variety of changes including portal and lobular inflammation, fat accumulation and Kupffer-cell hypertrophy is seen in extrahepatic conditions, especially febrile, inflammatory or widespread neoplastic diseases. Focal hepatocellular necroses may be found in the parenchyma. The distinction of these reactive changes from a mild form of chronic hepatitis or from residual acute hepatitis requires clinical information. The latter may sometimes be suspected from a predominantly perivenular location of inflammation and liver-cell loss. Reactive changes near space-occupying lesions such as metastatic tumours are discussed in **Chapter 1 (see Fig. 1.5)**.

The liver in pregnancy

In normal pregnancy there are no specific light microscopic findings in the liver. Electron microscopic changes reported in late pregnancy include giant mitochondria with paracrystalline inclusions, increase in the number of peroxisomes and proliferation of smooth endoplasmic reticulum.[316]

Liver disease in pregnancy is rare and falls into three categories[317]:

1   **Liver disease unique to pregnancy.** The four conditions included in this category[318-320] are **acute fatty liver of pregnancy (AFLP)**, **pre-eclampsia/ eclampsia**, the **HELLP syndrome (haemolysis, elevated liver enzymes and low platelets)** and **intrahepatic cholestasis of pregnancy (ICP)**.

2 **Intercurrent liver disease during pregnancy**. Viral hepatitis and cholelithiasis are examples. Hepatocellular carcinoma, including the fibrolamellar variety,[321] occurs rarely. **Viral hepatitis** is the most common form of liver disease encountered in pregnancy.

3 **Pre-existing liver disease in the pregnant patient**. Chronic hepatitis B viral infection and autoimmune hepatitis with or without cirrhosis are examples.

Jaundice and elevated serum aminotransferases are important aspects of the clinical presentation of liver disease in pregnancy. The following discussion is limited to those diseases unique to pregnancy.

Acute fatty liver of pregnancy

This uncommon and serious complication of pregnancy develops in the last weeks of gestation[322–324] and in certain cases is due to gene mutations affecting mitochondrial fatty acid oxidation enzymes.[325,326] Steatosis involves the greater part of each acinus, usually leaving a thin and incomplete rim of normal hepatocytes around the portal tracts.[327,328] The fat is mainly in the form of fine droplets, as in Reye's syndrome and other examples of microvesicular steatosis.[329] Large fat vacuoles of the kind seen in alcoholic liver disease are scanty, and the cause of the hepatocellular swelling and pallor may not be readily apparent on examination of paraffin sections (**Fig. 15.26**). PAS and trichrome stains are sometimes more helpful than H&E for identifying the small fat vacuoles. Fat staining of frozen sections makes the diagnosis clear, and a piece of the biopsy specimen should therefore be kept for frozen sectioning in patients with unexplained jaundice in late pregnancy. Inflammatory cells, mostly lymphocytes, are prominent in some examples and may lead to confusion with acute viral hepatitis,[330] in which microvesicular steatosis is not seen. In more severe examples of AFLP there is loss of hepatocytes leading to approximation of portal tracts. Fibrin deposits are occasionally demonstrable in hepatic sinusoids. One series showed cholestasis, extramedullary haemopoiesis and giant mitochondria[328] in some patients. With rare exceptions,[331] AFLP does not recur in subsequent pregnancies.

**Figure 15.26
Acute fatty liver
of pregnancy.**
Swollen pale-staining
hepatocytes are seen
around a terminal
hepatic venule (V).
The edge of a portal
tract with a mild
lymphocytic infiltrate
is seen at the upper
left corner. No large
fat vacuoles are seen.
(Postmortem liver,
H&E.)

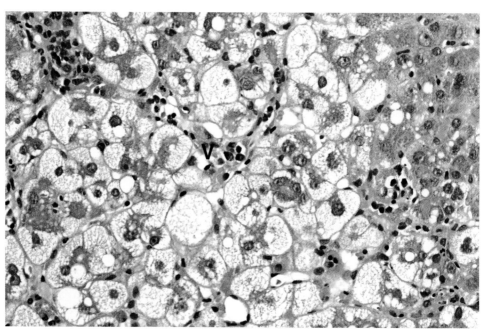

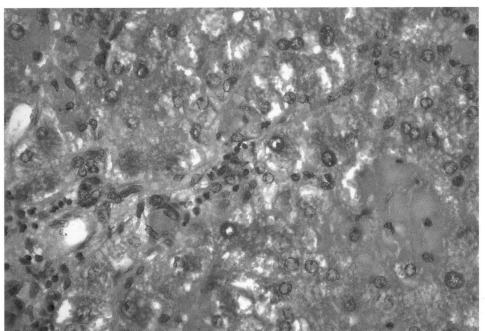

**Figure 15.27
Pre-eclampsia/
eclampsia.**
Fibrin is seen within
the periportal
sinusoids at lower
right. (Needle biopsy,
H&E.)

Pre-eclampsia/eclampsia

Hypertension, proteinuria, peripheral oedema and occasional coagulation abnormalities in pregnancy constitute pre-eclampsia, or eclampsia if convulsions and hyperreflexia are also present. Liver involvement is unusual, but may be manifested by elevated levels of serum aminotransferases and/or alkaline phosphatase. The incidence of pre-eclampsia is increased in patients with acute fatty liver.[330] The liver in pre-eclampsia shows fibrin thrombi in portal vessels and periportal sinusoids (**Fig. 15.27**) associated with necrosis and haemorrhage in more severe cases.[332,333] The identity of the fibrin can be established by phosphotungstic acid–haematoxylin staining or immunofluorescence.[334] These changes are not seen in all patients. Infarction, haematoma and rupture of the liver[335] are complications.

HELLP syndrome

This syndrome is exceedingly uncommon in pregnancy[322,336] and is seen in 20% of patients with severe pre-eclampsia.[318] Liver biopsy changes range from non-specific portal inflammation and glycogenated hepatocyte nuclei[322,337–339] to the periportal fibrin and necrosis seen in pre-eclampsia.[318] One study demonstrated a relationship between maternal AFLP and HELLP syndrome and a mitochondrial fatty acid γ-oxidation disorder with 3-hydroxyacyl-CoA dehydrogenase deficiency in their offspring.[340] Two of the children in the study had severe fatty change, necrosis and early nodules at autopsy.

Intrahepatic cholestasis of pregnancy

Pruritus, with or without cholestatic jaundice, may develop in late pregnancy and recur in subsequent pregnancies. It regresses after delivery. Liver biopsy shows little apart from canalicular cholestasis, most severe in perivenular areas.[332] Minor hepatocellular changes and inflammation are attributable to the cholestasis itself. Portal inflammation is absent or mild. No histological abnormalities are detectable between pregnancies, but the jaundice has been shown to return on administration of oral contraceptives.[341] Concomitant ICP and AFLP have been reported.[342] Some 15% of cases are accounted for by mutations in the multidrug resistance 3 (*MDR3*) bile transport gene.[343-346] Gallstone disease and hepatitis C virus infection are also associated with ICP, both before and after pregnancy.[347]

References

1   Bravo AA, Sheth SG, Chopra S. Liver biopsy. N Engl J Med 2001;344:495–500.

2   Burt AD. Liver pathology associated with diseases of other organs or systems. In: Burt AD, Portmann BC, Ferrell LD, editors. Pathology of the Liver. 5th ed. Edinburgh: Churchill Livingstone/Elsevier; 2007. p. 881–932 [Ch. 17].

3   Holtz T, Moseley RH, Scheiman JM. Liver biopsy in fever of unknown origin. A reappraisal. J Clin Gastroenterol 1993;17:29–32.

4   Sandor M, Weinstock JV, Wynn TA. Granulomas in schistosome and mycobacterial infections: a model of local immune responses. Trends Immunol 2003;24:44–52.

5   Lefkowitch JH. Hepatic granulomas. J Hepatol 1999;30:40–5.

6   Ferrell LD. Hepatic granulomas: a morphologic approach to diagnosis. Surg Pathol 1990;3:87–106.

7   Denk H, Scheuer PJ, Baptista A, et al. Guidelines for the diagnosis and interpretation of hepatic granulomas. Histopathology 1994;25:209–18.

8   Drebber U, Kasper H-U, Ratering J, et al. Hepatic granulomas: histological and molecular pathological approach to differential diagnosis – a study of 442 cases. Liver Int 2008;28:828–34.

9   Fauci AS, Wolff SM. Granulomatous hepatitis. In: Popper H, Schaffner F, editors. Progress in Liver Diseases, vol. V. New York: Grune & Stratton; 1976. p. 609–21 [Ch. 36].

10 Gaya DR, Thorburn KA, Oien KA, et al. Hepatic granulomas: a 10 year single centre experience. J Clin Pathol 2003;56:850–3.

11 Guckian JC, Perry JE. Granulomatous hepatitis: an analysis of 63 cases and review of the literature. Ann Intern Med 1966;65:1081–100.

12 Ishak KG. Granulomas of the liver. In: Ioachim HL, editor. Pathology of Granulomas. New York: Raven Press; 1983. p. 307–70.

13 Hunt J, Gordon FD, Jenkins RL, et al. Sarcoidosis with selective involvement of a second liver allograft: report of a case and review of the literature. Mod Pathol 1999;12:325–8.

14 Israel HL, Margolis ML, Rose LJ. Hepatic granulomatosis and sarcoidosis. Further observations. Dig Dis Sci 1984;29:353–6.

15 Hercules HD, Bethlem NM. Value of liver biopsy in sarcoidosis. Arch Pathol Lab Med 1984;108:831–4.

16 Ishak KG. Sarcoidosis of the liver and bile ducts. Mayo Clin Proc 1998;73:467–72.

17 Epstein MS, Devaney KO, Goodman ZD, et al. Liver disease in sarcoidosis. Hepatology 1990;12:839A.

18 Devaney K, Goodman ZD, Epstein MS, et al. Hepatic sarcoidosis. Clinicopathologic features in 100 patients. Am J Surg Pathol 1993;17:1272–80.

19 Maddrey WC, Johns CJ, Boitnott JK, et al. Sarcoidosis and chronic hepatic disease: a clinical and pathologic study of 20 patients. Medicine 1970;49:375–95.

20 Tekeste H, Latour F, Levitt RE. Portal hypertension complicating sarcoid liver disease: case report and review of the literature. Am J Gastroenterol 1984;79:389–96.

21 Moreno-Merlo F, Wanless IR, Shimamatsu K, et al. The role of granulomatous phlebitis and thrombosis in the pathogenesis of cirrhosis and portal hypertension in sarcoidosis. Hepatology 1997;26:554–60.

22 Rudzki C, Ishak KG, Zimmerman HJ. Chronic intrahepatic cholestasis of sarcoidosis. Am J Med 1975;59:373–87.

23 Bridges RA, Berendes H, Good RA. A fatal granulomatous disease of childhood. Am J Dis Child 1959;97:387–408.

24 Ishak KG, Sharp HL. Metabolic errors and liver disease. In: MacSween RNM, Anthony PP, Scheuer PJ, et al., editors. Pathology of the Liver. 3rd ed. Edinburgh: Churchill Livingstone; 1994. p. 123–218 [Ch. 4].

25 Nakhleh RE, Glock M, Snover DC. Hepatic pathology of chronic granulomatous disease of childhood. Arch Pathol Lab Med 1992;116:71–5.

26 Hussain N, Feld JJ, Kleiner DE, et al. Hepatic abnormalities in patients with chronic granulomatous disease. Hepatology 2007;45:675–83.

27 Feld JJ, Hussain N, Wright EC, et al. Hepatic involvement and portal hypertension predict mortality in chronic granulomatous disease. Gastroenterology 2008;134:1917–26.

28 Ardeniz O, Cunningham-Rundles C. Granulomatous disease in common variable immunodeficiency. Clin Immunol 2009;133:198–207.

29 Malamut G, Ziol M, Suarez F, et al. Nodular regenerative hyperplasia: the main liver disease in patients with primary hypogammaglobulinemia and hepatic abnormalities. J Hepatol 2008;48:74–82.

30 Daniels JA, Torbenson M, Vivekanandan P, et al. Hepatitis in common variable immunodeficiency. Hum Pathol 2009;40:484–8.

31 Fukushima K, Ueno Y, Kanegane H, et al. A case of severe recurrent hepatitis with common variable immunodeficiency. Hepatol Res 2008;38:415–20.

32 Emile JF, Sebagh M, Ferray C, et al. The presence of epithelioid granulomas in hepatitis C virus-related cirrhosis. Hum Pathol 1993;24:1095–7.

33 Barceno R, Sanroman AL, Del Campo S, et al. Posttransplant liver granulomatosis associated with hepatitis C? Transplantation 1998;65:1494–5.

34 Vakiani E, Hunt KK, Mazziotta RM, et al. Hepatitis C-associated granulomas after liver transplantation: morphologic spectrum and clinical implications. Am J Clin Pathol 2007;127:128–34.

35 Goldin RD, Levine TS, Foster GR, et al. Granulomas and hepatitis C. Histopathology 1996;28:265–7.

36 Asano K, Tada S, Matsumoto T, et al. A novel bacterium *Achromobacter xylosoxidans* as a cause of liver abscess: three case reports. J Hepatol 2005;43:362–5.

37 McMaster KR, Hennigar GR. Drug-induced granulomatous hepatitis. Lab Invest 1981;44:61–73.

38 Kurumaya H, Kono N, Nakanuma Y, et al. Hepatic granulomata in long-term hemodialysis patients with hyperaluminumemia. Arch Pathol Lab Med 1989;113:1132–4.

39 Ballestri M, Baraldi A, Gatti AM, et al. Liver and kidney foreign bodies granulomatosis in a patient with malocclusion, bruxism and worn dental prostheses. Gastroenterology 2001;121:1234–8.

40 Leong ASY, Disney APS, Gove DW. Spallation and migration of silicone from blood-pump tubing in patients on hemodialysis. N Engl J Med 1982;306:135–40.

41 Yao-Chang L, Tomashefski J, McMahon JT, et al. Mineral-associated hepatic injury: a report of seven cases with X-ray microanalysis. Hum Pathol 1991;22:1120–7.

42 Tjwa M, De Hertogh G, Neuville B, et al. Hepatic fibrin-ring granulomas in granulomatous hepatitis: report of four cases and review of the literature. Acta Clin Belg 2001;56:341–8.

43 Bernstein M, Edmondson HA, Barbour BH. The liver lesion in Q-fever. Clinical and pathologic features. Arch Intern Med 1965;116:491–8.

44 Pellegrin M, Delsol G, Auvergnat JC, et al. Granulomatous hepatitis in Q fever. Hum Pathol 1980;11:51–7.

45 Hofmann CE, Heaton JW Jr. Q fever hepatitis: clinical manifestations and pathological findings. Gastroenterology 1982;83:474–9.

46 Qizilbash AH. The pathology of Q fever as seen on liver biopsy. Arch Pathol Lab Med 1983;107:364–7.

47 Srigley JR, Vellend H, Palmer N, et al. Q-fever. The liver and bone marrow pathology. Am J Surg Pathol 1985;9:752–8.

48 Marazuela M, Moreno A, Yebra M, et al. Hepatic fibrin-ring granulomas. A clinicopathologic study of 23 patients. Hum Pathol 1991;22:607–13.

49 Vanderstigel M, Zafrani ES, Lejonc JL, et al. Allopurinol hypersensitivity syndrome as a cause of hepatic fibrin-ring granulomas. Gastroenterology 1986;90:188–90.

50 Lobdell DH. 'Ring' granulomas in cytomegalovirus hepatitis. Arch Pathol Lab Med 1987;111:881–2.

51 Nenert M, Mavier P, Dubuc N, et al. Epstein–Barr virus infection and hepatic fibrin-ring granulomas. Hum Pathol 1988;19:608–10.

52 Moreno A, Marazuela M, Yebra M, et al. Hepatic fibrin-ring granulomas in visceral leishmaniasis. Gastroenterology 1988;95:1123–6.

53 Ponz E, García-Pagán JC, Bruguera M, et al. Hepatic fibrin-ring granulomas in a patient with hepatitis A. Gastroenterology 1991;100:268–70.

54 Ruel M, Sevestre H, Henry-Biabaud E, et al. Fibrin ring granulomas in hepatitis A. Dig Dis Sci 1992;37:1915–17.

55 De Bayser L, Roblot P, Ramassamy A, et al. Hepatic fibrin-ring granulomas in giant cell arteritis. Gastroenterology 1993;105:272–3.

56 Murphy E, Griffiths MR, Hunter JA, et al. Fibrin-ring granulomas: a non-specific reaction to liver injury? Histopathology 1991;19:91–3.

57 Simon HB, Wolff SM. Granulomatous hepatitis and prolonged fever of unknown origin: a study of 13 patients. Medicine 1973;52:1–21.

58 Knox TA, Kaplan MM, Gelfand JA, et al. Methotrexate treatment of idiopathic granulomatous hepatitis. Ann Intern Med 1995;122:592–5.

59 Zoutman DE, Ralph ED, Frei JV. Granulomatous hepatitis and fever of unknown origin. An 11-year experience of 23 cases with three years' follow-up. J Clin Gastroenterol 1991;13:69–75.

60 Lucas SB. Other viral and infectious diseases and HIV-related liver disease. In: Burt AD, Portmann BC, Ferrell LD, editors. MacSween's Pathology of the Liver. 5th ed. Edinburgh: Churchill Livingstone/Elsevier; 2007. p. 443–92 [Ch. 9].

61 Huerre MR, Lan NT, Marianneau P, et al. Liver histopathology and biological correlates in five cases of fatal dengue fever in Vietnamese children. Virchows Arch 2001;438:107–15.

62 Elisaf M, Stefanaki S, Repanti M, et al. Liver involvement in hemorrhagic fever with renal syndrome. J Clin Gastroenterol 1993;17:33–7.

63 Klotz O, Belt TH. The pathology of the liver in yellow fever. Am J Pathol 1930;6:663–89.

64 Vieira WT, Gayotto LC, de Lima CP, et al. Histopathology of the human liver in yellow fever with special emphasis on the diagnostic role of the Councilman body. Histopathology 1983;7:195–208.

65 Goodman ZD, Ishak KG, Sesterhenn IA. Herpes simplex hepatitis in apparently immunocompetent adults. Am J Clin Pathol 1986;85:694–9.

66 Jacques SM, Qureshi F. Herpes simplex virus hepatitis in pregnancy: a clinicopathologic study of three cases. Hum Pathol 1992;23:183–7.

67 Carmichael GP Jr, Zahradnik JM, Moyer GH, et al. Adenovirus hepatitis in an immunosuppressed adult patient. Am J Clin Pathol 1979;71:352–5.

68 Varki NM, Bhuta S, Drake T, et al. Adenovirus hepatitis in two successive liver transplants in a child. Arch Pathol Lab Med 1990;114:106–9.

69 Phillips MJ, Glendis LM, Paucell S, et al. Syncytial giant-cell hepatitis. Sporadic hepatitis with distinctive pathologic features, a severe clinical course, and paramyxoviral features. N Engl J Med 1991;324:455–60.

70 Micchelli STL, Thomas D, Boitnott JK, et al. Hepatic giant cells in hepatitis C virus (HCV) mono-infection and HCV/HIV co-infection. J Clin Pathol 2008;61:1058–61.

71 Potenza L, Luppi M, Barozzi P, et al. HHV-6A in syncytial giant-cell hepatitis. N Engl J Med 2008;359:593–602.

72 Devaney K, Goodman ZD, Ishak KG. Postinfantile giant-cell transformation in hepatitis. Hepatology 1992;16:327–33.

73 Lau J, Koukoulis G, Mieli-Vergani G, et al. Syncytial giant-cell hepatitis – a specific disease entity? J Hepatol 1992;15:216–19.

74 Finegold MJ, Carpenter RJ. Obliterative cholangitis due to cytomegalovirus: a possible precursor of paucity of intrahepatic bile ducts. Hum Pathol 1982;13:662–5.

75 Chang M-H, Huang H-H, Huang E-S, et al. Polymerase chain reaction to detect human cytomegalovirus in livers of infants with neonatal hepatitis. Gastroenterology 1992;103:1022–5.

76 Theise ND, Conn M, Thung SN. Localization of cytomegalovirus antigens in liver allografts over time. Hum Pathol 1993;24:103–8.

77 Vanstapel MJ, Desmet VJ. Cytomegalovirus hepatitis: a histological and immunohistochemical study. Appl Pathol 1983;1:41–9.

78 Clarke J, Craig RM, Saffro R, et al. Cytomegalovirus granulomatous hepatitis. Am J Med 1979;66:264–9.

79 Snover DC, Horwitz CA. Liver disease in cytomegalovirus mononucleosis: a light microscopical and immunoperoxidase study of six cases. Hepatology 1984;4:408–12.

80 Kilpatrick ZM. Structural and functional abnormalities of liver in infectious mononucleosis. Arch Intern Med 1966;117:47–53.

81 Chang MY, Campbell WG Jr. Fatal infectious mononucleosis. Association with liver necrosis and herpes-like virus particles. Arch Pathol 1975;99:185–91.

82 Lebovics E, Thung SN, Schaffner F, et al. The liver in the acquired immunodeficiency syndrome: a clinical and histologic study. Hepatology 1985;5:293–8.

83 Glasgow BJ, Anders K, Layfield LJ, et al. Clinical and pathologic findings of the liver in the acquired immune deficiency syndrome (AIDS). Am J Clin Pathol 1985;83:582–8.

84 Dworkin BM, Stahl RE, Giardina MA, et al. The liver in acquired immune deficiency syndrome: emphasis on patients with intravenous drug abuse. Am J Gastroenterol 1987;82:231–6.

85 Schneiderman DJ, Arenson DM, Cello JP, et al. Hepatic disease in patients with the acquired immune deficiency syndrome (AIDS). Hepatology 1987;7:925–30.

86 Lebovics E, Dworkin BM, Heier SK, et al. The hepatobiliary manifestations of human immunodeficiency virus infection. Am J Gastroenterol 1988;83:1–7.

87 Wilkins MJ, Lindley R, Dourakis SP, et al. Surgical pathology of the liver in HIV infection. Histopathology 1991;18:459–64.

88 Stone VE, Bounds BC, Muse VV, et al. Case 29-2009: an 81-year-old man with weight loss, odynophagic, and failure to thrive. N Engl J Med 2009;361:1189–98.

89 Bach N, Theise ND, Schaffner F. Hepatic histopathology in the acquired immunodeficiency syndrome. Semin Liver Dis 1992;12:205–12.

90 Lefkowitch JH. The liver in AIDS. Semin Liver Dis 1997;17:335–44.

91 Lefkowitch JH. Pathology of AIDS-related liver disease. Dig Dis 1994;12:321–30.

92 Forsmark CE. AIDS and the gastrointestinal tract. Postgrad Med 1993;93:143–52.

93 Clark SJ, Creighton S, Portmann B, et al. Acute liver failure associate with antiretroviral treatment for HIV: a report of six cases. J Hepatol 2002;36:295–301.

94 Spengler U, Lichterfeld M, Rockstroh JK. Antiretroviral drug toxicity – a challenge for the hepatologist? J Hepatol 2002;36:283–94.

95 Sulkowski MS, Mehta SH, Torbenson M, et al. Hepatic steatosis and antiretroviral drug use among adults coinfected with HIV and hepatitis C virus. AIDS 2005;19:585–92.

96 Núñez M. Clinical syndromes and consequences of antiretroviral-related hepatotoxicity. Hepatology 2010;52:1143–55.

97 Scoazec JY, Feldmann G. Both macrophages and endothelial cells of the human hepatic sinusoid express the CD4 molecule, a receptor for the human immunodeficiency virus. Hepatology 1990;12:505–10.

98 Housset C, Lamas E, Courgnaud V, et al. Presence of HIV-1 in human parenchymal and non-parenchymal liver cells in vivo. J Hepatol 1993;19:252–8.

99 Steffan A-M, Lafon M-E, Gendrault J-L, et al. Primary cultures of endothelial cells from the human liver sinusoid are permissive for human immunodeficiency virus type 1. Proc Natl Acad Sci USA 1992;89:1582–6.

100 Housset C, Boucher O, Girard PM, et al. Immunohistochemical evidence for human immunodeficiency virus-1 infection of liver Kupffer cells. Hum Pathol 1990;21:404–8.

101 Lafon M-E, Kirn A. Human immunodeficiency virus infection of the liver. Semin Liver Dis 1992;12:197–204.

102 Witzleben CL, Marshall GS, Wenner W, et al. HIV as a cause of giant cell hepatitis. Hum Pathol 1988;19:603–5.

103 Molina J-M, Welker Y, Ferchal F, et al. Hepatitis associated with primary HIV infection. Gastroenterology 1992;102:739–46.

104 Palella FJ, Delaney KM, Moorman AC, et al. Declining morbidity and mortality among patients with advanced human immunodeficiency virus infection. N Engl J Med 1998;338:853–60.

105 Surgers L, Lacombe K. Hepatotoxicity of new antiretrovirals: a systematic review. Clin Res Hepatol Gastroenterol 2013;37:126–33.

106 Doherty AR, Ferrell LD, Morse CG, et al. Hepatic pigment accumulation in HIV patients on HAART therapy. Mod Pathol 2011;24(Suppl. 1s):Abstract 1522, 359A.

107 Hofman V, Marty P, Perrin C, et al. The histological spectrum of visceral leishmaniasis caused by Leishmania infantum MON-1 in acquired immune deficiency syndrome. Hum Pathol 2000;31:75–84.

108 Kahn DG, Garfinkle JM, Klonoff DC, et al. Cryptosporidial and cytomegaloviral hepatitis and cholecystitis. Arch Pathol Lab Med 1987;111:879–81.

109 Beaugerie L, Teilhac M-F, Deluol A-M, et al. Cholangiopathy associated with Microsporidia infection of the common bile duct mucosa in a patient with HIV infection. Ann Intern Med 1992;117:401–2.

110 Pol S, Romana C, Richard S, et al. Enterocytozoon bieneusi infection in acquired-immunodeficiency syndrome-related sclerosing cholangitis. Gastroenterology 1992;102:1778–81.

111 Pol S, Romana CA, Richard S, et al. Microsporidia infection in patients with the human immunodeficiency virus and unexplained cholangitis. N Engl J Med 1993;328:95–9.

112 Greene JB, Sidhu GS, Lewin S, et al. Mycobacterium avium-intracellulare: a cause of disseminated life-threatening infection in homosexuals and drug abusers. Ann Intern Med 1982;97:539–46.

113 Orenstein MS, Tavitian A, Yonk B, et al. Granulomatous involvement of the liver in patients with AIDS. Gut 1985;26:1220–5.

114 Gordon SC, Reddy KR, Gould EE, et al. The spectrum of liver disease in the acquired immunodeficiency syndrome. J Hepatol 1986;2:475–84.

115 Nakanuma Y, Liew CT, Peters RL, et al. Pathologic features of the liver in acquired immune deficiency syndrome (AIDS). Liver 1986;6:158–66.

116 Stevens A. Micro-organisms. In: Bancroft JD, Stevens A, editors. Theory and Practice of Histological Techniques. 2nd ed. Edinburgh: Churchill Livingstone; 1982. p. 278–96 [Ch. 15].

117 Kuper SWA, May JR. Detection of acid-fast-organisms in tissue sections by fluorescence microscopy. J Pathol Bacteriol 1960;79:59–68.

118 Poblete RB, Rodriguez K, Foust RT, et al. *Pneumocystis carinii* hepatitis in the acquired immunodeficiency syndrome (AIDS). Ann Intern Med 1989;110:737–8.

119 Margulis SJ, Honig CL, Soave R, et al. Biliary tract obstruction in the acquired immunodeficiency syndrome [published erratum appears in *Ann Intern Med* 1986 Oct; 105(4): 634]. Ann Intern Med 1986;105:207–10.

120 Cello J. Human immunodeficiency virus-associated biliary tract disease. Semin Liver Dis 1992;12:213–18.

121 Bouche H, Housset C, Dumont J-L, et al. AIDS-related cholangitis: diagnostic features and course in 15 patients. J Hepatol 1993;17:34–9.

122 Czapar CA, Weldon-Linne CM, Moore DM, et al. Peliosis hepatis in the acquired immunodeficiency syndrome. Arch Pathol Lab Med 1986;110:611–13.

123 Boylston AW, Cook HT, Francis ND, et al. Biopsy pathology of acquired immune deficiency syndrome (AIDS). J Clin Pathol 1987;40:1–8.

124 Perkocha LA, Geaghan SM, Yen TSB, et al. Clinical and pathological features of bacillary peliosis hepatis in association with human immunodeficiency virus infection. N Engl J Med 1990;323:1581–6.

125 Garcia-Tsao G, Panzini L, Yoselevitz M, et al. Bacillary peliosis hepatis as a cause of acute anemia in a patient with the acquired immunodeficiency syndrome. Gastroenterology 1992;102:1065–70.

126 Tappero JW, Koehler JE, Berger TG, et al. Bacillary angiomatosis and bacillary splenitis in immunocompetent adults. Ann Intern Med 1993;118:363–5.

127 Koehler JE, Sanchez MA, Garrido CS, et al. Molecular epidemiology of bartonella infections in patients with bacillary angiomatosis–peliosis. N Engl J Med 1997;337:1876–83.

128 Caccamo D, Pervez NK, Marchevsky A. Primary lymphoma of the liver in the acquired immunodeficiency syndrome. Arch Pathol Lab Med 1986;110:553–5.

129 Beral V, Peterman T, Berkelman R, et al. AIDS-associated non-Hodgkin lymphoma. Lancet 1991;337:805–9.

130 Newell A, Francis N, Nelson M. Hepatitis and HIV: interrelationship and interactions. Br J Clin Pract 1995;49:247–51.

131 Horvath J, Raffanti SP. Clinical aspects of the interactions between human immunodeficiency virus and the hepatotropic viruses. Clin Infect Dis 1994;18:339–47.

132 Petrovic LM. HIV/HCV co-infection: histopathologic findings, natural history, fibrosis, and impact of antiretroviral treatment: a review article. Liver Int 2007;27:598–606.

133 Colin J-F, Cazals-Hatem D, Loriot MA, et al. Influence of human immunodeficiency virus infection on chronic hepatitis B in homosexual men. Hepatology 1999;29:1306–10.

134 Collier J, Heathcote J. Hepatitis C viral infection in the immunosuppressed patient. Hepatology 1998;27:1–6.

135 Di Martino V, Rufat P, Boyer N, et al. The influence of human immunodeficiency virus coinfection on chronic hepatitis C in injection drug users: a long-term retrospective cohort study. Hepatology 2001;34:1193–9.

136 Lichtenstein DR, Makadon HJ, Chopra S. Fulminant hepatitis B and delta virus coinfection in AIDS. Am J Gastroenterol 1992;87:1643–7.

137 Housset C, Pol S, Carnot F, et al. Interactions between human immunodeficiency virus-1, hepatitis delta virus and hepatitis B virus infections in 260 chronic carriers of hepatitis B virus. Hepatology 1992;15:578–83.

138 Puius YA, Dove LM, Brust DG, et al. Three cases of autoimmune hepatitis in HIV-infected patients. J Clin Gastroenterol 2008;42:424–9.

139 O'Leary JG, Zachary K, Misdraji J, et al. De novo autoimmune hepatitis during immune reconstitution in an HIV-infected patient receiving highly active antiretroviral therapy. Clin Infect Dis 2008;46:e12–14.

140 Crum-Cianflone N, Dilay A, Collins G, et al. Nonalcoholic fatty liver disease among HIV-infected persons. J AIDS 2009;50:464–73.

141 Bissuel F, Bruneel F, Habersetzer F, et al. Fulminant hepatitis with severe lactate acidosis in HIV-infected patients on didanosine therapy. J Int Med 1994;235:367–72.

142 Olano JP, Borucki MJ, Wen JW, et al. Massive hepatic steatosis and lactic acidosis in a patient with AIDS who was receiving zidovudine. Clin Infect Dis 1995;21:973–6.

143 Freiman JP, Helfert KE, Hamrell MR, et al. Hepatomegaly with severe steatosis in HIV-seropositive patients. AIDS 1993;7:379–85.

144 Sterling RK, Smith PG, Brunt EM. Hepatic steatosis in human immunodeficiency virus. A prospective study in patients without viral hepatitis, diabetes, or alcohol, abuse. J Clin Gastroenterol 2013;47:182–7.

145 Ingiliz P, Valantin M-A, Duvivier C, et al. Liver damage underlying unexplained transaminase elevation in human immunodeficiency virus-1 mono-infected patients on antiretroviral therapy. Hepatology 2009;49:436–42.

146 Tateo M, Sebagh M, Bralet M-P, et al. A new indication for liver transplantation: nodular regenerative hyperplasia in human immunodeficiency virus-infected patients. Liver Transplant 2008;14:1194–8.

147 Mallet V, Blanchard P, Verkarre V, et al. Nodular regenerative hyperplasia is a new cause of chronic liver disease in HIV-infected patients. AIDS 2007;21:187–92.

148 Osick LA, Lee T-P, Pedemonte MB, et al. Hepatic amyloidosis in intravenous drug abusers and AIDS patients. J Hepatol 1993;19:79–84.

149 Kossaifi T, Dupon M, Le Bail B, et al. Perisinusoidal cell hypertrophy in a patient with acquired immunodeficiency syndrome. Arch Pathol Lab Med 1990;114:876–9.

150 Kahn E, Greco A, Daum F, et al. Hepatic pathology in pediatric acquired immunodeficiency syndrome. Hum Pathol 1991;22:1111–19.

151 Duffy LF, Daum F, Kahn E, et al. Hepatitis in children with acquired immune deficiency syndrome. Histopathologic and immunocytologic features. Gastroenterology 1986;90:173–81.

152 Ross JS, Del Rosario A, Bui HX, et al. Primary hepatic leiomyosarcoma in a child with the acquired immunodeficiency syndrome. Hum Pathol 1992;23:69–72.

153 Turck WP, Howitt G, Turnberg LA, et al. Chronic Q fever. Q J Med 1976;45:193–217.

153a Young EJ, Roushan MRH, Shafae S, et al. Liver histology of acute brucellosis caused by *Brucella melitensis*. Hum Pathol 2014;45:2023–8.

154 Cervantes F, Bruguera M, Carbonell J, et al. Liver disease in brucellosis. A clinical and pathological study of 40 cases. Postgrad Med J 1982;58:346–50.

155 Khosla SN. Typhoid hepatitis. Postgrad Med J 1990;66:923–5.

156 De Brito T, Trench Vieira W, D'Agostino Dias M. Jaundice in typhoid hepatitis: a light and electron microscopy study based on liver biopsies. Acta Hepatol Gastroenterol 1977;24:426–33.

157 Nasrallah SM, Nassar VH. Enteric fever: a clinicopathologic study of 104 cases. Am J Gastroenterol 1978;69:63–9.

158 Pais P. A hepatitis like picture in typhoid fever. Br Med J Clin Res 1984;289:225–6.

159 Lamps LW, Gray GF, Scott MA. The histologic spectrum of hepatic cat scratch disease. A series of six cases with confirmed *Bartonella henselae* infection. Am J Surg Pathol 1996;20:1253–9.

160 Thudi KR, Kreikemeier JT, Phillips NJ, et al. Cat scratch disease causing hepatic masses after liver transplant. Liver Int 2007;27:145–8.

161 Asada Y, Hayashi T, Sumiyoshi A, et al. Miliary tuberculosis presenting as fever and jaundice with hepatic failure. Hum Pathol 1991;22:92–4.

162 Alvarez SZ, Carpio R. Hepatobiliary tuberculosis. Dig Dis Sci 1983;28:193–200.

163 Essop AR, Posen JA, Hodkinson JH, et al. Tuberculosis hepatitis: a clinical review of 96 cases. Q J Med 1984;53:465–77.

164 Pottipati AR, Dave PB, Gumaste V, et al. Tuberculous abscess of the liver in acquired immunodeficiency syndrome. J Clin Gastroenterol 1991;13:549–53.

165 Alcantra-Payawal DE, Matsumura M, Shiratori Y, et al. Direct detection of *Mycobacterium tuberculosis* using polymerase chain reaction assay among patients with hepatic granuloma. J Hepatol 1997;27:620–7.

166 Hunt JS, Silverstein MJ, Sparks FC, et al. Granulomatous hepatitis: a complication of BCG immunotherapy. Lancet 1973;2:820–1.

167 Bodurtha A, Kim YH, Laucius JF, et al. Hepatic granulomas and other hepatic lesions associated with BCG immunotherapy for cancer. Am J Clin Pathol 1974;61:747–52.

168 Proctor DD, Chopra S, Rubenstein SC, et al. Mycobacteremia and granulomatous hepatitis following initial intravesical bacillus Calmette-Guérin instillation for bladder carcinoma. Am J Gastroenterol 1993;88:1112–15.

169 Case records of the Massachusetts General Hospital. Case 29-1998. N Engl J Med 1998;339:831–7.

170 Karat AB, Job CK, Rao PS. Liver in leprosy: histological and biochemical findings. BMJ 1971;1:307–10.

171 Chen TS, Drutz DJ, Whelan GE. Hepatic granulomas in leprosy. Their relation to bacteremia. Arch Pathol Lab Med 1976;100:182–5.

172 Terry SI, Hanchard B, Brooks SE, et al. Prevalence of liver abnormality in early syphilis. Br J Vener Dis 1984;60:83–6.

173 Murray FE, O'Loughlin S, Dervan P, et al. Granulomatous hepatitis in secondary syphilis. Irish J Med Sci 1990;159:53–4.

174 Sobel HJ, Wolf EH. Liver involvement in early syphilis. Arch Pathol 1972;93:565–8.

175 Fehér J, Somogyi T, Timmer M, et al. Early syphilitic hepatitis. Lancet 1975;2:896–9.

176 Romeu J, Rybak B, Dave P, et al. Spirochetal vasculitis and bile ductular damage in early hepatic syphilis. Am J Gastroenterol 1980;74:352–4.

177 Veeravahu M. Diagnosis of liver involvement in early syphilis. A critical review. Arch Intern Med 1985;145:132–4.

178 De Brito T, Machado MM, Montans SD, et al. Liver biopsy in human leptospirosis: a light and electron microscopy study. Virchows Arch Pathol Anat Physiol 1967;342:61–9.

179 De Brito T, Penna DO, Hoshino S, et al. Cholestasis in human leptospirosis: a clinical, histochemical, biochemical and electron microscopy study based on liver biopsies. Beitr Pathol 1970;140:345–61.

180 Ferreira Alves VA, Vianna MR, Yasuda PH, et al. Detection of leptospiral antigen in the human liver and kidney using an immunoperoxidase staining procedure. J Pathol 1987;151:125–31.

181 Goellner MH, Agger WA, Burgess JH, et al. Hepatitis due to recurrent Lyme disease. Ann Intern Med 1988;108:707–8.

182 Zanchi A, Gingold AR, Theise ND, et al. Necrotizing granulomatous hepatitis as an unusual manifestation of Lyme disease. Dig Dis Sci 2007;52:2629–32.

183 Thaler M, Pastakia B, Shawker TH, et al. Hepatic candidiasis in cancer patients: the evolving picture of the syndrome. Ann Intern Med 1988;108:88–100.

184 Lewis JH, Patel HR, Zimmerman HJ. The spectrum of hepatic candidiasis. Hepatology 1982;2:479–87.

185 Hassanein T, Perper JA, Tepperman L, et al. Liver failure occurring as a component of exertional heatstroke. Gastroenterology 1991;100:1442–7.

186 Jariwalla A, Tulloch BR, Fox H, et al. Disseminated histoplasmosis in an English patient with diabetes mellitus. BMJ 1977;1:1002–4.

187 Lanza FL, Nelson RS, Somayaji BN. Acute granulomatous hepatitis due to histoplasmosis. Gastroenterology 1970;58:392–6.

188 Smith JW, Utz JP. Progressive disseminated histoplasmosis. A prospective study of 26 patients. Ann Intern Med 1972;76:557–65.

189 Edmondson RP, Eykyn S, Davies DR, et al. Disseminated histoplasmosis successfully treated with amphotericin B. J Clin Pathol 1974;27:308–10.

190 Ridley DS. The laboratory diagnosis of tropical diseases with special reference to Britain: a review. J Clin Pathol 1974;27:435–44.

191 Williams AO, Lawson EA, Lucas AO. African histoplasmosis due to *Histoplasma duboisii*. Arch Pathol 1971;92:306–18.

192 Okudaira M, Straub M, Schwarz J. The etiology of discrete splenic and hepatic calcifications in an endemic area of histoplasmosis. Am J Pathol 1961;39:599–611.

193 Weinstein L. Bacterial hepatitis: a case report on an unrecognized cause of fever of unknown origin. N Engl J Med 1978;299:1052–4.

194 Engler S, Elsing C, Flechtenmacher C, et al. Progressive sclerosing cholangitis after shock: a new variant of vanishing bile duct disorders. Gut 2003;52:688–93.

195 Banks JG, Foulis AK, Ledingham IM, et al. Liver function in septic shock. J Clin Pathol 1982;35:1249–52.

196 Zimmerman HJ, Fang M, Utili R, et al. Jaundice due to bacterial infection. Gastroenterology 1979;77:362–74.

197 Lefkowitch JH. Bile ductular cholestasis: an ominous histopathologic sign related to sepsis and 'cholangitis lenta'. Hum Pathol 1982;13:19–24.

198 Vyberg M, Poulsen H. Abnormal bile duct epithelium accompanying septicaemia. Virchows Arch [A] 1984;402:451–8.

199 Riely CA, Dean PJ, Park AL, et al. A distinct syndrome of liver disease with multisystem organ failure associated with bile ductular cholestasis. Hepatology 1989;10:739A.

200 Ishak KG, Rogers WA. Cryptogenic acute cholangitis – association with toxic shock syndrome. Am J Clin Pathol 1981;76:619–26.

201 Weitberg AB, Alper JC, Diamond I, et al. Acute granulomatous hepatitis in the course of acquired toxoplasmosis. N Engl J Med 1979;300:1093–6.

202 Andres TL, Dorman SA, Winn W Jr, et al. Immunohistochemical demonstration of Toxoplasma gondii. Am J Clin Pathol 1981;75:431–4.

203 Conley FK, Jenkins KA, Remington JS. Toxoplasma gondii infection of the central nervous system. Use of the peroxidase–antiperoxidase method to demonstrate toxoplasma in formalin fixed, paraffin embedded tissue sections. Hum Pathol 1981;12:690–8.

204 Pounder DJ. Malarial pigment and hepatic anthracosis [letter]. Am J Surg Pathol 1983;7:501–2.

205 Brenard R, Dumortier P, Del Natale M, et al. Black pigments in the liver related to gold and titanium deposits. A report of four cases. Liver Int 2007;27: 408–13.

206 Editorial: tropical splenomegaly syndrome. Lancet 1976;i:1058–9.

207 Daneshbod K. Visceral leishmaniasis (kala-azar) in Iran: a pathologic and electron microscopic study. Am J Clin Pathol 1972;57:156–66.

208 Maltz G, Knauer CM. Amebic liver abscess: a 15-year experience. Am J Gastroenterol 1991;86:704–10.

209 Mokhtari M, Kumar PV. Amebic liver abscess: fine needle aspiration diagnosis. Acta Cytol 2014;58:225–8.

210 Dunn MA, Kamel R. Hepatic schistosomiasis. Hepatology 1981;1:653–61.

211 Andrade ZA. Hepatic schistosomiasis. Morphological aspects. In: Popper H, Schaffner F, editors. Progress in Liver Diseases, vol. II. New York: Grune & Stratton; 1965. p. 228–42 [Ch. 16].

212 Lucas SB. Other viral and infectious diseases. In: MacSween RNM, Anthony PP, Scheuer PJ, et al., editors. Pathology of the Liver. 3rd ed. Edinburgh: Churchill Livingstone; 1994. p. 269–316 [Ch. 7].

213 Andrade ZA, Peixoto E, Guerret S, et al. Hepatic connective tissue changes in hepatosplenic schistosomiasis. Hum Pathol 1992;23:566–73.

214 Canto AL, Sesso A, De Brito T. Human chronic Mansonian schistosomiasis-cell proliferation and fibre formation in the hepatic sinusoidal wall: a morphometric, light and electron-microscopy study. J Pathol 1977;123:35–44.

215 Grimaud JA, Borojevic R. Chronic human schistosomiasis mansoni. Pathology of the Disse's space. Lab Invest 1977;36:268–73.

216 Lyra LG, Reboucas G, Andrade ZA. Hepatitis B surface antigen carrier state in hepatosplenic schistosomiasis. Gastroenterology 1976;71:641–5.

217 Nash TE, Cheever AW, Ottesen EA, et al. Schistosome infections in humans: perspectives and recent findings. Ann Intern Med 1982;97:740–54.

218 Sun T. Pathology and immunology of Clonorchis sinensis infection in the liver. Ann Clin Lab Sci 1984;14:208–15.

219 Ona FV, Dytoc JNT. Clonorchis-associated cholangiocarcinoma: a report of two cases with unusual manifestations. Gastroenterology 1991;101:831–9.

220 Hartley JP, Douglas AP. A case of clonorchiasis in England. BMJ 1975;3:575.

221 Acosta-Ferreira W, Vercelli-Retta J, Falconi LM. Fasciola hepatica human infection. Histopathological study of sixteen cases. Virchows Arch [A] 1979;383:319–27.

222 Jones EA, Kay JM, Milligan HP, et al. Massive infection with Fasciola hepatica in man. Am J Med 1977;63: 836–42.

223 Drury RAB. Larval granulomata in the liver. Gut 1962;3:289–94.

224 Rubio-Tapia A, Murray JA. The liver in celiac disease. Hepatology 2007;46:1650–8.

225 Gogos CA, Nikolopoulou V, Zolota V, et al. Autoimmune cholangitis in a patient with celiac disease: a case report and review of the literature. J Hepatol 1999;30:321–4.

226 MacSween RNM, Burt AD. Liver pathology associated with diseases of other organs. In: MacSween RNM, Anthony PP, Scheuer PJ, et al., editors. Pathology of the Liver. 3rd ed. Edinburgh: Churchill Livingstone; 1994. p. 713–64 [Ch. 17].

227 Saint-Marc Girardin MF, Zafrani ES, Chaumette MT, et al. Hepatic granulomas in Whipple's disease. Gastroenterology 1984;86:753–6.

228 Everett GD, Mitros FA. Eosinophilic gastroenteritis with hepatic eosinophilic granulomas. Report of a case with 30-year follow-up. Am J Gastroenterol 1980;74:519–21.

229 Lai H-C, Lin C-C, Cheng K-S, et al. Increased incidence of gastrointestinal cancers among patients with pyogenic liver abscess: a population-based cohort study. Gastroenterology 2014;146:129–37.

230 Eade MN, Cooke WT, Brooke BN, et al. Liver disease in Crohn's colitis. A study of 21 consecutive patients having colectomy. Ann Intern Med 1971;74:518–28.

231 Shorvon PJ. Amyloidosis and inflammatory bowel disease. Am J Dig Dis 1977;22:209–13.

232 Quigley EMM, Zetterman RK. Hepatobiliary complications of malabsorption and malnutrition. Semin Liver Dis 1988;8:218–28.

233 Shepherd HA, Selby WS, Chapman RW, et al. Ulcerative colitis and persistent liver dysfunction. Q J Med 1983;52:503–13.

234 Haworth AC, Manley PN, Groll A, et al. Bile duct carcinoma and biliary tract dysplasia in chronic ulcerative colitis. Arch Pathol Lab Med 1989;113:434–6.

235 Fleming KA, Boberg KM, Glaumann H, et al. Biliary dysplasia as a marker of cholangiocarcinoma in primary sclerosing cholangitis. J Hepatol 2001;34:360–5.

236 Wee A, Ludwig J, Coffey RJ Jr, et al. Hepatobiliary carcinoma associated with primary sclerosing cholangitis and chronic ulcerative colitis. Hum Pathol 1985;16:719–26.

237 Mir-Madjlessi SH, Farmer RG, Sivak MV Jr. Bile duct carcinoma in patients with ulcerative colitis. Relationship to sclerosing cholangitis: report of six cases and review of the literature. Dig Dis Sci 1987;32:145–54.

238 Blackstone MO, Nemchausky BA. Cholangiographic abnormalities in ulcerative colitis associated pericholangitis which resemble sclerosing cholangitis. Am J Dig Dis 1978;23:579–85.

239 Wee A, Ludwig J. Pericholangitis in chronic ulcerative colitis: primary sclerosing cholangitis of the small bile ducts? Ann Intern Med 1985;102:581–7.

240 Tsui WMS, Wong KF, Tse CCH. Liver changes in reactive haemophagocytic syndrome. Liver 1992;12:363–7.

241 de Kerguenec C, Hillaire S, Molinié V, et al. Hepatic manifestations of hemophagocytic syndrome: a study of 30 cases. Am J Gastroenterol 2001;96:852–7.

242 Tristano AG. Macrophage activation syndrome: a frequent but under-diagnosed complication associated with rheumatic diseases. Med Sci Monit 2008;14:RA27–36.

243 Billiau AD, Roskams T, Van Damme-Lombaerts R, et al. Macrophage activation syndrome: characteristic findings on liver biopsy illustrating the key role of activated IFN-γ-producing lymphocytes and IL-6- and TNF-α-producing macrophages. Blood 2005;105:1648–51.

244 Bihl F, Emmenegger U, Reichen J, et al. Macrophage activating syndrome is associated with lobular hepatitis and severe bile duct injury with cholestasis. J Hepatol 2006;44:1208–12.

245 Aledort LM, Levine PH, Hilgartner M, et al. A study of liver biopsies and liver disease among hemophiliacs. Blood 1985;66:367–72.

246 Colombo M, Mannucci PM, Carnelli V, et al. Transmission of non-A, non-B hepatitis by heat-treated factor VIII concentrate. Lancet 1985;ii:1–4.

247 Hay CR, Preston FE, Triger DR, et al. Progressive liver disease in haemophilia: an understated problem? Lancet 1985;1:1495–8.

248 Bianchi L, Desmet VJ, Popper H, et al. Histologic patterns of liver disease in hemophiliacs, with special reference to morphologic characteristics of non-A, non-B hepatitis. Semin Liver Dis 1987;7:203–9.

249 Lefkowitch JH, Mendez L. Morphologic features of hepatic injury in cardiac disease and shock. J Hepatol 1986;2:313–27.

250 Craig CEH, Quaglia A, Dhillon AP. Extramedullary haematopoiesis in massive hepatic necrosis. Histopathology 2004;45:518–25.

251 Ludwig J, Gross JB, Perkins JD, et al. Persistent centrilobular necroses in hepatic allografts. Hum Pathol 1990;21:656–61.

252 Collins RH, Anastasi J, Terstappen LWMM, et al. Brief report: donor-derived long-term multilineage hematopoiesis in a liver-transplant recipient. N Engl J Med 1993;328:762–5.

253 Gilson TP, Bendon RW. Megakaryocytosis of the liver in a trisomy 21 stillbirth. Arch Pathol Lab Med 1993;117:738–9.

254 Ruchelli ED, Uri A, Dimmick JE, et al. Severe perinatal liver disease and Down syndrome: an apparent relationship. Hum Pathol 1991;22:1274–80.

255 Arai H, Ishida A, Nakajima W, et al. Immunohistochemical study on transforming growth factor-beta 1 expression in liver fibrosis of Down's syndrome with transient abnormal myelopoiesis. Hum Pathol 1999;30:474–6.

256 Youssef WI, Tavill AS. Connective tissue diseases and the liver. J Clin Gastroenterol 2002;35:345–9.

257 Keshavarzian A, Rentsch R, Hodgson HJF. Clinical implications of liver biopsy findings in collagen–vascular disorders. J Clin Gastroenterol 1993;17:219–26.

258 Matsumoto T, Kobayashi S, Shimizu H, et al. The liver in collagen diseases: pathologic study of 160 cases with particular reference to hepatic arteritis, primary biliary cirrhosis, autoimmune hepatitis and nodular regenerative hyperplasia of the liver. Liver 2000;20:366–73.

259 De Santis M, Crotti C, Selmi C. Liver abnormalities in connective tissue diseases. Best Prac Res Clin Gastroenterol 2013;27:543–51.

260 Gocke DJ, Hsu K, Morgan C, et al. Association between polyarteritis and Australia antigen. Lancet 1970;2:1149–53.

261 Levo Y, Gorevic PD, Kassab HJ, et al. Liver involvement in the syndrome of mixed cryoglobulinemia. Ann Intern Med 1977;87:287–92.

262 Misiani R, Bellavita P, Fenili D, et al. Hepatitis C virus infection in patients with essential mixed cryoglobulinemia. Ann Intern Med 1992;117:573–7.

263 Agnello V, Chung RT, Kaplan LM. A role for hepatitis C virus infection in type II cryoglobulinemia. N Engl J Med 1992;327:1490–5.

264 Peña LR, Nand S, De Maria N, et al. Hepatitis C virus infection and lymphoproliferative disorders. Dig Dis Sci 2000;45:1854–60.

265 Long R, James O. Polymyalgia rheumatica and liver disease. Lancet 1974;1:77–9.

266 Litwack KD, Bohan A, Silverman L. Granulomatous liver disease and giant cell arteritis. Case report and literature review. J Rheumatol 1977;4:307–12.

267 Gossmann HH, Dolle W, Korb G, et al. Liver changes in giant-cell arteritis: temporal arteritis and rheumatic polymyalgia (author's transl.). [German.]. Deutsche Med Wochenschr 1979;104:1199–202.

268 Leong AS, Alp MH. Hepatocellular disease in the giant-cell arteritis/polymyalgia rheumatica syndrome. Ann Rheum Dis 1981;40:92–5.

269 Rao R, Pfenniger K, Boni A. Liver function tests and liver biopsies in patients with rheumatoid arthritis. Ann Rheum Dis 1975;34:198–9.

270 Mills PR, MacSween RN, Dick WC, et al. Liver disease in rheumatoid arthritis. Scottish Med J 1980;25:18–22.

271 Mills PR, Sturrock RD. Clinical associations between arthritis and liver disease. Ann Rheum Dis 1982;41:295–307.

272 Smits JG, Kooijman CD. Rheumatoid nodules in liver [letter]. Histopathology 1986;10:1211–13.

273 Thorne C, Urowitz MB, Wanless I, et al. Liver disease in Felty's syndrome. Am J Med 1982;73:35–40.

274 Reynolds WJ, Wanless IR. Nodular regenerative hyperplasia of the liver in a patient with rheumatoid vasculitis: a morphometric study suggesting a role for hepatic arteritis in the pathogenesis. J Rheumatol 1984;11:838–42.

275 Murray-Lyon IM, Thompson RP, Ansell ID, et al. Scleroderma and primary biliary cirrhosis. BMJ 1970;1:258–9.

276 Reynolds TB, Denison EK, Frankl HD, et al. Primary biliary cirrhosis with scleroderma, Raynaud's phenomenon and telangiectasia. New syndrome. Am J Med 1971;50:302–12.

277 Feldmann G, Maurice M, Husson JM, et al. Hepatocyte giant mitochondria: an almost constant lesion in systemic scleroderma. Virchows Arch [A] 1977;374:215–27.

278 Runyon BA, LaBrecque DR, Anuras S. The spectrum of liver disease in systemic lupus erythematosus. Report of 33 histologically-proved cases and review of the literature. Am J Med 1980;69:187–94.

279 Matsumoto T, Yoshimine T, Shimouchi K, et al. The liver in systemic lupus erythematosus: pathologic analysis of 52 cases and review of Japanese autopsy registry data. Hum Pathol 1992;23:1151–8.

280 Gibson T, Myers AR. Subclinical liver disease in systemic lupus erythematosus. J Rheumatol 1981;8:752–9.

281 Miller MH, Urowitz MB, Gladman DD, et al. The liver in systemic lupus erythematosus. Q J Med 1984;53:401–9.

282 Chowdhary VR, Crowson CS, Poterucha JJ, et al. Liver involvement in systemic lupus erythematosus: case review of 40 patients. J Rheumatol 2008;35:1–6.

283 Robertson SJ, Higgins RB, Powell C. Malacoplakia of liver: a case report. Hum Pathol 1991;22:1294–5.

284 Marshall JB, Ravendhran N, Sharp GC. Liver disease in mixed connective tissue disease. Arch Intern Med 1983;143:1817–18.

285 Chopra S, Rubinow A, Koff RS, et al. Hepatic amyloidosis. A histopathologic analysis of primary (AL) and secondary (AA) forms. Am J Pathol 1984;115:186–93.

286 Buck FS, Koss MN. Hepatic amyloidosis: morphologic differences between systemic AL and AA types. Hum Pathol 1991;22:904–7.

287 Looi L-M, Sumithran E. Morphologic differences in the pattern of liver infiltration between systemic AL and AA amyloidosis. Hum Pathol 1988;19:732–5.

288 Wright JR, Calkins E, Humphrey RL. Potassium permanganate reaction in amyloidosis. A histologic method to assist in differentiating forms of this disease. Lab Invest 1977;36:274–81.

289 Shirahama T, Skinner M, Cohen AS. Immunocytochemical identification of amyloid in formalin-fixed paraffin sections. Histochemistry 1981;72:161–71.

290 Falk RH, Comenzo RL, Skinner M. The systemic amyloidoses. N Engl J Med 1997;337:898–909.

291 Rubinow A, Koff RS, Cohen AS. Severe intrahepatic cholestasis in primary amyloidosis: a report of four cases and a review of the literature. Am J Med 1978;64:937–46.

292 Finkelstein SD, Fornasier VL, Pruzanski W. Intrahepatic cholestasis with predominant pericentral deposition in systemic amyloidosis. Hum Pathol 1981;12:470–2.

293 Case records of the Massachusetts General Hospital. Case 50-1987. N Engl J Med 1987;317:1520–31.

294 Agaram N, Shia J, Klimstra DS, et al. Globular hepatic amyloid: a diagnostic peculiarity that bears clinical significance. Hum Pathol 2005;36:845–9.

295 Makhlouf HR, Goodman ZD. Globular hepatic amyloid: an early stage in the pathway of amyloid formation. A study of 20 new cases. Am J Surg Pathol 2007;31:1615–21.

296 Droz D, Noel LH, Carnot F, et al. Liver involvement in nonamyloid light chain deposits disease. Lab Invest 1984;50:683–9.

297 Kirkpatrick CJ, Curry A, Galle J, et al. Systemic kappa light chain deposition and amyloidosis in multiple myeloma: novel morphological observations. Histopathology 1986;10:1065–76.

298 Smith NM, Malcolm AJ. Simultaneous AL-type amyloid and light chain deposit disease in a liver biopsy: a case report. Histopathology 1986;10:1057–64.

299 Bruguera M. Liver involvement in porphyria. Semin Dermatol 1986;5:178–85.

300 Fakan F, Chlumská A. Demonstration of needle-shaped hepatic inclusions in porphyria cutanea tarda using the ferric ferricyanide reduction test. Virchows Arch [A] 1987;411:365–8.

301 Cortés JM, Oliva H, Paradinas FJ, et al. The pathology of the liver in porphyria cutanea tarda. Histopathology 1980;4:471–85.

302 Campo E, Bruguera M, Rodés J. Are there diagnostic histologic features of porphyria cutanea tarda in liver biopsy specimens? Liver 1990;10:185–90.

303 Lefkowitch JH, Grossman ME. Hepatic pathology in porphyria cutanea tarda. Liver 1983;3:19–29.

304 Nagy Z, Kószo F, Pár A, et al. Hemochromatosis (HFE) gene mutations and hepatitis C virus infection as risk factors for porphyria cutanea tarda in Hungarian patients. Liver Int 2004;24:16–20.

305 Bonkovsky HL, Poh-Fitzpatrick M, Pimstone N, et al. Porphyria cutanea tarda, hepatitis C and HFE gene mutations in North America. Hepatology 1998;27:1661–9.

306 Bulaj ZJ, Phillips JD, Ajioka RS, et al. Hemochromatosis genes and other factors contributing to the pathogenesis of porphyria cutanea tarda. Blood 2000;95:1565–71.

307 Fargion S, Piperno A, Cappellini MD, et al. Hepatitis C virus and porphyria cutanea tarda: evidence of a strong association. Hepatology 1992;16:1322–6.

308 Herrero C, Vicente A, Bruguera M, et al. Is hepatitis C virus infection a trigger of porphyria cutanea tarda? Lancet 1993;341:788–9.

309 DeCastro M, Sánchez J, Herrera JF, et al. Hepatitis C virus antibodies and liver disease in patients with porphyria cutanea tarda. Hepatology 1993;17:551–7.

310 Bonkovsky H, Poh-Fitzpatrick M, Tattrie C, et al. Porphyria cutanea tarda and hepatitis C in the USA. Hepatology 1996;24:486A.

311 Gisbert JP, García-Buey L, Pajares JM, et al. Prevalence of hepatitis C virus infection in porphyria cutanea tarda: systematic review and meta-analysis. J Hepatol 2003;39:620–7.

312 Fargion S, Fracanzani AL. Prevalence of hepatitis C virus infection in porphyria cutanea tarda. J Hepatol 2003;39:635–8.

313 Klatskin G, Bloomer JR. Birefringence of hepatic pigment deposits in erythropoietic protoporphyria. Specificity of polarization microscopy in the identification of hepatic protoporphyrin deposits. Gastroenterology 1974;67:294–302.

314 Bloomer JR, Phillips MJ, Davidson DL, et al. Hepatic disease in erythropoietic protoporphyria. Am J Med 1975;58:869–82.

315 Bonkovsky HL, Schned AR. Fatal liver failure in protoporphyria. Synergism between ethanol excess and the genetic defect. Gastroenterology 1986;90:191–201.

316 Pérez V, Gorodisch S, Casavilla F, et al. Ultrastructure of human liver at the end of normal pregnancy. Am J Obstet Gynecol 1971;110:428–31.

317 Hay JE. Liver disease in pregnancy. Hepatology 2008;47:1067–76.

318 Riely CA. Liver disease in the pregnant patient. Am J Gastroenterol 1999;94:1728–32.

319 Wakim-Fleming J, Zein NN. The liver in pregnancy: disease vs. benign changes. Cleveland Clin J Med 2005;72:713–21.

320 Schutt VA, Minuk GY. Liver diseases unique to pregnancy. Best Pract Res Clin Gastroenterol 2007;21:771–92.

321 Kroll D, Mazor M, Zirkin H, et al. Fibrolamellar carcinoma of the liver in pregnancy. A case report. J Reprod Med 1991;36:823–7.

322 Schorr-Lesnick B, Lebovics E, Dworkin B, et al. Liver diseases unique to pregnancy. Am J Gastroenterol 1991;86:659–70.

323 Samuels P, Cohen AW. Pregnancies complicated by liver disease and liver dysfunction. Obstet Gynecol Clin North Am 1992;19:745–63.

324 Kaplan MM. Acute fatty liver of pregnancy. N Engl J Med 1985;313:367–70.

325 Sibai BM. Imitators of severe preeclampsia. Obstet Gynecol 2007;109:956–66.

326 Ibdah JA. Acute fatty liver of pregnancy: an update on pathogenesis and clinical implications. World J Gastroenterol 2006;46:7397–404.

327 Burroughs AK, Seong NH, Dojcinov DM, et al. Idiopathic acute fatty liver of pregnancy in 12 patients. Q J Med 1982;51:481–97.

328 Rolfes DB, Ishak KG. Acute fatty liver of pregnancy: a clinicopathologic study of 35 cases. Hepatology 1985;5:1149–58.

329 Sherlock S. Acute fatty liver of pregnancy and the microvesicular fat diseases. Gut 1983;24:265–9.

330 Riely CA. Acute fatty liver of pregnancy. Semin Liver Dis 1987;7:47–54.

331 Schoeman MN, Batey RG, Wilcken B. Recurrent acute fatty liver of pregnancy associated with a fatty-acid oxidation defect in the offspring. Gastroenterology 1991;100:544–8.

332 Rolfes DB, Ishak KG. Liver disease in toxemia of pregnancy. Am J Gastroenterol 1986;81:1138–44.

333 Rolfes DB, Ishak KG. Liver disease in pregnancy. Histopathology 1986;10:555–70.

334 Arias F, Mancilla-Jimenez R. Hepatic fibrinogen deposits in pre-eclampsia. Immunofluorescent evidence. N Engl J Med 1976;295:578–82.

335 Cheung H, Hamzah H. Liver rupture in pregnancy: a typical case? Singapore Med J 1992;33:89–91.

336 Schorr-Lesnick B, Dworkin B, Rosenthal WS. Hemolysis, elevated liver enzymes, and low platelets in pregnancy (HELLP syndrome). A case report and literature review. Dig Dis Sci 1991;36:1649–52.

337 Weinstein L. Syndrome of hemolysis, elevated liver enzymes, and low platelet count: a severe consequence of hypertension in pregnancy. Am J Obstet Gynecol 1982;142:159–67.

338 Weinstein L. Preeclampsia/eclampsia with hemolysis, elevated liver enzymes, and thrombocytopenia. Obstet Gynecol 1985;66:657–60.

339 Baca L, Gibbons RB. The HELLP syndrome: a serious complication of pregnancy with hemolysis, elevated levels of liver enzymes, and low platelet count. Am J Med 1988;85:590–1.

340 Ibdah JA, Bennett MJ, Rinaldo P, et al. A fetal fatty-acid oxidation disorder as a cause of liver disease in pregnant women. N Engl J Med 1999;340:1723–31.

341 Adlercreutz H, Tenhunen R. Some aspects of the interaction between natural and synthetic female sex hormones and the liver. Am J Med 1970;49:630–48.

342 Vanjak D, Moreau R, Roche-Sicot J, et al. Intrahepatic cholestasis of pregnancy and acute fatty liver of pregnancy. An unusual but favorable association? Gastroenterology 1991;100:1123–5.

343 Dixon PH, Weerasekera N, Linton KJ, et al. Heterozygous *MDR3* missense mutation associated with intrahepatic cholestasis of pregnancy: evidence for a defect in protein trafficking. Hum Mol Genet 2000;9:1209–17.

344 Schneider G, Paus TC, Kullak-Ublick GA, et al. Linkage between a new splicing site mutation in the MDR3 alias ABCB4 gene and intrahepatic cholestasis of pregnancy. Hepatology 2007;45:150–8.

345 Keitel V, Vogt C, Häussinger D, et al. Combined mutations of canalicular transporter proteins cause severe intrahepatic cholestasis of pregnancy. Gastroenterology 2006;131:624–9.

346 Floreani A, Carderi I, Paternoster D, et al. Intrahepatic cholestasis of pregnancy: three novel MDR3 gene mutations. Aliment Pharmacol Ther 2006;23:1649–53.

347 Marschall H-U, Shemer EW, Ludvigsson JF, et al. Intrahepatic cholestasis of pregnancy and associated hepatobiliary disease: a population-based cohort study. Hepatology 2013;58:1385–91.

General reading

Flamm SL. Granulomatous liver disease. Clin Liver Dis 2012;16:387–96.

Gaya DR, Thorburn KA, Oien KA, et al. Hepatic granulomas: a 10 year single center experience. J Clin Pathol 2003;56:850–3.

Lucas SB, Zaki SR, Portmann BC. Other viral and infectious diseases and HIV-related liver disease. In: Burt AD, Portmann BC, Ferrell LD, editors. Macsween's Pathology of the Liver. 6th ed. Edinburgh: Churchill Livingstone/ Elsevier; 2012. p. 403–66.

Quaglia A, Burt AD, Ferrell LD, et al. Systemic disease. In: Burt AD, Portmann BC, Ferrell LD, editors. Macsween's Pathology of the Liver. 6th ed. Edinburgh: Churchill Livingstone/Elsevier; 2012. p. 935–86.

Sandor M, Weinstock JV, Wynn TA. Granulomas in schistosome and mycobacterial infections: a model of local immune responses. Trends Immunol 2003;24:44–52.

Sartin JS, Walker RC. Granulomatous hepatitis: a retrospective review of 88 cases at the Mayo Clinic. Mayo Clin Proc 1991;66:914–18.

The Liver in Organ Transplantation

Introduction

The pathologist is often asked to examine liver biopsies obtained to evaluate liver dysfunction in transplant patients, including recipients of liver, renal and bone marrow grafts. For liver transplantation, liver biopsy remains the diagnostic 'gold standard' when jaundice and allograft dysfunction develop, since biochemical tests do not adequately discriminate between rejection and other conditions that may develop in the allograft.[1] Moreover, even when serum liver function tests are normal, histological abnormalities (including rejection lesions) may be present.[2,3] At the time of harvesting or engraftment, the donor liver may also require assessment, sometimes by frozen section, for lesions that may determine whether or not the graft can be used, and that can affect the postoperative course and appearance of subsequent posttransplantation biopsies. This chapter reviews the histopathological features of liver transplant rejection and other conditions affecting the allograft. The concluding sections discuss liver disease in recipients of renal and bone marrow transplants.

Liver transplantation

Assessment of the donor liver

The source of the donor allograft is an important consideration when evaluating liver biopsies obtained prior to transplantation, after graft revascularisation or at later times. Biopsies from potential living donors in apparent good health may disclose conditions such as steatohepatitis or primary biliary cirrhosis (PBC), which disqualifies their candidacy.[4] Living donor left- or right-lobe grafts, if small in relation to the recipient's size, may show cholestasis or congestion associated with ascites, prolonged coagulation parameters and impaired metabolic function immediately after transplantation (**small-for-size syndrome**[5]) due to problems in venous drainage[6] and portal hyperperfusion.[5] Postoperative portal tract biliary obstructive changes may also be present due to ischaemia or mechanical obstruction of the large bile ducts associated with this type of procedure.[7] Cadaveric livers are subject to preservation (ischaemia/reperfusion) injury[8] after harvesting and transport to the site of surgery, which in early baseline biopsies is evident as variable degrees of perivenular necrosis, liver-cell ballooning and/or apoptosis. The increased risk of postoperative biliary strictures and bile leaks with 'donation after cardiac death' grafts[9] should be kept in mind if cholestasis and features of biliary obstruction are seen in a posttransplantation biopsy. If an allograft is used from a donor with known chronic hepatitis B or C ('extended donor criteria'), a baseline biopsy warrants careful attention to the grade and stage of the chronic hepatitis (**see Ch. 9**) for later comparison with subsequent biopsies. Allograft biopsies obtained soon after transplantation sometimes disclose an unsuspected condition in the donor, such as α_1-antitrypsin deficiency, iron overload or amyloidosis.[10]

Frozen section of potential donor livers may be requested to exclude pre-existing disease. Pathologists providing frozen-section coverage should be aware of three common reasons why frozen sections are requested: (1) *to determine whether steatosis is present*, and its degree; (2) *to exclude changes of chronic hepatitis* if the donor is known to be positive for antibodies to hepatitis B core antigen but negative for surface antigen (i.e. possible occult hepatitis B), or is positive for hepatitis C virus (HCV); and (3) *to evaluate a mass* found in the donor liver. Concern about a substantially **fatty liver** is based on the increased incidence of **primary graft dysfunction** or **non-function** when this is present.[11] The transplant surgeon may be concerned about significant steatosis when the donor liver appears yellow, has rounded edges and shows no surface capsular scratch marks (foci of capsular collagen rupture and disruption, thought to be a procurement phenomenon due to proximity to ice crystals).[12,13] The degree of macrovesicular (large droplet) fatty change should be categorised according to the percentage of parenchymal involvement as absent, mild (<30%), moderate (30–60%) or marked (>60%).[14,15] Transplant surgeons have considered the last category unsuitable for use because of the high risk of primary dysfunction or non-function associated with severe steatosis.[11,15] Microvesicular (small-droplet) fat is held not to be a contraindication, however,[16] but if it is substantial, it should also be graded and merits discussion with the transplant team since it may delay return of hepatic function and clinical recovery.[17] Diffuse portal mononuclear inflammatory cell infiltrates in donors with markers of hepatitis B or C viral infection support the presence of **chronic hepatitis**. The significance of this finding needs to be considered by the transplant team. With regard to **mass lesions** in the donor liver, demonstration of a malignant or metastatic tumour is an obvious contraindication to its use. However, the features of benign lesions such as focal nodular hyperplasia (**see Ch. 11**) are important to recognise since they are often encountered in this setting.

The liver allograft biopsy: general considerations

> **Box 16.1** Pathological considerations in the transplant liver
>
> Graft rejection
>   Humoral (hyperacute)
>   Acute (cellular)
>   Chronic (ductopenic)
>
> Functional cholestasis
>
> Preservation injury
>
> Bile duct obstruction
>
> Thrombosis of hepatic artery or portal vein
>
> Infections and sepsis
>
> Drug toxicity
>
> Recurrence of original disease
>
> **Neoplastic disease**
>
> Posttransplant lymphoproliferative disease
>
> Hepatocellular carcinoma

Needle liver biopsies are obtained as part of a liver transplantation protocol or because of clinical deterioration.[18] Discussion with the clinical team and careful review of pertinent radiographic, biochemical and microbiological findings are critical to biopsy interpretation and institution of appropriate therapy. Serial biopsies may be necessary to resolve difficult diagnostic problems.

There are many causes of allograft injury in addition to rejection (**Box 16.1**) and these should be considered in the context of the time elapsed since transplantation[19] (**Fig. 16.1**). For several weeks following transplantation, **functional cholestasis** may be present and must, if possible, be distinguished from the cholestasis of acute rejection, bile-duct obstruction, hepatitis, drug toxicity and sepsis. Bile is present within hepatocytes and canaliculi. This impairment of bile flow can be explained by exposure of the donor liver to cold ischaemia and reperfusion injury ('preservation injury') with resultant damage to liver-cell organelles.[20] Liver-cell death due to preservation injury actually shows features of

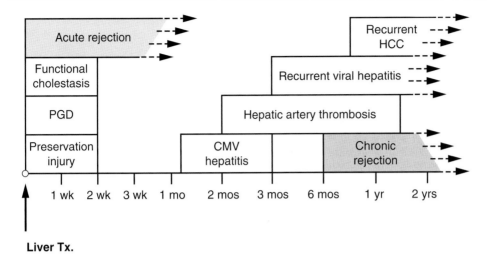

Figure 16.1 Timeline of pathological lesions after liver transplantation.
Common posttransplantation problems are shown correlated with the approximate time frame in which they develop. Hatched arrows indicate the potential for the condition to develop at a later time. CMV, cytomegalovirus; HCC, hepatocellular carcinoma; PGD, primary graft dysfunction, Tx, transplantation.

both necrosis and apoptosis ('necrapoptosis').[21] Early postoperative cholestasis may also be due to a 'small-for-size' graft.[22] Cholestasis may be accompanied by **hepatocellular balloning** in perivenular regions (**Fig. 16.2**) or in a diffuse distribution.[23,24] In the absence of frank perivenular necrosis, ballooning does not confer an unfavourable prognosis.[23] Hypoperfusion liver damage in the perioperative period may result in necrosis in periportal or perivenular regions and sometimes an irregular subcapsular band of infarction.[25] If the donor liver is fatty, rupture of hepatocytes affected by preservation injury may rarely cause sinusoidal engorgement by lipid vacuoles (**lipopeliosis**)[26] (**Fig. 16.3**).

In evaluating posttransplant biopsies, special attention should be paid to the portal tracts, the major sites of rejection lesions. The type of cellular infiltrate, the bile ducts, portal-vein branches and hepatic arterioles are examined to distinguish rejection from other conditions with portal tract pathology, particularly **bile-duct obstruction**, **recurrent viral hepatitis**, **drug toxicity** and immunosuppression-related **lymphoproliferative disease** (see Differential diagnosis in transplant biopsies, below). The perivenular region also requires inspection for possible preservation injury, cholestasis or inflammation, and for necroinflammation which may accompany portal tract lesions in more severe cases of acute rejection.[27] The lobular parenchyma shows few alterations in rejection apart from cholestasis and the occasional apoptotic bodies and scattered liver-cell mitoses which develop as the allograft equilibrates to the appropriate size for the recipient. As a result, in cases where confusion arises in the interpretation of portal changes, it is important to evaluate the lobular parenchyma carefully for evidence of intercurrent diseases such as viral or drug hepatitis. *The pathologist should always bear in mind that a given biopsy may show superimposed features attributable to several different posttransplantation complications.*

Graft rejection

The histopathological lesions of liver allograft rejection have been well characterised[28–32] and are classified as **humoral rejection, acute (cellular) rejection** and **chronic (ductopenic) rejection**, as recommended by an international working party which met in 1994.[27] Acute and chronic rejection are the most common forms seen in clinical practice.

Figure 16.2 Liver-cell ballooning after transplantation.
A liver biopsy obtained in week 2 following transplant shows ballooning of hepatocytes in a perivenular area. Intracellular cholestasis is visible. (Needle biopsy, H&E.)

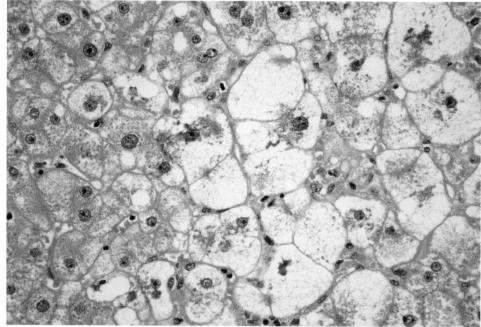

Figure 16.3 Lipopeliosis.
The enlarged empty spaces in this perivenular region represent ruptured and coalescent lipid vacuoles within sinusoids. This developed due to necrosis and rupture of steatotic hepatocytes following allograft preservation injury. A Kupffer-cell foreign-body reaction engulfing the lipid is present (arrow). (Needle biopsy, H&E.)

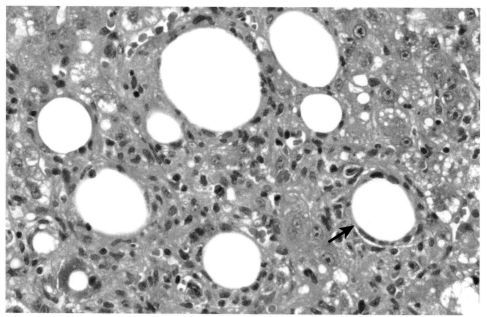

Antibody-mediated (humoral) rejection

Antibody-mediated rejection is rare after liver transplantation and has been best studied in recipients of ABO-incompatible allografts. Microvascular damage evolves over the first few hours after transplantation, consisting of sinusoidal infiltrates of neutrophilic leukocytes, fibrin and red blood cells associated with focal haemorrhages. This progresses to portal and periportal oedema with coagulative and haemorrhagic necrosis and a ductular reaction over the next few days[33] **(Fig. 16.4)**. Immunofluorescent studies show linear deposits of IgG or IgM, complement fractions C1q, C3 and C4 and fibrinogen in arterial

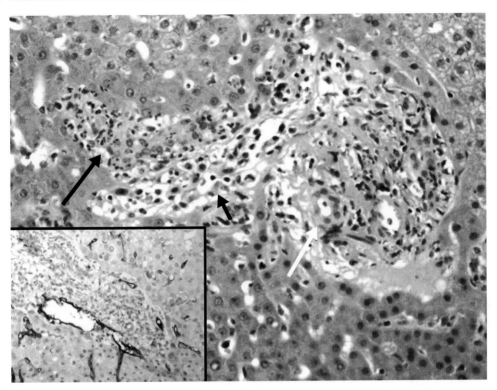

Figure 16.4 Antibody-mediated rejection after ABO-incompatible liver transplantation.
There is mild portal tract oedema with an early periportal ductular reaction and increased neutrophils (long arrow) in this 1 week postoperative allograft biopsy. The portal-vein branch (short arrow) is infiltrated by lymphocytes and eosinophils within the lumen. The relatively normal-appearing native bile duct (white arrow) and artery are seen at right. Inset: C4d immunohistochemical staining shows strong positivity in the portal vein and adjacent inlet vessels. (Allograft needle biopsy, H&E; inset: C4d-specific immunohistochemistry.)

walls.[27,34] The graft may remain stable in some patients for the first few days, however, possibly because of Kupffer-cell protection against the effects of circulating antibodies.[35] Graft failure within 2–4 weeks is associated with a progressive and marked rise in serum aminotransferase activity. The liver appears mottled and cyanotic at gross examination. Recipients of ABO-unmatched livers may also develop **graft-versus-host haemolysis**, associated with erythrophagocytosis and **Kupffer-cell siderosis**.[36] A potential role for antibody-mediated rejection is sometimes considered in the ABO-compatible recipient with early or late allograft dysfunction/failure who has high-titre donor-specific antibodies.[37–39] Endothelial cell hypertrophy involving portal veins and capillaries (and sometimes arterioles) accompanied by intraluminal lymphocytes and eosinophils adherent and embedded into the endothelium are helpful diagnostic features.[39a] The appropriate methodology for demonstrating C4d deposition in such cases (immunohistochemistry vs immunofluorescence) has been controversial, in part owing to differing results with these techniques (i.e. specific immunoperoxidase staining for C4d using paraffin-embedded sections may demonstrate strong portal vein and microvessel positivity[39b] **(Fig. 16.4, inset)**, while immunofluorescence shows a sinusoidal distribution of positivity).

Acute (cellular) rejection

Acute (cellular) rejection, the most common form of rejection, is a cell-mediated immune injury directed at bile-duct epithelium and the endothelium of portal-vein branches and

**Figure 16.5
Acute rejection.**
Heterogeneous portal inflammation consisting of lymphocytes, plasma cells and scattered neutrophils infiltrates the bile duct (between arrows) and the portal-vein branch at top. (Needle biopsy, H&E.)

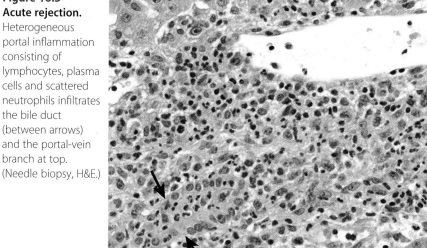

terminal hepatic venules. This usually occurs within the first month to 6 weeks after transplantation,[40] but may be seen later if immunosuppression is lowered or discontinued. The characteristic histological **triad** of cellular rejection includes **portal inflammation**, **bile-duct damage** and **endotheliitis (endothelialitis)**. Endotheliitis is not present in all cases. The portal inflammatory lesion is typically heterogeneous, with lymphocytes predominating among plasma cells, neutrophils and, occasionally, large lymphoid cells, some in mitosis (**Fig. 16.5**). Eosinophils are often abundant (**Fig. 16.6**), which is a very helpful diagnostic sign that acute rejection is present.[41,42]

Bile ducts are surrounded and infiltrated by immune cells and damage to their epithelium takes the form of variation in nuclear size, vacuolation of cytoplasm, regions of cell stratification or cell loss and irregularity of duct outlines (**Figs 16.5–16.7**). Endotheliitis comprises attachment of lymphoid cells to the endothelium of portal-vein branches or terminal hepatic venules, variable degrees of endothelial damage, subendothelial inflammation (**Figs 16.5 and 16.6**) and lifting off of endothelial cells from the underlying vein wall (**Fig. 16.8**). Sinusoidal endotheliitis is occasionally also present. Mild focal endotheliitis is sometimes found in association with hypoperfusion damage in baseline biopsies, but extensive endotheliitis in the postoperative period is very characteristic of rejection.[28] Necrosis of perivenular hepatocytes, accompanied by endotheliitis of terminal hepatic venules and expansive portal inflammatory lesions involving the periportal parenchyma, is indicative of severe acute rejection.[43] **Central perivenulitis (central venulitis)** – characterised by endotheliitis of terminal venules, drop-out and apoptosis of nearby hepatocytes (sometimes with focal sinusoidal congestion and dilatation) – often presages later episodes of acute rejection and chronic ductopenic rejection.[44–46] Central perivenulitis is a common expression of rejection in paediatric allografts.[47] It is sometimes the chief manifestation of rejection, with few or no portal tract changes, as **isolated central perivenulitis**[48] in both paediatric and adult allografts, many months or longer after transplantation (see Late liver allograft dysfunction, below).

Descriptive and semi-quantitative **grading of acute rejection** can effectively be accomplished using the scoring system presented in the Banff international consensus

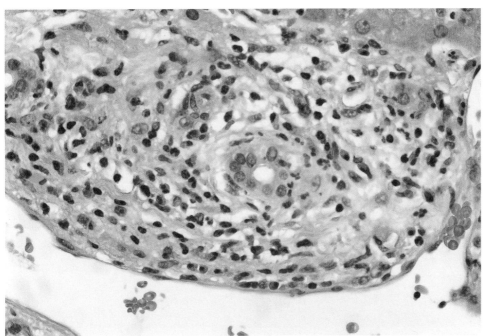

Figure 16.6
Acute rejection.
The portal tract infiltrate is rich in eosinophils. The portal-vein branch at bottom shows endotheliitis, with subendothelial lymphocytes and eosinophils. (Needle biopsy, H&E.)

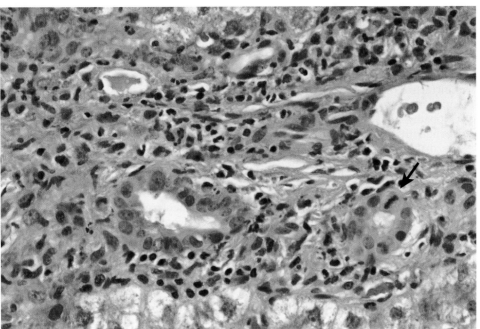

Figure 16.7
Acute rejection.
A damaged bile duct, cut twice in this portal tract, shows irregular epithelium with mild nuclear pleomorphism. Neutrophils are admixed with lymphocytes around and above the duct at left. The duct profile at right shows a mitotic figure (arrow). (Needle biopsy, H&E.) (Case kindly provided by Dr Jurgen Ludwig, Rochester, MN, USA.)

document[43] (**Table 16.1**). Using the semi-quantitative approach of assigning a numerical score to each component of the acute rejection triad, a total **Rejection Activity Index (RAI)** can be conveyed in the biopsy report. Alternatively, a simpler global assessment of the biopsy as showing indeterminate, mild, moderate or severe changes of acute rejection can be used (**Table 16.2**). The choice of grading system, as with grading and staging for chronic hepatitis, should be made after discussion with clinicians.

Figure 16.8
Endotheliitis in
acute rejection.
An efferent vein
shows lymphocytic
infiltration of its wall.
The endothelium is
focally lifted off the
underlying vein wall
and partially
destroyed. (Needle
biopsy, H&E.)

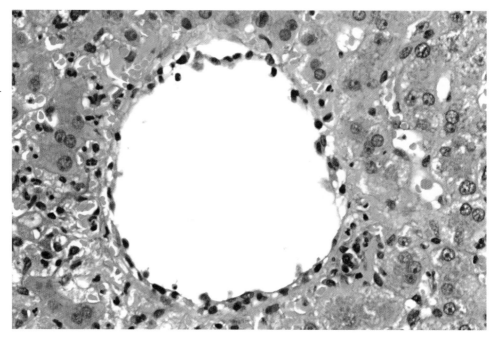

Chronic (ductopenic) rejection

Chronic (ductopenic) rejection ('vanishing bile-duct syndrome') is defined as obliterative vasculopathy and loss of bile ducts occurring 60 days or longer after transplantation.[27,49] The incidence of chronic rejection in liver transplant patients has declined to less than 5% in some series[50–52] as immunosuppression regimens have improved. In most cases, vasculopathy and ductopenia occur together, but in a minority they can be present independently.[53]

The diagnosis of chronic rejection can be problematic even for experienced hepatic pathologists,[54,55] particularly in the early stages.[27] Atrophy, nuclear pleomorphism and pyknosis of small ducts (bile-duct 'dystrophy') often precede frank ductopenia.[56] If such bile duct dystrophic and senescent changes are widespread, clinical jaundice may be prolonged over many weeks and associated with prominent centrilobular cholestasis and hepatocyte ballooning on liver biopsy (**Fig. 16.9**). The centrilobular changes may be mistaken for drug-induced liver injury, but careful inspection of the bile ducts usually clarifies the cause to be pervasive rejection-related duct injury. The presence of ductopenia is established when a formal count of small bile ducts and hepatic artery branches within portal tracts demonstrates loss of bile ducts from over 50% of portal tracts (**Fig. 16.10**). Progressive bile-duct loss results from a destructive cholangitis, which in most cases stems from bouts of acute rejection that are not controlled by immunosuppression. Cytokeratin immunostaining may help identify remnants of bile-duct epithelium.[31] Portal tract hepatic arterioles may also be lost.[49] Over time, portal inflammation becomes sparse and bile ducts disappear from the majority of portal tracts, usually without a ductular reaction[49] (**Fig. 16.10**). Episodes of acute rejection with increased inflammation and endotheliitis may develop superimposed on changes of chronic rejection. The pathology report in chronic rejection should therefore include consideration of the following points[49]: (1) whether acute rejection is present; (2) the degree of bile-duct loss in portal tracts; (3) the presence of perivenular necrosis or fibrosis; and (4) the degree of hepatic arteriole loss in relation to the total number of portal tracts.

Table 16.1 Banff grading scheme for acute rejection*

Category	Criteria	Score
Portal inflammation	Mostly lymphocytic inflammation involving, but not noticeably expanding, a minority of the triads	1
	Expansion of most or all of the triads, by a mixed infiltrate containing lymphocytes with occasional blasts, neutrophils and eosinophils	2
	Marked expansion of most or all of the triads by a mixed infiltrate containing numerous blasts and eosinophils with inflammatory spillover into the periportal parenchyma	3
Bile-duct inflammation damage	A minority of the ducts are cuffed and infiltrated by inflammatory cells and show only mild reactive changes, such as increased nucleus–cytoplasm ratio of the epithelial cells	1
	Most or all of the ducts are infiltrated by inflammatory cells. More than an occasional duct shows degenerative changes such as nuclear pleomorphism, disordered polarity and cytoplasmic vacuolisation of the epithelium	2
	As above for 2, with most or all of the ducts showing degenerative changes or focal luminal disruption	3
Venous endothelial inflammation	Subendothelial lymphocytic infiltration involving some, but not most, of the portal and/or hepatic venules	1
	Subendothelial infiltration involving most or all of the portal and/or hepatic venules	2
	As above for 2, with moderate or severe perivenular inflammation that extends into the perivenular parenchyma and is associated with perivenular hepatocyte necrosis	3

Note: total score = sum of components. Criteria that can be used to score liver allograft biopsies with acute rejection are as defined in the World Gastroenterology Consensus Document.
*The Rejection Activity Index (RAI) is the sum of the scores for each of the three components of acute rejection. RAI ≥ 4 (mild), RAI ≥ 6 (moderate or severe).
Reproduced from International Panel. Banff schema for grading liver allograft rejection: an international consensus document. *Hepatology* 1997; **25**: 658–663.

The presence of obliterative vasculopathy (rejection arteriopathy) may be more difficult to demonstrate on needle biopsies, since the characteristic subintimal accumulations of foamy histiocytes and myointimal cells predominantly affect the large-calibre arteries of the liver hilum[53,57] (**Fig. 16.11**). However, foam-cell lesions can sometimes be demonstrated in medium-sized portal arterioles present in biopsies and occasionally in portal veins and sinusoids (**Fig. 16.12**). The presence of arteriopathy in most cases must be inferred when perivenular ischaemic necrosis and fibrosis are seen in liver biopsies obtained in the appropriate time frame of chronic rejection. Demonstration of perivenular necrosis in repeated biopsies indicates a poor prognosis.[58] Mismatch of recipient and donor histocompatibility antigens, activation of the complement membrane attack complex and

Table 16.2 Descriptive terminology for acute rejection

Global assessment*	Criteria
Indeterminate	Portal inflammatory infiltrate that fails to meet the criteria for the diagnosis of acute rejection (see text)
Mild	Rejection infiltrate in a minority of the triads that is generally mild and confined within the portal spaces
Moderate	Rejection infiltrate, expanding most or all of the triads
Severe	As above for moderate, with spillover into periportal areas and moderate-to-severe perivenular inflammation that extends into the hepatic parenchyma and is associated with perivenular hepatocyte necrosis

Note: global assessment of rejection grade is made on a review of the biopsy and after the diagnosis of rejection has been established.
*Verbal description of mild, moderate or severe acute rejection could also be labelled as grades I, II and III, respectively. Reproduced from International Panel. Banff schema for grading liver allograft rejection: an international consensus document. *Hepatology* 1997; **25**: 658–663.

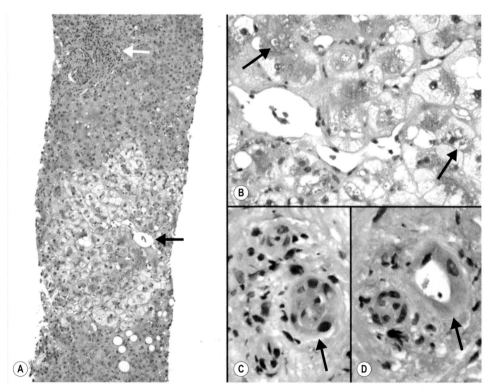

Figure 16.9 Prolonged acute rejection with extensive bile-duct injury, centrilobular cholestasis and hepatocyte ballooning.
A: Marked cholestasis and hepatocyte ballooning are present in the centrilobular region (black arrow) and reflect the extensiveness of rejection-related bile-duct injury. The portal tract at top (white arrow) shows rejection-related inflammation. **B:** Marked cholestasis within bile canaliculi (arrows) and hepatocyte has resulted in prominent liver-cell ballooning. **C:** The interlobular bile duct (arrow) is dysmorphic, with altered nuclear size and chromaticity as well as dyspolarity. **D:** This severely dystrophic (senescent) bile duct (arrow) shows a highly simplified structure composed of only a few cells with disparate nuclear features. (Allograft needle biopsy, H&E.)

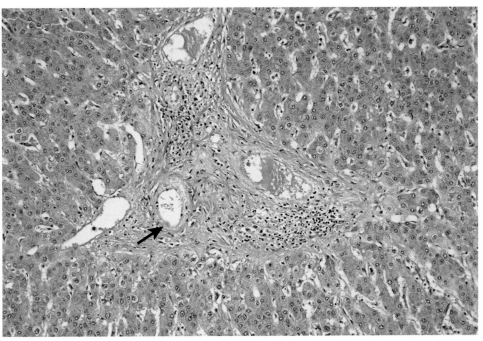

Figure 16.10 Chronic (ductopenic) rejection.
A hepatic artery branch (arrow) is present in the portal tract but the corresponding interlobular bile duct has disappeared as a result of rejection. A sparse lymphocytic infiltrate remains. (Explanted donor liver, H&E.) (Case kindly provided by Dr Jurgen Ludwig, Rochester, MN, USA.)

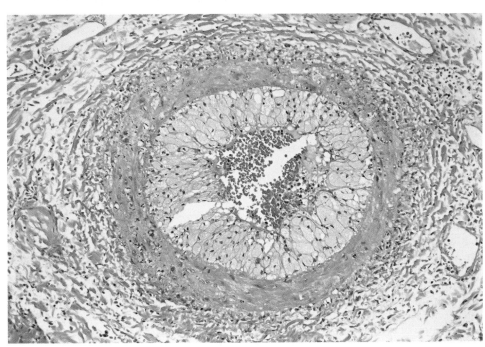

Figure 16.11 Rejection arteriopathy.
A hilar artery from a transplant liver removed because of rejection shows an accumulation of subintimal foam cells. (Explanted donor liver, H&E.) (Case kindly provided by Dr Jurgen Ludwig, Rochester, MN, USA.)

**Figure 16.12
Sinusoidal foam
cells in transplant
rejection.**
Months after
transplantation, foam
cells may be
deposited in
large-calibre arteries
and also within
hepatic sinusoids.
(Needle biopsy, H&E.)

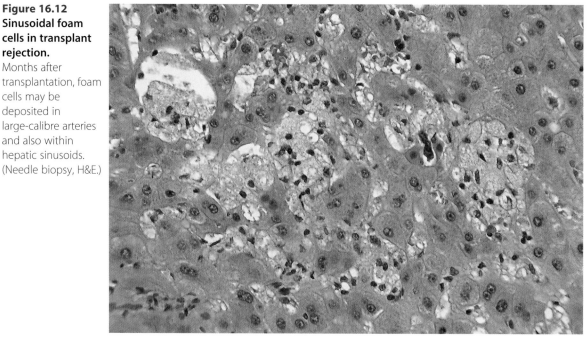

persistent cytomegalovirus (CMV) infection in the allograft have been invoked in the pathogenesis of bile-duct loss and arteriopathy.[31,59-63]

Chronic rejection usually leads to irreversible graft failure, although some patients may recover.[31,64] The late stage characteristically shows marked cholestasis and bile-duct loss, portal and periportal fibrosis, perivenular fibrosis and variable numbers of bridging fibrous septa linking portal tracts or central veins to portal tracts. Cirrhosis develops after liver transplantation in only a minority of patients and is typically due to recurrent or acquired viral hepatitis, rather than chronic rejection[65] (see Recurrent disease, below).

Other causes of graft dysfunction

Infection

CMV is a common pathogen in liver allografts; most cases of CMV hepatitis occur 4–8 weeks after transplant.[66] Typical intranuclear and cytoplasmic CMV inclusions (**see Ch. 15**) can be found in hepatocytes, bile-duct epithelium (**see Fig. 15.5**) and endothelial cells. CMV infection should be suspected when small **microabscess**-like foci of necrosis with an infiltrate of neutrophils are present (**Fig. 16.13**). Smaller collections of parenchymal neutrophils ('**mini-microabscesses**') are occasionally seen in patients without CMV infection, apparently without adverse effects on the graft.[67] CMV infection may also lead to formation of epithelioid granulomas. Immunohistochemical staining for CMV antigens is a sensitive method of demonstrating occult infection.[68]

Epstein–Barr virus infection should be considered if portal tracts and sinusoids contain a preponderance of atypical lymphocytes and immunoblasts.[69-71] The possibility that as yet unidentified hepatitis viruses may cause posttransplantation liver dysfunction has been considered.[72]

Infection by **Gram-negative bacilli** may produce hepatocellular and canalicular cholestasis or, with sepsis, the more unusual picture of inspissated bile in periportal bile ductules ('bile ductular cholestasis') (**see Ch. 15 and Fig. 15.12**). Cholestasis due to infection and/

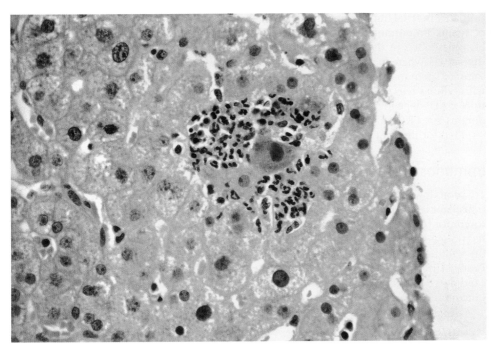

Figure 16.13
Cytomegalovirus hepatitis.
A microabscess-like cluster of neutrophils surrounds a hepatocyte with a smudged intranuclear inclusion. (Needle biopsy, H&E.)

or sepsis must be distinguished from that seen in bile-duct obstruction and rejection. Assessment of portal tract changes as well as results of microbiological studies are important in making these distinctions. Culture and special stains of liver biopsy specimens that show microabscesses or granulomas are the best means of documenting **bacterial, fungal or other infections.**[73]

Biliary obstruction

Perihilar bile leaks ('bilomas'), anastomotic strictures[74] and, less commonly, bile cast syndrome[75] may develop following transplant, with associated cholestasis and portal tract changes of obstruction (**see Ch. 5**) on biopsy. There may be residual portal and periportal fibrosis with a ductular reaction after prior episodes of obstruction and decompression by biliary stenting which should be taken into account when interpreting later allograft biopsies.

Thrombosis

Thrombosis of the hepatic artery[76,77] or portal vein[78] (the latter particularly in children) may develop within the first few weeks or months of transplantation, leading to infarction of the liver (**see Ch. 12**). Needle biopsy specimens may not be representative owing to the irregular distribution of infarcted liver parenchyma. Thrombosis, stricture or foam-cell arteriopathy of perihilar arteries may cause necrosis, stricture or cholangiectases of perihilar bile ducts due to impaired duct perfusion.[79] Liver biopsy in such cases may show features of biliary obstruction.[79]

Drug toxicity

The therapeutic regimen for immunosuppression in liver transplant patients includes several potentially hepatotoxic agents. **Azathioprine** hepatotoxicity has been reported primarily in renal transplant patients (see Renal transplantation, below). Elevated activities of serum aminotransferases with **sinusoidal congestion** and **perivenular necrosis** have been described in liver transplant patients treated with this drug,[80] and **veno-occlusive disease** elsewhere in the graft should be suspected, even if not demonstrated in the biopsy sample. There may also be **fibrosis of terminal hepatic venules**, particularly in patients with cellular rejection and endotheliitis.[81] **Ciclosporin** may cause **cholestasis**[82] by inhibition of ATP-dependent bile-salt transport.[83,84] Although a similar mechanism of cholestasis obtains for **FK 506**, hepatotoxicity is rare, probably due to the lower dose of FK 506 required for immunosuppression.[85,86]

Immunosuppression withdrawal

Titration downward and cessation of immunosuppression have been undertaken in some transplant recipients with apparently stable allografts in the hope of achieving **operational tolerance** (defined as 'a phenotype of tolerance with an immune response or deficit that has no significant clinical impact'[87]). Since rejection and other changes may develop during the withdrawal process,[87–90] liver biopsy in this setting remains diagnostically important. Protocol pre-weaning biopsies are recommended as a critical baseline for determining candidacy for immunosuppression withdrawal and for monitoring its complications and outcomes.[87]

Recurrent disease

Many of the diseases for which liver transplantation is performed have the potential to recur,[91] including viral hepatitis, malignant tumours, alcoholic and non-alcoholic steatohepatitis,[92–94] Budd–Chiari syndrome and variants of veno-occlusive disease,[95] autoimmune hepatitis (AIH), PBC and primary sclerosing cholangitis (PSC).[96–98] The diagnosis of recurrent disease on liver biopsy can be controversial because some of these pretransplant disorders have histopathological features which overlap with those seen in rejection or posttransplantation biliary obstruction.

Although the incidence of **recurrent viral hepatitis** in patients transplanted for severe liver disease due to hepatitis B, C and D varies at different transplantation centres, without prophylactic therapy it is an expected outcome in most cases. There are varied histopathological expressions of **recurrent hepatitis B**, including acute hepatitis, chronic hepatitis, cirrhosis, a carrier state with minimal histological disease and fibrosing cholestatic hepatitis[99,100] (see below). Recurrent hepatitis B may evolve from chronic hepatitis to cirrhosis within a year after transplantation.[101] Hepatitis B and D (delta) antigens can be demonstrated by immunohistochemistry in allografts as early as 1–3 weeks after transplantation.[101] For patients with **co-infection by hepatitis B and hepatitis D** in the native liver, recurrence may follow a variable course. In some patients, delta virus recurs without demonstrable hepatitis B virus (HBV) replication (absence of HBV core antigen on immunohistochemistry) or histological evidence of hepatitis.[102] Once HBV replication recurs and core antigen is present in the allograft, chronic hepatitis may then be seen on biopsy.[103] A minority of patients with recurrent hepatitis B infection may show a **fibrosing cholestatic hepatitis** with large numbers of ground-glass inclusions, 'cytopathic' liver-cell ballooning, cholestasis and a network of periportal fibrosis[100,104–108] (**Figs 16.14 and 16.15**). This pattern of disease recurrence is associated with a high rate of graft failure.

Recurrent hepatitis C after transplantation results in a characteristic sequence of pathological changes.[109] Within the first several months, increased numbers of apoptotic bodies appear, an important histological marker of recurrence[110] (**Fig. 16.16**). Their number and close proximity within the lobule far exceed that seen in acute rejection alone. Steatosis is often present and variable in degree, sometimes severe when genotype 3 infection recurs.[111] Increased lobular necroinflammation and liver-cell ballooning[112] follow and by 6 months to 1 year the portal lesion of recurrent chronic hepatitis becomes established.

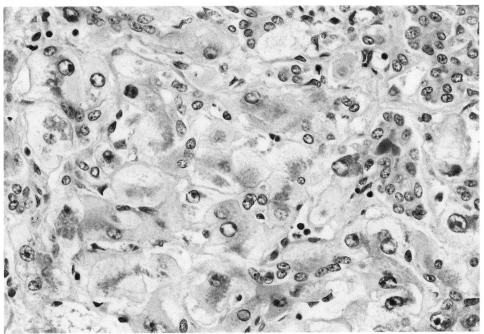

Figure 16.14 Fibrosing cholestatic hepatitis. Hepatocytes are swollen and many contain ground-glass inclusions. A bile thrombus is seen to the right of centre. (Explanted donor liver, H&E.) (Case kindly provided by Dr Bernard Portmann, London, UK.)

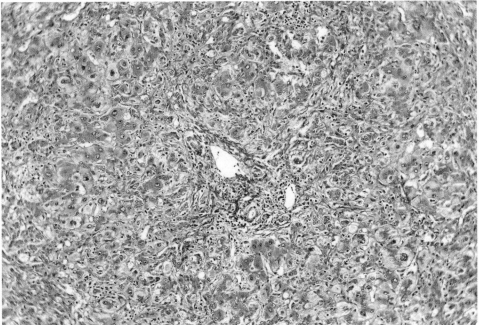

Figure 16.15 Fibrosing cholestatic hepatitis. Trichrome stain from the case depicted in **Figure 17.12** shows an intricate network of fibrosis emanating from the portal tract (centre). (Explanted donor liver, trichrome.) (Case kindly provided by Dr Bernard Portmann, London, UK.)

This is manifested by the presence of lymphoid aggregates or follicles (sometimes an isolated finding in the first few months after transplant), lymphocytic or lymphoplasma-cytic inflammation and variable degrees of interface hepatitis. The disease is frequently mild.[113,114] Polarisation of lymphoplasmacytic infiltrates towards the edges of the portal tracts and periportal regions supports the diagnosis of recurrent chronic hepatitis C, in contrast to acute rejection, where the infiltrates are more centrally localised around the

**Figure 16.16
Early recurrent
hepatitis C after
transplantation.**
The numerous
acidophilic
(apoptotic) bodies
shown here were
the earliest
histopathological
evidence of
recurrent hepatitis C
in this case. (Needle
biopsy, H&E.)

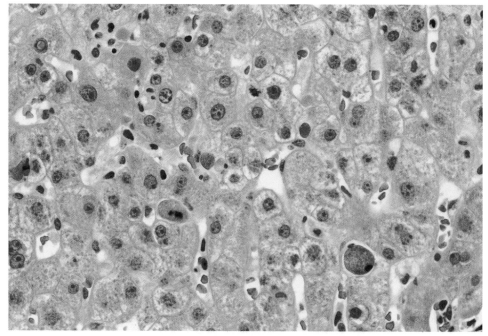

**Figure 16.17
Cholestatic
recurrent chronic
hepatitis C.**
The portal tract
shows mild chronic
inflammation and
fibrosis, with a
prominent periportal
ductular reaction
(arrowheads). Inset:
Hepatocytes show
considerable
ballooning,
cytopathic damage
and cholestasis.
(Needle biopsy, H&E.)

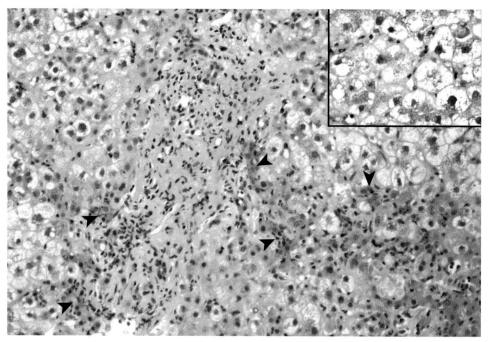

bile ducts and portal-vein branches. A ductular reaction is sometimes present in combination with the features of chronic hepatitis and correlates with advancing fibrosis.[114a] (**Fig. 16.17**). In the more serious form of recurrent hepatitis C known as **fibrosing cholestatic hepatitis C (FCH-C)**, the portal tracts show exceptionally prominent ductular reaction with scattered neutrophils in association with portal and periportal stellate fibrosis.

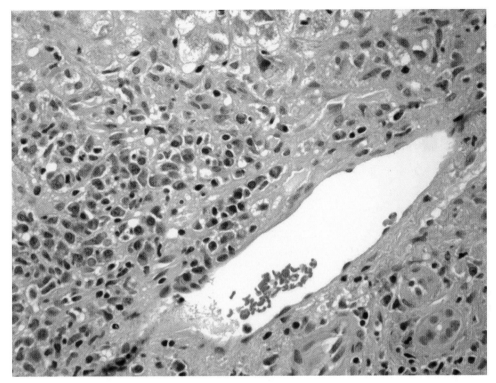

Figure 16.18 Plasma cell hepatitis after recurrence of chronic hepatitis C.
A plasma cell-predominant infiltrate with active interface hepatitis expands the portal tract outward. This unusual lesion is sometimes triggered by interferon administration and is thought to be an atypical rejection response ('alloimmune rejection') with a worrisome prognosis. The lower right corner shows a normal-appearing bile duct and portal-vein branch without damage from rejection.

Parenchymal cholestasis and liver-cell ballooning are typically striking (**Fig. 16.17, inset**) and are attributed to direct cytopathic effects of the virus.[114b] Overall, the combination of features resembles those seen in fibrosing cholestatic hepatitis B.[115] Serum bilirubin and HCV titres are usually high.[116,117] Trichrome stain often accentuates the ductular reaction in FCH-C, which can be further highlighted with cytokeratin 7 or 19 immunostains. Other forms of severe recurrent hepatitis C show confluent necrosis, liver-cell ballooning, bridging fibrosis and cirrhosis.[116,117] Occasional cases of recurrent chronic hepatitis C show **plasma cell hepatitis** with a preponderance of plasma cells in portal and periportal regions resembling AIH, often with accompanying lymphoplasmacytic central perivenulitis[118] (**Fig. 16.18**). This picture sometimes follows a reduction in immunosuppression or introduction of interferon therapy[119,120] and appears to be a variant form of *alloimmune* rejection[121] with a worse outcome.[122] Such complex cases warrant discussion with the clinical team. Distinction of recurrent chronic hepatitis C from acute rejection is often a considerable diagnostic problem,[109,123] especially compounded when evidence of both processes is present in a given biopsy. Many histological parameters must therefore be evaluated (**Table 16.3**). The major pathological process should be emphasised in the pathology report whenever possible.

Following transplantation for **PBC**, serum antimitochondrial antibodies may persist or recur, liver function tests (particularly serum alkaline phosphatase activity) may worsen and liver biopsy may demonstrate recurrent damage to bile ducts.[124] Florid bile-duct lesions and adjacent epithelioid granulomas are the most useful histological signs of recurrent disease. Ductular reaction and progressive copper deposition are other helpful

Table 16.3 Comparative features of acute rejection versus recurrent chronic hepatitis C

Feature	Acute rejection	Recurrent hepatitis C
Lobular necroinflammation	No	Yes
Apoptotic bodies	Few	Many
Cholestasis	Mild	May be marked
Interface hepatitis	No (unless severe)	Often
Lymphoid aggregates/follicles	No	Yes
Portal inflammation	Heterogeneous	Lymphocytes, plasma cells
Fat	No (except with corticosteroid therapy)	Yes (genotype 3 especially)
Ductular reaction	No	Variable (common in cholestatic type)
Central venulitis	Often, diffuse	Uncommon, focal
Bile-duct damage	Yes, diffuse	Focal or none
Portal/periportal fibrosis	No	Often

features. There may also be portal lymphoid aggregates and mononuclear inflammation as well as ductopenia, but these can also be seen in HCV infection and rejection. If there is uncertainty, HCV infection should be serologically excluded. Recurrent PBC can progress to cirrhosis within several years.[125] **AIH** with high levels of serum globulins and typical liver biopsy features has also been reported in patients transplanted for PBC.[126] AIH with high biochemical and histological activity pretransplantation may presage recurrence in the allograft.[127]

Recurrence of **PSC** after transplantation is reported[128] but has been controversial, because the radiological and histopathological features of PSC resemble those seen in biliary complications of the transplant procedure, such as biliary stricture due to hepatic artery thrombosis and bile-duct or choledochojejunostomy-anastomotic obstruction.[91] Biopsy features of cholestasis and portal obstructive changes therefore require cautious interpretation in the context of radiological and other data. Fibro-obliterative lesions (**see Ch. 5**) are more specific for recurrence,[128] but are infrequently found in biopsies.[97] Perihilar xanthogranulomatous cholangitis in the explanted PSC liver (**see Ch. 5**) has been associated with increased posttransplantation morbidity and mortality.[129]

Studies of patients transplanted for AIH are at variance with regard to the incidence of recurrence.[91] An abrupt rise in serum aminotransferases, detectable autoantibodies, hypergammaglobulinaemia and portal inflammation with interface hepatitis on biopsy are consistent with recurrent disease. Lobular hepatitis may be the first sign of recurrence.[72] In children, recurrent AIH may be an aggressive disease resulting in cirrhosis and retransplantation.[130]

Recurrence of **alcoholic** or **non-alcoholic fatty liver disease** may be manifested by steatosis and steatohepatitis after transplantation.[131] Immunosuppression agents (e.g. corticosteroids, calcineurin inhibitors) and weight gain contribute to recurrent or new metabolic syndrome in adults and in children.[132–136] Steatosis, steatohepatitis and cirrhosis also are seen after transplantation for progressive familial intrahepatic cholestasis type 1.[137]

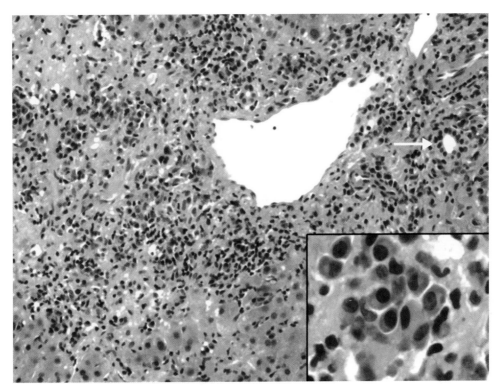

Figure 16.19 *De novo* **autoimmune hepatitis.**
Liver dysfunction developed 3 years after liver transplantation for alcoholic cirrhosis in this case and the allograft biopsy showed marked plasma cell infiltrates (inset) within portal tracts and periportal regions, with extensive interface hepatitis. The bile duct (white arrow) and portal vein branch to its left appear normal. Centrilobular necroinflammation with increased plasma cells was also present. (Allograft needle biopsy, H&E.) (Case kindly provided by Dr Glen Friedman, Las Palmas Medical Center, El Paso, Texas.)

De novo autoimmune hepatitis

Children and adults who have undergone liver transplantation for conditions other than AIH infrequently (<6%) develop *de novo* AIH several years or more after transplantation, with elevated serum immunoglobulin levels and a variety of autoantibodies.[96-98] The major histological criteria consist of interface hepatitis with substantial activity and abundant plasma cells (**Fig. 16.19**) and plasma cell-enriched centrilobular necroinflammation.[138] Paediatric cases may also show prominent lobular necroinflammation and apoptosis without interface hepatitis or plasma cell enrichment.[98b]

A related, severe form of posttransplant liver disease, **graft dysfunction mimicking AIH**,[139] can result in graft loss.

Neoplastic disease

Posttransplant lymphoproliferative disease (PTLD), chiefly B-cell lymphoma in lymph nodes and extranodal sites, is a complication of immunosuppression in patients with organ transplants. Special studies are important in determining whether the PTLD is polymorphic or monomorphic according to the current World Health Organization classification.[140] B-cell lymphoma in the liver has been reported as early as 2 months after liver transplantation[141] but usually occurs 1 year or more after adult liver transplantation and

**Figure 16.20
Posttransplant
lymphoprolifera-
tive disease.**
The portal tract at
left is infiltrated and
overrun by a
proliferation of
lymphoid cells. Inset:
The cytological
features are
consistent with a
high-grade, large
B-cell lymphoma.
Flow cytometry,
immunohistochemi-
cal staining and
gene rearrangement
studies are
undertaken
for further
characterisation of
the lymphoid
infiltrates. (Needle
biopsy, H&E.)

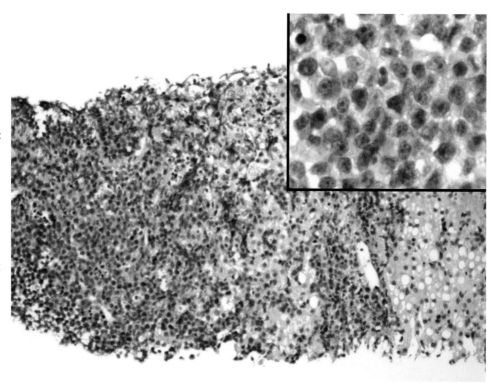

within a year in children.[140] Lymphoma usually originates in recipient lymphoid tissue, but rarely it may be derived from donor lymphoid tissue present in the allograft.[142] Hepatic involvement consists of diffuse lymphoma nodules or portal tract infiltration by lymphoma cells (**Fig. 16.20**). Biopsy demonstration of Epstein–Barr virus, which is involved in the pathogenesis of most cases of PTLD,[140] is helpful in distinguishing this from rejection.[143] *De novo*[144,145] or recurrent[146] **hepatocellular carcinoma** has also developed in patients transplanted for chronic hepatitis B and C, even after viral clearance.[147]

Late liver allograft dysfunction

Most transplant recipients with abnormal liver function tests or symptoms at 1 year or later after transplantation show biopsy changes related to recurrent disease or biliary stricture.[148] However, as with earlier biopsies, several pathological processes may be evident, and helpful histological guidelines for sorting these out have been provided by the Banff Working Group.[148] Examination for changes of acute or chronic rejection is always important. Particular attention should be paid to perivenular regions since certain cases of ongoing or late acute rejection may be confined to these areas as **isolated central perivenulitis**[48,149,150] (**Fig. 16.21**). The changes are similar to those of central perivenulitis earlier after transplantation, but there may also be perivenular fibrosis and possible evolution to ductopenic rejection. The degree of terminal venule involvement and associated perivenular hepatocyte drop-out and necrosis in isolated central perivenulitis should be specifically described in the diagnosis.[148]

Late biopsies sometimes show non-specific portal or lobular lymphocytic infiltrates of uncertain aetiology in the absence of more diagnostic changes of rejection. Unexplained periportal fibrosis in paediatric allograft biopsies several years after transplant has also been reported.[3] A small number of late paediatric and adult allograft biopsies

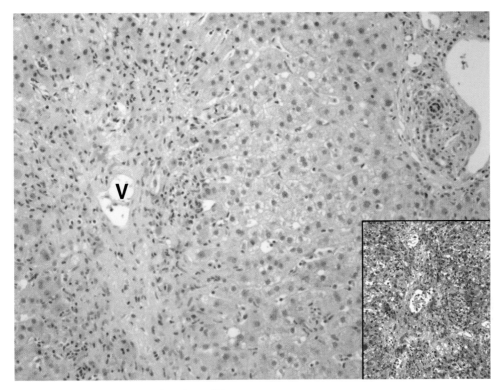

Figure 16.21 Isolated central perivenulitis.
The rejection lesion in this 1-year posttransplant biopsy chiefly involves terminal venules (V) where lymphocytic infiltrates, congestion and perivenular fibrosis are seen. The portal tract at upper right is relatively spared, with only sparse lymphocytes and no bile-duct or portal-vein damage. (Needle biopsy, H&E.) Inset: Connective tissue stain highlights the collagenous scar surrounding the venule. (Trichrome stain.)

show histological changes of chronic hepatitis or cirrhosis that are unexplained by chronic hepatitis B or C or AIH. These instances of **'idiopathic posttransplantation hepatitis'** **(IPTH)** may represent a variant form of chronic rejection.[97,151] Another consideration in IPTH is chronic hepatitis E virus (HEV) infection (whether recurrent, reactivated or newly acquired in the donor liver), which should be excluded with serological studies of HEV RNA as well as IgM and IgG anti-HEV antibodies.[152,153,153a,153b]

Differential diagnosis in transplant biopsies

Most problems in biopsy interpretation after liver transplantation arise in distinguishing rejection from other conditions (**Table 16.4**). It should be kept in mind that rejection and other allograft disorders can coexist. Difficult pathological problems are usually resolved by discussion with clinicians, assessment of viral serologies and microbial culture results, and review of drug therapy. When necessary, patency of vascular or biliary anastomoses may need to be radiologically demonstrated.

While **endotheliitis** may be seen in several forms of liver disease,[154] when it is found in combination with bile-duct damage and a mixed portal inflammatory infiltrate the diagnosis of acute rejection is usually clear. Endotheliitis involving central veins (**central venulitis**) sometimes presents diagnostic difficulties.[47] Regular involvement of most central veins in a biopsy specimen favours rejection or the less common development of *de novo*

Table 16.4 Differential diagnostic features in transplant biopsies

Histological feature	Rejection	Condition			
		Recurrent HBV	Recurrent HCV	Biliary obstruction	Ischaemia
Cholestasis	+/–	Unusual (except in fibrosing cholestatic hepatitis)	Unusual	Yes	No
Portal inflammation					
Mixed (L, P, N, E)*	Yes	+/–	+/–	No	No
Lymphocytes, plasma cells	+/–	Yes	Yes	No	No
Neutrophils	+/–	No	No	Yes	No
Bile duct damage	Yes	Unusual	Yes	No	No
Endotheliitis	Yes	Unusual	Unusual	No	Occasional
Zone 3 necrosis	Yes, if chronic	No	No	No	Yes
Sinusoidal inflammation	No	+/–	++	No	No
Apoptotic bodies	+/–	+	+++	No	No

+/– indicates a feature which is not characteristic, but which may sometimes be present.
*Mixed portal inflammation includes lymphocytes (L), plasma cells (P), neutrophils (N) and eosinophils (E).
HBV, HCV, hepatitis B, C virus.

AIH. Central venulitis due to viral and drug hepatitis is more irregular in distribution. **Bile-duct damage** represents a more difficult histological problem, because it is a feature seen in rejection, chronic hepatitis C and PBC. Portal tract lymphoid aggregates, numerous apoptotic bodies, interface hepatitis and prominent sinusoidal inflammation support the diagnosis of chronic hepatitis C. As noted earlier, the presence of a granulomatous, destructive cholangitis in a hepatitis C-seronegative patient transplanted for PBC is important evidence of recurrent PBC.

Neutrophils may be seen in the vicinity of damaged bile ducts in rejection (**Fig. 16.5**) and should not be mistaken for evidence of biliary obstruction. Obstruction can usually be excluded if portal tract oedema and ductular reaction are absent. **Eosinophils** are often prominent in rejection but can be seen in fewer numbers in recurrent viral hepatitis or AIH. Subendothelial eosinophils in portal-vein branches favour rejection. Drug hepatitis as a cause of eosinophil infiltrates may need consideration when there is antibiotic prophylaxis with sulfa agents such as trimethoprim–sulfamethoxazole, but the parenchymal changes of acute hepatitis usually help to distinguish this from rejection. **Plasma cells** in small numbers are often present in acute rejection infiltrates, but are also seen admixed with lymphocytes as periportal interface hepatitis in recurrent diseases such as chronic hepatitis B or C or AIH. Interface hepatitis with large numbers of plasma cells in clusters in biopsies from transplant recipients without such antecedent native liver diseases suggests possible *de novo* AIH, which should be further substantiated by the presence of serum autoantibodies and elevated γ-globulin level. Posttransplant recurrent chronic hepatitis C with plasma-cell infiltrates (plasma cell hepatitis) was discussed earlier.

Cholestasis may pose significant diagnostic problems because of several potential causes,[22] including biliary obstruction, rejection and sepsis. In biopsies obtained early (1–2 weeks) after transplantation, cholestasis is usually functional in nature. Small-for-size living donor grafts may also develop cholestasis. Cholestasis accompanied by portal oedema and a ductular reaction should prompt an assessment of the biliary anastomosis. Fibrosing cholestatic hepatitis may mimic such biliary obstructive features, but oedema is typically absent and the hepatocyte swelling and apoptosis accompanying the cholestasis usually clarify that there is recurrent severe HBV or HCV infection. In such cases, clinical exclusion of biliary obstruction is also typically undertaken. The distinctive pattern of 'bile ductular cholestasis' is usually associated with sepsis. Rarely, one or two visibly damaged bile ducts may contain inspissated bile in cases of prolonged, refractory rejection.

Steatosis of large-droplet type in posttransplant biopsies may be due to several factors, including corticosteroid immunosuppression and recurrent HCV infection. Genotype 3 reinfection particularly may result in severe fatty change.[111] Considerable fat also develops in allografts of children transplanted for progressive familial intrahepatic cholestasis type 1.[155]

HBV-negative recipients of liver and other transplants occasionally develop **ground-glass-like hepatocellular inclusions** that are periodic acid–Schiff-positive and represent an abnormal form of glycogen.[156–158] These should be distinguished from other types of ground-glass inclusions (**see Ch. 4**).[159]

Renal transplantation

Patients who have undergone renal transplantation are exposed to many viruses capable of causing acute or chronic hepatitis, particularly hepatitis B[160] and hepatitis C.[161] Steatosis, chronic hepatitis and cirrhosis are often found on biopsy.[162] Fibrosing cholestatic hepatitis is infrequently seen in recipients with chronic hepatitis C.[163] There may be lesions related to administration of potentially hepatotoxic drugs such as azathioprine, which may cause cholestasis, veno-occlusive disease, nodular regenerative hyperplasia and other lesions.[80,164–166] Cirrhosis develops in a small proportion of patients. Incrimination of a single aetiological agent is often difficult. Transfusions may cause substantial siderosis involving both hepatocytes and macrophages.[167,168] Vascular lesions following renal transplantation include narrowing or occlusion of efferent veins,[169] peliosis hepatis[170] and non-cirrhotic portal hypertension.[171] Portal hypertension associated with dilatation of sinusoids in acinar zones 2 and 3, with eventual development of fibrosis or cirrhosis, has also been reported.[172]

Patients who have been treated by **haemodialysis** may have birefringent material, probably derived from silicone tubing, in portal tracts. In some instances this material gives rise to a giant-cell or granulomatous reaction.[173–175] Haemodialysis patients often have Kupffer-cell siderosis.

Bone marrow transplantation

Graft recipients are liable to liver damage from graft-versus-host disease (GVHD), chemotherapy-related sinusoidal obstruction syndrome/veno-occlusive disease, infection and idiosyncratic drug jaundice. Siderosis is often present because of prior transfusions. **GVHD** involving the liver has varying histological features depending on the stage of evolution.[176–178] The most characteristic features of acute (less than 90 days after transplant) GVHD are **bile-duct damage** and **cholestasis**.[176,177] The ducts often appear attenuated, tapering and stretched lengthwise. The duct epithelium is irregular, with vacuolated or acidophilic cytoplasm, nuclear pleomorphism and multilayering, and increased

Figure 16.22 Graft-versus-host disease.
The bile-duct epithelium shows dyspolarity and attenuation. A small apoptotic nuclear fragment is seen at top (arrowhead) near an intracellular degenerative vacuole. The surrounding lymphocytic infiltrate is relatively mild. (Needle biopsy, H&E.)

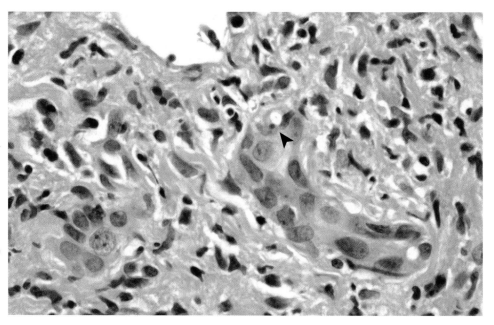

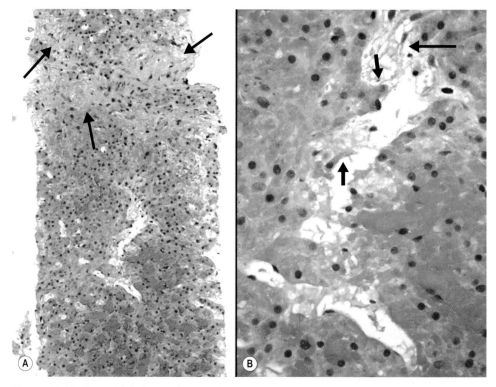

Figure 16.23 Sinusoidal obstruction syndrome.
A: There is marked congestion and several venules and nearby sinusoids contain plugs of young fibrous tissue (arrows). The terminal venule at centre is injured. The injury was attributed to recent busulphan conditioning chemotherapy prior to hematopoietic stem-cell transplantation for leukaemia. **B:** The endothelium of this terminal venule is partially denuded and detached (long arrow) with extrusion of hepatocytes into the vessel lumen (short arrows). (Needle biopsy, H&E.)

nucleus–cytoplasm ratio[176,179] (**Fig. 16.22**). Lymphocytes infiltrate the portal tracts and duct epithelium, but are sparse. In early GVHD (less than 35 days), duct changes are less apparent and numerous parenchymal acidophilic bodies may be present.[176] Endotheliitis is uncommon, in comparison with acute liver allograft rejection. In **chronic GVHD** (after 90 days) there is progressive bile-duct dystrophy and senescence, ductopenia and portal fibrosis.[180] The clinical and radiological picture may mimic intrahepatic PSC.[181] Rarely, there are parenchymal changes of an acute hepatitis.[182,183] Cirrhosis of biliary type may finally develop.[184] Chemotherapy for leukaemia/lymphoma may damage sinusoidal endothelium leading to **sinusoidal obstruction syndrome/veno-occlusive disease**[185] (also discussed in **Ch. 12**). Such cases show variable perivenular or more diffuse sinusoidal congestion with disruption and effacement of endothelium, intravasation of erythrocytes into the space of Disse and patchy fibrosis of sinusoids and terminal venules[186] (**Fig. 16.23**). Eosinophilic cytoplasmic inclusions in hepatocytes of patients dying after bone marrow transplantation have been described.[187]

References

1 Henley KS, Lucey MR, Appelman HD, et al. Biochemical and histopathological correlation in liver transplant: the first 180 days. Hepatology 1992;16:688–93.

2 Abraham SC, Poterucha JJ, Rosen CB, et al. Histologic abnormalities are common in protocol liver allograft biopsies from patients with normal liver function tests. Am J Surg Pathol 2008;32:965–73.

3 Ekong UD, Melin-Aldana H, Seshadri R, et al. Graft histology characteristics in long-term survivors of pediatric liver transplantation. Liver Transpl 2008;14:1582–7.

4 Minervini MI, Ruppert K, Fontes P, et al. Liver biopsy findings from healthy potential living liver donors: reasons for disqualification, silent diseases and correlation with liver injury tests. J Hepatol 2009;50:501–10.

5 Demetris AJ, Kelly DM, Eghtesad B, et al. Pathophysiologic observations and histopathologic recognition of the portal hyperperfusion or small-for-size syndrome. Am J Surg Pathol 2006;30:986–93.

6 Kasahara M, Takada Y, Fujimoto Y, et al. Impact of right lobe with middle hepatic vein graft in living-donor liver transplantation. Am J Transplant 2005;5:1339–46.

7 Ayata G, Pomfret E, Pomposelli JJ, et al. Adult-to-adult live donor liver transplantation: a short-term clinicopathologic study. Hum Pathol 2001;32:814–22.

8 Gaffey MJ, Boyd JC, Traweek ST, et al. Predictive value of intraoperative biopsies and liver function tests for preservation injury in orthotopic liver transplantation. Hepatology 1997;25:184–9.

9 de Vera ME, Lopez-Solis R, Dvorchik I, et al. Liver transplantation using donation after cardiac death donors: long-term follow-up from a single center. Am J Transplant 2009;9:773–81.

10 Pungpapong S, Krishna M, Abraham SC, et al. Clinicopathologic findings and outcomes of liver transplantation using grafts from donors with unrecognized and unusual diseases. Liver Transpl 2006;12:310–15.

11 Verran D, Kusyk T, Painter D, et al. Clinical experience gained from the use of 120 steatotic donor livers for orthotopic liver transplantation. Liver Transpl 2003;9:500–5.

12 Yersiz H, Lee C, Kaidas FM, et al. Assessment of hepatic steatosis by transplant surgeon and expert pathologist: a prospective double-blind evaluation of 201 donor livers. Liver Transpl 2013;19:437–49.

13 Brunt EM. Surgical assessment of significant steatosis in donor livers: the beginning of the end for frozen-section analysis? Liver Transpl 2013;19:360–1.

14 Bzeizi KI, Jalan R, Plevris JN, et al. Primary graft dysfunction after liver transplantation: from pathogenesis to prevention. Liver Transpl Surg 1997;3:137–48.

15 Trevisani F, Colantoni A, Caraceni P, et al. The use of donor fatty liver for liver transplantation: a challenge or a quagmire? J Hepatol 1996;24:114–21.

16 Fishbein TM, Fiel MI, Emre S, et al. Use of livers with microvesicular fat safely expands the donor pool. Transplantation 1997;64:248–51.

17 Sharkey FE, Lytvak I, Prihoda TJ, et al. High-grade microsteatosis and delay in hepatic function after orthotopic liver transplantation. Hum Pathol 2011;42:1337–42.

18 Eggink HF, Hofstee N, Gips CH, et al. Histopathology of serial graft biopsies from liver transplant recipients. Am J Pathol 1984;114:18–31.

19 Ludwig J, Lefkowitch JH. Histopathology of the liver following transplantation. In: Maddrey WC, Schiff ER, Sorrel MF, editors. Transplantation of the Liver. 3rd ed. Philadelphia: Lippincott Williams & Wilkins; 2001. p. 229–50, [Ch. 15].

20 Williams JW, Vera S, Peters TG, et al. Cholestatic jaundice after hepatic transplantation. A nonimmunologically mediated event. Am J Surg 1986;151:65–70.

21 Jaeschke H, LeMasters JJ. Apoptosis versus oncotic necrosis in hepatic ischemia/reperfusion injury. Gastroenterology 2003;125:1246–57.

22 Ben-Ari Z, Pappo O, Mor E. Intrahepatic cholestasis after liver transplantation. Liver Transpl 2003;9:1005–18.

23 Ng IOL, Burroughs AK, Rolles K, et al. Hepatocellular ballooning after liver transplantation: a light and electronmicroscopic study with clinicopathological correlation. Histopathology 1991;18:323–30.

24 Goldstein NS, Hart J, Lewin KJ. Diffuse hepatocyte ballooning in liver biopsies fromorthotopic liver transplant patients. Histopathology 1991;18:331–8.

25 Russo PA, Yunis EJ. Subcapsular hepatic necrosis in orthotopic liver allografts. Hepatology 1986;6:708–13.

26 Cha I, Bass N, Ferrell LD. Lipopeliosis. An immunohistochemical and clinicopathologic study of five cases. Am J Surg Pathol 1994;18:789–95.

27 International Working Party. Terminology for hepatic allograft rejection. Hepatology 1995;22:648–54.

28 Snover DC, Sibley RK, Freese DK, et al. Orthotopic liver transplantation: a pathological study of 63 serial liver biopsies from 17 patients with special reference to the diagnostic features and natural history of rejection. Hepatology 1984;4:1212–22.

29 Demetris AJ, Lasky S, Van Thiel DH, et al. Pathology of hepatic transplantation: a review of 62 adult allograft recipients immunosuppressed with a cyclosporine/steroid regimen. Am J Pathol 1985;118:151–61.

30 Hubscher SG. Histological findings in liver allograft rejection – new insights into the pathogenesis of hepatocellular damage in liver allografts. Histopathology 1991;18:377–83.

31 Freese DK, Snover DC, Sharp HL, et al. Chronic rejection after liver transplantation: a study of clinical, histopathological and immunological features. Hepatology 1991;13:882–91.

32 Wiesner RH, Ludwig J, Krom RAF, et al. Hepatic allograft rejection: new developments in terminology, diagnosis, prevention, and treatment. Mayo Clin Proc 1993;68:69–79.

33 Haga H, Egawa H, Shirase T, et al. Periportal edema and necrosis as diagnostic histological features of early humoral rejection in ABO-incompatible liver transplantation. Liver Transpl 2004;10:16–27.

34 Demetris AJ, Jaffe R, Tzakis A, et al. Antibody-mediated rejection of human orthotopic liver allografts. A study of liver transplantation across ABO blood group barriers. Am J Pathol 1988;132:489–502.

35 Wardle EN. Kupffer cells and their function. Liver 1987;7:63–75.

36 Clavien P-A, Camargo CA, Cameron R, et al. Kupffer cell erythrophagocytosis and graft-versus-host hemolysis in liver transplantation. Gastroenterology 1996;110:1891–6.

37 Banff 2013 meeting report: inclusion of C4d-negative antibody-mediated rejection and antibody-associated arterial lesions. Am J Transplant 2014;14:272–83.

38 Kozlowski T, Andreoni K, Schmitz J, et al. Sinusoidal C4d deposits in liver allografts indicate an antibody-mediated response: diagnostic considerations in the evaluation of liver allografts. Liver Transpl 2012;18:641–58.

39 Taner T, Stegall MD, Heimbach JK. Antibody-mediated rejection in liver transplantation: current controversies and future directions. Liver Transpl 2014;20:514–27.

39a O'Leary JG, Shiller SM, Bellamy C, et al. Acute liver allograft antibody-mediated rejection: an inter-institutional study of significant histopathological features. Liver Transplant 2014;20:1244–55.

39b Salah A, Fujimoto M, Yoshizawa A, et al. Application of complement component 4d immunohistochemistry to ABO-compatible and ABO-incompatible liver transplantation. Liver Transpl 2014;20:200–9.

40 Wiesner RH, Demetris AJ, Belle SH, et al. Acute hepatic allograft rejection: incidence, risk factors and impact on outcome. Hepatology 1998;28:638–45.

41 DeGroen PC, Kephart GM, Gleich GJ, et al. The eosinophil as an effector cell of the immune response during hepatic allograft rejection. Hepatology 1994;20:654–62.

42 Nagral A, Ben-Ari Z, Dhillon AP, et al. Eosinophils in acute cellular rejection in liver allografts. Liver Transpl Surg 1998;4:355–62.

43 International Panel. Banff schema for grading liver allograft rejection: an international consensus document. Hepatology 1997;25:658–63.

44 Khettry U, Backer A, Ayata G, et al. Centrilobular histopathologic changes in liver transplant biopsies. Hum Pathol 2002;33:270–6.

45 Lovell MO, Speeg KV, Halff GA, et al. Acute hepatic allograft rejection: a comparison of patients with and without centrilobular alterations during first rejection episode. Liver Transpl 2004;10:369–73.

46 Sundaram SS, Melin-Aldana H, Neighbors K, et al. Histologic characteristics of late cellular rejection, significance of centrilobular injury, and long-term outcome in pediatric liver transplant patients. Liver Transpl 2006;12:58–64.

47 Demetris AJ. Central venulitis in liver allografts: considerations of differential diagnosis. Hepatology 2001;33:1329–30.

48 Hübscher SG. Central perivenulitis: a common and potentially important finding in late posttransplant liver biopsies. Liver Transpl 2008;14:596–600.

49 International Panel. Update of the international Banff schema for liver allograft rejection: working recommendations for the histopathologic staging and reporting of chronic rejection. Hepatology 2000;31:792–9.

50 Weisner RH, Batts KP, Krom RAF. Evolving concepts in the diagnosis, pathogenesis and treatment of chronic hepatic allograft rejection. Liver Transpl Surg 1999;5:388–400.

51 Wiesner RH, Demetris AJ, Seaberg EC. Chronic hepatic allograft rejection: defining clinical risk factors and assessing impact on graft outcome. Hepatology 1998;28:314A.

52 Ludwig J, Hashimoto E, Porayko MK, et al. Failed allografts and causes of death after orthotopic liver transplantation from 1985 to 1995: decreasing prevalence of irreversible hepatic allograft rejection. Liver Transpl Surg 1996;2:185–91.

53 McCaughan GW, Bishop GA. Atherosclerosis of the liver allograft. J Hepatol 1997;27:592–8.

54 Demetris AJ, Belle SH, Hart J, et al. Intraobserver and interobserver variation in the histopathological assessment of liver allograft rejection. Hepatology 1991;14:751–5.

55 Thung SN, Gerber MA. Histological features of liver allograft rejection: do you see what I see? Hepatology 1991;14:949–51.

56 Sebagh M, Blakolmer K, Falissard B, et al. Accuracy of bile duct changes for the diagnosis of chronic liver allograft rejection: reliability of the 1999 Banff schema. Hepatology 2002;35:117–25.

57 Liu G, Butany J, Wanless IR, et al. The vascular pathology of human hepatic allografts. Hum Pathol 1993;24:182–8.

58 Ludwig J, Gross JB, Perkins JD, et al. Persistent centrilobular necroses in hepatic allografts. Hum Pathol 1990;21:656–61.

59 Arnold JC, Portmann BC, O'Grady JG, et al. Cytomegalovirus infection persists in the liver graft in the vanishing bile duct syndrome. Hepatology 1992;16:285–92.

60 Donaldson PT, Alexander GJM, O'Grady J, et al. Evidence for an immune response to HLA Class I antigens in the vanishing-bile duct syndrome after liver transplantation. Lancet 1987;1:945–8.

61 O'Grady JG, Alexander GJM, Sutherland S, et al. Cytomegalovirus infection and donor/recipient HLA antigens: interdependent co-factors in pathogenesis of vanishing bile duct syndrome after liver transplantation. Lancet 1988;2:302–5.

62 Lautenschlager I, Höckerstedt K, Jalanko H, et al. Persistent cytomegalovirus in liver allografts with chronic rejection. Hepatology 1997;25:190–4.

63 Conti F, Grude P, Calmus Y, et al. Expression of the membrane attack complex of complement and its inhibitors during human liver allograft transplantation. J Hepatol 1997;27:881–9.

64 Hubscher SG, Buckels JAC, Elias E, et al. Vanishing bile-duct syndrome following liver transplantation – is it reversible? Transplantation 1991;51:1004–10.

65 Tabatabai L, Lewis WD, Gordon F, et al. Fibrosis/cirrhosis after orthotopic liver transplantation. Hum Pathol 1999;30:39–47.

66 Seehofer D, Rayes N, Tullius SG, et al. CMV hepatitis after liver transplantation: incidence, clinical course, and long-term follow-up. Liver Transpl 2002;8:1138–46.

67 MacDonald GA, Greenson JK, DelBuono EA, et al. Mini-microabscess syndrome in liver transplant patients. Hepatology 1997;26:192–7.

68 Theise ND, Conn M, Thung SN. Localization of cytomegalovirus antigens in liver allografts over time. Hum Pathol 1993;24:103–8.

69 Alshak NS, Jimenez AM, Gedebou M, et al. Epstein–Barr virus infection in liver transplantation patients: correlation of histopathology and semiquantitative Epstein–Barr virus-DNA recovery using polymerase chain reaction. Hum Pathol 1993;24:1306–12.

70 Markin RS. Manifestations of Epstein–Barr virus-associated disorders in liver. Liver 1994;14:1–13.

71 Hubscher SG, Williams A, Davison SM, et al. Epstein–Barr virus in inflammatory diseases of the liver and liver allografts: an in situ hybridization study. Hepatology 1994;20:899–907.

72 Pessoa MG, Terrault NA, Ferrell LD, et al. Hepatitis after liver transplantation: the role of the known and unknown viruses. Liver Transpl Surg 1998;4:461–8.

73 Blair JE, Kusne S. Bacterial, mycobacterial, and protozoal infections after liver transplantation – Part I. Liver Transpl 2005;11:1452–9.

74 Wojcicki M, Milkiewicz P, Silva M. Biliary tract complications after liver transplantation: a review. Dig Surg 2008;25:245–57.

75 Paik WH, Lee SH, Ryu JK, et al. Long-term clinical outcomes of biliary cast syndrome in liver transplant recipients. Liver Transpl 2013;19:275–82.

76 Hertzler GL, Millikan WJ. The surgical pathologist's role in liver transplantation. Arch Pathol Lab Med 1991;115:273–82.

77 Oh C-K, Pelletier SJ, Sawyer RG, et al. Uni- and multi-variate analysis of risk factors for early and late hepatic artery thrombosis after liver transplantation. Transplantation 2001;71:767–72.

78 Harper PL, Edgar PR, Luddington RJ, et al. Protein C deficiency and portal thrombosis in liver transplantation in children. Lancet 1988;2:924–7.

79 Ludwig J, Batts KP, MacCarty RL. Ischemic cholangitis in hepatic allografts. Mayo Clin Proc 1992;67:519–26.

80 Sterneck M, Wiesner R, Ascher N, et al. Azathioprine hepatotoxicity after liver transplantation. Hepatology 1991;14:806–10.

81 Dhillon AP, Burroughs AK, Hudson M, et al. Hepatic venular stenosis after orthotopic liver transplantation. Hepatology 1994;19:106–11.

82 Gulbis B, Adler M, Ooms HA, et al. Liver-function studies in heart-transplant recipients treated with cyclosporin A. Clin Chem 1988;34:1772–4.

83 Kadmon M, Klünemann C, Böhme M, et al. Inhibition by cyclosporin A of adenosine triphosphate-dependent transport from the hepatocyte into bile. Gastroenterology 1993;104:1507–14.

84 Arias IM. Cyclosporin, the biology of the bile canaliculus, and cholestasis. Gastroenterology 1993;104:1558–60.

85 Thomson AW. FK-506 enters the clinic. Immunol Today 1990;11:35–6.

86 Fung JJ, Todo S, Tzakis A, et al. Current status of FK 506 in liver transplantation. Transplant Proc 1991;23:1902–5.

87 Banff Working Group on Liver Allograft Pathology. Importance of liver biopsy findings in immunosuppression management: biopsy monitoring and working criteria for patients with operational tolerance. Liver Transpl 2012;18:1154–70.

88 Benítez C, Londoño M-C, Miquel R, et al. Prospective multicentre clinical trial of immunosuppressive drug withdrawal in stable adult liver transplant recipients. Hepatology 2013;58:1824–35.

89 Levitsky J. Immunosuppression withdrawal following liver transplantation: the older, the wiser...but maybe too late. Hepatology 2013;58:1529–32.

90 Feng S, Ekong UD, Lobritto SJ, et al. Complete immunosuppression withdrawal and subsequent allograft function among pediatric recipients of parental living donor liver transplants. JAMA 2012;307:283–93.

91 Davern TJ, Lake JR. Recurrent disease after liver transplantation. Semin Gastrointest Dis 1998;9:86–109.

92 Kim WR, Poterucha JJ, Porayko MK, et al. Recurrence of nonalcoholic steatohepatitis following liver transplantation. Transplantation 1996;62:1802–5.

93 Molloy RM, Komorowski R, Varma RR. Recurrent nonalcoholic steatohepatitis and cirrhosis after liver transplantation. Liver Transpl Surg 1997;3:177–8.

94 Carson K, Washington MK, Treem WR, et al. Recurrence of nonalcoholic steatohepatitis in a liver transplant recipient. Liver Transpl Surg 1997;3:174–6.

95 Fiel MI, Schiano TD, Klion FM, et al. Recurring fibro-obliterative venopathy in liver allografts. Am J Surg Pathol 1999;23:734–7.

96 Duclos-Vallee J-C, Sebagh M. Recurrence of autoimmune disease, primary sclerosing cholangitis, primary biliary cirrhosis, and autoimmune hepatitis after liver transplantation. Liver Transpl 2009;15:S25–34.

97 Hübscher SG. What is the long-term outcome of the liver allograft? J Hepatol 2011;55:702–17.

98 Liberal R, Longhi MS, Grant CR, et al. Autoimmune hepatitis after liver transplantation. Clin Gastroenterol Hepatol 2012;10:346–53.

98b Pongpaibul A, Venick RS, McDiarmid SV, et al. Histopathology of de novo autoimmune hepatitis. Liver Transplant 2012;18:811–18.

99   Walker N, Apel R, Kerlin P, et al. Hepatitis B virus infection in liver allografts. Am J Surg Pathol 1993;17:666–77.

100 Lucey MR, Graham DM, Martin P, et al. Recurrence of hepatitis B and delta hepatitis after orthotopic liver transplantation. Gut 1992;33:1390–6.

101 ten Kate FJW, Schalm SW, Willemse PJA, et al. Course of hepatitis B and D virus infection in auxiliary liver grafts in hepatitis B-positive patients. A light-microscopic and immunohistochemical study. J Hepatol 1992;14:168–75.

102 Ottobrelli A, Marzano A, Smedile A, et al. Patterns of hepatitis delta virus reinfection and disease in liver transplantation. Gastroenterology 1991;101:1649–55.

103 David E, Rahier J, Pucci A, et al. Recurrence of hepatitis D (delta) in liver transplants: histopathological aspects. Gastroenterology 1993;104:1122–8.

104 Davies SE, Portmann BC, O'Grady JG, et al. Hepatic histological findings after transplantation for chronic hepatitis B virus infection, including a unique pattern of fibrosing cholestatic hepatitis. Hepatology 1991;13:150–7.

105 O'Grady JG, Smith HM, Davies SE, et al. Hepatitis B virus reinfection after orthotopic liver transplantation. Serological and clinical implications. J Hepatol 1992;14:104–11.

106 Benner KG, Lee RG, Keeffe EB, et al. Fibrosing cytolytic liver failure secondary to recurrent hepatitis B after liver transplantation. Gastroenterology 1992;103:1307–12.

107 Lau JYN, Bain VG, Davies SE, et al. High-level expression of hepatitis B viral antigens in fibrosing cholestatic hepatitis. Gastroenterology 1992;102:956–62.

108 Phillips MJ, Cameron R, Flowers MA, et al. Post-transplant recurrent hepatitis B viral liver disease. Viral-burden, steatoviral, and fibroviral hepatitis B. Am J Pathol 1992;140:1295–308.

109 Demetris AJ, Eghtesad B, Marcos A, et al. Recurrent hepatitis C in liver allografts. Prospective assessment of diagnostic accuracy, identification of pitfalls, and observations about pathogenesis. Am J Surg Pathol 2004;28:658–69.

110 Saxena R, Crawford JM, Navarro VJ, et al. Utilization of acidophil bodies in the diagnosis of recurrent hepatitis C infection after orthotopic liver transplantation. Mod Pathol 2002;15:897–903.

111 Gordon FD, Pomfret EA, Pomposelli JJ, et al. Severe steatosis as the initial histologic manifestation of recurrent hepatitis C genotype 3. Hum Pathol 2004;35:636–8.

112 Guerrero RB, Batts KP, Burgart LJ, et al. Early detection of hepatitis C allograft reinfection after orthotopic liver transplantation: a molecular and histologic study. Mod Pathol 2000;13:229–37.

113 Ferrell LD, Wright TL, Roberts J, et al. Hepatitis C viral infection in liver transplant recipients. Hepatology 1992;16:865–76.

114 Böker KHW, Dalley G, Bahr MJ, et al. Long-term outcome of hepatitis C virus infection after liver transplantation. Hepatology 1997;25:203–10.

114a Prakoso E, Tirnitz-Parker JEE, Clouston AD, et al. Analysis of the intrahepatic ductular reaction and progenitor cell responses in hepatitis C virus recurrence after liver transplantation. Liver Transplant 2014;20:1508–19.

114b Moreira RK, Salomao M, Verna EC, et al. The hepatitis aggressiveness score (HAS): a novel classification system for post-liver transplantation recurrent hepatitis C. Am J Surg Pathol 2013;37:104–13.

115 Dickson RC, Caldwell SH, Ishitani MB, et al. Clinical and histologic patterns of early graft failure due to recurrent hepatitis C in four patients after liver transplantation. Transplantation 1996;61:701–5.

116 Taga SA, Washington MK, Terrault N, et al. Cholestatic hepatitis C in liver allografts. Liver Transpl Surg 1998;4:304–10.

117 Schluger LK, Sheiner PA, Thung SN, et al. Severe recurrent cholestatic hepatitis C following orthotopic liver transplantation. Hepatology 1996;23:971–6.

118 Khettry U, Huang W-Y, Simpson MA, et al. Patterns of recurrent hepatitis C after liver transplantation in a recent cohort of patients. Hum Pathol 2007;38:443–52.

119 Berardi S, Lodato F, Gramenzi A, et al. High incidence of allograft dysfunction in liver transplanted patients treated with pegylated-interferon alpha-2b and ribavirin for hepatitis C recurrence: possible de novo autoimmune hepatitis? Gut 2007;56:237–42.

120 Levitsky J, Fiel MI, Norvell JP, et al. Risk for immune-mediated graft dysfunction in liver transplant recipients with recurrent HCV infection treated with pegylated interferon. Gastroenterology 2012;142:1132–9.

121 Demetris AJ, Sebagh M. Plasma cell hepatitis in liver allografts: variant of rejection or autoimmune hepatitis? Liver Transpl 2008;14:750–5.

122 Ward SC, Schiano TD, Thung SN, et al. Plasma cell hepatitis in hepatitis C virus patients post-liver transplantation: case control study showing poor outcome and predictive features in the liver explant. Liver Transpl 2009;15:1826–33.

123 Souza P, Prihoda TJ, Hoyumpa AM, et al. Morphologic features resembling transplant rejection in core biopsies of native livers from patients with hepatitis C. Hum Pathol 2009;40:92–7.

124 Sylvestre PB, Batts KP, Burgart LJ, et al. Recurrence of primary biliary cirrhosis after liver transplantation: histologic estimate of incidence and natural history. Liver Transpl 2003;9:1086–93.

125 Hubscher SG, Elias E, Buckels JAC, et al. Primary biliary cirrhosis. Histological evidence of disease recurrence after liver transplantation. J Hepatol 1993;18:173–84.

126 Khettry U, Anand N, Faul PN, et al. Liver transplantation for primary biliary cirrhosis: a long-term pathologic study. Liver Transpl 2003;9:87–96.

127 Montano-Loza AJ, Mason AL, Ma M, et al. Risk factors for recurrence of autoimmune hepatitis after liver transplantation. Liver Transpl 2009;15:1254–61.

128 Graziadei IW, Wiesner RH, Batts KP, et al. Recurrence of primary sclerosing cholangitis following liver transplantation. Hepatology 1999;29:1050–6.

129 Keaveny AP, Gordon FD, Goldar-Najari A, et al. Native liver xanthogranulomatous cholangiopathy in primary sclerosing cholangitis: impact ono posttransplant outcome. Liver Transpl 2004;10:115–22.

130 Birnbaum AH, Benkov KJ, Pittman NS, et al. Recurrence of autoimmune hepatitis in children after liver transplantation. J Pediatr Gastroenterol Nutr 1997;25:20–5.

131 Malik SM, deVera ME, Fontes P, et al. Recurrent disease following liver transplantation for nonalcoholic steatohepatitis cirrhosis. Liver Transpl 2009;15:1843–51.

132 Bianchi G, Marchesini G, Marzocchi R, et al. Metabolic syndrome in liver transplantation: relation to etiology and immunosuppression. Liver Transpl 2008;14:1648–54.

133 Patil DT, Yerian LM. Evolution of non-alcoholic fatty liver disease recurrence after liver transplantation. Liver Transpl 2012;18:1147–53.

134 Watt KD. Metabolic syndrome: is immunosuppression to blame? Liver Transpl 2011;17:S38–42.

135 Lunati ME, Grancini V, Agnelli F, et al. Metaoblic syndrome after liver transplantation: short-term prevalence and pre- and post-operative risk factors. Dig Liver Dis 2013;45:833–9.

136 Perito ER, Lau A, Rhee S, et al. Posttransplant metabolic syndrome in children and adolescents after liver transplantation: a systematic review. Liver Transpl 2012;18:1009–28.

137 Miyagawa-Hayashino A, Egaqa H, Yorifuji T, et al. Allograft steatohepatitis in progressive familial intrahepatic cholestasis type 1 after living donor liver transplantation. Liver Transpl 2009;15:610–18.

138 Sebagh M, Casstillo-Rama M, Axoulay D, et al. Histologic findings predictive of a diagnosis of de novo autoimmune hepatitis after liver transplantation in adults. Transplantation 2013;96:1–9.

139 Heneghan MA, Portmann BC, Norris SM, et al. Graft dysfunction mimicking autoimmune hepatitis following liver transplantation in adults. Hepatology 2001;34:464–70.

140 Leblond V, Choquet S. Lymphoproliferative disorders after liver transplantation. J Hepatol 2004;40:728–35.

141 Palazzo JP, Lundquist K, Mitchell D, et al. Rapid development of lymphoma following liver transplantation in a recipient with hepatitis B and primary hemochromatosis. Am J Gastroenterol 1991;88:102–4.

142 Spiro IJ, Yandell DW, Li C, et al. Brief report: lymphoma of donor origin occurring in the porta hepatis of a transplanted liver. N Engl J Med 1993;329:27–9.

143 Lones MA, Shintaku IP, Weiss LM, et al. Posttransplant lymphoproliferative disorder in liver allograft biopsies: a comparison of three methods for the demonstration of Epstein–Barr virus. Hum Pathol 1997;28:533–9.

144 Luketic VA, Shiffman ML, McCall JB, et al. Primary hepatocellular carcinoma after orthotopic liver transplantation for chronic hepatitis B infection. Ann Intern Med 1991;114:212–13.

145 Saxena R, Ye MQ, Emre S, et al. De novo hepatocellular carcinoma in a hepatic allograft with recurrent hepatitis C cirrhosis. Liver Transpl Surg 1999;5:81–2.

146 McPeake JR, O'Grady JG, Zaman S, et al. Liver transplantation for primary hepatocellular carcinoma: tumor size and number determine outcome. J Hepatol 1993;18:226–34.

147 Morita K, Taketoni A, Soejima Y, et al. De novo hepatocellular carcinoma in a liver graft with sustained hepatitis C virus clearance after living donor liver transplantation. Liver Transpl 2009;15:1412–16.

148 Banff Working Group. Liver biopsy interpretation for causes of late liver allograft dysfunction. Hepatology 2006;44:489–501.

149 Krasinskas AM, Demetris AJ, Poterucha JJ, et al. The prevalence and natural history of untreated isolated central perivenulitis in adult allograft livers. Liver Transpl 2008;14:625–32.

150 Abraham SC, Freese DK, Ishitani MB, et al. Significance of central perivenulitis in pediatric liver transplantation. Am J Surg Pathol 2008;32:1479–88.

151 Shaikh OS, Demetris AJ. Idiopathic posttransplantation hepatitis? Liver Transpl 2007;13:943–6.

152 Unzueta A, Rakela J. Hepatitis E infection in liver transplant recipients. Liver Transpl 2014;20:15–24.

153 Grewal P, Kamili S, Motamed D. Chronic hepatitis E in an immunocompetent patient: a case report. Hepatology 2014;59:347–8.

153a Behrendt P, Steinmann E, Manns MP, et al. The impact of hepatitis E in the liver transplant setting. J Hepatol 2014;61:1418–29.

153b Protzer U, Bohm F, Longerich T, et al. Molecular detection of hepatitis E virus (HEV) in liver biopsies after liver transplantation. Mod Pathol 2015; [Epub ahead of print].

154 Nonomura A, Mizukami Y, Matsubara F, et al. Clinicopathological study of lymphocyte attachment to endothelial cells (endothelialitis) in various liver diseases. Liver 1991;11:78–88.

155 Lykavieris P, van Mil S, Cresteil D, et al. Progressive familial intrahepatic cholestasis type 1 and extrahepatic features: no catch-up of stature growth, exacerbation of diarrhea, and appearance of liver steatosis after liver transplantation. J Hepatol 2003;39:447–52.

156 Lefkowitch JH, Lobritto SJ, Brown RS Jr, et al. Ground-glass, polyglucosan-like hepatocellular inclusions: a 'new' diagnostic entity. Gastroenterology 2006;131:713–18.

157 Bejarano PA, Garcia MT, Rodriguez MM, et al. Liver glycogen bodies: ground-glass hepatocytes in transplanted patients. Virchows Arch 2006;449:539–45.

158 Wisell J, Boitnott J, Haas M, et al. Glycogen pseudoground glass change in hepatocytes. Am J Surg Pathol 2006;30:1085–90.

159 Vázquez JJ. Ground glass hepatocytes: light and electron microscopy. Characterization of the different types. Histol Histopathol 1990;5:379–86.

160 Degos F, Degott C. Hepatitis in renal transplant recipients. J Hepatol 1989;9:114–23.

161 Chan T-M, Lok ASF, Cheng IKP, et al. A prospective study of hepatitis C virus infection among renal transplant recipients. Gastroenterology 1993;104:862–8.

162 Rao KV, Anderson WR, Kasiske BL, et al. Value of liver biopsy in the evaluation and management of chronic liver disease in renal transplant recipients. Am J Med 1993;94:241–50.

163 Delladetsima JK, Boletis JN, Makris F, et al. Fibrosing cholestatic hepatitis in renal transplant recipients with hepatitis C virus infection. Liver Transpl Surg 1999;5:294–300.

164 Sopko J, Anuras S. Liver disease in renal transplant recipients. Am J Med 1978;64:139–46.

165 Ware AJ, Luby JP, Hollinger B, et al. Etiology of liver disease in renal-transplant patients. Ann Intern Med 1979;91:364–71.

166 Weir MR, Kirkman RL, Strom TB, et al. Liver disease in recipients of long-functioning renal allografts. Kidney Int 1985;28:839–44.

167 Rao KV, Anderson WR. Hemosiderosis: an unrecognized complication in renal allograft recipients. Transplantation 1982;33:115–17.

168 Rao KV, Anderson WR. Hemosiderosis and hemochromatosis in renal transplant recipients. Clinical and pathological features, diagnostic correlations, predisposing factors, and treatment. Am J Nephrol 1985;5:419–30.

169 Marubbio AT, Danielson B. Hepatic veno-occlusive disease in a renal transplant patient receiving azathioprine. Gastroenterology 1975;69:739–43.

170 Degott C, Rueff B, Kreis H, et al. Peliosis hepatis in recipients of renal transplants. Gut 1978;19:748–53.

171 Nataf C, Feldmann G, Lebrec D, et al. Idiopathic portal hypertension (perisinusoidal fibrosis) after renal transplantation. Gut 1979;20:531–7.

172 Gerlag PG, Lobatto S, Driessen WM, et al. Hepatic sinusoidal dilatation with portal hypertension during azathioprine treatment after kidney transplantation. J Hepatol 1985;1:339–48.

173 Krempien B, Bommer J, Ritz E. Foreign body giant cell reaction in lungs, liver and spleen. A complication of long term haemodialysis. Virchows Arch A Pathol Anat Histol 1981;392:73–80.

174 Leong AS, Disney AP, Gove DW. Refractile particles in liver of haemodialysis patients [letter]. Lancet 1981;1:889–90.

175 Parfrey PS, O'Driscoll JB, Paradinas FJ. Refractile material in the liver of haemodialysis patients [letter]. Lancet 1981;1:1101–2.

176 Shulman HM, Sharma P, Amos D, et al. A coded histologic study of hepatic graft-versus-host disease after human bone marrow transplantation. Hepatology 1988;8:463–70.

177 McDonald GB, Shulman HM, Sullivan KM, et al. Intestinal and hepatic complications of human bone marrow transplantation. Part I. Gastroenterology 1986;90:460–77.

178 McDonald GB, Shulman HM, Sullivan KM, et al. Intestinal and hepatic complications of human bone marrow transplantation. Part II. Gastroenterology 1986;90:770–84.

179 Snover DC, Weisdorf SA, Ramsay NK, et al. Hepatic graft versus host disease: a study of the predictive value of liver biopsy in diagnosis. Hepatology 1984;4:123–30.

180 Shulman HM, Kleiner D, Lee SJ, et al. Histopathologic diagnosis of chronic graft-versus-host disease: National Institutes of Health consensus development project on criteria for clinical trials in chronic graft-versus-host disease. II. Pathology Working Group report. Biol Blood Marrow Transplant 2006;12:31–47.

181 Geubel AP, Cnudde A, Ferrant A, et al. Diffuse biliary tract involvement mimicking primary sclerosing cholangitis after bone marrow transplantation. J Hepatol 1990;10:23–8.

182 Strasser SI, Shulman HM, Flowers ME, et al. Chronic graft-versus-host disease of the liver: presentation as an acute hepatitis. Hepatology 2000;32:1265–71.

183 Malik AH, Collins RH Jr, Saboorian MH, et al. Chronic graft-*versus*-host disease after hematopoietic cell transplantation presenting as an acute hepatitis. Am J Gastroenterol 2001;96:588–90.

184 Knapp AB, Crawford JM, Rappeport JM, et al. Cirrhosis as a consequence of graft–versus-host disease. Gastroenterology 1987;92:513–19.

185 DeLeve LD, Shulman HM, McDonald GB. Toxic injury to hepatic sinusoids: sinusoidal obstruction syndrome (veno-occlusive disease). Semin Liver Dis 2002;22:27–42.

186 Shulman HM, Fisher LB, Schoch HG, et al. Venoocclusive disease of the liver after marrow transplantation: histological correlates of clinical signs and symptoms. Hepatology 1994;19:1171–80.

187 Zubair I, Herrera GA, Pretlow TG, et al. Cytoplasmic inclusions in hepatocytes of bone marrow transplant patients: light and electron microscopic characterization. Am J Clin Pathol 1985;83:65–8.

General reading

Adeyi O, Fischer SE, Guindi M. Liver allograft pathology: approach to interpretation of needle biopsies with clinicopathological correlation. J Clin Pathol 2010;63:47–74.

Banff Working Group. Liver biopsy interpretation for causes of late liver allograft dysfunction. Hepatology 2006;44:489–501.

Carbone M, Neuberger JM. Autoimmune liver disease, autoimmunity and liver transplantation. J Hepatol 2014;60:210–23.

Demetris AJ, Crawford JM, Minervini MI, et al. Transplantation pathology of the liver. In: Odze RD, Goldblum JR, editors. Surgical Pathology of the GI Tract, Liver, Biliary Tract, and Pancreas. 2nd ed. Philadelphia, PA: Saunders/Elsevier, 2009. p. 1169–230.

Hübscher S. What is the long-term outcome of the liver allograft? J Hepatol 2011;55:702–11.

Hübscher SG, Clouston AD. Transplantation pathology. In: Burt AD, Portmann BC, Ferrell LD, editors. MacSween's Pathology of the Liver. 6th ed. Edinburgh: Churchill Livingstone/Elsevier, 2012. p. 853–934.

International Panel. Banff schema for grading liver allograft rejection: an international consensus document. Hepatology 1997;25:658–63.

International Panel. Update of the international Banff schema for liver allograft rejection: working recommendations for the histopathologic staging and reporting of chronic rejection. Hepatology 2000;31:792–9.

Electron Microscopy and Other Techniques

Introduction

This chapter will focus primarily on the role of transmission electron microscopy (TEM) in the assessment of liver ultrastructure and disease. It also describes, in brief, the principles and uses of other methodologies. The special conditions required for tissue processing in each of these techniques (**Table 17.1**) should be carefully planned for in advance of obtaining specimens. Use of newer 'molecular fixatives' (in lieu of traditional formalin) for liver specimens is a recent option for improving RNA and DNA preservation while also allowing tissue embedding in paraffin (thereby obviating the need for snap freezing, use of OCT compound and other special procedures).[1] Molecular fixatives also produce quality routine and immunohistochemical staining results that are comparable to formalin-fixed specimens.[1] While some of these methods are not universally available in pathology departments, other departments at one's institution or at other centres of investigation may be consulted in cases of particular diagnostic or research interest. Procedures for fixation and processing for TEM are available in several of the General reading references at the end of the chapter.

Electron microscopy of liver biopsies

TEM continues to provide important information about the normal cellular and extracellular constituents of the liver and their alterations in disease. Recent interest in the relationships between the various sinusoidal cells of the liver has benefited from TEM studies,[2,3] as has investigations of hepatic progenitor cells.[4] Data from standard TEM studies can be enhanced by the application of immunohistochemical stains (see Immunoelectron microscopy, below), digitised three-dimensional computer reconstructions[5-7] and morphometry. TEM is sometimes limited by the lack of specificity of certain ultrastructural changes and the problem of sampling error in lesions that may not be uniformly distributed. The first of these limitations is well illustrated in cholestasis; various features of cholestasis such as loss of canalicular microvilli are easily recognised under the electron microscope, but many causes produce these changes. Sampling error can sometimes be reduced by the combination of light and electron microscopy in a single instrument.[8]

In diagnostic work TEM should be seriously considered under five circumstances:

1   *To establish the nature of an inborn error of metabolism.* In a number of storage diseases the ultrastructural changes are diagnostic or give an indication of the type of disease to be considered.[9,10] Specific features are seen, for example, in type II glycogenosis, in Gaucher's disease and in Niemann–Pick disease

Table 17.1 Liver tissue processing for various techniques

Technique	Tissue preparation
Transmission electron microscopy	Glutaraldehyde fixation
Scanning electron microscopy	Perfusion fixation; critical point drying; coating with gold or platinum
Immunoelectron microscopy	Glutaraldehyde/paraformaldehyde fixation
Immunoperoxidase of tissue sections	Fixation in 10% neutral formalin or alternative fixative
Immunoperoxidase and immunofluorescence of frozen sections	Snap freeze after embedding in OCT compound*
In situ hybridisation	Snap freeze after embedding in OCT compound*
Flow cytometry	Fresh tissue
Confocal laser scanning microscopy	Snap freeze after embedding in OCT compound*
Laser capture microdissection	Conventional tissue sections for light microscopy
Gene array analysis	Snap freeze in liquid nitrogen*; store at −80°C

OCT, optimal cutting temperature.
*Use of molecular fixatives allows paraffin embedding of tissue in lieu of snap freezing. See reference 1.

(**Fig. 17.1**). Storage diseases can and should often be diagnosed by other, usually biochemical, methods, but even then electron microscopy can reduce the period of investigation by drawing attention to a likely diagnosis. Electron microscopy may show whether a liver-cell pigment is lipofuscin or the pigment of the Dubin–Johnson syndrome (**Fig. 17.2**), and can therefore be helpful when this syndrome is suspected but not fully proved by light microscopy.[11] In some patients with Wilson's disease characteristic changes may be seen in liver-cell mitochondria (see below).

2 *To establish the presence of viral infection.* Electron microscopy of liver biopsies may prove to be important when serological test results or cultures for suspected viral infection are unavailable or incomplete. Both intranuclear and intracytoplasmic virions may be identified by the appearances of their spherical or hexagonal capsids, dense core material, surface envelopes and paracrystalline and lattice-like arrays. These features can be compared with published micrographs for identification of the candidate virion.[12,13] For example, some adult patients with the unusual finding of giant-cell hepatitis on routine light microscopy have been shown to have paramyxovirus-like particles in the liver as a result of electron microscopic studies of biopsy material.[14,15] Electron microscopy can also be applied to cell cultures, as shown in a study demonstrating 50–90 nm hepatitis C virions.[16] Glutaraldehyde fixation of biopsy specimens is preferred, but viral particles can also be identified in formalin-fixed tissues which are washed and then processed for electron microscopy.

3 *To establish the nature of a tumour of doubtful histogenesis.* The ultrastructural features of many tumours, including neuroendocrine tumours and malignant

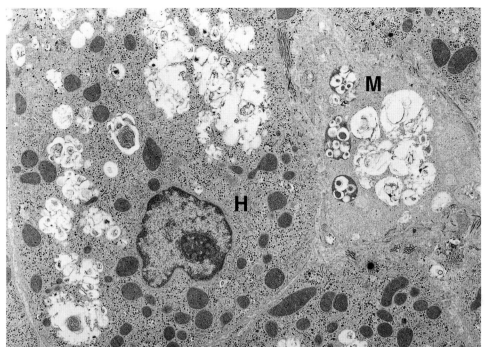

Figure 17.1 Liver tissue from a patient with Niemann–Pick disease. Macrophages (M) and hepatocytes (H) contain abundant vacuoles in which there are lamellar lipid inclusions. (Needle biopsy, lead citrate; ×4600.)

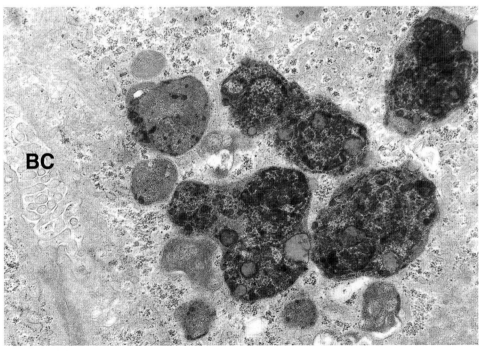

Figure 17.2 Dubin–Johnson syndrome. Large, characteristically complex dense bodies are seen near a bile canaliculus (BC). (Needle biopsy, lead citrate; ×18 900.)

Figure 17.3 Amiodarone-induced phospholipidosis. An enlarged lysosome (*), resembling a myelin figure, contains densely packed, concentrically arranged osmiophilic lipids, thought to represent drug–lipid complexes. A smaller membranous whorl (arrowhead) is seen in the cytoplasm. L, lipid. (Ferrocyanide, ×38,000.) (Illustration kindly provided by Dr S Poucell and Professor MJ Phillips, Toronto, Canada.)

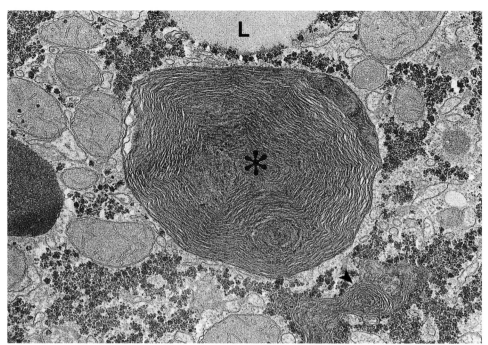

melanomas, help in making a firm diagnosis.[17] The more obvious features such as neurosecretory granules in neuroendocrine tumours survive paraffin embedding; re-embedding of paraffin material for electron microscopy should therefore be considered.

4   *To establish the presence of specific drug-related changes.* In liver damage due to a small number of drugs, including perhexiline maleate[18] and amiodarone,[19–22] hepatocytes contain lysosomes filled with lamellar phospholipid material (**Fig. 17.3**).

5   *To provide material for research.* Electron microscopy offers wide potential for research into human liver disease, and it may be that future research will increase the diagnostic value of electron microscopy in this field. If liver biopsy is performed in a patient having a disease with potentially helpful or interesting ultrastructural features, small pieces of the specimen can be embedded for electron microscopy and stored indefinitely in block form. The extent to which this is done clearly depends on the resources of the particular laboratory.

Whenever electron microscopy of a liver biopsy specimen is considered, the laboratory should be contacted beforehand and arrangements made for collection and fixation of the specimen at the bedside. Proper processing of the tissue, including optimal fixation, provides the basis for accurate analysis of ultrastructural changes.

The normal liver and examples of ultrastructural changes in disease

The following description of the liver under the TEM is a general one. It should be noted that the quality of fixation will influence the appearance of cells and organelles. The labels in the description of normal liver refer to **Figures 17.4** and **17.5**.

Several cell types are found in the hepatic lobules. The hepatocytes or parenchymal cells are separated from the sinusoidal endothelial cells by the space of Disse, in which there

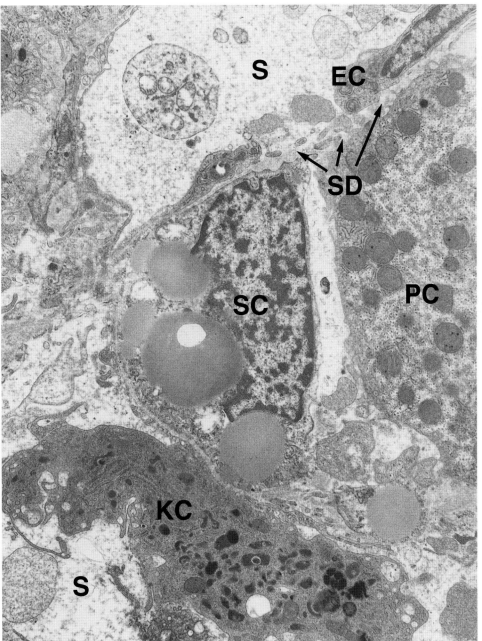

Figure 17.4
Normal human liver.
At the edge of a liver-cell plate the parenchymal cell (PC) is separated from the sinusoidal lumen (S) by an endothelial cell (EC) and Kupffer cell (KC). SC, stellate cell; SD, space of Disse. (Needle biopsy, lead citrate, ×10 000.)

are collagen fibres and stellate cells, formerly known as perisinusoidal cells, Ito cells or fat-storing cells. Within the sinusoidal lumen are Kupffer cells, the hepatic macrophages and large granular lymphocytes (also called pit cells) with natural killer activity.

Hepatocyte (liver cell, parenchymal cell)

Hepatocytes have similar features in different lobular regions but vary in detailed structure. For example, there are more lysosomes and mitochondria in periportal than in perivenular hepatocytes, while the converse is true for the smooth-surfaced endoplasmic reticulum.

Figure 17.5 Normal human liver.
Two parenchymal cells have formed a bile canaliculus (BC) delimited by junctional complexes (JC). Lysosomes (Ly) have varying density: the darker ones correspond to lipofuscin, as seen under the light microscope. N, nucleus; M, mitochondria; Gly, glycogen; RER, rough-surfaced endoplasmic reticulum; G, Golgi apparatus. (Needle biopsy, lead citrate, ×24 000.)

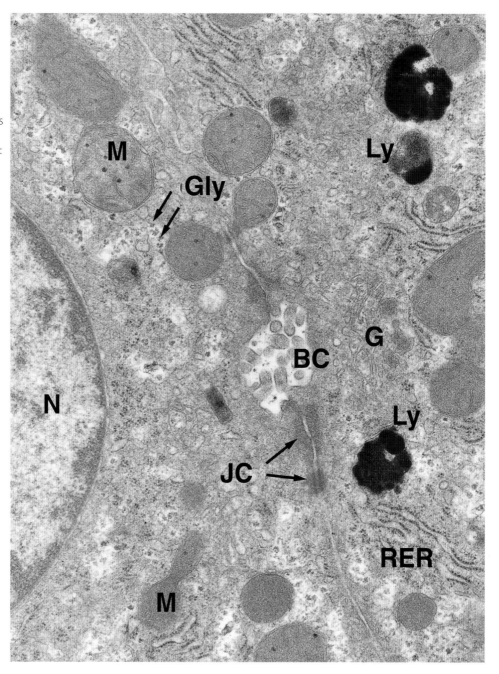

The hepatocyte is a highly polarised cell with surfaces facing the space of Disse, other hepatocytes and the bile canaliculus. The plasma membrane is specialised in these three areas. Many microvilli project into the space of Disse and into the bile canaliculus. This is a potential space formed by two or three hepatocytes in normal liver, and sometimes more in disease. The intercellular membrane of the hepatocyte is relatively smooth and forms several types of intercellular junctions.

The nucleus

The nucleus is normally limited by a double membrane, the nuclear envelope, which is continuous with the rough-surfaced endoplasmic reticulum. The nuclear envelope has small pores which are thought to serve as a route of communication between the nucleoplasm and the cytoplasm. Within the nucleus there is irregularly distributed chromatin, and a nucleolus is often visible.

Structural changes

Large amounts of monoparticulate glycogen are seen in some adult hepatocyte nuclei in diabetes mellitus and in insulin resistance, in children and also in type I glycogen storage disease. In type B hepatitis, core virus particles are seen (**Fig. 17.6**). Intranuclear virions are also seen in infections due to cytomegalovirus, herpesvirus, echovirus and adenovirus.

Mitochondria

Mitochondria are the sites of oxidative enzyme activity, and are involved in the metabolism of amino acids, lipids and carbohydrates. There are an average of 2200 mitochondria within the hepatocyte.[23] A smooth outer limiting membrane and an inner membrane with deep infoldings, the cristae, give the mitochondria a characteristic appearance. The inner membrane surrounds the mitochondrial matrix which contains many dense granules.

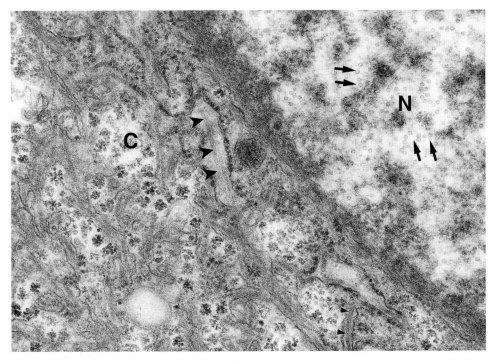

Figure 17.6 Hepatocyte in hepatitis B surface material (HBsAg)-positive chronic hepatitis.
In the nucleus (N) there are numerous core particles (arrows). The cytoplasm (C) contains irregularly shaped cisternae of the endoplasmic reticulum in which there are tubules (arrowheads), the morphological *in situ* counterpart of surface antigen. Glycogen rosettes are also visible in the cytoplasm at left. (Needle biopsy, lead citrate, ×45 000.)

Figure 17.7
Wilson's disease.
Hepatocyte
cytoplasm with
mitochondria
showing dilatation of
intracristal spaces
(arrowheads). Some
are microcystic and
their contents are
finely granular (*).
Dense granules are
prominent.
(Ferrocyanide,
×11 400.) (Illustration
kindly supplied by
Professor MJ Phillips
and Ms JS Patterson,
Toronto, Canada.)

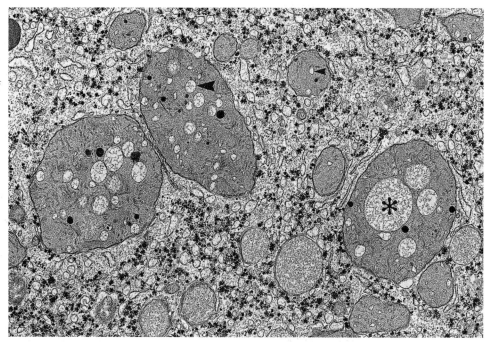

Structural changes

Cristae of atypical shape, crystalline inclusions and enlarged or unusually scanty granules are found in a wide variety of conditions, and sometimes also in normal liver. Giant mitochondria are seen most often in alcoholic liver disease[24] but are also found in non-alcoholic fatty liver disease[25] and other conditions.[26] Immunohistochemistry and immunoelectron microscopy can assist in their detection.[27] They are frequently found in patients with systemic sclerosis.[28] In the early stages of Wilson's disease mitochondria show variation in shape, increased electron density, widening of the spaces between membranes, vacuolation, enlargement of matrix granules and deposition of crystalline material[29,30] (**Fig. 17.7**). Three types of Wilsonian mitochondria are described which show intrafamilial concordance.[31] Abnormal, swollen and irregular mitochondria are found in hepatocytes in Reye's syndrome[32] and other microvesicular fat syndromes.[33] Highly irregular mitochondria are also seen in mitochondriopathies where there is respiratory chain dysfunction due to defects in mitochondrial DNA (mitochondrial depletion and deletion syndromes) (**Fig. 17.8**). Affected neonates and infants may have liver failure and cholestasis in combination with neurological or neuromuscular disease[34-37] (neurohepatopathy) (**see Ch. 13, Fig. 13.17**).

Endoplasmic reticulum

This is an important site of protein synthesis and transport. It also contains enzymes involved in drug and steroid metabolism. Morphologically, the endoplasmic reticulum is a cisternal membrane-bound system continuous with the nuclear envelope. It is the morphological counterpart of the microsomes. Two main types of endoplasmic reticulum can be recognised. The **rough-surfaced endoplasmic reticulum** is studded with ribosomes and is often arranged in a lamellar pattern. The **smooth-surfaced endoplasmic reticulum** lacks ribosomes and has a tubular or vesicular appearance.

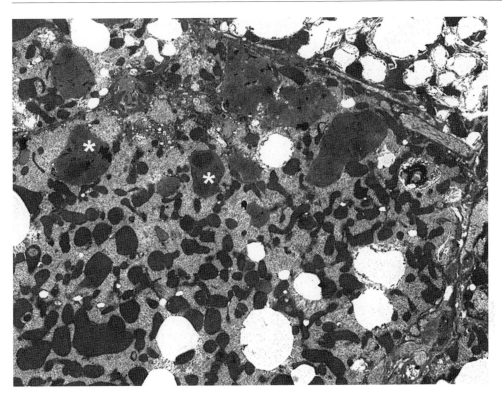

Figure 17.8 Mitochondriopathy.
Markedly pleomorphic mitochondria are present and show abnormal branching and tapering, marked enlargement and unusually large, dark osmiophilic matrix densities (mitochondria shown at *). Microvesicular fat vacuoles are also present. Genetic analysis of this infant with neurological deficits, liver failure and cholestasis demonstrated a mitochondrial DNA depletion syndrome. (Needle biopsy, osmium tetroxide.)

Structural changes

Dilatation, degranulation, vesiculation and proliferation of the endoplasmic reticulum can be seen in many conditions. Some of these 'changes' are also influenced by the fixation procedure, making them difficult to evaluate. Their accurate quantification requires carefully controlled processing conditions and morphometric analysis. However, in α_1-antitrypsin deficiency the dilatation of endoplasmic reticulum is striking, and finely granular material accumulates in the cisternae (**Fig. 17.9**). In chronic type B hepatitis the cisternae are also dilated and contain tubular structures representing the surface material of the hepatitis B virus (**Fig. 17.6**), and sometimes complete Dane particles.

Lysosomes

Lysosomes are organelles that carry many different lytic enzymes and are involved in the breakdown of proteins, carbohydrates and lipids. **Primary lysosomes** are small vesicles containing enzymes, but not yet involved in catabolic processes. **Secondary lysosomes** are membrane-bound, often irregularly shaped electron-dense bodies in which the breakdown processes take place. When undigested residues accumulate and enzyme activity is diminished, the secondary lysosomes are called residual bodies. These are the lipofuscin granules. All types of secondary lysosomes tend to be concentrated around the bile canaliculi.

Figure 17.9
α₁-Antitrypsin deficiency.
In this parenchymal cell the cisternae of the endoplasmic reticulum (ER) are dilated and filled with finely granular material. M, mitochondrion. (Needle biopsy, lead citrate; ×16 000.)

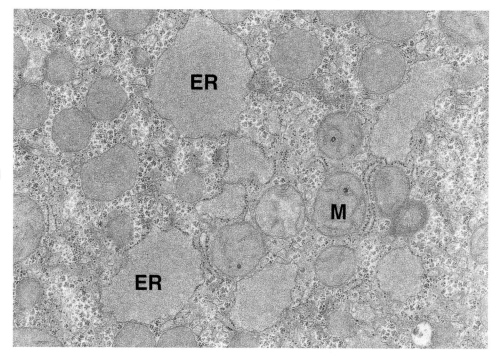

Structural changes

Lysosomes accumulate iron pigment in various forms of iron overload, including hereditary haemochromatosis.[38] They can be strikingly enlarged in inborn errors of metabolism, such as Niemann–Pick disease (**Fig. 17.1**) and type II glycogenosis, or show characteristic changes, such as in the Dubin–Johnson syndrome (**Fig. 17.2**). Lamellar and reticular inclusions are seen within them in acquired, drug-related phospholipidosis.[17–21]

Peroxisomes

These are round or oval bodies with an even, granular matrix bounded by a single membrane. Human peroxisomes infrequently have a nucleoid, whereas this is often seen in other species. They are most numerous in perivenular hepatocytes. They contain numerous oxidative enzymes and are involved in β-oxidation of long-chain fatty acids and synthesis of bile acids and prostaglandins. Their catalase enzyme mediates conversion of peroxide to water.

Structural changes

Peroxisomes are absent in Zellweger's syndrome (cerebro-hepato-renal syndrome).[39] In alcoholic and drug hepatitis, catalase content of peroxisomes is decreased[38] and they show irregular shapes.[39–41] Increased numbers of peroxisomes are seen in alcoholic and drug hepatitis[40] as well as in cirrhosis.[42]

Golgi apparatus

The Golgi apparatus is a membranous system involved in excretory functions of the cell. It contains enzymes such as glycosyl transferases and is involved in glycoprotein metabolism. Morphologically it is composed of small groups of flattened sacs with associated vesicles.

Structural changes

The appearance of the Golgi apparatus is influenced by fixation, and changes are therefore difficult to quantify, but dilatation is evident in regenerating liver and in hepatocellular carcinoma. Electron-dense liposomes accumulate in the system during the development of fatty liver.

Cell sap (cytosol)

The soluble portion of the cytoplasm (cell sap) contains variable amounts of glycogen, free ribosomes, microtubules, intermediate filaments and microfilaments. A few lipid droplets and scanty iron-containing granules are also seen.

Structural changes

Ferritin particles accumulate in iron storage disorders.[38] Fat droplets are numerous in fatty liver, but the amount of fat varies greatly with the patient's state of nutrition. Core particles of hepatitis B virus can be identified in the cytoplasm in many cases of chronic type B hepatitis. Cytoplasmic crystalline inclusions are seen both in normal and in diseased livers. In alcoholic hepatitis, the Mallory–Denk bodies found in ballooned hepatocytes are composed of accumulations of cytokeratin and other proteins in the form of filaments (**Fig. 17.10**).

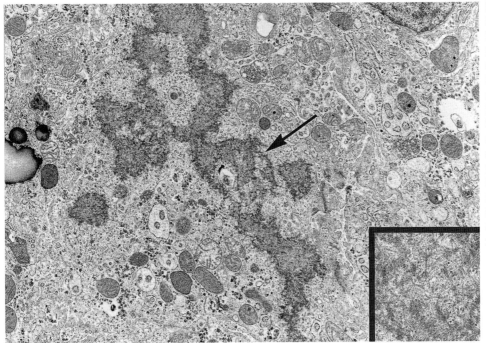

**Figure 17.10
Mallory–Denk
bodies.**
Irregular electron-dense material (arrow) is seen in the cytoplasm of a hepatocyte. The fibrillar nature of the material is evident at the higher magnification shown in the inset. (Needle biopsy, uranyl acetate and lead citrate; ×8600; inset: ×27 000.)

Bile canaliculus

The bile canaliculus measures approximately 0.75 µm and is formed by membranes of several contiguous hepatocytes which are joined by tight junctions.[43] Surface microvilli covered with a thin glycoprotein coat project into the canalicular lumen. Actin filaments are present within the microvilli and extend downward into a pericanalicular web also composed of actin, functioning in canalicular contraction.

Structural changes

Alterations in the bile canaliculus are similar in many forms of cholestasis. Loss of microvilli, formation of surface membrane blebs and disorganisation of the pericanalicular actin filament web are common features. In the cholestasis related to preservation injury after liver transplantation, for example, ischaemia and reperfusion injury result in canalicular dilatation, loss of microvilli and compaction of actin filaments.[44] Intracanalicular bile appears as electron-dense filamentous material. Coarsely granular canalicular bile ('Byler bile') is a characteristic of progressive familial intrahepatic cholestasis type 1 (Byler disease) seen in Amish children[45] (**Fig. 17.11**).

Glycogen

Glycogen particles are normally distributed throughout the cytoplasm among other organelles, but are often near the smooth endoplasmic reticulum. Monoparticulate

Figure 17.11 Progressive familial intrahepatic cholestasis, type 1 (PFIC-1).
The dilated bile canaliculus (BC) contains coarsely granular bile ('Byler bile'), a feature associated with cholestasis in Amish children. The canaliculus is delimited by several junctional complexes (arrows) and has a reduced number of microvilli. (Needle biopsy, lead citrate; ×24 475.) (Illustration kindly provided by Dr AS Knisely, Galveston, TX, USA.)

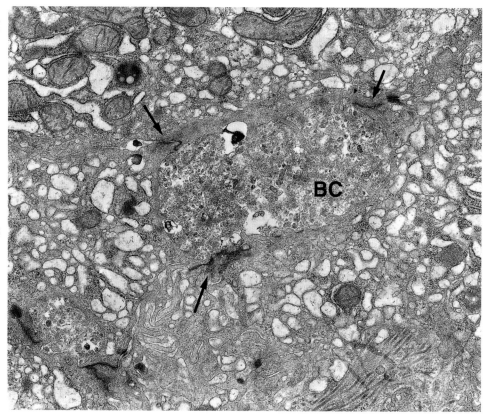

glycogen (beta) particles are deeply osmiophilic 7–18-nm polygonal granules. However, the most common type of glycogen granules seen in normal hepatocytes are 200-nm glycogen rosettes (alpha particles) which consist of aggregates of monoparticulate granules (**Fig. 17.6**).

Structural changes

Glycogen storage diseases[46] (glycogenoses) and certain cases of poorly controlled diabetes ('glycogenic hepatopathy'; **see Ch. 7**) show excessive cytoplasmic glycogen granules within distended hepatocytes. Pools of monoparticulate glycogen displace mitochondria and other organelles towards the cell membrane (**Fig. 17.12**), resulting in the light microscopic appearance of thickened, plant-like hepatocyte membranes. In type II glycogenosis, intra-lysosomal glycogen deposits are present, while intranuclear glycogen is a feature of glycogenosis type Ia (as well as diabetes, insulin resistance, childhood and Wilson's disease). Ground-glass-like cytoplasmic inclusions of abnormal glycogen granules in hepatocytes may be seen in adult polyglucosan body disease,[47] in Lafora disease[48] (myoclonus epilepsy) and in certain recipients of organ transplants.[49]

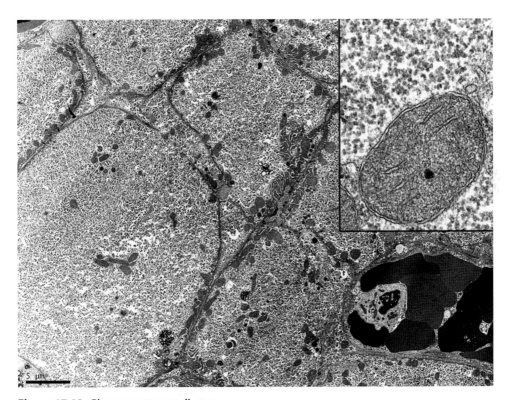

Figure 17.12 Glycogen storage disease.
Several hepatocytes are seen in this field, each of which shows pools of monoparticulate glycogen within the cytoplasm and displacement of most mitochondria and other organelles towards the cell membranes. This type of glycogenosis is seen in several types of glycogen storage disease, including type I (von Gierke's disease). Inset: High magnification shows monoparticulate glycogen particles (each particle approximately 7–18 nm in diameter), with a normal-appearing mitochondrion nearby for size comparison. (Needle biopsy, osmium tetroxide.)

Kupffer cell

The Kupffer cell has an irregular outline, with many finger-like protrusions of the cell surface by which it anchors to endothelial cells. It is rich in phagocytic vacuoles (phagosomes), lysosomes and mitochondria, while the endoplasmic reticulum is only moderately well developed. The nucleus is irregular in shape, with a tendency for the chromatin to be concentrated at the nuclear periphery.

Structural changes

Hypertrophied Kupffer cells can be seen in all conditions of parenchymal cell destruction (e.g. hepatitis) and in pigment overload (e.g. cholestasis, siderosis). Many storage disorders affect the Kupffer cells; in Niemann–Pick disease, for example, both Kupffer cells and hepatocytes are enlarged and filled with vacuoles containing accumulated sphingomyelin (**Fig. 17.1**).

Endothelial cell

The endothelial cell is a flattened cell with a smooth surface, showing small fenestrae organised into sieve plates which provide direct communication between the sinusoidal lumen and the space of Disse.[50] Fenestrae show open and multifolded labyrinth-like configurations.[51] The cytoplasmic volume is relatively small. Many micropinocytotic vesicles can be seen beneath the plasma membrane.

Structural changes

In hepatitis and other conditions, endothelial cells undergo several changes, including the accumulation of iron-rich siderosomes and the formation of basement membrane material on the aspect of the cells facing the space of Disse.[52] In patients with chronic viral hepatitis and acquired immunodeficiency syndrome (AIDS), **tubuloreticular structures** and **cylindrical confronting cisternae** develop within the rough endoplasmic reticulum of endothelial cells and sometimes within Kupffer cells, stellate cells (see below) and lymphocytes.[53,54] Tubuloreticular structures are reticular aggregates of branching tubules within the cisternae of the endoplasmic reticulum and sometimes the perinuclear envelope. Cylindrical confronting cisternae are cylinders of fused membranous lamellae derived from two or more cisternae of endoplasmic reticulum, one inside the other. They appear to be a result of increased endogenous levels of α- and β-interferon. Membrane-bound dense bodies, seen on light microscopy as diastase–periodic acid–Schiff (PAS)-positive cytoplasmic granules, are sometimes present in chronic hepatitis B and C and autoimmune hepatitis[55] (**see Fig. 9.12**).

Stellate cell

The stellate cell, previously known as the Ito cell, fat-storing cell, perisinusoidal cell or lipocyte, is a major storage site for vitamin A. In liver injury, it becomes a transitional cell or myofibroblast-like cell capable of synthesising collagen types I, III and IV as well as laminin.[56] Stellate cells are located within the space of Disse (**see Fig. 7.6**) and have conspicuous rough endoplasmic reticulum, a large Golgi apparatus and large lipid droplets containing vitamin A. In alcoholic liver disease, hypervitaminosis A and methotrexate toxicity, stellate cells undergo hyperplasia and are associated with increased collagen fibres within the space of Disse. Multivesicular stellate cells with numerous lipid droplets have been reported in primary biliary cirrhosis.[57]

Pit cell (large granular lymphocyte)

This cell is located within the sinusoidal lumen, preferentially in the periportal region compared to acinar zone 3.[58] Its surface uropodia and pseudopodia are often in close contact with endothelial cells or Kupffer cells. The nucleus is dense, eccentrically located in the cell and indented. The cell's name derives from its characteristic electron-dense, membrane-bound granules of cytotoxic enzymes which resemble 'pits' or pips in fruit. The cytoplasm contains profiles of rough endoplasmic reticulum, a well-developed Golgi apparatus, centrioles and occasional rod-cored vesicles. Pit cells function as natural killer cells and have been identified in autoimmune hepatitis and in increased numbers in livers with malignant tumours.[59]

Immunoelectron microscopy

The principles employed in immunohistochemical staining of liver biopsy sections for light microscopy (see Immunohistochemistry, below) can be adapted for use in electron microscopy.[60] Following fixation of the specimen in a mixture of glutaraldehyde and para-formaldehyde, the tissue is treated with borohydride, cryoprotected and frozen for storage. Thick sections of 20–40 μm are later cut from the thawed samples and stained by either a direct or indirect immunoperoxidase method.[61] The stained sections are then postfixed in osmium tetroxide, dehydrated and embedded in Epon. Under the electron microscope, electron-dense immunoreactive material is seen at the site of the target antigen.

Availability of a wide variety of monoclonal and polyclonal antibodies to tissue antigens and receptors has greatly expanded investigations of interactions of hepatocytes with immune cells and with the extracellular matrix. Intercellular adhesion molecules, histo-compatibility antigens and interferon receptors are among the potential list of antigens that can be studied by immunoelectron microscopy.[62-64] An example of this technique is shown in **Figure 17.13**, which demonstrates the upregulation of the type A receptor for tumour necrosis factor on hepatocyte membranes in a patient with chronic hepatitis B.[65]

Scanning electron microscopy

The three-dimensional structure of the liver can be assessed by scanning electron micros-copy of specially prepared tissues,[66] or even of sections from paraffin blocks[67] (**Fig. 17.14**). X-ray microanalysis may be combined with the scanning technique and is useful in ele-mental analysis. Laboratories with scanning electron microscopes are best equipped to provide details on appropriate tissue fixation, critical point drying and coating of speci-mens with gold or platinum. Scanning electron microscopy is useful in examining bile ducts[68] and resin casts of hepatic vasculature.[69-72]

Immunohistochemistry

Immunohistochemical techniques are widely available in pathology laboratories and the methods for both immunoperoxidase stains and immunofluorescence microscopy are covered in standard textbooks.[73] The utility of immunostains for specific keratins in the catalogue of Moll[74] and, particularly, of cytokeratins 7 and 20 in determining the histogen-esis of tumours[75] is widely recognised and is also important in the evaluation of hepatic neoplasms. Specific immunostains for the diagnosis of hepatocellular carcinoma and other hepatobiliary tumours are discussed in detail in **Chapter 11 (see Fig. 11.18)**. Demonstra-tion of hepatitis B viral antigens in the context of chronic hepatitis and cirrhosis is

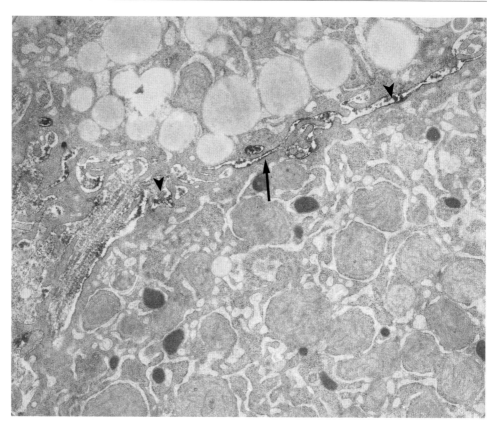

Figure 17.13 Type A receptor for tumour necrosis factor (TNF).
A case of hepatitis B virus-positive chronic hepatitis stained with monoclonal antibody Utr-1 (directed against type A receptor of TNF) shows positive staining on the membranes of two adjacent hepatocytes in a discontinuous pattern (arrow) and in the intercellular space (arrowheads). (Immunoelectron microscopy, ×18 400.) (Illustration kindly provided by Drs VJ Desmet, R Volpes, J Van den Oord and R De Vos, Leuven, The Netherlands.)

addressed in **Chapter 9**. Other viruses such as cytomegalovirus can also be studied immunohistochemically (e.g. post liver transplantation).[76] Cytokeratin 7 immunostain has special value for the identification of native bile ducts, the ductular reaction and hepatic progenitor cells and their derivatives, and is therefore discussed in many sections of this book. The use of ubiquitin immunostain for Mallory–Denk bodies and combined cytokeratin 8 and 18 immunohistochemistry for damaged and ballooned hepatocytes in steatohepatitis is outlined in **Chapter 7**. There is a large and growing menu of immunohistochemical stains for potential use in day-to-day liver biopsy practice as well as for research studies on liver pathobiology. These are mentioned throughout the course of this book and can be updated by consulting PubMed and other internet resources.

Gene array, gene sequencing and molecular analysis

The recent elucidation of the human genome and the expanded availability of many techniques for analysing gene expression patterns and signatures as well as mutational sequences have had an enormous impact on basic science and clinical studies in

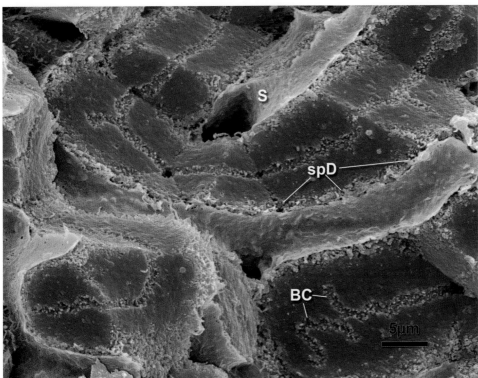

Figure 17.14
Colourised
scanning electron
micrograph of liver.
Sinusoids (S) (light
pink) course
between the hepatic
cords (green). The
network of bile
canaliculi (BC) is well
demonstrated. Note
the narrow space of
Disse (spD) between
the sinusoidal
endothelial lining
cells and the surfaces
of hepatocytes.
(Micrograph kindly
provided by Jackie
Lewin, UCL Medical
School, London, UK.)

hepatology. Various types of liver specimens can be used for genomic and molecular analysis, including fresh tissue, formalin-fixed and paraffin-embedded tissue,[77] touch imprints[78] and archival tissue blocks, provided that their DNA and RNA are sufficiently well preserved. The liver transcriptosome expresses some 25–40% of the 39 000 genes in the human genome[79] and their expression patterns and alterations can be studied by gene microarray analysis and other methods. Combining techniques, such as *in situ* hybridisation with laser capture microdissection and polymerase chain reaction, can increase the sensitivity of the analysis, according to certain studies.[80] Genome-wide studies identify gene signatures that can be implicated in the pathogenesis of diverse liver diseases such as chronic hepatitis C and non-alcoholic fatty liver disease.[81] Sanger sequencing[82] and 'next-gen' (deep) sequencing methods can now be utilised to characterise the types of gene mutations present in specific tumours as a component of personalised genomic medicine and to provide targeted therapy[83] An example of this type of sequencing analysis, in this instance for *KRAS* mutation, is shown in **Figure 17.15**.

Other techniques

Special investigations, such as confocal microscopy, *in situ* hybridisation, polymerase chain reaction and laser capture microdissection, are now widely used in pathology departments and other biomedical venues and can also be implemented for evaluating liver specimens. These procedures require specific fixation and other procedural conditions, as indicated in **Table 17.1**. The reader is encouraged to consult the numerous publications available through PubMed, other internet sources and textbooks for additional details on methodology and potential areas of investigation.

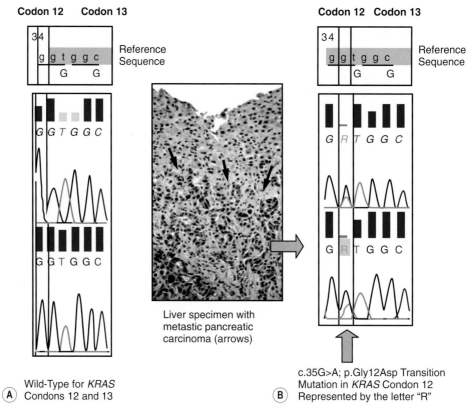

Codon 12   Codon 13

Reference Sequence

Codon 12   Codon 13

Reference Sequence

G G T G G C

G G T G G C

Liver specimen with metastic pancreatic carcinoma (arrows)

G R T G G C

G R T G G C

(A) Wild-Type for *KRAS*
Condons 12 and 13

(B) c.35G>A; p.Gly12Asp Transition Mutation in *KRAS* Condon 12 Represented by the letter "R"

Figure 17.15 Direct DNA-PCR di-deoxyterminator sequencing of codons 12 and 13 of the *KRAS* gene on paraffin-embedded, microdissected tissue from selected liver metastases. **A:** This wild-type *KRAS* sequence of codons 12 and 13 was found in a poorly differentiated colorectal adenocarcinoma metastasis to segment 4 of the liver in a 60-year-old female with a history of colorectal adenocarcinoma of the left colon and a previous history of liver metastases. **B:** This tumour had a mutant *KRAS* sequence which demonstrated the following transition mutation (at yellow arrow) affecting base pair 35 in codon 12: c.35G>A; p.Gly12Asp. This mutation was found in a poorly differentiated adenocarcinoma liver metastasis in a 62-year-old male patient with a history of pancreatic adenocarcinoma (a portion of the resected tumour is shown to the left of the *KRAS* sequence).

References

1   Staff S, Kujala P, Karhu R, et al. Preservation of nucleic acids and tissue morphology in paraffin-embedded clinical samples: comparison of five molecular fixatives. J Clin Pathol 2013;66:807–10.

2   Burt AD, Le Bail B, Balabaud C, et al. Morphologic investigation of sinusoidal cells. Semin Liver Dis 1993;13:21–38.

3   Rieder H, Meyer zum Büschenfelde K-H, Ramadori G. Functional spectrum of sinusoidal endothelial liver cells. Filtration, endocytosis, synthetic capacities and intercellular communication. J Hepatol 1992;15:237–50.

4   Xiao J-C, Ruck P, Adam A, et al. Small epithelial cells in human liver cirrhosis exhibit features of hepatic stem-like cells: immunohistochemical, electron microscopic and immunoelectron microscopic findings. Histopathology 2003;42:141–9.

5   Nagore N, Howe S, Boxer L, et al. Liver cell rosettes: structural differences in cholestasis and hepatitis. Liver 1989;9:43–51.

6   Nagore N, Howe S, Scheuer PJ. The three-dimensional liver. In: Popper H, Schaffner F, editors. Progress in Liver Diseases, vol. IX. Philadelphia, PA: WB Saunders; 1989. p. 1–10.

7   Ludwig J, Ritman EL, LaRusso NF, et al. Anatomy of the human biliary system studied by quantitative computer-aided three-dimensional imaging techniques. Hepatology 1998;27:893–9.

8   Jones S, Chapman SK, Crocker PR, et al. Combined light and electron microscope in routine histopathology. J Clin Pathol 1982;35:425–9.

9   Spycher MA. Electron microscopy: a method for the diagnosis of inherited metabolic storage diseases. Electron microscopy in diagnosis. Pathol Res Pract 1980;167:118–35.

10   Ishak KG, Sharp HL. Metabolic errors and liver disease. In: MacSween RNM, Anthony PP, Scheuer PJ, et al., editors. Pathology of the Liver. 3rd ed. Edinburgh: Churchill Livingstone; 1994. p. 123–218, [Ch. 4].

11   Toker C, Trevino N. Hepatic ultrastructure in chronic idiopathic jaundice. Arch Pathol 1965;80:453–60.

12   Miller SE. Detection and identification of viruses by electron microscopy. J Electron Microsc Tech 1986;4:265–301.

13   Phillips MJ, Poucell S, Patterson J, et al. The Liver. An Atlas and Text of Ultrastructural Pathology. New York: Raven Press; 1987.

14   Phillips MJ, Glendis LM, Paucell S, et al. Syncytial giant-cell hepatitis. Sporadic hepatitis with distinctive pathologic features, a severe clinical course, and paramyxoviral features. N Engl J Med 1991;324:455–60.

15   Fimmel CJ, Guo L, Compans RW, et al. A case of syncytial giant cell hepatitis with features of a paramyxoviral infection. Am J Gastroenterol 1998;93:1931–7.

16   Lazaro CA, Chang M, Tang W, et al. Hepatitis C virus replication in transfected and serum-infected cultured human fetal hepatocytes. Am J Pathol 2007;170:478–89.

17   Lloreta-Trull J, Serrano S. The current role of electron microscopy in the diagnosis of epithelial and epithelioid tumors. Semin Diagn Pathol 2003;20:46–59.

18   Pessayre D, Bichara M, Degott C, et al. Perhexiline maleate-induced cirrhosis. Gastroenterology 1979;76:170–7.

19   Poucell S, Ireton J, Valencia-Mayoral P, et al. Amiodarone-associated phospholipidosis and fibrosis of the liver. Light, immunohistochemical, and electron microscopic studies. Gastroenterology 1984;86:926–36.

20   Simon JB, Manley PN, Brien JF, et al. Amiodarone hepatotoxicity simulating alcoholic liver disease. N Engl J Med 1984;311:167–72.

21   Pirovino M, Müller O, Zysset T, et al. Amiodarone-induced hepatic phospholipidosis: correlation of morphological and biochemical findings in an animal model. Hepatology 1988;8:591–8.

22   Lewis JH, Ranard RC, Caruso A, et al. Amiodarone hepatotoxicity: prevalence and clinicopathologic correlations among 104 patients. Hepatology 1989;9:679–85.

23   Rohr HP, Lüthy J, Gudat F, et al. Stereology: a new supplement to the study of human liver biopsy specimens. In: Popper H, Schaffner F, editors. Progress in Liver Diseases, vol. V. New York: Grune & Stratton; 1976. p. 24–34.

24   Uchida T, Kronborg I, Peters RL. Alcoholic hyalin-containing hepatocytes – a characteristic morphologic appearance. Liver 1984;4:233–43.

25   Caldwell SH, de Freitas AR, Park SH, et al. Intramitochondrial crystalline inclusions in nonalcoholic steatohepatitis. Hepatology 2009;49:1888–95.

26   Chedid A, Jao W, Port J. Megamitochondria in hepatic and renal disease. Am J Gastroenterol 1980;73:319–24.

27   Foschini MP, Macchia S, Losi L, et al. Identification of mitochondria in liver biopsies. A study by immunohistochemistry, immunogold and Western blot analysis. Virchows Arch 1998;433:267–73.

28   Feldmann G, Maurice M, Husson JM, et al. Hepatocyte giant mitochondria: an almost constant lesion in systemic scleroderma. Virchows Arch A Pathol Anat Histol 1977;374:215–27.

29   Sternlieb I. Evolution of the hepatic lesion in Wilson's disease (hepatolenticular degeneration). In: Popper H, Schaffner F, editors. Progress in Liver Diseases, vol. IV. New York: Grune & Stratton; 1972. p. 511–25, [Ch. 29].

30   Scheinberg IH, Sternlieb I. Wilson's disease. Major Problems in Internal Medicine XXIII. Philadelphia, PA: WB Saunders; 1984.

31   Sternlieb I. Fraternal concordance of types of abnormal hepatocellular mitochondria in Wilson's disease. Hepatology 1992;16:728–32.

32   Tonsgard JH. Effect of Reye's syndrome serum on the ultrastructure of isolated liver mitochondria. Lab Invest 1989;60:568–73.

33   Lichtenstein GR, Kaiser LR, Tuchman M, et al. Fatal hyperammonemia following orthotopic lung transplantation. Gastroenterology 1997;112:236–40.

34   Karadimas CL, Vu TH, Holve SA, et al. Navajo neurohepatopathy is caused by a mutation in the MPV17 gene. Am J Hum Genet 2006;79:544–8.

35   Spinazzola A, Santer R, Akman OH, et al. Hepatocerebral form of mitochondrioal depletion syndrome. Novel MPV17 mutations. Arch Neurol 2008;65:1108–13.

36   El-Hattab AW, Li F-Y, Schmitt E, et al. MPV17-associated hepatocerebral mitochondrial DNA depletion syndrome: new patients and novel mutations. Mol Genet Metab 2010;99:300–8.

37   Labarthe F, Dobbelaere D, Devisme L, et al. Clinical, biochemical and morphological features of hepatocerebral syndrome with mitochondrial DNA depletion due to deoxyguanosine kinase deficiency. J Hepatol 2005;43:333–41.

38   Iancu TC, Deugnier Y, Halliday JW, et al. Ultrastructural sequences during liver iron overload in genetic hemochromatosis. J Hepatol 1997;27:628–38.

39   Mooi WJ, Dingemans KP, Van Den Bergh Weerman MA, et al. Ultrastructure of the liver in cerebrohepatorenal syndrome of Zellweger. Ultrastruct Pathol 1983;5:135–44.

40   De Craemer D, Kerckaert I, Roels F. Hepatocellular peroxisomes in human alcoholic and drug-induced hepatitis: a quantitative study. Hepatology 1991;14:811–17.

41   Sternlieb I, Quintana N. The peroxisomes of human hepatocytes. Lab Invest 1977;36:140–9.

42   De Craemer D, Pauwels M, Roels F. Peroxisomes in cirrhosis of the human liver: a cytochemical, ultrastructural and quantitative study. Hepatology 1993;17:404–10.

43   Arias IM, Che M, Gatmaitan Z, et al. The biology of the bile canaliculus, 1993. Hepatology 1993;17:318–29.

44   Cutrin JC, Cantino D, Biasi F, et al. Reperfusion damage to the bile canaliculi in transplanted human liver. Hepatology 1996;24:1053–7.

45   Bull LN, Carolton VEH, Stricker NL, et al. Genetic and morphological findings in progressive familial intrahepatic cholestasis (Byler disease [PFIC-1] and Byler syndrome): evidence for heterogeneity. Hepatology 1997;26:155–64.

46 Hicks J, Wartchow E, Mierau G. Glycogen storage diseases: a brief review and update on clinical features, genetic abnormalities, pathologic features, and treatment. Ultrastruct Pathol 2011;35:183–96.

47 Hajdu CH, Lefkowitch JH. Adult polyglucosan body disease: a rare presentation with chronic liver disease and ground-glass hepatocellular inclusions. Semin Liver Dis 2011;31:223–9.

48 Nishimura RN, Ishak KG, Reddick R, et al. Lafora disease: diagnosis by liver biopsy. Ann Neurol 1980;8:409–15.

49 Lefkowitch JH, Lobritto SJ, Brown RS Jr, et al. Ground-glass, polyclucosan-like hepatocellular inclusions: a "new" diagnostic entity. Gastroenterology 2006;131:713–18.

50 Horn T, Lyon H, Christoffersen P. The blood hepatocytic barrier: a light microscopical, transmission and scanning electron microscopic study. Liver 1986;6:233–45.

51 Braet F, Riches J, Geerts W, et al. Three-dimensional organization of fenestrae labyrinths in liver sinusoidal endothelial cells. Liver Int 2009;29:603–13.

52 Bardadin KA, Scheuer PJ. Endothelial cell changes in acute hepatitis. A light and electron microscopic study. J Pathol 1984;144:213–20.

53 Schaff Z, Hoofnagle JH, Grimley PM. Hepatic inclusions during interferon therapy in chronic viral hepatitis. Hepatology 1986;6:966–70.

54 Luu J, Bockus D, Remington F, et al. Tubuloreticular structures and cylindrical confronting cisternae: a review. Hum Pathol 1989;20:617–27.

55 Iwamura S, Enzan H, Saibara T, et al. Appearance of sinusoidal inclusion-containing endothelial cells in liver disease. Hepatology 1994;20:604–10.

56 Friedman SL. The cellular basis of hepatic fibrosis. N Engl J Med 1993;328:1828–35.

57 Cameron RG, Neuman MG, Shear N, et al. Multivesicular stellate cells in primary biliary cirrhosis. Hepatology 1997;26:819–22.

58 Luo D, Vanderkerken K, Bouwens L, et al. The number and distribution of hepatic natural killer cells (pit cells) in normal rat liver: an immunohistochemical study. Hepatology 1995;21:1690–4.

59 Bouwens L, Wisse E. Pit cells in the liver. Liver 1992;12:3–9.

60 De Vos R, De Wolf-Peeters C, van den Oord JJ, et al. A recommended procedure for ultrastructural immunohistochemistry on small human tissue samples. J Histochem Cytochem 1985;33:959–64.

61 Elia JM. Immunohistopathology. A Practical Approach to Diagnosis. Chicago, IL: ASCP Press; 1990.

62 Volpes R, van den Oord JJ, Desmet VJ. Can hepatocytes serve as 'activated' immunomodulating cells in the immune response? J Hepatol 1992;16:228–40.

63 Horiike N, Onji M, Kumon I, et al. Intercellular adhesion molecule-1 expression on the hepatocyte membrane of patients with chronic hepatitis B and C. Liver 1993;13:10–14.

64 Volpes R, van den Oord JJ, De Vos R, et al. Expression of interferon-gamma receptor in normal and pathological human liver tissue. J Hepatol 1991;12:195–202.

65 Volpes R, van den Oord JJ, De Vos R, et al. Hepatic expression of type A and type B receptors for tumor necrosis factor. J Hepatol 1992;14:361–9.

66 Vonnahme F-J. The Human Liver. A Scanning Electron Microscopic Atlas. Basel: Karger; 1993.

67 Ishak KG. Applications of scanning electron microscopy to the study of liver disease. In: Popper H, Schaffner F, editors. Progress in Liver Diseases, vol. VIII. Orlando, FL: Grune & Stratton; 1986. p. 1–32.

68 Petersen C, Grasshoff S, Luciano L. Diverse morphology of biliary atresia in an animal model. J Hepatol 1998;28:603–7.

69 Haratake J, Hisaoka M, Furuta A, et al. A scanning electron microscopic study of postnatal development of rat peribiliary plexus. Hepatology 1991;14:1196–200.

70 Haratake J, Hisaoka M, Yamamoto O, et al. Morphological changes of hepatic microcirculation in experimental rat cirrhosis: a scanning electron microscopic study. Hepatology 1991;13:952–6.

71 Gaudio E, Pannarale L, Onori P, et al. A scanning electron microscopic study of liver microcirculation disarrangement in experimental rat cirrhosis. Hepatology 1993;17:477–85.

72 Terada T, Ishida F, Nakanuma Y. Vascular plexus around intrahepatic bile ducts in normal livers and portal hypertension. J Hepatol 1989;8:139–49.

73 Dabbs DJ. Diagnostic Immunohistochemistry: Theranostic and Genomic Applications. Philadelphia: Elsevier Saunders; 2013.

74 Moll R, Franke WW, Schiller D, et al. The catalog of human cytokeratins: pattern of expression in normal epithelia, tumors and cultured cells. Cell 1982;31:11–24.

75 Wang NP, Zee S, Zarbo RJ, et al. Coordinate expression of cytokeratins 7 and 20 defines unique subsets of carcinomas. Appl Immunohistochem 1995;3:99–107.

76 Theise ND, Conn M, Thung SN. Localization of cytomegalovirus antigens in liver allografts over time. Hum Pathol 1993;24:103–8.

77 Hoshida Y, Villanueva A, Kobayashi M, et al. Gene expression in fixed tissues and outcome in hepatocellular carcinoma. N Engl J Med 2008;359:1995–2004.

78 Dogan S, Becker JC, Rekhtman N, et al. Use of touch imprint cytology as a simple method to enrich tumor cells for molecular analysis. Cancer Cytopathol 2013;121:354–60.

79 Shackel NA, Gorrell MD, McCaughan GW. Gene array analysis and the liver. Hepatology 2002;36:1313–25.

80 Horner SM. Defining the spatial relationship between hepatitis C virus infection and interferon-stimulated gene induction in the human liver. Hepatology 2014;59:2065–7.

81 Smalling RL, Delker DA, Zhang Y, et al. Genome-wide transcriptome analysis identifies novel gene signatures implicated in human chronic liver disease. Am J Physiol Gastrointest Liver Physiol 2013;305:G364–74.

82 Sanger F, Coulson AR. A rapid method for determining sequences in DNA by primed synthesis with DNA polymerase. J Mol Biol 1975;94:441–8.

83 Karagkounis G, Torbenson MS, Daniel HD, et al. Incidence and prognostic impact of KRAS and BRAF mutation in patients underoing liver surgery for colorectal metastases. Cancer 2013;119:4137–44.

General reading

Dabbs DJ. Diagnostic Immunohistochemistry: Theranostic and Genomic Applications. Philadelphia: Elsevier Saunders; 2013.

Ghadially FN. Ultrastructural Pathology of the Cell and Matrix. 3rd ed. London: Butterworths; 1988.

Phillips MJ, Poucell S, Patterson J, et al. The Liver. An Atlas and Text of Ultrastructural Pathology. New York: Raven Press; 1987.

Shackel NA, Gorrell MD, McCaughan GW. Gene array analysis and the liver. Hepatology 2002;36:1313–25.

Smedsrod B, Le Couteur D, Ikejima K, et al. Hepatic sinusoidal cells in health and disease: update from the 14th International Symposium. Liver Int 2009;29:490–9.

Staff S, Kujala P, Karhu R, et al. Preservation of nucleic acids and tissue morphology in paraffin-embedded clinical samples: comparison of five molecular fixatives. J Clin Pathol 2013;66:807–10.

Vonnahme F-J. The Human Liver. A Scanning Electron Microscopic Atlas. Basel: Karger; 1993.

Watson JD, Gilman M, Witkowski J, et al. Recombinant DNA. 2nd ed. New York: Scientific American Books; 1992.

Glossary

Note: Words in *italics* are defined elsewhere in the glossary.

Acidophil body (Figs 6.2, 16.16) A *hepatocyte* which has undergone apoptosis; now often referred to as an apoptotic body. See also *Councilman bodies*.

Acinus (Fig. 3.1) An anatomical unit based on blood supply, its three parenchymal zones containing successively less oxygenated blood. Zone 1 is nearest to the terminal portal vessels in a small portal tract.

Activity (Figs 9.7, 9.8) In histological terms, an expression of the degree of hepatocellular damage and associated inflammation. Especially used in chronic hepatitis and cirrhosis, in which it forms the basis of *grading*.

Apoptosis (Figs 6.2, 16.16) Shrinkage and fragmentation of cells, seen in the liver mainly in the form of densely stained rounded structures derived from hepatocytes but lying free outside the *liver-cell plates*.

Autoimmune hepatitis A form of hepatitis associated with high titres of autoantibodies in serum. Usually responds to immunosuppressive therapy.

Ballooning degeneration Swelling and rounding of hepatocytes, with loss of their normal polygonal shape. Different forms of ballooning are seen in viral hepatitis (Fig. 6.2) and *steatohepatitis* (Fig. 7.8C).

Bile canaliculus (Fig. 5.2) The tubular space formed between the biliary poles of two or three *hepatocytes*, or more in diseased liver. The canaliculus has no separate epithelial lining of its own.

Bile duct (Fig. 3.2) The smallest ducts, the interlobular bile ducts, are centrally located in small portal tracts and are usually accompanied by blood vessels. In practice they are sometimes difficult to distinguish from *bile ductules*, the transition being gradual.

Bile ductule and canal of Hering (Fig. 3.3) At the portal–parenchymal interface the canalicular system drains into the *canals of Hering* which are partly lined by hepatocytes and partly by biliary epithelial cells (*cholangiocytes*). These in turn connect with bile ductules, fully lined by biliary epithelium.

Bile extravasate (Fig. 5.9) Leakage of bile from a duct into the connective tissue of the portal tract, occasionally seen in large bile-duct obstruction.

Bile infarct (Fig. 5.4) An area of liver-cell death in a cholestatic liver; often periportal, whereas canalicular *cholestasis* is mainly perivenular. Bile staining is variable and may be absent. Bile infarcts are easily mistaken for accumulations of foamy macrophages.

Bile lake An accumulation of bile outside a *liver-cell plate*.

Bile thrombus (Fig. 5.2) Synonymous with bile plug: the accumulation of visible bile in a *bile canaliculus*.

Bilirubinostasis A term sometimes used for histological cholestasis.

Bridging fibrosis (Fig. 7.21) Linking of portal tracts and/or efferent venules by fibrous tissue.

Bridging necrosis (Fig. 6.9) Confluent hepatocellular necrosis and *collapse* linking vascular structures; usually and preferably confined to linking of portal tracts to efferent venules.

Canals of Hering (Fig. 3.3) Structures lined partly by *hepatocytes* and partly by bile ductular epithelium. They are a probable site of *progenitor cells*.

Central perivenulitis (Fig. 16.21) A feature of liver transplant rejection in which efferent venules are targeted by lymphocytes and other effector immune cells. Dropout and *apoptosis* of perivenular *hepatocytes* and focal congestion are also frequently present. This common manifestation of paediatric allograft rejection is sometimes present in combination with classical portal tract rejection changes and occasionally is seen late (>1 year after transplantation) as the isolated expression of rejection.

Ceroid pigment (Fig. 6.5) Brown pigment in macrophages, found after hepatocellular injury; rich in oxidised lipids and PAS-positive after diastase digestion. Distinct from *lipofuscin*.

Cholangiocyte Epithelial cell of the biliary tract.

Cholate stasis (Fig. 5.10) A term sometimes used for chronic *cholestasis*, on the assumption that the hepatocellular changes result from the accumulation of toxic bile salts. Also known as *precholestasis* or *pseudoxanthomatous change*.

Cholestasis (Fig. 5.2) In morphological terms, *bilirubinostasis* or visible bile in a section of liver. Also defined as failure of bile to reach the duodenum and biochemically as a type of jaundice with dark urine, pale stools, conjugated hyperbilirubinaemia and raised serum alkaline phosphatase level.

Cirrhosis The transformation of the normal hepatic architecture into nodules separated by *fibrosis*.

Collapse (Fig. 4.8) Condensation of pre-existing reticulin framework as a result of necrosis. May be followed by *fibrosis*.

Confluent necrosis (Fig. 8.4) Death of groups of adjacent *hepatocytes*.

Councilman bodies *Hepatocytes* which have undergone *apoptosis*. The term is best restricted to yellow fever, the disease in which they were described by Dr Councilman.

Disse space (Fig. 17.4) The space between the sinusoidal endothelium and *hepatocytes*; contents include extracellular matrix and *hepatic stellate cells*.

Ductopenia (Figs 13.6, 16.10) Loss of significant numbers of interlobular *bile ducts*. Causes include rejection of liver grafts, graft-versus-host disease, primary biliary cirrhosis, primary sclerosing cholangitis and drug injury. Diseases characterised by ductopenia are known as *vanishing bile duct syndromes*.

Ductular proliferation Use of this term is discouraged for the reason given in the next definition.

Ductular reaction (Fig. 4.13) A reaction of ductular phenotype, seen as an increase in ductular structures. This may be the result of proliferation of pre-existing ductules, but the new structures could also arise from biliary metaplasia of *hepatocytes* or from transformation of *progenitor cells*.

Dysmetabolic hepatic iron overload (DHIO) (Fig. 7.12) *Siderosis* of *Kupffer cells* and/or *hepatocytes* due to insulin resistance and its effects on iron homeostasis. Most often evident histologically as iron overload in the setting of macrovesicular *steatosis* in non-alcoholic fatty liver disease.

Dysplasia (Figs 10.8, 10.9) A change in the size, nucleus:cytoplasm ratio and/or nuclear appearances of *hepatocytes*, usually in chronic hepatitis and *cirrhosis*. Large-cell and small-cell types are described. Also known as large- and small-cell change.

Fat-storing cells *Hepatic stellate cells*.

Fatty liver disease Includes both *steatosis* and *steatohepatitis*, as in alcoholic fatty liver disease (AFLD) and non-alcoholic fatty liver disease (NAFLD).

Feathery degeneration (Fig. 5.3) A type of liver-cell injury in *cholestasis*, attributed to toxic effects of bile salts. Affected *hepatocytes*, often single cells lying within normal *parenchyma*, are swollen and have pale-staining feathery cytoplasm.

Fibrosis Formation of new collagen fibres. It may follow *collapse* of pre-existing connective tissue framework or arise *de novo*.

Focal necrosis (Fig. 9.8) Death of *hepatocytes*, singly or in small groups. Because of the rapid disappearance of the dead cells, focal necrosis is usually recognised by the presence of inflammatory cells and by a break in continuity of a *liver-cell plate* rather than by the presence of necrotic tissue.

Follicle See *lymphoid follicle*.

Glycogen vacuolation See *nuclear vacuolation*.

Grading Semi-quantitative scoring of the various processes comprising hepatocellular damage and inflammation, usually in chronic hepatitis. Numerical assessment of histological activity.

Granuloma (Fig. 15.1) A focal accumulation of epithelioid cells, which are modified macrophages with abundant cytoplasm and often curved, elongated nuclei. To be distinguished from simple accumulations of macrophages.

Ground-glass hepatocytes (Fig. 9.13) *Hepatocytes* with a well-defined, lightly eosinophilic homogeneous area occupying much of the cytoplasm. The most common form is seen in the livers of patients infected with the hepatitis B virus.

Haemochromatosis (See also *siderosis*.) A condition in which hepatic *fibrosis* and *cirrhosis* ultimately develop as a result of iron overload. The common form, hereditary haemochromatosis, is usually the result of mutations of the *HFE* gene on chromosome 6.

Hepatic stellate cells (Figs 7.6, 17.4) Cells containing vacuoles rich in vitamin A, lying within the *Disse space*. In pathological conditions, they are able to transform into myofibroblasts and produce extracellular matrix components. Previously used synonyms include *fat-storing cells*, *Ito cells*, *lipocytes*, *parasinusoidal cells* and *perisinusoidal cells*.

Hepatocytes Liver cells.

Interface hepatitis (Figs 9.3, 9.4) Death of *hepatocytes* at the interface of connective tissue and *parenchyma* in chronic liver disease, accompanied by inflammatory-cell infiltration. Characteristic of chronic hepatitis and synonymous with the older term *piecemeal necrosis.*

Ito cells *Hepatic stellate cells.*

Kupffer cells The resident macrophages of the liver, straddling the sinusoidal lumens.

Limiting plate The layer of *hepatocytes* next to a portal tract.

Lipocytes *Hepatic stellate cells.*

Lipofuscin (Fig. 3.6) Pigmented granular material in *hepatocytes*, of lysosomal origin and most abundant at the biliary poles of the cells. Found in normal liver in greatly varying amounts.

Liver-cell plates (Fig. 3.5) Interconnecting walls of *hepatocytes*, one cell thick in adults. Thicker plates are found in children and in regenerating liver.

Lobular activity (Fig. 9.8) Inflammation and hepatocellular damage deep within the lobules, in contrast to *interface hepatitis.*

Lobule (Fig. 3.1) An anatomical unit with an efferent (centrilobular) vein at its centre and portal tracts peripherally.

Lupoid hepatitis An old term for *autoimmune hepatitis*, no longer in use.

Lymphoid follicle (Figs 9.16, 9.17) A structured accumulation of lymphocytes resembling the follicles of normal lymph nodes.

Mallory bodies (Figs 7.17, 17.10) Irregular, dense cytoplasmic inclusions with a cytokeratin component, often in the form of strands or garlands. Electron microscopy reveals a filamentous structure.

Massive necrosis (Figs 4.13D, 6.12) *Multilobular necrosis* involving a substantial part of the whole liver. This usually leads to severe liver insufficiency.

Metabolic syndrome The association of insulin resistance with central (truncal) obesity, diabetes mellitus, hyperlipidaemia and systemic arterial hypertension. Non-alcoholic fatty liver disease (NAFLD) is considered the hepatic expression of the metabolic syndrome.

Multilobular necrosis (Figs 4.13D, 6.12) Confluent necrosis involving the whole of several adjacent lobules. The clinical effects are variable, depending on the extent of the lesion.

Non-alcoholic steatohepatitis (NASH) (Fig. 7.22) A form of hepatitis resembling alcoholic *steatohepatitis* but associated with other causes such as obesity, diabetes or drugs.

Nuclear vacuolation (Fig. 7.13) Empty *hepatocyte* nuclei in paraffin sections. May be due to glycogen accumulation, lipid or invagination of cytoplasm. Glycogen nuclei, common in the young, the obese and the diabetic, are typically enlarged and have prominent nuclear membranes. The glycogen may be demonstrable histochemically but is often lost during processing.

Panacinar necrosis (Fig. 6.12) Necrosis of an entire *acinus.*

Panlobular necrosis (Fig. 6.12) Necrosis of an entire *lobule.*

Parasinusoidal cells *Hepatic stellate cells.*

Parenchyma The specialised tissue of the liver, as opposed to the connective tissue. Often used loosely to describe the contents of the *lobules* as opposed to the portal tracts.

Periportal The part of the hepatic *lobule* or *acinus* next to a small portal tract.

Perisinusoidal cells *Hepatic stellate cells.*

Piecemeal necrosis *Interface hepatitis* is now often used for this process, because it almost certainly involves *apoptosis* rather than, or as well as, necrosis.

Polyploidy (Fig. 3.9) The coexistence of different classes of nuclei containing multiple sets of chromosomes (e.g. quadriploid, octaploid); a normal state in adult human liver.

Portal triad (Fig. 3.2) The triad of artery, vein and *bile duct* present in most portal tracts.

Precholestasis (Fig. 5.10) See *cholate stasis.*

Progenitor cell A partly committed cell capable of producing a range of specialised cell types. In the liver, progenitor cells are probably located in *bile ductules* or *canals of Hering*. See also *stem cell.*

Pseudoacini *Rosettes.*

Pseudoxanthomatous change (Fig. 5.10) See *cholate stasis.*

Regeneration (Fig. 10.6) Loosely used to describe hepatocellular hyperplasia following injury or loss. Not easily recognised in conventional sections because of low mitotic rate; characterised by increase in the thickness of the cell plates.

Rosettes (Figs 4.11, 9.9, 9.18) In liver pathology this term refers to a change of the normal plate pattern of *hepatocytes* to glandular structures formed by several *hepatocytes*. Different types of rosette formation are seen in *cholestasis* and in chronic hepatitis.

Septa (Figs 10.15, 10.16) Walls of fibrous tissue, seen in two-dimensional sections as lines or bands. Septa may be formed by *collapse* ('passive septa'), by new fibre formation ('active septa') or by both.

Siderosis The presence of stainable iron in any component of liver tissue. The many causes of siderosis include several diseases under the heading of *haemochromatosis*, in which progressive iron accumulation leads to *fibrosis* and *cirrhosis*. However, at an early stage of hereditary *haemochromatosis* there is iron deposition without *fibrosis*.

Sinusoidal obstruction syndrome (Fig. 16.23) Circulatory obstruction within hepatic sinusoids and efferent venules following endothelial damage due to myeloablative chemotherapy or exposure to toxins such as pyrrolizine alkaloids. The term is often used as an alternative to veno-occlusive disease.

Spotty necrosis Widespread, but patchy hepatocellular necrosis, typical of acute hepatitis.

Staging The semi-quantitative assessment of structural changes including *fibrosis* and *cirrhosis*.

Steatohepatitis (Fig. 7.16) A form of hepatitis characterised by *steatosis*, hepatocellular *ballooning*, *Mallory bodies* and pericellular *fibrosis*.

Steatosis (Figs 7.1, 7.2) The accumulation of excess lipid in *hepatocytes*.

Stellate cells See *hepatic stellate cells*.

Stem cell A self-renewing cell with the potential to give rise to a variety of cells, including *progenitor cells*.

Vanishing bile duct syndromes Disorders characterised by loss of *bile ducts* leading to *ductopenia* (paucity of ducts) with consequent *cholestasis*.

Index

Page numbers followed by 'f' indicate figures, 't' indicate tables, and 'b' indicate boxes.